# Medical Radiology

## Diagnostic Imaging

*Series Editors*

Albert L. Baert
Maximilian F. Reiser
Hedvig Hricak
Michael Knauth

*Editorial Board*

For further volumes:
http://www.springer.com/series/4354

Michele Bertolotto · Carlo Trombetta

Editors

# Scrotal Pathology

Foreword by
M. F. Reiser

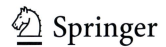 Springer

*Editors*
Michele Bertolotto, MD
Department of Radiology
University of Trieste
Ospedale di Cattinara
Strada di Fiume 447
34149 Trieste
Italy
e-mail: bertolot@units.it

Carlo Trombetta, MD
Department of Urology
University of Trieste
Ospedale di Cattinara
Strada di Fiume 447
34149 Trieste
Italy
e-mail: trombcar@units.it

ISSN 0942-5373
ISBN 978-3-642-12455-6          e-ISBN 978-3-642-12456-3
DOI 10.1007/978-3-642-12456-3
Springer Heidelberg Dordrecht London New York

Library of Congress Control Number: 2011935746

*Cover design:* eStudio Calamar, Berlin/Figueres

Printed on acid-free paper

Springer is part of Springer Science+Business Media (www.springer.com)

*Genoa (Italy)*
*is the city where we were born*
*is our beginning (or "starting point" ?)*
*and it continues to provoke us a particular feeling*
*like that so well described by John Keats (1795–1821)*

*"Yet do I sometimes feel a languishment*
*For skies Italian, and an inward groan*
*To sit upon an Alp as on a throne*
*And half forget what world or worldling meant"*

Michele Bertolotto
Carlo Trombetta

# Foreword

Scrotal pathologies play an important role in the daily clinical practice. In order to correctly diagnose the medical condition of patients with scrotal disorders, it is important to know the clinical evidence and use the imaging modalities in the best possible way. This volume of the Diagnostic Imaging series therefore integrates the clinical and the imaging perspective.

It is to the merit of M. Bertolotto and C. Trombetta to present a monograph on this topic in which the scrotal anatomy, the clinical methods as well as the range of related disorders are thoroughly described by distinguished experts. It is as such the first comprehensive practical guide on scrotal pathology. On behalf of the series editors I would like to thank M. Bertolotto and C. Trombetta as well as the contributing authors for their excellent work.

We are confident that this reference book will be indispensable for urologists, radiologists and other medical doctors. Due to the fact that it is structured according to the major clinical symptoms such as acute scrotal pain, scrotal lumps, the infertile man and the undescended testis—which are covered separately for adults and children where necessary—the reader will easily find his way.

This monograph will certainly also facilitate the cooperation between radiologists and other medical doctors, especially urologists, by describing their respective diagnostic and therapeutic approaches.

Munich, May 2011                                           M. F. Reiser

# Preface

Evaluation of patients with scrotal pathologies, either children or adults, is one of the commonest situations in the daily clinical practice. While management of these patients usually requires imaging, correct interpretation of imaging features always needs integration with history and clinical features. Unfortunately, radiologists often have a superficial knowledge of what urologists really need from imaging studies, while clinicians, even those performing ultrasound, themselves often have insufficient knowledge of the diagnostic capabilities offered by the latest generation ultrasound equipment and by other imaging methods.

At the university hospital of Trieste, urologists and radiologists have been working together for several years, performing imaging studies and sharing clinical information. We are highly convinced that before starting any diagnostic imaging procedure, regardless of the urological or radiological background, the patient has to be investigated by means of careful evaluation of the medical history, and a complete orthostatic and clinostatic physical examination. This is easy to be performed due to the great external accessibility to the scrotal content. Also, data of hormonal assessment on the patient, and results of sperm analysis are often useful for the correct interpretation of imaging features.We finally believe that all the different specialists that apply scrotal pathologies must know the current diagnostic possibilities offered by the different imaging modalities, and the advantages provided by the use of newest equipment.

A large amount of high-quality original investigations and review articles are available which cover virtually all arguments in clinics, imaging and management of scrotal disease. To the best of our knowledge, however, no comprehensive books have been recently published on this field. This lack is often felt in the clinical practice and has consequences for the optimum management of the patients: not surprisingly, it was Prof. Emanuele Belgrano, the chairman of our Urological Department, who was first convinced that there was a real demand for a monograph addressing this topic, and first suggested to us to combine our expertise and edit a book considering all aspects of diagnosis and management of scrotal pathologies.

We are pleased to serve as the editors of this book. It is addressed not only to radiologists and urologists primary involved in urogenital imaging, but also to graduate students, and to all clinicians who need a reference book for managing scrotal problems during their everyday clinical work.

As commonly occurs in the clinical practice, in this book the different pathologies are arranged according to their clinical presentation. Since in many cases diseases are essentially different in children and in adults, a separate presentation is provided. We arranged the chapters with this practical approach in mind, and with the aim to provide useful information to specialists with different backgrounds. Each topic is introduced by clinical chapters in which symptoms, useful clinical tests, clinical management, and outcomes are fully described. Thereafter, imaging features are fully described and illustrated.

This volume is an expression of the efforts of distinguished experts throughout the world. The contributing authors bring a wealth of international experience in clinics and imaging of scrotal disease. All have provided excellent contributions, representing their broad experience, and the current clinical applications in their own practices. We are greatly indebted to them for their enthusiastic commitment and support. Without them, this book would not have been possible.

We are grateful to Professor Hedvig Hricak, Professor Maximilian F. Reiser, Medical Radiology series editor, and to Ute Heilmann, PhD, Editorial Director, Clinical Medicine at Springer, for entrusting us to be the editors of this volume. We are also grateful to Ms. Daniela Brandt at Springer for her support in prepairing this book.

We hope that this book will be a useful resource to our collegues primary interested in scrotal pathology, as well as to those who are not experts in this field, but encounter scrotal diseases during their daily medical workup. We hope, in particular, that it will stimulate, motivate, and inspire radiologists and urologists to apply in this field integrating knowledge of imaging modalities and clinical features. We believe that our patients will benefit both from an integrated approach to scrotal problems, and from an optimal use of the different diagnostic tools.

Michele Bertolotto
Carlo Trombetta

# Contents

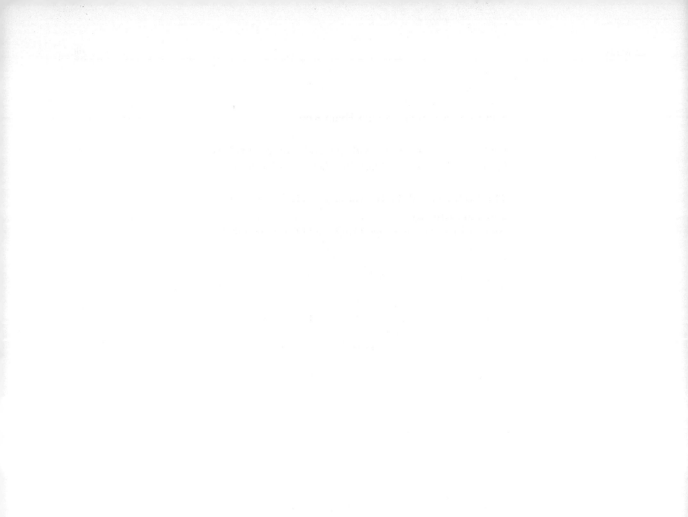

# Abbreviations

| | |
|---|---|
| 3D US | 3 Dimensional Ultra Sound |
| 18FDG | 18fluoro-2-deoxy-D-glucose |
| AAST | American Association for Surgery and Trauma |
| ACTH | Adreno Cortico Tropic Hormone |
| ADC | Apparent Diffusion Coefficient |
| AMH | Anti Müllerian Hormone |
| ART | Advanced Reproductive Techniques |
| ATP | Adenosine Three Phosphate |
| AVM | Arterio Venous Malformation |
| AZF | A Zoospermia Factor |
| CAIS | Complete Androgen Insensitivity Syndrome |
| CASA system | Computer Aided Sperm Analysis |
| CBAVD | Congenital Bilateral Absence of the Vas Deferens |
| CEUS | Contrast-Enhanced Ultrasonography |
| CFTR | Cystic Fibrosis Transmembrane Regulator |
| CIS | Carcinoma In Situ |
| CMUT | Capacitive Micromachined Ultrasonic Elements |
| CUAVD | Congenital Unilateral Absence of the Vas Deferens |
| DHT | Di Hydro Testosterone |
| DVD | Digital Versatile Disc |
| DXA | Dual energy X-ray Absorptiometry |
| EAU | European Association of Urology |
| ECD | Eco-Color-Doppler |
| ED | Erectile Dysfunction |
| EDV | End Diastolic Velocity |
| EOH | Early Onset of Hypogonadism |
| FIVET | Fecundation In Vitro and Embryo Transfer |
| FNA | Fine Needle Aspiration |
| FSH | Follicle-Stimulating Hormone |
| GnRH | Gonadotropin Releasing Hormone |
| HCG | Human Chorionic Gonadotropin |
| HIF | Hypoxia-Inducible Factor |
| HIV | Human Immunodeficiency Virus |
| ICSI | Intracytoplasmatic Sperm Injection |
| INSL | Insuline-Like Hormone |
| IVF | In Vitro Fertilization |
| LH | Luteinizing Hormone |
| LOH | Late Onset of Hypogonadism |
| MAGI | Male Accessory Glands Infection |
| MESA | Microsurgical Epididymal Sperm Aspiration |

| | |
|---|---|
| MIP | Maximum Intensity Projection |
| MIS | Müllerian Inhibiting Substances |
| MRA | Magnetic Resonance Arteriography |
| MRI | Magnetic Resonance Imaging |
| MRV | Magnetic Resonance Venography |
| NOA | Non Obstructive Azoospermia |
| NPT | Non-Palpable Testis |
| PAN | PolyArteritis Nodosa |
| PDGF | Plateled-Derived Growth Factor |
| PESA | Percutaneous Epididymal Sperm Aspiration |
| PET | Positron Emission Tomography |
| PI | Pulsatility Index |
| PRF | Pulse Repetition Frequency |
| PRL | Prolactin |
| PSA | Prostate-Specific Antigen |
| PSV | Peak Systolic Velocity |
| PW Doppler | Pulsed Wave Doppler |
| RCT | Random Controlled Trial |
| RI | Resistance Index |
| RPLND | Retro Peritoneal Lymph Node Dissection |
| SCOS | Sertoli Cell Only Syndrome |
| SHBG | Sex-Hormone Binding Globulin |
| SIEDY | Structured Interview on Erectile DYsfunction |
| SLE | Systemic Lupus Erythematosus |
| SNR | Signal to Noise Ratio |
| Spd\tub | Spermatidis\tub\ |
| SSRI | Selective Serotonin Reuptake Inhibitors |
| STD | Sexual Transmitted Infection |
| T | Testosterone |
| TBC | Tuberculosis |
| TDS | Testicular Disgenesis Syndrome |
| TE | Eco Time |
| TeFNA | Testicular Fine Needle Aspiration |
| TESA | Testicular Sperm Aspiration |
| TESE | Testicular Sperm Extraction |
| TGF | Transforming Growth Factor |
| Tin | Intratubarian germ cell neoplasia |
| TRUS | TRansurethral Ultra Sonography |
| TSE | Turbo Spin Echo |
| TSH | Thyroid-Stimulating Hormone |
| TURED | Transurethral Resection of the Ejaculatory Ducts |
| TURP | Trans Urethral Resection of the Prostate |
| UDT | Un Descended Testis |
| US | Ultra Sonography |
| VE | Vaso Epidydimostomy |
| VEGF | Vasculare Endothelial Growth Factor |
| VEOH | Very Early Onset Hypogonadism |
| WHO | World Health Organization |

# Instrumentation, Technical Requirements: US

Michele Bertolotto, Carlo Martinoli, and Lorenzo E. Derchi

## Contents

**Abstract**

Ultrasound is the first imaging modality in virtually all patients with scrotal disease, and has been widely used in this field by radiologists and urologists, since its introduction in the clinical practice. Image quality, however, improved substantially in last years due to the development of new broadband high frequency probes and digital equipment. Increased spatial resolution and doppler sensitivity allow excellent depiction of the scrotal content and full evaluation of the testicular and extratesticular vasculature. New imaging modalities are available, some of which have already established clinical role, with others requiring clinical validation. This chapter introduces technical features of modern ultrasound equipment and their application to scrotal ultrasound. Specific topics discussed are characteristics of newest broadband small-part transducers, extended field of view facilities, compounding techniques, 3D US, and adaptive filtering.

## 1 Introduction

Latest-generation beam forming technologies and use of new broadband high-frequency probes improved significantly the quality of ultrasound imaging, particularly in the examination of superficial structures.

Even though scrotal structures have been successfully investigated, since many years using less performing equipment, scrotal ultrasonography has gained many benefits from the introduction of these technologies. Improved spatial and contrast resolution

M. Bertolotto (✉)
Department of Radiology, University of Trieste,
Ospedale di Cattinara, Strada di Fiume 447,
34124 Trieste, Italy
e-mail: bertolot@units.it

C. Martinoli · L. E. Derchi
Dicmi-Radiologia, University of Genova,
Largo R. Benzi 8, 16132 Genoa, Italy

M. Bertolotto and C. Trombetta (eds.), *Scrotal Pathology,* Medical Radiology. Diagnostic Imaging,
DOI: 10.1007/174_2011_168, © Springer-Verlag Berlin Heidelberg 2012

allow evaluating with excellent detail normal and pathological structures generally of less than 1 mm such as, for instance, intact and disrupted tunica albuginea in trauma patients. Increased color doppler sensitivity for slow flow allows full evaluation of testicular vasculature also in children and in hypoperfused testis.

This chapter will review the main advances in ultrasound technology and address the clinical impact that they have had or are likely to have in the future, in imaging scrotal disease.

## 1.1    Broadband Transducers

The transducer is an essential element of ultrasound equipment, responsible for generation of the ultrasound beam and for detection of returning echoes. It greatly influences spatial resolution, penetration and signal-to-noise ratio.

Many factors including material, mechanical and electrical construction, and the external mechanical and electrical load conditions, influence the behavior of the transducer. Manufacturers strive to provide innovative transducer technology that results in the highest-quality axial and lateral resolution with improved depth penetration. Today's ultrasound transducers are broadband probes that image for detail at higher frequencies and use lower frequencies for better depth penetration.

The main components of a modern transducer are the array of active elements, the matching layers, and the absorbing backing material (Claudon et al. 2002).

The active elements are piezoelectric components that convert electrical energy to ultrasonic energy and then receive back ultrasonic energy and convert it to electrical energy. To get as much energy out of the transducer as possible, an impedance matching is placed between the active elements and the face of the transducer. Optimal impedance matching is achieved by sizing the matching layers so that their thickness is 1/4 of the desired wavelength. This keeps waves that were reflected within the matching layers in phase when they exit the layers. The backing material supporting the active elements has a great influence on the damping characteristics of a transducer. Using a backing material with an impedance similar to that of the active elements, will produce the most effective damping. Such a transducer will have a wider

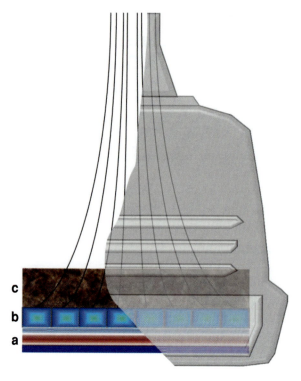

**Fig. 1** Architecture of an ultrasound transducer. Matching layers (**a**) are placed between the piezoelectric components (**b**) and the face of the transducer. The absorbing backing material (**c**) is placed at the rear face of the transducer

bandwidth resulting in higher sensitivity. Transducers also incorporate a wear plate to protect the matching layers and active elements from scratching (Fig. 1).

Research in transducer technology has been focused on the development of piezoelectric elements with lower acoustic impedances and greater electromechanical coupling coefficients (Szabo and Lewin 2007), as well as on improving the characteristics of absorbing backing layers and quarter-wave impedance matching layers. Currently, transducer arrays are formed by ceramic polymer composite elements. A variety of technical solutions have been applied to improve their mechanical characteristics. In particular, piano-concave elements can be used to provide a uniform elevation plane radiation pattern both in the near and in the far field (Jedrzejewicz 1999). Similar results have been obtained producing multi-layered piezoelectric elements (Whittingham 1999a) or shaping the elements in other suitable ways. These refinements led to the use of very short pulses, increased bandwidth, and better intrinsic collimation of the ultrasound beam (Fig. 2).

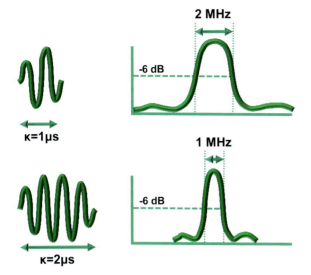

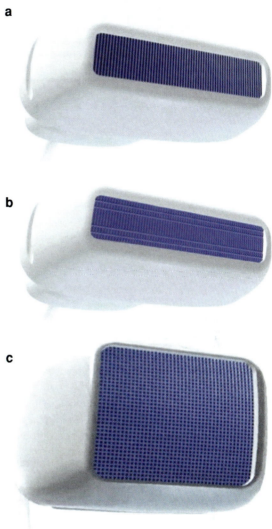

**Fig. 2** Relationship between spatial pulse length and frequency spectrum. Intensity versus time diagrams (*left illustrations*) illustrate two pulses with different length κ of 1 μs and 2 μs, respectively, and the corresponding spectrum of frequency of 2 MHz and 1 MHz, respectively. The longer pulse (2 μs) generates a narrower bandwidth (1 MHz). (The bandwidth is measured between the 6 dB points of each side of the spectrum)

## 1.2    "1.5D" Matrix Transducers

Whereas considerable efforts have been undertaken in the recent years to improve axial and lateral resolution of ultrasound images by means of sofisticated dynamic focusing techniques, relatively poor attention has been paid until recently to reduce slice thickness of the ultrasound beam. Focusing on the z-plane is commonly obtained by means of acoustic lenses with fixed focal length. As a consequence, resolution of less than 1 mm is currently obtained into the scan plane, whereas slice thickness of several mm are commonly encountered outside the focal zone. As a consequence, some artifacts occur which may have practical consequences in imaging the scrotum as well. If the curvature of a small lesion in z-plane is comparable or smaller than the slice thickness, tissues outside the lesion can be displayed into the scan plane producing noise and blurring of the lesion profile (Rizzatto 1999). For instance, small testicular cysts may present blurred contours and low-level echoes inside, simulating solid lesions, and leading to unnecessary orchidectomy.

Electronic control of focusing in both lateral and elevation directions can be obtained using the

**Fig. 3** Types of ultrasound transducers. **a** Conventional linear array with one row of elements. **b** "1.5D" matrix transducer with five rows of elements. **c** "2D" matrix transducer with similar number of elements in both rows and columns

so-called 1.5D matrix arrays. In these transducers, the single row of long piezoelectric elements found in a conventional probe is replaced by more layers (three to seven) incorporated into a single thin layer to produce parallel rows of short elements. The slice thickness of the ultrasound beam is improved by performing dynamic focusing in the elevation plane, which leads to excellent contrast resolution and image uniformity throughout the entire field of view, and to the reduction of partial volume averaging artifacts in both shallow regions and in the far field (Fig. 3).

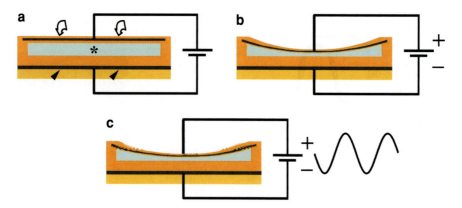

**Fig. 4** Diagram illustrating the working principle of a CMUT element. **a** CMUT consists in a parallel plate capacitor having a top movable electrode (*curved arrows*) and a bottom fixed electrode (*arrowheads*). The intervening dielectric medium (*asterisks*) is air or vacuum. **b** When a static voltage is placed between the two electrodes, the membrane is attracted to the substrate. **c** When an alternate voltage is superimposed, the membrane oscillates, generating an ultrasound beam

## 1.3 "2D" Matrix Transducers

The 2D arrays are matrix with similar number of active elements in both rows and columns which allow unrestricted control of focusing and beam formation over a scan volume (Fig. 3). They provide very thin slice thickness with excellent axial, lateral and elevation resolution, allow simultaneous visualization of different planes in real time, and are capable of unrestricted eletronic scanning in 3D. Although a substantial amount of work has been done in the area of ultrasonic imaging during the past decade, high performance commercially available 2D arrays have been introduced only recently. Besides high cost, the main problems arising for the 2D matrix transducers at megahertz frequencies are small size and huge count of the elements, high electrical impedance, low sensitivity, bad SNR, and slower data acquisition rate. The major technological difficulty that still remains is the high density of the interconnections among the thousands of elements which form the probe (Eames and Hossack 2008; Wygant et al. 2008). The high performance 2D matrix transducers with these characteristics which are available in the market are designed for imaging abdominal organs, but functioning high-frequency prototypes are ready to enter the market in the next future. In scrotal imaging, they might have a role especially in imaging infertile men, since they allow very accurate volume measurements, and improved parametric analysis of testicular flows, both using conventional color/power doppler techniques, and microbubble specific modes.

## 1.4 CMUT Matrix Transducers

Matrix transducers made of capacitive micromachined ultrasonic elements (CMUT) are now in an advanced stage of development, and well-functioning prototypes have been produced (Caronti et al. 2006). These transducers use capacitors instead of piezoelectric elements to generate and detect ultrasound waves. In brief, the CMUT element is a parallel plate capacitor having two electrodes and an intervening dielectric medium (either vacuum or air gap) (Fig. 4). The top electrode (membrane) is movable, and the bottom electrode (backplate) is fixed. When a static voltage is placed between the two electrodes, the membrane is attracted to the substrate by coulombic forces. When an alternate voltage is superimposed, the membrane will move in response to the signal and an ultrasonic wave is generated and launched into the environment (Caliano et al. 2005). CMUT matrix transducers have the potential to outperform conventional piezoelectric transducers in terms of bandwidth, sensitivity, and electromechanical coupling efficiency (Novell et al. 2009). The main advantages compared to piezoelectric transducers are the better acoustic matching to the propagation medium, resulting in wider immersion bandwidth and improved image resolution, the ease of fabrication, the ability to be integrated with electronic circuits on the same wafer, and the expected reduction of production costs. This technology, in particular, has a great potential for production of high performance 2D arrays with a large number of elements working at a

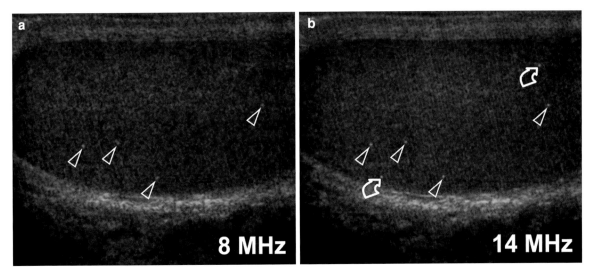

**Fig. 5** Multiple frequency transducers. Longitudinal ultrasound images of the testis obtained with a 8–15 MHz multiple frequency transducer by setting the center frequency, respectively, at 8 MHz (**a**) and at 14 MHz (**b**). With the 8 MHz setting, four testicular microliths are identified in the ultrasound view (*arrowheads*). Shifting on the higher frequencies of the bandwidth penetration slightly reduces, but two additional microliths are identified (*curved arrows*), as a result of increased spatial resolution

wide range of elevated frequencies (Wygant et al. 2008). They, therefore, have a great potential for real-time 3D high resolution imaging of superficial structures at reasonable cost (Oralkan et al. 2003; Wygant et al. 2009).

## 1.5 Transducer Selection and Handling

A variety of linear array transducers is currently available in the frequency range used for scrotal ultrasound imaging. Selection of the most appropriate transducer primarily depends on the frequency but is also related to other factors. Compared to small transducers, for instance, larger probes tend to have a large near field beam width leading to a poor lateral resolution at shallow depths. Higher frequency narrow transducers are, therefore, preferred when imaging very superficial structures, while lower frequency larger probes might be best suited deeper.

During scrotal ultrasound examination, probe handling has need of maximum stability over the region of interest; compression is not required, and the mobility of the probe to cover the region of interest is considerably less than in other studies. As pathologic findings may be small in size and are evaluated by placing the probe over a curvilinear

surface, stability of the transducer is a key factor for high quality examinations. In our experience, the best grip to obtain probe stability can be obtained by placing the ulnar fingers (long, ring, little) directly on the patient's skin while holding the probe with the radial fingers (so that the probe hangs between the thumb and the index finger). This grip allows easy translation of the probe along its short axis at a given angle minimizing rotational changes.

## 1.6 Multiple Frequency and Wide-band Imaging

In broadband transducers, the high frequency components of the spectrum tend to increase the intensity of the ultrasound beam in the most superficial regions and in the focal zone, whereas the low frequency components extend the penetration depth (Whittingham 1999b). In multiple frequency imaging, the available broad bandwidth is subdivided into multiple frequency steps for transmission and reception of sound waves: these transducers enable selection of the optimal frequency range in a given scanning plane, as though two or more independent transducers, each with a different center frequency, were available (Fig. 5).

Other systems use the entire transducer bandwidth for the transmitted pulse and then adjust the receiver bandwidth to lower frequencies as deeper depths are sampled. These systems give increased flexibility to the ultrasound examination, enabling the same transducer to change the image acquisition parameters during scanning based on the desired clinical information.

## 1.7 Coded Transmission

The issue of maximizing penetration depth retaining or enhancing spatial resolution constitutes one of the major challenges in ultrasound imaging. Compared to earlier transducers, modern broadband probes provide better axial resolution without changing the emission frequency. In principle, however, short pulses suffer attenuation to a greater extent and are characterized by less penetration than long pulses. Moreover, use of higher frequency beam increase spatial and contrast resolution of ultrasound images, and therefore, the possibility to increase penetration of high frequency pulses would be advisable for both, imaging of abdominal organs and of superficial structures.

The simplest way to increase penetration of short pulses is to increase the acoustic power of the ultrasound beam, because signal from deeper tissue regions can be recorded over the noise threshold. However, concerns about potential and undesirable side effects, in particular related to acoustic cavitation, set limits on the possibility of overcoming the frequency dependent attenuation by increasing peak acoustic amplitudes of the waves probing the tissue. Moreover, low amplitudes are mandatory when pulses for contrast specific non-destructive modes are designed, in order to limit microbubble destruction.

A substantial effort has been done by the different manufacturers of ultrasound machines to overcome limitations of peak acoustic amplitude by using coded pulses (Lewandowski and Nowicki 2008; Huang and Li 2007; Huang and Li 2006; Chiao and Hao 2005). Basically, the principle of coded transmission is similar to that of amplitude, frequency, and phase modulation used since many decades in telecommunications. A carrier wave is used to convey information by varying its instantaneous amplitude, frequency, or phase. Since the characteristics of the carrier are known, the information can be recovered during the reception phase using appropriate filtering algorithms (Fig. 6).

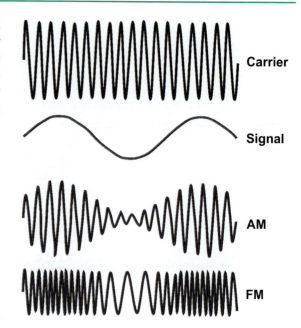

**Fig. 6** Principle of amplitude and phase modulation. The information (Signal) is conveyed over a carrier wave by varying its instantaneous value of amplitude (amplitude modulation, AM), or its instantaneous value of frequency (frequency modulation FM)

Coded transmission offers two major advantages over conventional ultrasound beam forming. Coded pulses can be readily recognized from random noise, and pulses with increased average power can be driven within the tissue without increasing the peak acoustic amplitude. As a consequence, a significant improvement of the signal-to-noise ratio is obtained and frequency-dependent attenuation is reduced. Higher ultrasound frequencies can be used for ultrasound imaging both with abdominal and small part applications, enclosing scrotal imaging, resulting in increased spatial and contrast resolution (Nowicki et al. 2004).

## 1.8 Adaptive Filtering

In addition to spatial and frequency compounding, several high end equipment implement adaptive filters to further reduce the amount of speckle and other sources of noise in ultrasound images. These complex algorithms analyze the local features of image texture, and recognize regions with different speckle patterns (Noble 2010; Wu et al. 2008). Distinct low-pass and edge enhancement filters are, therefore, applied in the different portions of the image.

Several adaptive filtering techniques have been developed and applied to medical ultrasound imaging. The major challenge is to obtain maximum speckle suppression in real time without significant frame rate reduction, while avoiding structure creation, and preserving edge details and information associated with real objects. Results are very encouraging: it appears that the visual perception of features such as small discrete structures, subtle fluctuations in mean echo level and changes in image texture may be enhanced relative to that for unprocessed images (Meuwly et al. 2003; Barr et al. 2009).

Image segmentation process starts searching for proper seed regions having the speckle pattern expected for the different tissues. To find a proper seed region, an initially assumed seed region is successively contracted according to previously selected criteria. Once the seed regions are determined, the next step is to grow them based on measures of local homogeneity and similarity of the neighboring region.

The design of adaptive filters is complex, since the criteria used to start and guide image segmentation cannot be established unequivocally. Speckle patterns expected for the different portions of the image, for instance fluid and solid tissues, are calculated by the manufacturer using algorithms that simulate the interaction between the ultrasound beam and the different body tissues. The patterns obtained through simulations are then customized performing measurements in real tissues with true ultrasound machines. Latest generation equipment have been customized to recognize speckle pattern of fluid and of several solid tissues such as liver, kidney, and fat.

As regards scrotal imaging, use of adaptive filtering results in artifact reduction, especially in areas containing fluid. It also results in brighter, more continuous boundaries while maintaining the image's integrity. Depiction of the tunica albuginea and of subtle anatomical features is improved. Variations in the echogenicity of various regions of the tissue are easier to see because the user's eyes are not distracted by speckle and other sources of noise.

## 1.9 New Sonographic Modes

Technologic innovations in ultrasound have resulted in improved diagnostic performance for the evaluation of superficial structures. Some of them have a role for ultrasound scrotal imaging as well, in particular, wide-band doppler imaging, and compounding. Other innovations can be useful in selected cases.

### 1.9.1 Wide-band Doppler Imaging

The ability of newest equipment to detect low flow states in superficial tissues improved significantly the diagnostic performance of doppler techniques in imaging scrotal disorders. In ultrasound, scrotal imaging with high sensitivity for slow flows and good signal resolution is essential, for instance, to evaluate the prepuberal testis, suspected ischemic conditions, and hypovascular scrotal lesions. Besides color, power, and PW doppler modes, other doppler modalities are now available. Directional power doppler US, for instance, encodes flow direction in real time with a two-color scale but estimates the signal intensity, as does the conventional power doppler mode. This system should add the advantages of better sensitivity and lower dependence on angle of the power mode to estimation of flow direction.

In modern ultrasound equipment, doppler signal is recorded using wide-band techniques, which are designed to take advantage of the characteristics of high frequency, broadband transducers (Brands and Hoeks 1992). Unlike conventional doppler systems, in which a long burst pulse containing a large number of cycles are used, broadband doppler technology makes use of short pulses with a significant improvement in frame rate and axial resolution. Actually, use of broadband doppler technology with high-frequency probes also has potential limitations. When short pulses with wide frequency spectra are transmitted and received, and the number of ultrasound wave transmissions and receptions in the same direction is reduced in order to increase the frame rate, the doppler spectra become wider. A wider doppler spectrum results in greater superimposition of clutter (tissue echoes) and blood flow, which are difficult to separate out using a wall filter. This problem can cause reduction in doppler signal sensitivity, and significant motion artifacts. Moreover, higher frequencies are attenuated with depth, producing bandwidth narrowing and central frequency shift towards the lower frequencies. Although this phenomenon exists also for narrow-band doppler acquisition, it is much more pronounced using wide-band techniques.

High performance signal processing algorithms have been developed to avoid reduction in doppler

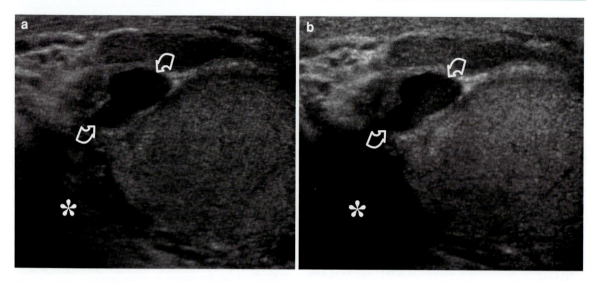

**Fig. 7** Use of tissue harmonic imaging in scrotal ultrasound. **a** Conventional scan and **b** corresponding harmonic image showing reduced artifacts (*asterisks*) and better depiction of the fluid level in a spermatocele (*curved arrows*) in the harmonic image

signal sensitivity, increase penetration, and improve separation between doppler signal and clutter (Brands and Hoeks 1992). To ensure penetration and improve doppler signal sensitivity, the center frequency is swept according to the depth during signal reception, and appropriate waveform shaping is obtained using complex mean frequency estimators which provide a better separation of signal from clutter compared to conventional wall filters.

Design and performance of mean frequency estimators is crucial. Several parameters must be considered when processing the signal, the most important of which are the noise level, mean frequency, bandwidth, and power of both the doppler signal and the stationary component over a given time window. A variety of algorithms with different characteristics have been implemented on ultrasound machines by the different manufacturers. Their quality and robustness account for most of differences in the quality of doppler signal observed in modern equipment.

### 1.9.2 Tissue Harmonic Imaging

Tissue harmonic imaging is based on the phenomenon of nonlinear distortion of an acoustic signal as it travels through the body. Harmonic waves are generated within the tissue and build up with depth to a point of maximal intensity before they decrease due to attenuation. This technique was originally thought to improve image quality during abdominal examinations of difficult patients (Choudhry et al. 2000; Oktar et al. 2003; Sodhi et al. 2005). With use of wide focal zones and broadband small part transducers, however, high intensity ultrasound waves are transmitted over a large portion of the image field when imaging superficial organs as well. Since increasingly higher frequencies are used, nonlinear distorsion of the acoustic signal occurs within few centimeters.

Different techniques such as frequency filtering, pulse inversion/phase cancellation, and coded harmonics can be used to process the received echoes so that only the returning high-frequency harmonic signal is used to produce the image, whereas signal from the fundamental frequencies are rejected.

Tissue harmonic imaging suffers less from some artifacts which affect conventional gray-scale ultrasound. In particular, noise from side lobe artifact in the near field and echo detection from multiple scattering events are reduced. This reduced noise is most likely responsible for the superiority of harmonic imaging over conventional gray-scale ultrasound in the visualization of cystic lesions and other structures containing fluid.

When imaging the scrotum, tissue harmonic imaging helps differentiate cysts from hypoechoic solid masses, and clarifies the content of cysts and other fluid collections helping differentiate artifact from true echogenic content such as vegetations, debris, hemorrhage, and septations (Fig. 7).

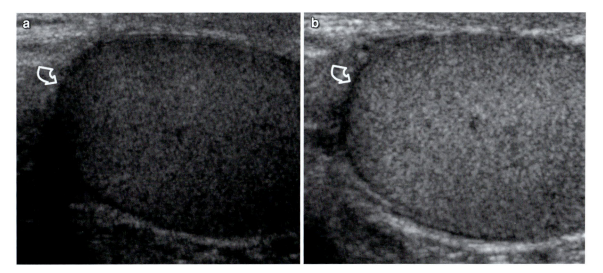

**Fig. 8** Spatial compound imaging. **a** Conventional scrotal scan and **b** corresponding compound image showing a more homogeneous echotexture, and improved depiction of the tunica albuginea and reduced artifacts especially at the poles (*curved arrow*)

### 1.9.3 Spatial Compounding

Careful evaluation of the normal tunica albuginea and of its changes is essential in several scrotal pathologies. Major problems exist, however, to evaluate thin curved interfaces with ultrasound because specular reflection and speckle artifacts may reduce their visibility.

Specular reflections produce discontinuities of curved interfaces, such as the tunica albuginea, which appear echogenic only when insonated at perpendicular angles. Speckle results from interference of the coherent waves produced by the elements of the transducer. It appears as subtle brightness fluctuations and small discontinuities of reflecting interfaces such as the tunica albuginea. Specular reflection and speckle artifacts may have profound repercussion in the clinical practice, for instance, in patients with scrotal trauma in whom small ruptures of the tunica albuginea may be overlooked. Moreover, edge shadowing artifacts are generated distal to smooth, curved interfaces such as cysts, spermatoceles, and the testis itself that may partially mask the anatomic structures below.

Spatial compound imaging is highly effective to overcome these limitations. In this technique, electronic steering is used to image the same tissue multiple times from different directions and echoes from these multiple acquisitions are averaged together in real-time into a single composite image (Hangiandreou 2003; Entrekin et al. 2001). The advantages of compound mode are many, including reduction of image artifacts (e.g., speckle, clutter, noise, angle-generated artifacts), sharper delineation of tissue interfaces and better discrimination of lesions over the background as well as improvement in detail resolution and image contrast. In scrotal imaging, an improved delineation of structures composed of specular echoes is obtained, such as the tunica albuginea testis (Fig. 8). This derives from the fact that when the tunica is investigated, a synthetic image is obtained from frames collected at different angles, and larger portions of this curved interface are insonated perpendicularly. Moreover, compared to the single frames, several images are averaged to obtain the compound image, resulting in improved signal-to-noise ratio. Since speckle artefacts depend on the direction of the ultrasound beam, frames obtained from different view angles have different speckle patterns, which average out when combined in the compound image. Finally, edge shadows resulting from curved boundaries are suppressed because they reflect only weakly at oblique angle.

### 1.9.4 Frequency Compounding

Beside beam direction and tissue characteristics, speckle pattern depends also on the frequency of the ultrasound beam. Imaging modalities have been developed that use emission of two different bands of frequencies to obtain distinct images, which are averaged to decorrelate speckle and improve signal-to-noise ratio (Oktar et al. 2003). The disadvantage of

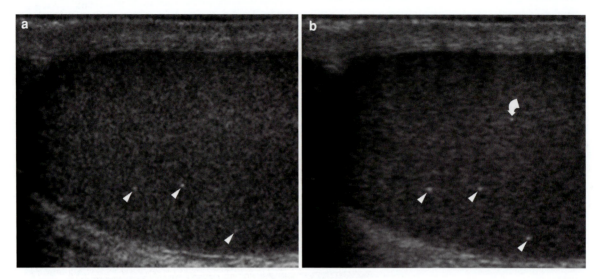

**Fig. 9** Frequency compound imaging. **a** Conventional scan and **b** corresponding frequency compound image showing a more homogeneous testicular echotexture, and increased conspicuity of microliths (*arrowheads*) due to speckle reductions which results in improved contrast resolution. One microlith (*curved arrow*) is visible on the compound image only

frequency compounding over spatial compounding is that only speckle is reduced, while specular reflection and angle generated artifacts are not significantly affected. Moreover, the transmission band of the probe is reduced to obtain emission of beams centered at different frequencies, resulting in reduced spatial resolution (Fig. 9).

### 1.9.5 Three-Dimensional (3D) Imaging

Currently, mechanical 3D probes are available for volume imaging of the superficial structures (Prager et al. 2010). These transducers sweep the ultrasound beam throughout the tissue volume by tilting the scanhead with a mechanized drive along the z-axis. During this procedure, serial slices are recorded resulting in a pyramid-shaped volume scan. Mechanically swept 3D probes are larger than standard probes, heavier and more difficult to handle.

The major limitations of these probes are limited spatial resolution along the z-axis and intrinsically limited frame rate. In fact, besides the technical complexity of manufacturing rapidly moving mechanisms, errors are performed during reconstruction of the volumetric image which increase dramatically at higher angular speed, resulting in missing parts and geometric distortion (Cao et al. 2010).

The forthcoming introduction of high performance 2D matrix array with thousands of active elements in the frequency range suitable for analysis of superficial tissues is providing a significant improvement in ergonomic use and image quality of volume ultrasound imaging (Prager et al. 2010). These probes are substantially smaller and lighter than mechanically driven arrays, and a better spatial resolution is achievable at higher frame rates.

Following volume scan acquisition, reconstructed slices can be displayed according to longitudinal, transverse, and coronal planes. Each plane can be oriented within the volume block for detailed analysis by parallel or rotational shifting around any of the three spatial axes. Data can also be displayed as true 3D images using various rendering algorithms, including maximum intensity projection (MIP), transparent, surface and doppler rendering (Prager et al. 2010; Kim et al. 2010). Doppler signal measurement and quantification over the entire volume is possible using dedicated software, providing accurate vascular mapping. Parametric analysis of tissue perfusion over the entire volume is becoming commercially available.

Three-Dimensional ultrasound is opening new interesting perspectives for evaluation of scrotal pathologies as well. Elwagdy et al. (2007) claim that 3D ultrasound is an important addition to conventional gray-scale ultrasound, offering new diagnostic means of differentiating benign from malignant scrotal lesions. Indeed, definition of margins, echo pattern, and actual extension of both extratesticular

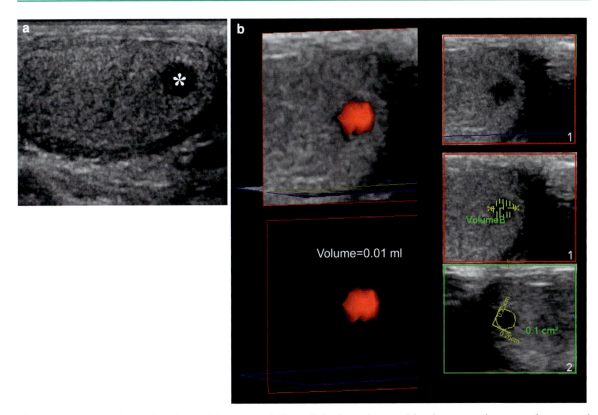

**Fig. 10** Three-dimensional imaging. Volume acquisition using a dedicated mechanical 3D probe. **a** Conventional ultrasound image showing a small testicular lesion (*asterisks*). **b** Lesion volume and its changes can be accurately measured using the data of the volume scan processed with a dedicated commercially available software

and intratesticular masses is improved, with reduced operator dependency. Detailed study of the 3D vascular supply of the lesions and surrounding tissues helps identification of isoechoic lesions (Elwagdy et al. 2007). Among the possible fields of application of 3D ultrasound in scrotal imaging volume measurements, assessment of diffuse pathological conditions, and of perfusion changes are especially promising. Accurate measurement of testicular volume is important in assessing pubertal development and testicular function. Using conventional transducers, testicular volume can be determined accurately by measuring the dimensions of the testis along three orthogonal axes and applying the ellipsoid formula. However, the results obtained have been reported to be underestimates of true testicular volume, and empirical formulas which approximate more closely the true testicular volume have been suggested (Sakamoto et al. 2008). Use of 2D matrix transducers has been associated with substantial reduction in volumetric errors (Elliott 2008). Similarly, accurate

volume measurement can be obtained for testicular and extratesticular lesions managed conservatively, improving the capability to assess their growth rate (Fig. 10). Progression of pathologies involving large portions of the testis, such as testicular microlithiasis, can be evaluated effectively during the follow up by direct comparison of volume datasets obtained at different time intervals. Variation of the amount of calcifications, and of associated parenchyma inhomogeneities can be assessed, which is difficult to establish subjectively. Finally, an increasing concern is rising over the role of impaired testicular microcirculation in infertile male (Unsal et al. 2007; Tarhan et al. 2003; Gat et al. 2005). Herwig et al. (2007) showed that mapping of testicular perfusion at color doppler interrogation in patients suffering from azoospermia may improve the chances of sperm retrieval during testicular sperm extraction (TESE) procedures. This evaluation is improved using 3D probes, and it is conceivable that further improvement will be possible with parametric quantification of the entire testicular microcirculation on volume data obtained after microbubble injection.

### 1.9.6 Elastographic Imaging

Ultrasound tissue elasticity imaging is a research area of increasing interest. Reason for the use of elastographic modes stems from the existence of large differences in stiffness between surrounding normal and pathologic tissues that may otherwise possess similar image contrasts with conventional gray-scale ultrasound imaging (Fig. 11).

Approaches used to attain information on elastic properties of tissues are based on comparison of raw ultrasound (radiofrequency) data while changing the external force applied to tissues. Depending on the characteristics of the mechanical stimuli applied, quasi-static and dynamic modes are distinguished (Varghese 2009). The former makes use of small movements of the ultrasound probe, or other stimuli causing small amounts of tissue deformation (about 1%). Echo-signals acquired before and after tissue distortion are compared with a variety of algorithms to build up a map of movement, which is related to the stiffness of tissues. The latter obtain information on tissue elasticity by sending shear waves within the tissue and measuring velocity variation of them (Varghese 2009).

At present, several different commercial ultrasound system manufacturers offer quasi-static modes on their clinical systems for imaging of superficial structures. Dynamic modes have been currently implemented for imaging abdominal tissues.

Algorithms for displacement and strain estimation have progressed over the last two decades (Varghese 2009). Only the axial strain distribution was initially considered, namely, tissue displacement along the insonification and deformation direction. Then, more complex methods have been developed that consider also tissue deformation perpendicular to the beam propagation direction within the scan plane (2D tracking), and tissue deformation perpendicular to the scan plane (3D tracking). This latter method allows tracking the complete displacement vector, and therefore, the components of the strain tensor, which is computed from the time gradient of the displacement vector.

Most commercial clinical ultrasound systems implement strain imaging modes. The strain tensor distribution, however, does not indicate the absolute elastic properties of tissue, because it is significantly dependent on the applied deformation or stress distribution. Many investigators are focusing on the estimation of the Young modulus in tissue, which if estimated accurately would provide an absolute or quantitative distribution of the underlying tissue elastic properties. However, there are many challenges that have to be addressed for accurate estimation of the Young's modulus (Varghese 2009) because additional information is necessary on both the boundary conditions during the applied deformation, and on the local stress distribution in tissue. Unfortunately, these parameters are generally unknown, and therefore, a reliable calculation of Young's modulus distribution is impossible using the current technology.

Strain imaging of breast lesions has been widely reported in literature (Kumm and Szabunio 2010; Zhi et al. 2010; Thomas et al. 2010; Cho et al. 2010). In fact, many breast lesions are superficial and are known to be significantly stiffer than surrounding normal breast tissue. Invasive cancers in the breast are well depicted as areas of stiffness in the strain images. Also cysts present typical features on strain images. Besides breast imaging, applications of elasticity modes have been investigated in imaging thyroid gland, lymph nodes, and prostate. Other possible applications are evaluation of stiffness increase of thrombi with age, and stiffness variation of uterine cervix in pregnant women.

Since most testicular lesions are palpable, elasticity imaging has not been widely applied in this field. It must still be established whether strain mode adds useful diagnostic information to gray-scale ultrasound and lesion palpation in the setting of scrotal imaging. Preliminary investigation claims that elasticity imaging can be used as an additional method for detecting pathologic tissue alterations, since changes of elasticity pattern seems to be related to volume and function (Schurich et al. 2009). Another possible application is to support the ultrasound diagnosis of benign abnormality when a soft mass, not completely characterized at gray-scale ultrasound is demonstrated in the appropriate clinical setting (Shah et al. 2010). In particular, complex cystic benign lesions might be differentiated from solid tumors. Also evaluation of lesion mobility may have a role to differentiate between benign masses loosely attached to background normal tissue and malignant lesions. Elastographic parameters may also be potentially used to estimate the fluid content in tissues, and to differentiate between normal and edematous tissues (Konofagou et al. 2001; Righetti et al. 2007), with

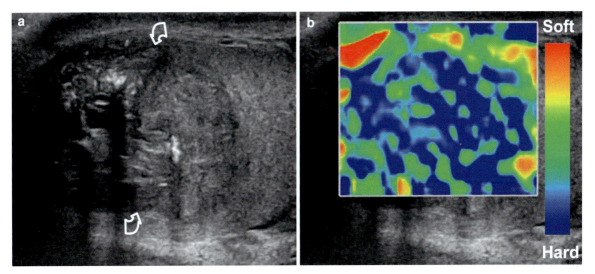

**Fig. 11** Elastographic imaging. **a** Conventional grey-scale image showing a testicular mass (*curved arrows*). **b** Corresponding elastographic image showing that the mass is harder (*imaged in blue*) than the surrounding testicular parenchyma (*imaged in green/red*). (By courtesy of M. Valentino, Bologna, Italy)

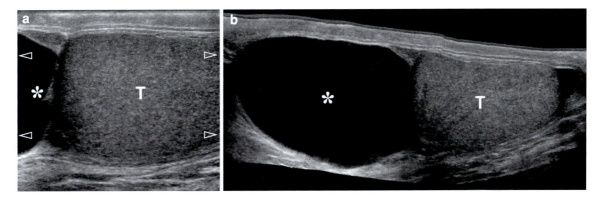

**Fig. 12** Extended field of view technology. **a** Using conventional rectangular field of view, the testis (*T*) and spermatocele (*asterisks*) cannot be displayed in its full extent: part of them (*arrowheads*) are out of the field of view of the ultrasound image. **b** Corresponding extended field of view image shows the testis and spermatocele in their full extent

potential application in imaging many scrotal pathologies as well, such as inflammation, and ischemia.

## 1.10    Extended Field of View

Ultrasound images have a field of view which is limited by the probe width. During the study, the examiner moves the probe over the area of interest to acquire information on large volumes of tissue and reconstructs in his/her mind the spatial relationships within the scanned area by memorizing many frames (Weng et al. 1997). This is a distinct disadvantage of ultrasound compared to other imaging methods, and is a major drawback in conveying the information of the study to clinicians. The extended field of view mode, also called panoramic imaging, has been developed to overcome these limitations. It allows the reconstruction of wide images by progressive addition of data during a hand sweep of the target in real time with a conventional probe.

The reconstruction process is based on the fact that image features of a given frame and the next frame

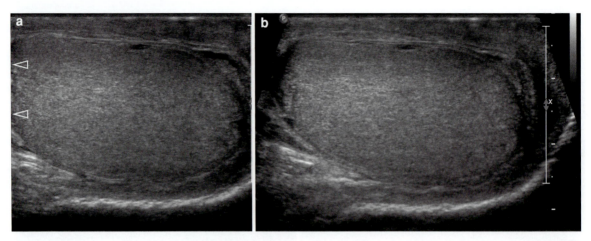

**Fig. 13** Wide field of view technology. **a** Using conventional rectangular field of view the testis cannot be displayed in its full extent: part of it (*arrowheads*) is out of the field of view of the ultrasound image. Accurate measurement of testicular size cannot be taken. **b** Corresponding wide (*trapezoidal*) field of view image shows the testis in its full extent

are very similar, except that the second image is slightly shifted or rotated relative to the first one. Successive frames are registered and blended with the previous ones based on autocorrelation algorithms. Accurate distance or size measurements of large organs are possible using the panoramic mode. As determined on phantoms, geometric measurement is accurate to within <5%.

In scrotal imaging panoramic mode provides accurate data because of the absence of respiratory movements or pulsatility of large vessels. It allows accurate measurement of testicular diameters overcoming the limitation of high frequency transducers that often have an array of elements shorter than 4 cm, and cannot, therefore, be used to measure directly the longitudinal diameter of many adult testes. Moreover, extended field of view imaging can show abnormalities such as large fluid collections, masses, and traumatic lesions in all their extent, in association with the appropriate landmarks (Fig. 12).

### 1.11 Wide Field of View

This mode makes use of the beam steering function to increase the lateral size of the ultrasound image in the far field. The resultant trapezoid shape of the field of view allows reproduction in their full extent of targets larger than the rectangular field of view of the transducer. Similar to panoramic imaging this function is useful in scrotal imaging as well to measure accurately testes and other lesions whose size exceeds the length of the transducer (Fig. 13).

## References

Barr RG, Maldonado RL, Georgian-Smith D (2009) Comparison of conventional, compounding, computer enhancement, and compounding with computer enhancement in ultrasound imaging of the breast. Ultrasound Q 25:129–134

Brands PJ, Hoeks AP (1992) A comparison method for mean frequency estimators for doppler ultrasound. Ultrason Imaging 14:367–386

Caliano G, Carotenuto R, Cianci E et al (2005) Design, fabrication and characterization of a capacitive micromachined ultrasonic probe for medical imaging. IEEE Trans Ultrason Ferroelectr Freq Control 52:2259–2269

Cao J, Karadayi K, Managuli R et al (2010) Reconstruction error in 3D ultrasound imaging with mechanical probes. In: Jan D.h. Stephen A.M. (eds.) SPIE, 762903

Caronti A, Caliano G, Carotenuto R et al (2006) Capacitive micromachined ultrasonic transducer (CMUT) arrays for medical imaging. Microelectron J 37:770–777

Chiao RY, Hao X (2005) Coded excitation for diagnostic ultrasound: a system developer's perspective. IEEE Trans Ultrason Ferroelectr Freq Control 52:160–170

Cho N, Moon WK, Kim HY et al (2010) Sonoelastographic strain index for differentiation of benign and malignant nonpalpable breast masses. J Ultrasound Med 29:1–7

Choudhry S, Gorman B, Charboneau JW et al (2000) Comparison of tissue harmonic imaging with conventional US in abdominal disease. Radiographics 20:1127–1135

Claudon M, Tranquart F, Evans DH et al (2002) Advances in ultrasound. Eur Radiol 12:7–18

Eames MD, Hossack JA (2008) Fabrication and evaluation of fully-sampled, two-dimensional transducer array for "sonic window" imaging system. Ultrasonics 48:376–383

Elliott ST (2008) Volume ultrasound: the next big thing? Br J Radiol 81:8–9

Elwagdy S, Razmy S, Ghoneim S et al (2007) Diagnostic performance of three-dimensional ultrasound extended imaging at scrotal mass lesions. Int J Urol 14:1025–1033

Entrekin RR, Porter BA, Sillesen HH et al (2001) Real-time spatial compound imaging: Application to breast, vascular, and musculoskeletal ultrasound. Semin Ultrasound CT MR 22:50–64

Gat Y, Zukerman Z, Chakraborty J et al (2005) Varicocele, hypoxia and male infertility. Fluid mechanics analysis of the impaired testicular venous drainage system. Hum Reprod 20:2614–2619

Hangiandreou NJ (2003) AAPM/RSNA physics tutorial for residents. Topics in US: B-mode US: Basic concepts and new technology. Radiographics 23:1019–1033

Herwig R, Tosun K, Schuster A et al (2007) Tissue perfusion-controlled guided biopsies are essential for the outcome of testicular sperm extraction. Fertil Steril 87:1071–1076

Huang SW, Li PC (2006) Arbitrary waveform coded excitation using bipolar square wave pulsers in medical ultrasound. IEEE Trans Ultrason Ferroelectr Freq Control 53:106–116

Huang SW, Li PC (2007) Binary code design for high-frequency ultrasound. IEEE Trans Ultrason Ferroelectr Freq Control 54:947–956

Jedrzejewicz T (1999) System architecture for various image reconstruction and processing techniques. Eur Radiol 9 (Suppl 3):S334–337

Kim HC, Yang DM, Jin W et al (2010) Relation between total renal volume and renal function: Usefulness of 3D sonographic measurements with a matrix array transducer. AJR Am J Roentgenol 194:W186–W192

Konofagou EE, Harrigan TP, Ophir J et al (2001) Poroelastography: Imaging the poroelastic properties of tissues. Ultrasound Med Biol 27:1387–1397

Kumm TR, Szabunio MM (2010) Elastography for the characterization of breast lesions: Initial clinical experience. Cancer Control 17:156–161

Lewandowski M, Nowicki A (2008) High frequency coded imaging system with RF. IEEE Trans Ultrason Ferroelectr Freq Control 55:1878–1882

Meuwly JY, Thiran JP, Gudinchet F (2003) Application of adaptive image processing technique to real-time spatial compound ultrasound imaging improves image quality. Invest Radiol 38:257–262

Noble JA (2010) Ultrasound image segmentation and tissue characterization. Proc Inst Mech Eng H 224:307–316

Novell A, Legros M, Felix N et al (2009) Exploitation of capacitive micromachined transducers for nonlinear ultrasound imaging. IEEE Trans Ultrason Ferroelectr Freq Control 56:2733–2743

Nowicki A, Secomski W, Trots I et al (2004) Extending penetration depth using coded ultrasonography. Bull Pol Ac Tech 52:215–220

Oktar SO, Yucel C, Ozdemir H et al (2003) Comparison of conventional sonography, real-time compound sonography, tissue harmonic sonography, and tissue harmonic compound sonography of abdominal and pelvic lesions. AJR Am J Roentgenol 181:1341–1347

Oralkan O, Cheng C-H, Johnson J et al (2003) Volumetric Ultrasound Imaging Using 2D CMUT Arrays. IEEE Trans Ultrason Ferroelect Freq Contr 50:1581–1594

Prager RW, Ijaz UZ, Gee AH et al (2010) Three-dimensional ultrasound imaging. Proc Inst Mech Eng H 224:193–223

Righetti R, Garra BS, Mobbs LM et al (2007) The feasibility of using poroelastographic techniques for distinguishing between normal and lymphedematous tissues in vivo. Phys Med Biol 52:6525–6541

Rizzatto G (1999) Evolution of ultrasound transducers: 1.5 and 2D arrays. Eur Radiol 9(Suppl 3):S304–306

Sakamoto H, Ogawa Y, Yoshida H (2008) Relationship between testicular volume and varicocele in patients with infertility. Urology 71:104–109

Schurich M, Aigner F, Frauscher F, et al (2009) The role of ultrasound in assessment of male fertility. Eur J Obstet Gynecol Reprod Biol, 144(Suppl 1):S192–198

Shah A, Lung PF, Clarke JL et al (2010) Re: new ultrasound techniques for imaging of the indeterminate testicular lesion may avoid surgery completely. Clin Radiol 65: 496–497

Sodhi KS, Sidhu R, Gulati M et al (2005) Role of tissue harmonic imaging in focal hepatic lesions: Comparison with conventional sonography. J Gastroenterol Hepatol 20:1488–1493

Szabo TL, Lewin PA (2007) Piezoelectric materials for imaging. J Ultrasound Med 26:283–288

Tarhan S, Gumus B, Gunduz I et al (2003) Effect of varicocele on testicular artery blood flow in men color doppler investigation. Scand J Urol Nephrol 37:38–42

Thomas A, Degenhardt F, Farrokh A et al (2010) Significant differentiation of focal breast lesions: Calculation of strain ratio in breast sonoelastography. Acad Radiol 17:558–563

Unsal A, Turgut AT, Taskin F et al (2007) Resistance and pulsatility index increase in capsular branches of testicular artery: Indicator of impaired testicular microcirculation in varicocele? J Clin Ultrasound 35:191–195

Varghese T (2009) Quasi-static ultrasound elastography. 4:323–338

Weng L, Tirumalai AP, Lowery CM et al (1997) US extended field of view imaging technology. Radiology 203:877–880

Whittingham TA (1999a) An overview of digital technology in ultrasonic imaging. Eur Radiol 9(Suppl 3):S307–311

Whittingham TA (1999b) Broadband transducers. Eur Radiol 9(Suppl 3):S298–303

Wu J, Kamath MV, Noseworthy MD et al (2008) Segmentation of images of abdominal organs. Crit Rev Biomed Eng 36:305–334

Wygant IO, Zhuang X, Yeh DT et al (2008) Integration of 2D CMUT arrays with front-end electronics for volumetric ultrasound imaging. IEEE Trans Ultrason Ferroelectr Freq Control 55:327–342

Wygant IO, Jamal NS, Lee HJ et al (2009) An integrated circuit with transmit beamforming flip-chip bonded to a 2D CMUT array for 3D ultrasound imaging. IEEE Trans Ultrason Ferroelectr Freq Control 56:2145–2156

Zhi H, Xiao XY, Yang HY et al (2010) Ultrasonic elastography in breast cancer diagnosis strain ratio vs 5-point scale. Acad Radiol 17(10):1227–33

# Instrumentation, Technical Requirements: MRI

Yuji Watanabe

## Contents

**Abstract**

This section of the chapter provides practical guide for MR examination of the scrotum and comprehensive description of clinical applications. The techniques used for scrotal MR imaging can be implemented with virtually any MR unit. Several technical points are described in obtaining high-resolution scrotal MR imaging: patient preparation, coil selection, respiratory compensation, imaging planes, pulse sequence design, fat suppression, multiple contrast, injection of contrast material, and the scanning order of pulse sequences. Image analysis is also described in the evaluation of testicular volume and perfusion. The scrotal MR imaging can be clinically applied for acute scrotal symptoms, intrascrotal masses, scrotal trauma, nonpalpable testis, infertility, etc. The recommended protocol of pulse sequences should include T1-weighted, FS-T2-weighted, and heavily T2-weighted imaging in the coronal plane. Some changes to the basic protocol should be made depending on the clinical settings. The dynamic subtraction contrast-enhanced MR imaging can be used to provide information about testicular perfusion with the use of dynamic subtraction contrast-enhanced technique.

## 1 Introduction

Magnetic resonance (MR) imaging has been thought to play a minor and questionable role in the evaluation of scrotal symptoms (Hricak et al. 1995;

Y. Watanabe (✉)
Department of Radiology, Kurashiki Central Hospital,
1-1-1-Miwa, Kurashiki 710-8602, Japan
e-mail: yw5904@kchnet.or.jp

M. Bertolotto and C. Trombetta (eds.), *Scrotal Pathology,* Medical Radiology. Diagnostic Imaging,
DOI: 10.1007/174_2011_169, © Springer-Verlag Berlin Heidelberg 2012

Trambert et al. 1990). Clinical application has been limited to a clinical setting when ultrasonography proves to be inadequate or inconclusive. However, with the use of dynamic subtraction contrast-enhanced technique, MR imaging can provide information about testicular perfusion due to its high sensitivity for contrast enhancement (Baker et al. 1987; Cheng et al. 1997; Costabile et al. 1993; Kodama et al. 2000; Landa et al. 1988; Watanabe et al. 2000).

When compared with the normal-side testis, torsion, infarction, and hemorrhagic necrosis of affected-side testis showed significant reductions in contrast enhancement, whereas tumors and orchitis showed significant increases (Watanabe et al. 2000). These findings lead MR imaging to a practical tool that relies on functional as well as anatomic assessments for improving diagnostic accuracy.

## 2    Static Magnetic Field Strength

The techniques used for the scrotal MR imaging (Watanabe et al. 2000) can be implemented with virtually any MR unit (Choyke 2000). There is no significant difference in the interpretation and quantification of scrotal images among scrotal imaging with any static magnetic field strength. Image quality and signal-to-noise ratio can be better with high-field-strength MR unit. However, imaging criteria at 1.5 T for image interpretation are applicable at other field strength 0.5, 1.0, and 3.0 T, etc. In contrast, the problem will be a susceptibility artifact, which causes signal loss or image distortion at the air–tissue interface especially found at high field strength such as 3.0 T. To minimize such a problem, it is recommended to use turbo spin echo pulse sequence, which can be less influenced by susceptibility artifact than gradient echo sequence.

The problem might be heating of the scrotum by high-magnetic-field-strength MR imaging which could affect spermatogenesis adversely. However, it was reported that the temperature recorded, when MR imaging with 1.5 T at relatively high specific absorption rates, produced a significant increase in scrotal skin temperature, which was below the threshold known to affect spermatogenesis in mammals (Shellock et al. 1990).

## 3    MR Imaging

Both T1- and T2-weighted turbo (fast) spin-echo sequences are essential for scrotal MR imaging. Contrast-enhancement and special techniques, such as dynamic subtraction contrast-enhanced MR imaging, can also be used in cases where further tissue characterization is needed or when patients present with acute scrotal pain. There are several points to be considered in obtaining high-resolution scrotal MR imaging: coil selection, respiratory compensation, imaging planes, pulse sequence design, multiple contrast, contrast enhancement, and fat suppression.

### 3.1    Coil Selection

A circular surface coil is recommended for best results in imaging the testis (Rholl et al. 1987). In the choice of a surface coil, patient age, size of scrotum and imaging coverage should be taken into consideration. A circular 17 cm coil is usually used for adolescents and adults. A small circular coil of 11or 8 cm is used for children and adolescents. A circular surface coil is recommended to be placed on a patient's lower pelvis and centered over the scrotum (Fig. 1).

### 3.2    Respiratory Compensation

Respiratory compensation may be used to reduce motion artifact. However, it takes a long scan time to obtain MR images with respiratory compensation. In patients with acute scrotal symptoms, it is required to shorten the imaging time as much as possible and not to use respiratory compensation. Image quality obtained without respiratory compensation can be high enough for the diagnosis (Frush and Sheldon 1998).

### 3.3    Preparation for Patients

Adequate support and positioning of the scrotum under the surface coil are key factors in obtaining diagnostic-quality MR images. Especially, the bilateral testes should be arranged to maintain nearly equal distance from the surface coil (Rholl et al. 1987; Baker et al. 1987).

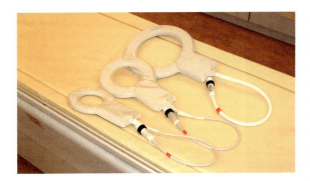

**Fig. 1** Surface coil. A variety of circular surface coils: 17, 11 and 8 cm in diameter

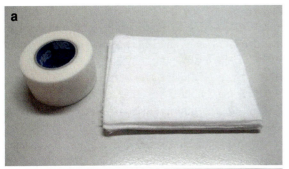

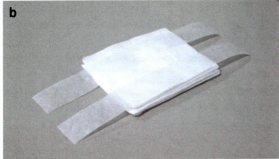

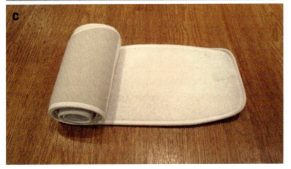

**Fig. 2** Stuff required for preparations. **a** Adhesive tape and towel. **b** Gauze. **c** Band with velcro tape

Before examination, stuffs such as adhesive tape, gauze, towel, and bands should be prepared for patients (Fig. 2). In practice, with the patient in the supine and feet-first position on the patient table, the penis is kept upward, covered with a light cloth such as gauze, and then taped against the abdominal wall (Fig. 3a). Towels or sponges are placed between the thighs to minimize motion artifact. The scrotum are then lifted up gently and fixed on the thighs. Then, bands are used to get the thighs as close as possible to keep the scrotum on the thighs. The surface coil is placed over the scrotum in a flat position, supported, and secured (Fig. 3b). To use parallel imaging technique, another surface coil could be placed under the bottom (van den Brink et al. 2003).

A peripheral intravenous line with a 21-gauge needle is placed into the subcutaneous veins of the forearm or antecubital fossa. Then, the patient should be brought into the bore of MR unit with the feet first (Fig. 3c).

The special attention should be paid to infant patients who require sedation in MR imaging. Infant patients are laid on the patient table gently and the surface coil is placed on the scrotum. No other preparations for the scrotum are necessary.

## 3.4 Imaging Plane and Coverage

The testes are usually examined in at least two planes, along the length and transverse axes (Fig. 4). Thus, the coronal and transaxial plane images are recommended to allow direct comparison of the two testes and evaluation of the spermatic cord. The coronal plane is ideal for imaging the scrotal contents, allowing complete visualization of all the important anatomic structures (Baker et al. 1987). The size and signal intensity of each testis and the epididymis are compared with those on the opposite side.

Optimal coverage of the scrotum is provided by thin sections (4–5 mm) with a 0.4–0.5 mm intersection gap and a 8–22 cm field of view (Table 1).

## 3.5 Pulse Sequence Design and Multiple Contrast

As shown in Table 1, there are a variety of pulse sequences and parameters used for scrotal imaging. Common pulse sequences used are turbo (fast) spin echo (TSE) (Hricak et al. 1995; Rholl et al. 1987; Baker et al. 1987). The advantages of this TSE sequence

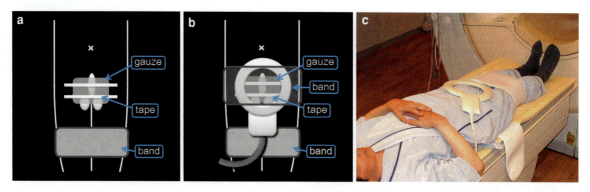

**Fig. 3** Preparation for patients. **a** Taping penis on the abdominal wall. **b** Placement of a surface coil on the scrotum. **c** Photograph of a patient going into the bore with the feet first

are (a) multiple contrast weightings such as T1- and T2-weighted imaging, (b) high-spatial resolution, (c) high signal-to-noise ratio with use of a surface coil.

Lengthy examination time may decrease patient comfort and acceptability, and increase patient movement, which can lead to degradation of image quality from motion artifact. To reduce scan time by accelerating image acquisition, parallel imaging techniques such as sensitivity encoding, simultaneous acquisition of spatial harmonics can be applied with another surface coil placed under the bottom (van den Brink et al. 2003).

T1-weighted imaging provides anatomical information of testis, epididymis, and spermatic cord, which show intermediate signal intensity areas delineated by high signal intensity area of surrounding fat tissue (Hricak et al. 1995).

T2-weighted imaging shows a variety of tissue contrast depending on the echo time (TE) (Watanabe et al. 2000, 2007). T2-weighted images obtained with TE of 100 ms yield standard T2-contrast between testes, epididymis, spermatic cord, and surrounding fat tissue. With chemical-selective fat suppression, testes show homogeneous high signal intensity area (Watanabe et al. 2000, 2007; Frush and Sheldon 1998). Spermatic cord and epididymis demonstrates very high and intermediate signal intensity area, respectively. Long TE such as 350 ms produces heavily T2-weighted images which clearly demonstrate intravaginal fluid collection as very high signal intensity area and depicts testes and epididymis as intermediate signal intensities.

T2*-weighted gradient echo sequence should be incorporated in MR imaging of patients suspected of having testicular torsion (Watanabe et al. 2007). This image is sensitive to susceptibility and important in the detection and characterization of lesions with short T2, such as acute hemorrhage (Bradley 1993; Hermier and Nighoghossian 2004).

Diffusion-weighted imaging of the scrotum may provide another information of testes about tissue characterization such as interstitial edema, capillary congestion, ischemic change, and degenerative change. Apparent diffusion coefficient (ADC) maps based on the diffusion-weighted images was reported to be useful for the early detection of testicular torsion in a rat model (Kaipia et al. 2005; Kangasniemi et al. 2001). Though diffusion-weighted imaging of the scrotum is still at a stage of investigation, it may be used for the detection of testicular torsion without contrast materials and for the evaluation of testicular dystrophy and degeneration in undescended testes and infertility.

Contrast-enhanced MR imaging gives additional information in scrotal disorders and facilitates diagnosis. It is helpful when findings at physical examination and ultrasound differ and when plain T1- and T2-weighted images are equivocal (Muller-Leisse et al. 1994). Especially, dynamic contrast-enhanced imaging with bolus infusion of contrast material provides important information about testicular perfusion (Watanabe et al. 2000, 2007).

## 3.6 Dynamic Subtraction Contrast-Enhanced MR Imaging

Contrast enhancement with special techniques called dynamic subtraction contrast-enhanced MR imaging contribute to the evaluation of testicular perfusion and further tissue characterization (Watanabe et al. 2000,

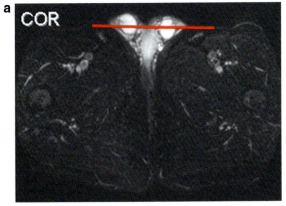

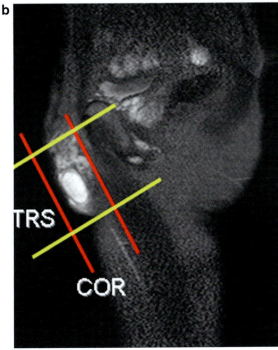

**Fig. 4** Imaging planes. **a** Coronal imaging plane depicted on the transaxial image. **b** Coronal and transaxial imaging planes depicted on the sagittal image

distinguishing torsion and trauma from other acute causes of pain (Choyke 2000).

In practice, the dynamic subtraction contrast-enhanced MR imaging is performed in the coronal plane. Fat-suppressed turbo spin echo sequence is recommended to obtain sufficient contrast enhancement of testis. Other scan parameters to achieve high image quality and appropriate temporal resolution of the scrotum are two signal acquisition, low–high k-space trajectory, 5–6 mm section thickness, 0.5–0.6 mm intersection gap, six slices, 180 mm field of view, 204 × 256 matrix, 50–60 s per sequence. Images are obtained before and after a rapid intravenous bolus injection of 0.1 mmol/kg of gadolinium-based paramagnetic contrast agents. The rapid injection of contrast agents is performed within 5 s, followed by flush of 20 ml physiological saline. Five imaging sets are consecutively acquired 15 s after the injection of contrast agents. First four imaging sets are obtained at no interval, except for that the last imaging set is obtained at an interval of 90 s after the end of the fourth imaging set. The actual examination time is approximately 6 min.

Then, the slice-by-slice subtraction is performed to obtain dynamic subtraction contrast-enhanced images. The data set obtained immediately before administration of contrast agents is used as a mask and subtracted from each of the five original data sets acquired after administration of contrast agents with commercially available software (Fig. 5).

## 3.7    The Scanning Order of Pulse Sequences

In general, non-contrast-enhanced images, such as T1- and T2-weighted images, should be first obtained, and then, contrast-enhanced images including dynamic subtraction contrast-enhanced imaging are subsequently obtained, if necessary. However, in patients with acute scrotal pain suspicious of testicular torsion, dynamic subtraction contrast-enhanced imaging can be first performed to provide information about testicular perfusion, which allows for accurate diagnosis of testicular torsion and prompt determination of treatment plan. Soon after knowing the results of testicular perfusion, fat-suppressed T2-weighted, heavily-T2-weighted and T2*-weighted images can be obtained. Though there may be minimal influence of administered contrast material on

2007). This technique can be implemented with virtually any MR unit. This method is simple, straightforward, and time efficient. Serial imaging is performed after a bolus injection of gadolinium-based paramagnetic contrast agents. Based on contrast enhancement of testis, testicular blood flow can be accurately assessed. The analysis of the enhancement profiles is simple enough to compare peak and upslope of enhancement between normal and affected testis. This MR technique should be useful in distinguishing tumors from nonmalignant lesions and in

**Table 1** Scrotal imaging: pulse sequence parameters

| Scan number | 1 | 2 | 3 | 3' | 4 | 5 | 5' | 6 | 6' | 7 | 8 | 8' |
|---|---|---|---|---|---|---|---|---|---|---|---|---|
| image contrast | Scout | T1WI | T2WI | T2WI | T2*WI | Heavily-T2WI | Heavily-T2WI | DWI | DWI | Dynamic subtraction CE | CE T1WI | CE T1WI |
| pulse sequence | TurboSE | TurboSE | TurboSE | TurboSE | FFE | TurboSE | TurboSE | SE-EPI | SE-EPI | TurboSE | TurboSE | TurboSE |
| imaging direction | three directions | coronal | coronal | transaxial | coronal | coronal | transaxial | coronal | transaxial | coronal | coronal | transaxial |
| TR | 192 ms | 500 ms | 3606 ms | 3568 ms | 522 ms | 5000 ms | 5593 ms | 1982 ms | 1764 ms | 466 ms | 500 ms | 500 ms |
| TE | 16 ms | 15 ms | 100 ms | 100 ms | 20 ms | 350 ms | 350 ms | 64 ms | 61 ms | 14 ms | 15 ms | 15 ms |
| Flip angle (degree) | 90 | 90 | 90 | 90 | 25 | 90 | 90 | 90 | 90 | 90 | 90 | 90 |
| Echo train length | 3 | 3 | 9 | 9 | | 65 | 65 | single-shot | single-shot | 3 | 3 | 3 |
| Field of view | 300 mm | 220 mm | 220 mm | 220 mm | 220 mm | 220 mm | 220 mm | 280 mm | 280 mm | 180 mm | 220 mm | 220 mm |
| Matrix | 192 | 204 × 256r | 192 × 256r | 192 × 256r | 204 × 256r | 256 × 256r | 256 × 256r | 128 × 256r | 128 × 256r | 204 × 256r | 204 × 256r | 204 × 256r |
| Section thickness | 10 mm | 4 mm | 4 mm | 4 mm | 4 mm | 4 mm | 4 mm | 5 mm | 5 mm | 6 mm | 4 mm | 4 mm |
| Intersection gap | 5 mm | 0.4 mm | 0.4 mm | 0.4 mm | 0.4 mm | 0.4 mm | 0.4 mm | 0.5 mm | 0.5 mm | 0.6 mm | 0.4 mm | 0.4 mm |
| Number of sections | 3 each | 16 | 16 | 16 | 16 | 16 | 16 | 15 | 15 | 6 | 16 | 16 |
| Breathing | rest | rest | rest | rest | rest | rest | rest | rest | rest | rest | rest | rest |
| Band width (Hz/pixel) | 107.2 | 210 | 71.5 | 71.5 | 217.1 | 183.4 | 214 | 21.4 | 37.9 | 145.8 | 210 | 221 |
| Fat suppression | – | – | SPIR | SPIR | – | – | – | SPIR | SPIR | SPIR | SPIR | SPIR |
| Number of signal acquisition | 2 | 3 | 3 | 3 | 2 | 4 | 4 | 8 | 8 | 2 | 3 | 3 |
| Acquisition time | 35.6 s | 2 min 4 s | 2 min 20 s | 2 min 19 s | 2 min 8 s | 2 min 30 s | 2 min 59 s | 1 min 53 s | 1 min 41 s | 52.2 s × 6 | 2 min 4 s | 2 min 4 s |
| Phase direction | | F-H | F-H | A-P | F-H | F-H | A-P | F-H | A-P | F-H | F-H | A-P |
| Other parameters | | | | | | | | Half scan 0.61 b = 800 | Half scan 0.61 b = 800 with SENSE | | | |

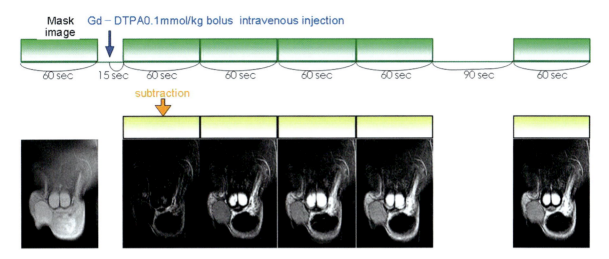

**Fig. 5** Diagram and images of the dynamic subtraction contrast-enhanced imaging. The green and yellow belts demonstrate the data acquisition and post-processing using subtraction technique, respectively. In the set of serial MR images obtained in a patient with testicular torsion, the twisted testis (*left*) shows no contrast enhancement and the normal testis (*right*) shows gradual increase in contrast enhancement

signal intensity, it is possible to evaluate the testicular damage such as hemorrhagic necrosis.

# 4 Image Analysis

## 4.1 Assessment of Contrast Enhancement

The dynamic subtraction contrast-enhanced images allow for visual assessment of testicular contrast enhancement (Fig. 5). The objective analysis of testicular enhancement can be performed with the contrast–enhancement profile curve as a function of time (Watanabe et al. 2000, 2007) (Fig. 6). Normal testes demonstrate slow and steady increase of contrast enhancement. Comparison of contrast enhancement between the right and left testes facilitate the evaluation of contrast enhancement of the affected-side testis with the unaffected-side testis serving as a normal control (Fig 6). The objective indexes used for the comparison are relative peak height(%) and relative mean slope(%) calculated from the contrast–enhancement profile curves as follows:

- Relative peak height (%) = maximum signal intensity of affected testis/that of unaffected testis × 100
- Relative mean slope (%) = upslope of enhancement during the first 3 minutes of affected testis/that of unaffected testis × 100

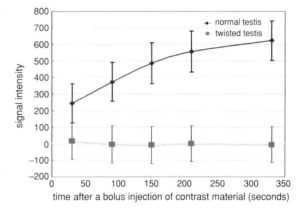

**Fig. 6** Time–intensity profile curve. The time–intensity profile curve obtained in a patient with testicular torsion reveal no contrast enhancement for the twisted testis and steady progressive increase in contrast enhancement for the normal testis

The increase in tissue signal intensity after contrast material enhancement, depends on the blood supply and the volume of the extravascular fluid in the tissue (Newhouse and Murphy 1981; Young et al. 1980). Both the relative peak height and relative mean slope can be very helpful not only in distinguishing testicular diseases from extratesticular diseases but also in dividing testicular diseases into two groups: one group of diseases with no or decreased contrast enhancement including testicular torsion, testicular infarction, traumatic testicular hemorrhagic necrosis, and testicular

**Table 2** Clinical applications and recommended protocol of pulse sequences

| | Clinical setting | Recommended protocol: the scanning order[a] | | |
|---|---|---|---|---|
| 1 | Acute scrotal symptoms | 3-4-5-7 | 7-4-3-5 | 7 |
| 2 | Intrascrotal masses | 2-3-5-3′-7-8-8′ | | |
| 3 | Scrotal trauma | 3-4-5-3′-7-8-8′ | | |
| 4 | Inguinal herniation | 2-3 | | |
| 5 | Nonpalpable (undescended) testis | 2-3-5-3′-7 | 2-3-5-3′ | 2-3-5-3′-6 |
| 6 | Infertility | 3-5-3′-5′-7 | 3-5-3′ | 3-5-3′-5′-6-6′ |
| 7 | Hydrocele | 3-5-3′-5′ | | |

[a] The numbers used are the scan number listed in Table 1

epidermoid cyst; and the other group of diseases with increased contrast enhancement including malignant testicular tumors and acute mumps orchitis (Watanabe et al. 2000; Terai et al. 2006).

## 4.2 Measurement of Testicular Volume

Testicular size can be determined with MR images by measuring the anteroposterior diameter on comparable transverse images of the left and right sides or by calculating testicular volume with the formula for an ellipsoid: $V = L \times W \times H \times 0.71$ (or 0.52), where $V$: volume, $L$: length, $W$: width, and $H$: height, as reported with ultrasound imaging (Oyen 2002; Paltiel et al. 2002). Although these measurements are not acquired routinely, they should be obtained in patients with varicocele, testicular atrophy, or acute scrotum to assess changes in testicular size. Testicular volume is approximately 1–2 cm$^3$ before the age of 12 years and reaches 4 cm$^3$ in pubertal males. In the peripubertal period, a difference of 3 mm in anteroposterior diameter is significant (Baud et al. 1998).

## 5 Clinical Applications and Protocol for Scrotal MR Imaging

The scanning protocol of pulse sequences recommended for the scrotal MR examinations should vary depending on the clinical settings. The basic protocol for the scrotal imaging should include T1-weighted, FS-T2-weighted, and heavily T2-weighted imaging in the coronal plane for a minimum requirement. Some changes to the basic protocol are necessary for the evaluation of the following pathology or clinical

symptoms (Table 2). The major clinical applications for MR imaging of the scrotum include the following.
1. *Acute scrotal symptoms suspicious of testicular torsion.* The recommended protocol should implement FS-T2-weighted, T2*-weighted, heavily T2-weighted and dynamic subtraction contrast-enhanced imaging in the coronal plane (Watanabe et al. 2000, 2007). Those pulse sequences are usually performed in the order of scan described above. Among these sequences, however, dynamic subtraction contrast-enhanced imaging can be first performed to promptly obtain information about testicular perfusion. When the contrast enhancement of the affected testis is found to be normal, possibilities of testicular torsion can be ruled out except for a case of spontaneous detorsion. Then, FS-T2-weighted imaging can be added to obtain anatomical and inside information of testis and surrounding testicular structures. When the affected testis shows no or little contrast enhancement, FS-T2-weighted, T2*-weighted, heavily T2-weighted images are required to obtain information about the presence or absence of hemorrhagic necrosis of testis and/or epidydimis. T1-weighted imaging is not always necessary and can be skipped.
2. *Intrascrotal masses* with need for differentiation between intra- and extratesticular masses as well as between malignant and benign masses and for local staging of testicular cancer: the recommended protocol should implement T1-weighted, FS-T2-weighted, heavily T2-weighted and dynamic subtraction contrast-enhanced imaging in the coronal plane, and contrast-enhanced FS-T1-weighted imaging in both the transaxial and coronal planes (Watanabe et al. 2000; Kim et al. 2007). FS-T2-

weighted and T1-weighted imaging is useful in the assignment of the lesion to the testis, epididymis, or other scrotal structure. Dynamic subtraction contrast-enhanced images are helpful in differentiating between malignant and benign tumors by demonstrating tissue vascularity of tumor. Contrast-enhanced FS-T1-weighted image is necessary for the local staging of teticular cancer such as extracapsular extension.

3. *Scrotal trauma.* The recommended protocol should implement FS-T2-weighted, heavily T2-weighted, T2*-weighted and dynamic subtraction contrast-enhanced imaging in the coronal plane, and contrast-enhanced FS-T1-weighted imaging in both the transaxial and coronal planes. Presence or absence of a hematocele and testicular rupture should be determined with MR imaging (Kim et al. 2007). T2*-weighted and dynamic subtraction contrast-enhanced images are important for demonstrating intra- or extra-testicular hematoma. Contrast-enhanced FS-T1-weighted image is also useful in the detection of capsular disruption.

4. *Inguinal and scrotal mass suspicious of inguinoscrotal herniation.* The recommended protocol should implement T1-weighted, FS-T2-weighted imaging in the coronal plane. T1-weighted image is very important to demonstrate fat tissue protruding through the inguinal canal (Shadbolt et al. 2001).

5. *Nonpalpable testis in the scrotum.* The recommended protocol should implement T1-weighted, FS-T2-weighted, and dynamic subtraction contrast-enhanced imaging in the coronal plane. Localization of the undescended testis can be done with T1-weighted and FS-T2-weighted images (Frush and Sheldon 1998; Shadbolt et al. 2001; Fritzsche et al. 1987; Kier et al. 1988; Tripathi et al. 1992). Possible degeneration or torsion of the undescended testis can be evaluated with heavily T2-weighted and dynamic subtraction contrast-enhanced images. Diffusion-weighted images may also be useful for this assessment. In case of intrapelvic testis, transaxial T1- and FS-T2-weighted images are obtained from the bottom of the scrotum to above the seminal vesicles. The examination should be extended to the lower poles of the kidneys when no testis is seen in the pelvis.

6. *Infertility.* The recommended protocol should implement FS-T2-weighted, heavily T2-weighted imaging in both the transaxial and coronal planes and dynamic subtraction contrast-enhanced imaging in the coronal plane. Atrophy and degeneration of intratesticular seminiferous tubules can be demonstrated with T2-weighted images (Jhaveri et al. 2010; Simpson et al. 2009). The relationship between varicoceles and infertility (Costabile et al. 1993) has been believed, and dynamic subtraction contrast-enhanced imaging could reveal subtle disruptions of the blood-testis barrier associated with infertility. Diffusion-weighted imaging may also provide information of testicular degenerative changes. However, further investigation should be needed.

7. *Hydrocele.* The recommended protocol should implement FS-T2-weighted, heavily T2-weighted imaging in both the transaxial and coronal planes. Fluid collection between the tunica vaginalis can be clearly demonstrated with heavily T2-weighted images.

# 6 Contraindications of MR Examination

In general, MR imaging is contraindicated for patients who have electrically, magnetically, or mechanically activated implants, such as cardiac pacemakers, implantable cardiac defibrillators, cochlear implants, neurostimulators, bone-growth stimulators, and implantable drug infusion pumps (Hricak et al. 1995; Shellock 1992). Ferromagnetic or metallic biomedical implants or foreign bodies (including various kinds of vascular clips, skin staples, prosthetic heart valves, and orthopedic implants and devices) are also under contraindication of MR imaging due to possible danger of dislodgement or movement (Hricak et al. 1995; Shellock and Crues 1988). In addition, such objects may be subject to heating and induction of electrical currents. In contrast, patients with non-ferromagnetic or minimally ferromagnetic implants or devices can safely undergo MR imaging.

# References

Baker LL, Hajek PC, Burkhard TK et al (1987a) MR imaging of the scrotum: pathologic conditions. Radiology 163:93–98

Baker LL, Hajek PC, Burkhard TK et al (1987b) MR imaging of the scrotum: normal anatomy. Radiology 163:89–92

Baud C, Veyrac C, Couture A et al (1998) Spiral twist of the spermatic cord: a reliable sign of testicular torsion. Pediatr Radiol 28:950–954

Bradley WG Jr (1993) MR appearance of hemorrhage in the brain. Radiology 189:15–26

Cheng HC, Khan MA, Bogdanov A Jr et al (1997) Relative blood volume measurements by magnetic resonance imaging facilitate detection of testicular torsion. Invest Radiol 32:763–769

Choyke PL (2000) Dynamic contrast-enhanced MR imaging of the scrotum: reality check. Radiology 217:14–15

Costabile RA, Choyke PL, Frank JA et al (1993) Dynamic enhanced magnetic resonance imaging of testicular perfusion in the rat. J Urol 149:1195–1197

Fritzsche PJ, Hricak H, Kogan BA et al (1987) Undescended testis: value of MR imaging. Radiology 164:169–173

Frush DP, Sheldon CA (1998) Diagnostic imaging for pediatric scrotal disorders. Radiographics 18:969–985

Hermier M, Nighoghossian N (2004) Contribution of susceptibility-weighted imaging to acute stroke assessment. Stroke 35:1989–1994

Hricak H, Hamm B, Kim B (1995) Imaging techniques, anatomy, artifacts and bioeffects: magnetic resonance imaging. Raven Press, New York

Jhaveri KS, Mazrani W, Chawla TP et al (2010) The role of cross-sectional imaging in male infertility: a pictorial review. Can Assoc Radiol J 61:144–155

Kaipia A, Ryymin P, Makela E et al (2005) Magnetic resonance imaging of experimental testicular torsion. Int J Androl 28:355–359

Kangasniemi M, Kaipia A, Joensuu R (2001) Diffusion weighted magnetic resonance imaging of rat testes: a method for early detection of ischemia. J Urol 166:2542–2544

Kier R, McCarthy S, Rosenfield AT et al (1988) Nonpalpable testes in young boys: evaluation with MR imaging. Radiology 169:429–433

Kim W, Rosen MA, Langer JE et al (2007) US MR imaging correlation in pathologic conditions of the scrotum. Radiographics 27:1239–1253

Kodama K, Yotsuyanagi S, Fuse H et al (2000) Magnetic resonance imaging to diagnose segmental testicular infarction. J Urol 163:910–911

Landa HM, Gylys-Morin V, Mattery RF et al (1988) Detection of testicular torsion by magnetic resonance imaging in a rat model. J Urol 140:1178–1180

Muller-Leisse C, Bohndorf K, Stargardt A et al (1994) Gadolinium-enhanced T1-weighted versus T2-weighted imaging of scrotal disorders: is there an indication for MR imaging? J Magn Reson Imaging 4:389–395

Newhouse JH, Murphy RX Jr (1981) Tissue distribution of soluble contrast: effect of dose variation and changes with time. Am J Roentgenol 136:463–467

Oyen RH (2002) Scrotal ultrasound. Eur Radiol 12:19–34

Paltiel HJ, Diamond DA, Di Canzio J et al (2002) Testicular volume: comparison of orchidometer and US measurements in dogs. Radiology 222:114–119

Rholl KS, Lee JK, Ling D et al (1987) MR imaging of the scrotum with a high-resolution surface coil. Radiology 163:99–103

Shadbolt CL, Heinze SB, Dietrich RB (2001) Imaging of groin masses: inguinal anatomy and pathologic conditions revisited. Radiographics 21:S261–S271

Shellock F (1992) Biologic effects and safety considertions. Raven Press, New York

Shellock FG, Crues JV (1988) High-field-strength MR imaging and metallic biomedical implants: an ex vivo evaluation of deflection forces. Am J Roentgenol 151:389–392

Shellock FG, Rothman B, Sarti D (1990) Heating of the scrotum by high-field-strength MR imaging. Am J Roentgenol 154:1229–1232

Simpson WL Jr, Rausch DR (2009) Imaging of male infertility: pictorial review. Am J Roentgenol, 192(Suppl 6):S98-107 (Quiz S108-111)

Terai A, Yoshimura K, Ichioka K et al (2006) Dynamic contrast-enhanced subtraction magnetic resonance imaging in diagnostics of testicular torsion. Urology 67:1278–1282

Trambert MA, Mattrey RF, Levine D et al (1990) Subacute scrotal pain: evaluation of torsion versus epididymitis with MR imaging. Radiology 175:53–56

Tripathi RP, Jena AN, Gulati P et al (1992) Undescended testis: evaluation by magnetic resonance imaging. Indian Pediatr 29:433–438

van den Brink JS, Watanabe Y, Kuhl CK et al (2003) Implications of SENSE MR in routine clinical practice. Eur J Radiol 46:3–27

Watanabe Y, Dohke M, Ohkubo K et al (2000) Scrotal disorders: evaluation of testicular enhancement patterns at dynamic contrast-enhanced subtraction MR imaging. Radiology 217:219–227

Watanabe Y, Nagayama M, Okumura A et al (2007) MR imaging of testicular torsion: features of testicular hemorrhagic necrosis and clinical outcomes. J Magn Reson Imaging 26:100–108

Young SW, Turner RJ, Castellino RA (1980) A strategy for the contrast enhancement of malignant tumors using dynamic computed tomography and intravascular pharmacokinetics. Radiology 137:137–147

# Anatomy of the Scrotum

Giovanni Liguori, Giangiacomo Ollandini, Renata Napoli,
Giorgio Mazzon, Miloš Petrovic, and Carlo Trombetta

## Contents

G. Liguori · G. Ollandini · R. Napoli ·
GiorgioMazzon · M. Petrovic · C. Trombetta (✉)
Department of Urology, University of Trieste,
Ospedale di Cattinara,
Strada di Fiume 447, Trieste 34124, Italy
e-mail: trombcar@units.it

**Abstract**

An adequate knowledge of normal anatomy of the scrotum and its content is mandatory to identify the structures during imaging evaluation, and to understand their modifications when pathologies occur. In this chapter anatomy of the scrotal wall, testis, and cord will be described with particular emphasis to the structures that are clinically relevant and can be better recognized at ultrasound and other imaging modalities.

## 1 Introduction

Among the male reproductive system, the scrotum, a thin external sac of skin, contains the two testes, the epididymes and part of the spermatic cord. The scrotum is a cutaneous pouch divided in its surface into two lateral portions. It is derived from the labioscrotal folds, which under the influence of testosterone, swell and fuse to form twin scrotal sacs. The point of fusion is the median raphe, which extends from the anus along the perineum to the ventral surface of the penis (Larsen 1993). Usually the two parts of the scrotum are not fully symmetrical: the left side hangs lower than the right, due to a greater length of left spermatic cord.

## 2 Scrotal Wall

The scrotal wall (Fig. 1) is composed of the following structures, listed from the superficial to the deep layers: rugated skin, superficial fascia, dartos tunica, external spermatic fascia, cremasteric fascia, and

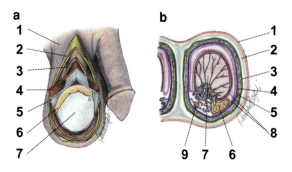

**Fig. 1** Layers of the scrotal wall. **a** Side view. **b** Transversal view. *1* skin, *2* dartos, *3* external spermatic fascia or cremasteric fascia, *4* cremaster muscle, *5* internal spermatic fascia or tunica vaginalis communis, *6* epididymis, *7* testis, *8* visceral and parietal layers of the tunica vaginalis *9* vas deferens

internal spermatic fascia. It varies from 2 to 8 mm in thickness (Leung et al. 1984). The system of different membranes inside the scrotum avoids testes from being injured due to blows or squeezes and acts as a covering and a protection to the testes: the testes lies suspended and loose in its cavity and are surrounded by several different layers in order to allow them a better mobility.

## 2.1 Skin

The skin of the scrotum is a brownish layer, usually thrown into folds or rugæ, which contains roots of scattered, crisp hairs that cover the scrotum surface. It is very elastic and capable of great distension, and on account of the looseness and amount of subcutaneous tissue, the scrotum becomes greatly enlarged in cases of edema, to which this part is especially liable as a result of its dependent position.

## 2.2 Dartos

The tunica dartos is a fat-free thin layer of smooth muscular fibers: it is a continuation of Scarpa's fascia which is a membranous layer of the subcutaneous tissue in the abdominal wall. The dartos divides the scrotum into two cavities, each containing one testis, through an inward septum that extends between the raphe and the under surface of the penis. In older males, the dartos muscle loses its tone, and tends to cause the scrotum to be smoother and to hang down

further. The tunica dartos acts to regulate the temperature of the testicles, which promotes spermatogenesis. It does this by expanding or contracting to wrinkle the scrotal skin. The dartos is closely united to the skin externally, but connected with the subjacent parts by delicate areolar tissue, upon which it glides with the greatest facility.

## 2.3 External Spermatic and Cremasteric Fascia

Prolonged downward around the surface of the cord and testis, the external spermatic fascia is a thin membrane, derived from the aponeurosis of the external oblique muscle. It is separated from the dartos by loose areolar tissue. The cremaster muscle consists of scattered bundles of muscular fibers connected together into a continuous covering by intermediate areolar tissue. It is a thin layer of skeletal muscle found in the inguinal canal and scrotum between the external and internal layers of spermatic fascia, surrounding the testis and spermatic cord. The cremaster muscle is a paired structure, there being one on each side of the body.

Anatomically, the lateral cremaster muscle originates from the internal oblique muscle, just superior to the inguinal canal, and the middle of the inguinal ligament. The medial cremaster muscle, which sometimes is absent, originates from the pubic tubercle and sometimes the lateral pubic crest. Both insert into the tunica vaginalis underneath the testis.

## 2.4 Internal Spermatic Fascia

The infundibuliform fascia (tunica vaginalis communis) is a thin layer, which loosely invests the cord; it is a continuation downward of the transversalis fascia.

## 3 Testis

The testes, or testicles, are two glandular organs, which secrete the semen, and are suspended in the scrotum by the spermatic cords. Usually, the left testis hangs lower than its fellow. They normally, complete their descent into the scrotum from their point of origin on the back wall of the abdomen in the seventh month after conception. At an early period of fetal life the testes are contained in the abdominal cavity, behind the peritoneum. Before birth they descend into the inguinal canal with the spermatic cord, and then into the scrotum, becoming invested in their course by coverings derived from the serous, muscular, and fibrous layers of the abdominal walls, as well as by the scrotum.

Testicular size depends on age and stage of sexual development. At birth, the testes measure approximately 1.5 cm in length and 1 cm in width. Before the age of 12 years testicular volume is around 1–2 cm$^3$. Clinically, a male individual is considered to have reached puberty once the testis achieves volume of 4 cm$^3$. On average, testes of adults are 3.8 cm long, 3 cm wide, and 2.5 cm deep and have a volume of 30 ml. The weight varies from 10.5 to 14 g (Leung et al. 1984). Testes are oval and have an oblique position in the scrotum: the upper extremity is directed forward and a little lateralward; the lower, backward and a little medialward; the anterior convex border looks forward and downward, the posterior or straight border, to which the cord is attached, backward and upward. Prepubertal testes are of low to medium echogenicity, whereas pubertal and postpubertal testes are of medium homogeneous echogenicity, reflecting the development of germ cell elements and tubular maturation (Siegel 1997).

Each testis is enclosed in a fibrous inextensible sac, the tunica albuginea. This sac is lined internally by the tunica vasculosa, which contains a network of blood vessels, held together by areolar tissue. The anterior border, lateral surfaces, and both extremities of the testis are convex, free, smooth, and invested by the visceral layer of the tunica vaginalis. The posterior border of the testis, to which the cord is attached, receives only a partial investment from that membrane and is covered by the epididymis on the lateral edge.

## 4    Tunica Vaginalis

The tunica vaginalis (tunica vaginalis propria testis) is a pouch of serous membrane that invests the testis, covered by a layer of endothelial cells in the inner surface. It derives from the saccus vaginalis of the peritoneum, which in the fetus preceded the descent of the testis from the abdomen into the scrotum. After its descent, the upper portion of the pouch becomes obliterated,

while the lower one remains as a shut sac, covering the surface of the testis. The tunica vaginalis is divided into two parts: the visceral and the parietal lamina. The visceral lamina (lamina visceralis) covers the greater part of the testis and epididymis. It reflects on to the internal surface of the scrotum from the posterior border of the gland. The parietal lamina (lamina parietalis) is larger than the visceral lamina, extending upward in front and on the medial side of the cord and reaching below the testis. The visceral and parietal laminæ set a virtual cavity inside the tunica vaginalis. Several pathological processes can involve this space, predominantly in the form of fluid collections. Hydroceles occur when serous fluid accumulates between the parietal and visceral layers of the tunica vaginalis. A small amount of fluid is normal and has been noted at sonography in up to 86% of asymptomatic men (Leung et al. 1984). When the tunica vaginalis does not become obliterated and still communicates with the peritoneum, an oblique inguinal hernia usually appears.

## 5    Tunica Albuginea

The tunica albuginea is an inextensible, fibrous layer that covers the testis composed of bundles of collagenous and smooth muscle elements which interlace in every direction. It is covered by the tunica vaginalis, except along the posterior border of the testis where the spermatic vessels enter the gland and at the epididymis. At ultrasound, the tunica albuginea can be seen as a thin echogenic line around the testis.

The mediastinum testis (corpus highmori) is an invagination of the tunica albuginea, from which multiple septa (trabeculae) arise dividing the testis into multiple (250–400) lobules (Fig. 2a). The mediastinum extends from the upper to near the lower extremity of the gland, and supports the vessels and ducts of the testis in their passage to and from the parenchima of the gland. At ultrasound, it is identified as an echogenic band of variable thickness and length extending in a caudocranial direction.

## 6    Structure of the Testis

The lobules are cone-shaped spaces that become narrower as they converge to the mediastinum and contains one to three convoluted seminiferous tubules

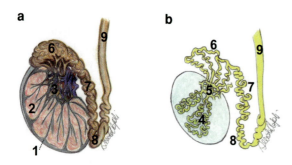

**Fig. 2** Anatomy of the testis and epididymis. **a** Longitudunal anatomical section. **b** Inner structure of the spermatic route. *1* tunica albuginea, *2* lobules, *3* mediastinum testis, *4* seminiferous tubules, *5*, rete testis, *6* head of the epididymis, *7* body of the epididymis, *8* tail of the epididymis, *9* vas deferens

(Fig. 2b). These are supported by loose connective tissue which contains somewhere groups of "interstitial cells" (Leydig cells) responsible for testosterone production. The total number of tubules is estimated at 840, and the average length of each is 70–80 cm. Their diameter range from 0.12 to 0.3 mm. Within the tubules spermatocytes and the supporting Sertoli cells give rise to sperm. The development of the spermatozoa begins around the inner extremities of the supporting cells. The nuclear portion of the spermatid, which is partly imbedded in the supporting cell, is differentiated in the head of the spermatozoön, while part of the cell protoplasm forms the middle piece and the tail is produced by an outgrowth from the double centriole of the cell. Ultimately the heads are liberated and the spermatozoa are set free (Gray 1918). In the apices of the lobules, the tubules become less convoluted, assume a nearly straight course, and unite together to form about twenty to thirty larger ducts, of about 0.5 mm in diameter, called tubuli recti. They enter the fibrous tissue of the mediastinum, and pass upward and backward, forming a close network of anastomosing tubes, called rete testis (Fig. 2b). The normal rete testis can be identified at high-frequency US in 18% of patients as a hypoechoic area with a striated configuration adjacent to the mediastinum testis (as opposed to the tubular ectasia of the rete testis when it is seen as fluid-filled dilated tubular structures) (Thomas and Dewbury 1993).

The rete testis terminates at the upper end of the mediastinum perforating the tunica albuginea with the ductuli efferentes (from 10 to 15). Their course is firstly straight, then the ducts become enlarged,

convoluted, and form a sort of conical masses, called the coni vasculosi, which together constitute the head of the epididymis. These multiple ducti converge within the body and tail of the epididym into a single larger duct (Hirsh 1995).

## 7 Epididymis

Sperm cells produced in the testes are transported to the epididymes, where they mature and are stored. Each epididymis has three regions (Fig. 2), called, respectively, the head (globus major), body, and tail (globus minor). The head is intimately connected with the upper end of the testis by means of the efferent ductules of the gland; the tail is connected with the lower end by cellular tissue, and a reflection of the tunica vaginalis. The body is attached to the posterior side of the testis and extends the length of the gland. The lateral surface, head and tail of the epididymis are free and covered by the serous membrane; the body is also completely invested by it, excepting along its posterior border; while between the body and the testis is a pouch, named the sinus of the epididymis (digital fossa). The smallest region is the tail, which begins at the point of separation of the epididymis from the testis. Sperm cells mature primarily in the head and body of the epididymis and are stored in the tail (Bostwick 1997). The epididymis is best evaluated in a longitudinal view when the epididymal head (globus major) can be seen as a pyramidal structure 5–12 mm in maximum length lying atop the superior pole of the testis. The head of the epididymis is usually isoechoic to the testis, and its echotexture may be coarser than that of the testis (Bree and Hoang 1996; Dambro et al. 1998). The narrow body of the epididymis (2–4 mm in diameter), when normal, is usually indistinguishable from the surrounding peritesticular tissue. The tail of the epididymis (globus minor) is approximately 2–5 mm in diameter and can be seen as a curved structure at the inferior pole of the testis, where it becomes the proximal portion of the ductus deferens.

## 8 Appendages

Testicular and epididymal appendages were once considered anatomic anomalies, however, some studies report that these structures are present in the majority of normal individuals. Such appendages are

**Fig. 3** Anatomical location of appendages. Epididimal appendage (*curved arrow*), testicular appendage (*arrow head*), paraepididymis (*arrow*), superior and inferior vas aberrans (*)

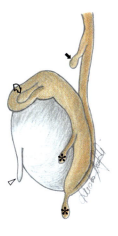

**Fig. 4** Vascularization of the testis and epididymis.
*1* internal iliac vessels,
*2* deferential vessels,
*3* inferior epigastrc vessels,
*4* external spermatic vessels,
*5* pampiniform plexus,
*6* internal spermatic vessels,
*7* internal spermatic fascia,
*8* cremasteric muscle,
*9* deferential vessels

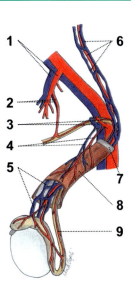

easily seen at scrotal ultrasound. When they are too long or pedunculated, appendages can twist around their own axis, causing very painful symptoms, simulating torsion of the spermatic cord (Favorito et al. 2004). There are also reports on tumors originated from these structures. Four testicular appendages have been described: the appendix testis, the appendix epididymis, the vas aberrans, and the paradidymis (Fig. 3). These are remnants of embryonic ducts (Trainer 1992).

## 8.1    Appendix Testis and Epididymis

The appendix testis (hydatid of morgagni) is a müllerian duct remnant and consists of fibrous tissue and blood vessels within an envelope of columnar epithelium (Bucci et al. 2002). It is attached to the upper pole of the testis in the groove between the testis and the epididymis. In postmortem studies, the appendix testis has been identified in 92% of testes unilaterally and in 69% bilaterally. The appendix epididymis is attached to the head of the epididymis and has been encountered unilaterally in 34% and bilaterally in 12% of testes in postmortem series (Rolnick et al. 1968).

## 8.2    Other Appendages

The vas aberrans is a blind tube that is occasionally present parallel to the first part of the vas deferens and that may communicate with the vas deferens or with

the epididymis. The paradidymis, also called parepididymis, is a small body, sometimes attached to the front of the lower part of the spermatic cord, above the head of the epididymis, composed of the remnants of tubules of the mesonephros (Murnaghan 1959).

## 9    Vascular Supply

The right and left spermatic arteries, branches of the abdominal aorta, arise just distal to the renal arteries and provide the primary vascular supply to the testes (Fig. 4). They enter the spermatic cord at the deep inguinal ring and divide into two main branches: testicular and epididymal artery. Testicular artery continues along the posterior surface of the testis, penetrating the tunica albuginea and building a vascular terminal system, made of capsular and intratesticular arteries, within the tunica vasculosa. Centripetal branches arising from the capsular arteries carry blood toward the mediastinum, where they divide to form the recurrent branches that carry blood away from the mediastinum into the testis. A transmediastinal arterial division of testicular artery is evident in approximately 50% of normal testes; it courses through the mediastinum to supply the capsular arteries and is usually accompanied by a large vein (Middleton and Bell 1993). The deferential artery, a branch of the superior vesicle artery, and the cremasteric artery, a branch of the inferior epigastric artery, supply the epididymis, vas deferens, and peritesticular tissue (Siegel 1994).

The number and locations of anastomoses vary between the testicular artery and its branches and between the artery to the vas deferens and the cremasteric artery. Branches of the pudendal artery supply the scrotal wall.

Venous anatomy of the scrotum is very complex (Dogra et al. 2003). The subcutaneous veins are divided into anterior and posterior scrotal veins. The former drain into the external pudendal veins, drained themselves into the major saphenous or directly into the femoral vein. The latter drain into the internal pudendal vessels through the deep dorsal vein of the penis. The deep venous system originates as a plexus, anatomically schematized into anterior and posterior pampiniform plexuses. This plexus runs with a pattern of a decreasing number of constituents into the spermatic funicle forming three main groups—anterior group: including the spermatic vein, intermediate group: including the ductus deferens vein (a layer of the internal spermatic fascia separate it from the anterior group); posterior group: including the cremasteric veins.

The anterior pampiniform plexus drains the blood coming from the testicle and the head of the epididymis. It is composed of 3–9 veins greatly connected with the deferential and cremasteric veins in a large amount of anastomoses. The normal size of these veins ranges from 0.5 to 1.5 mm in diameter, with the main draining vein being as large as 2 mm in diameter.

Beyond the internal inguinal orifice, the spermatic vein turns back into the retroperitoneum; here this vein can be single, double, or even multiple. On the left side, the spermatic vein connects with the left renal vein, whereas on the right side it drains directly into the vena cava. It is a propulsive-type vein, as mostly happens below the diaphragm. Most of these veins that drain blood against gravity, contain semilunar valves, forming membranous pouches, in order not to allow blood reflow. It is highly discussed in the scientific literature whether semilunar valves are present within the spermatic vein or not. There is no clear evidence of a role of the semilunar valves on varicocele's pathogenesis (Wishahi 1992).

The deferential, cremasteric, and external pudendal vein originate from the posterior pampiniform plexus and are highly connected with several anastomoses building a supplementary circulation system.

Whereas the contribution of deferential and cremasteric veins to the total amount of blood drainage is low, both in healthy and varicocele-suffering men, on the contrary, the external pudendal vein plays an important role, especially after the treatment of varicocele (ligation or sclerotization of the internal spermatic veins).

The deferential vein ascends with the deferential artery and duct within the spermatic cord and drains into the vesicoprosthatic plexus. Therefore, it is connected to the internal iliac vein: its preservation after varicocele correction prevents testicular congestion.

The cremasteric vein, (or external spermatic veins) runs into the posterior section of the deep venous system of the testis outside the funicle, and drains blood into the inferior epigastric or into the big saphenous vein to the external iliac vein.

Soon after originating from the pampiniformis plexus, the external pudendal vein runs on the side, to reach the big saphenous vein or the femoral vein directly draining blood into the external iliac vein.

The scrotal veins, a superficial venous system of the scrotum, drain into the external pudendal vein too, but they also communicate with the internal pudendal vein, reaching the internal iliac through the superficial veins of the perineum.

## 10  Spermatic Cord

The vas deferens, testicular artery, cremasteric artery, deferential artery, pampiniform plexuses, genitofemoral nerve, and lymphatic vessels compose the spermatic cord, which begin at the deep inguinal ring and descends vertically into the scrotum. The spermatic cord or funicle is an organ of cylindrical shape surrounded by adipose tissue and enveloped within three fasciae: the external spermatic fascia, an extension of the oblique muscle's aponevrosis; the cremasteric fascia and muscle, that is a continuation of the internal oblique muscle and its fascia; the internal spermatic fascia, extending from the transversalis fascia. The spermatic cord should be evaluated in every scrotal ultrasound examination. It lies just below the skin but can sometimes be difficult to discriminate it from surrounding soft tissue (Woodward et al. 2003).

# 11 Lymphatic Drainage

Lymph vessels are made of 4–8 collector ducts, that run aside to the spermatic vessels, and reach abdomino-aortic lymph nodes along aortic biforcation, until renal vessels. There is also a supplementary lymphatic pathway reaching the external iliac lymph nodes.

# 12 Innervation

The skin and dartos of the scrotum are largely supplied posteriorly by the posterior scrotal nerves and by branches of the pudendal nerve which supply the sensory innervation to the external genitalia. The perineal branches of the posterior femoral cutaneous nerves expand laterally toward the scrotum. Its anterior and upper part is supplied by the ilioinguinal and genitofemoral nerves, the ilioinguinal nerve originating from the lumbar plexus and descending through the superficial inguinal ring to form the anterior scrotal nerves. The genitofemoral nerve supplies both the skin and the cremasteric muscle (Yachia 2007).

# 13 Congenital Anomalies

Several scrotal congenital abnormalities may be recognized. Among them, abnormalities of the position of the scrotum, funicular abnormalities, as well as variation in the number and position of the testes should be considered.

## 13.1 Scrotal Transposition

The abnormal descent of the scrotum leads to scrotal transposition: in these cases the penis is lying sideways or behind the scrotum, or in the middle of it. The complete transposition of the scrotum, which represents the true ectopy is rare and is usually associated with other severe malformations, such as perineal hypospadias, absence of the urinary tract, polycystic kidneys, and imperforated anus.

## 13.2 Funicular Anomalies

The closure of the peritoneal-vaginal duct is a late event during embryonic development and its patency at birth is rather frequent, being present in 94% of infants. The complete or partial persistence of a patent peritoneal-vaginal duct may lead to three different diseases: hydrocele, cord cyst, and inguinal hernia. The accumulation of peritoneal fluid through the peritoneal-vaginal duct leads to formation of a congenital hydrocele. This event is particularly frequent at birth, but spontaneous closure of the duct during the first year of life leads to spontaneous resolution in most of cases (Garriga et al. 2009). If there is the overlap of inflammatory phenomena, the differential diagnosis with other causes of acute scrotum can be particularly difficult. The persistence of a hydrocele after two years of life expresses a condition that has no chance of spontaneous resolution.

A partial obliteration of the peritoneal-vaginal duct can lead to the formation of a cyst of the spermatic cord that may be present at every level, from the scrotum to the inguinal canal. The ultrasound diagnosis is usually easy, but particular attention should be given to the differential diagnosis of congenital hernia, a disease which is often associated.

## 13.3 Number Abnormalities of the Testis

Absence of one (monorchidism) or both (anorchidism) testes is a rare occurrence, reported in a variable percentage from 3.3 to 5.2% of patients operated on for cryptorchidism. The absence is unilateral in 80% of cases (Messina et al. 2000).

Before concluding for an absent testis, a careful instrumental evaluation is mandatory to eventually identify the missed testis elsewhere (testicular ectopy).

Poliorchidism is very rare compared to monorchidism or anorchidism. It is represented by the presence of a supernumerary testis, generated by an abnormal transverse division on embryonic gonad. The supernumerary gonad can be normal sized and may or may not be connected with the seminal ducts. In adults it can actively contribute to normal spermatogenesis (Smart 1972), but often, although histologically normal, their spermatogenesis is abnormal. Poliorchidism is very often associated with other anomalies, such as hydrocele, hernia (30% of cases) or cryptorchidism (50% of cases). The supernumerary testes are intrascrotal in approximately 75% of cases, presenting as painless scrotal masses. Of the remaining cases,

20% of the testes are inguinal and 5% retroperitoneal (Bostwick 1997).

## 13.4 Position Abnormalities of the Testis

Testicular ectopy is defined as the presence of the testicle outside the normal route of descent. Depending on the position, five ectopic sites can be generally recognized: superficial inguinal above the band of external oblique muscle, perineal, femoral or crural, contralateral (in which both testes are in the same inguinal channel), pelvic.

The undescended testis results in a pathological condition widely known, and called cryptorchidism. Cryptorchidism is an extremely common disease with an incidence of 3.4% in normal newborns and 30.3% in preterm ones. The undescended testis may be positioned anywhere along the normal path of descent. The most common location is in the inguinal canal (72%), followed by prescrotal (20%) and abdominal (8%) locations (Nguyen et al. 1999). The undescended testis is generally smaller and less echogenic than the normal testis.

The major complications of cryptorchidism are malignant degeneration, infertility, torsion, and bowel incarceration because of an associated indirect inguinal hernia. Orchiopexy of a cryptorchid testis is usually performed in patients between 1 and 10 years of age; orchiectomy is considered for postpubertal patients (Dogra et al. 2003).

## References

Bostwick DG (1997) Spermatic cord and testicular adnexa. In: Bostwick DG, Eble JN (eds) Urologic surgical pathology. Mosby, St Louis, pp 647–674

Bree RL, Hoang DT (1996) Scrotal ultrasound. Radiol Clin North Am 34:1183–1205

Bucci S, Liguori G, Buttazzi L et al (2002) Bilateral testicular carcinoma in patient with the persistent mullerian duct syndrome. J Urol 167:1790

Dambro TJ, Stewart RR, Barbara CA (1998) The scrotum. In: Rumack CM, Wilson SR, Charboneau JW (eds) Diagnostic ultrasound, 2nd edn. Mosby, St Louis, pp 791–821

Dogra VS, Gottlieb RH, Oka M et al (2003) Sonography of the scrotum. Radiology 227:18–36

Favorito LA, Cavalcante AG, Babinski MA (2004) Study on the incidence of testicular and epididymal appendages in patients with cryptorchidism. Int Braz J Urol 30:49–52

Garriga V, Serrano A, Marin A et al (2009) US of the tunica vaginalis testis: anatomic relationships and pathologic conditions. Radiographics 29:2017–2032

Gray H (1918) Anatomy of the human body. Lea & Febiger, Philadelphia

Hirsh AV (1995) The anatomical preparations of the human testis and epididymis in the Glasgow Hunterian Anatomical Collection. Hum Reprod Update 1:515–521

Larsen W (1993) Human embryology. Churchill Livingstone, New York

Leung ML, Gooding GA, Williams RD (1984) High-resolution sonography of scrotal contents in asymptomatic subjects. AJR Am J Roentgenol 143:161–164

Messina M, Ferrucci E, Zingaro P et al (2000) Epididymal anomalies in cryptorchidism and in peritoneal-vaginal duct persistence. A multicentric study. Minerva Urologica e Nefrologica 52:189–193

Middleton WD, Bell MW (1993) Analysis of intratesticular arterial anatomy with emphasis on transmediastinal arteries. Radiology 189:157–160

Murnaghan GF (1959) The appendages of the testis and epididymis: a short review with case reports. Br J Urol 31:190–195

Nguyen HT, Coakley F, Hricak H (1999) Cryptorchidism: strategies in detection. Eur Radiol 9:336–343

Rolnick D, Kawanoue S, Szanto P et al (1968) Anatomical incidence of testicular appendages. J Urol 100:755–756

Siegel BA (ed) (1994) Diagnostic ultrasonography test and syllabus (second series). American College of Radiology, Reston, pp 148–149

Siegel MJ (1997) The acute scrotum. Radiol Clin North Am 35:959–976

Smart RH (1972) Polyorchism with normal spermatogenesis. J Urol 107:278

Thomas RD, Dewbury KC (1993) Ultrasound appearances of the rete testis. Clin Radiol 47:121–124

Trainer TD (1992) Testis and the excretory duct system. In: Sternberg SS (ed) Histology for pathologists. Raven, New York, pp 744–746

Wishahi MM (1992) Anatomy of the spermatic venous plexus (pampiniform plexus) in men with and without varicocele: intraoperative venographic study. J Urol 147:1285–1289

Woodward PJ, Schwab CM, Sesterhenn IA (2003) From the archives of the AFIP: extratesticular scrotal masses: radiologic-pathologic correlation. Radiographics 23:215–240

Yachia D (2007) Surgical anatomy of the penis and scrotum. In: Yachia D (ed) Text atlas of penile surgery. Healthcare Informa, London, pp 1–8

# Clinical Evaluation of Scrotal Disease

Carlo Trombetta, Giorgio Mazzon, Giovanni Liguori, Stefano Bucci, Giangiacomo Ollandini, Sara Benvenuto, Giuseppe Ocello, Renata Napoli, and Emanuele Belgrano

## Contents

**Abstract**

The basic approach to the urological patient is still dependent on taking a complete history and an appropriate physical examination. A well-taken history frequently is sufficient to determine the correct diagnosis. Symptoms which have to be researched with attention are, in particular, pain, and sexual dysfunction. Physical examination should be performed conscientiously. Complete evaluation requires inspection of the breast, testis, vas deferens, and epididymis. In this chapter, those urologic symptoms and clinical signs which are apt to be brought to the physician's attention would be discussed.

## 1 Introduction

The ability of ultrasonography to diagnose the etiology of scrotal pathologies is high and actually unsurpassed. However, in the workup of any patient, the collection of a complete patient's history and of a well done physical examination are of paramount importance to determine the correct diagnosis.

## 2 Medical History

The medical history is the cornerstone of the evaluation of the urologic patient. A well-taken history frequently is sufficient to determine the correct diagnosis.

A complete history can be divided into the chief complaint and history of the present illness, the patient's past medical history, and the family history.

C. Trombetta (✉) · G. Mazzon · G. Liguori · S. Bucci · G. Ollandini · S. Benvenuto · G. Ocello · R. Napoli · E. Belgrano
Department of Urology, University of Trieste, Ospedale di Cattinara, Strada di Fiume 447, 34124 Trieste, Italy
e-mail: trombcar@units.it

Each segment can provide significant positive and negative findings that will contribute to the overall evaluation and treatment of the patient. During the interview of the patients, the symptoms which have to be researched with attention are, in particular, pain, and sexual dysfunction.

## 2.1 Pain

Scrotal pain may be either primary or referred. The testes arise embryologically in close proximity to the kidneys, for this reason pain arising in the kidneys or retroperitoneum may be referred to the testes (Dogra and Bhatt 2004). Conversely, the dull pain associated with an inguinal hernia could be referred to the scrotum.

Acute epididymitis and torsion of the testis or of the testicular appendaces are the most frequent pathologies that determine primary acute scrotal pain (Nickel et al. 2002). Because of the edema and pain associated with all these pathologies, it is frequently difficult to determine the real etiology of the pain (Abul et al. 2005). Alternatively, scrotal pain may result from inflammation of the scrotal wall itself. This may result from a simple infected hair follicle or sebaceous cyst, but it may also be secondary to a severe disease, such as Fournier's gangrene, which is a necrotizing infection involving perineum, penis, and scrotum that can rapidly progress and be fatal unless promptly recognized and treated.

Chronic scrotal pain is generally caused by non-inflammatory conditions such as a hydrocele or a varicocele. The pain is generally characterized as a dull, heavy sensation that does not radiate (Ciftci et al. 2004). However, also patients with testicular cancer may feel a chronic scrotal pain. For this reason physical examination of the scrotum is mandatory.

## 2.2 Sexual Dysfunction

Male sexual dysfunction is frequently used synonymously with erectile dysfunction, although it refers specifically to the inability to achieve and maintain an erection adequate for intercourse. Patients presenting with "impotence" should be questioned carefully to rule out other male sexual disorders, including loss of libido, absence of emission, absence of orgasm and,

most commonly, premature ejaculation (Lutz et al. 2005). Obviously, it is important to identify the precise problem before proceeding with further evaluation and treatment.

### 2.2.1 Loss of Libido

Because androgens have a major influence on sexual desire, a decrease of the libido may indicate androgen deficiency arising from either pituitary or testicular dysfunction. In this case, measurement of serum testosterone is indicated and, if abnormal, should be further evaluated by measurement of serum gonadotropins and prolactin. As the amount of testosterone required to maintain libido is usually less than that required for full stimulation of the prostate and seminal vesicles, patients with hypogonadism may also note decreased or absent ejaculation (Arver and Lehtihet 2009). Conversely, if semen volume is normal, it is less probable that endocrine factors would be responsible for loss of libido. A decrease in libido may also result from depression and a variety of medical illnesses that affect general health and well-being.

### 2.2.2 Erectile Dysfunction

Erectile dysfunction refers specifically to the inability to achieve and maintain an erection sufficient for intercourse. A careful history will often determine whether the problem is primarily psychogenic or organic. In men with psychogenic impotence, the condition frequently develops rather quickly, secondary to a precipitating event such as marital stress and change or loss of a sexual partner. In men with organic impotence, the condition usually develops more insidiously and frequently can be linked to advancing age or other underlying risk factors.

In evaluating men with erectile dysfunction, it is important to determine whether the problem exists in all situations (Bemelmans et al. 1991). Many men who report impotence may not be able to have intercourse with one partner but will be able with another. Similarly, it is important to determine whether men are able to achieve normal erections with alternative forms of sexual stimulation (e.g., masturbation, erotic videos). Finally, the patient should be asked whether he ever notes nocturnal or early morning erections. Generally, patients who are able to achieve adequate erections in some situations but not others have primarily psychogenic rather than organic impotence.

### 2.2.3 Failure to Ejaculate

An ejaculation may result from several causes: (a) androgen deficiency (b) sympathetic denervation (c) pharmacologic agents, and (d) bladder neck and prostatic surgery. Androgen deficiency results in decreased secretions from the prostate and seminal vesicles causing a reduction or loss of seminal volume. Sympathectomy or extensive retroperitoneal surgery, such as retroperitoneal lymphadenectomy for testicular cancer, may damage autonomic innervation of the prostate and seminal vesicles, resulting in absence of smooth muscle contraction and absence of seminal emission at time of orgasm. Moreover, a group of pharmacologic agents, particularly α-adrenergic antagonists, may interfere with bladder neck closure at time of orgasm and result in retrograde ejaculation. Similarly, previous bladder neck or prostatic urethral surgery, most commonly transurethral resection of the prostate, may interfere with bladder neck closure, resulting in retrograde ejaculation. Finally, retrograde ejaculation may develop spontaneously in medical diseases such as diabetes mellitus. Patients who complain of absence of ejaculation should be questioned regarding loss of libido or other symptoms of androgen deficiency, present medications, diabetes, and previous surgery.

### 2.2.4 Absence of Orgasm

An orgasmia is frequently psychogenic or caused by certain medications used to treat psychiatric diseases. Sometimes, however, anorgasmia may be due to decreased penile sensation owing to impaired pudendal nerve function. Most commonly, this occurs in patients with a peripheral neuropathy, in particular diabetic patients. Men with anorgasmia in association with decreased penile sensation should undergo vibratory testing of the penis and further neurologic evaluation as indicated (Rowland et al. 2010).

### 2.2.5 Premature Ejaculation

Men who complain of premature ejaculation should be questioned carefully, because this is obviously a very subjective symptom. Men with true premature ejaculation reach orgasm within less than 1 min after initiation of intercourse. This problem is almost always psychogenic and it's not an organic andrological disease.

The best treatment of patients with premature ejaculation requires an evaluation by a clinical psychologist or psychiatrist specialized in treatment of this problem and other psychological aspects of male sexual dysfunction. With counselling and appropriate modifications in sexual technique, this problem can usually be overcome. Alternatively, a group of molecules like sertraline or fluoxetine, which act as selective serotonin reuptake inhibitors (SSRI), have been demonstrated to be helpful in men with premature ejaculation (Rowland et al. 2010).

### 2.2.6 Hematospermia

Hematospermia refers to the presence of blood in the seminal fluid. It almost always results from nonspecific inflammation of the prostate and/or seminal vesicles and resolves spontaneously, usually within several weeks. It frequently occurs after a prolonged period of sexual abstinence, and we have observed it several times in men whose wives are in the final weeks of pregnancy.

If hematospermia persists beyond several weeks, patient needs a specific evaluation because, rarely, an underlying etiology will be identified (Leocadio and Stein 2009). A genital and rectal examination should be done to exclude the presence of testicular cancer, PSA test, and rectal examination should be done to exclude prostatic carcinoma, and urinary cytology should be done to exclude the possibility of transitional cell carcinoma of the prostate. It should be emphasized, however, that hematospermia almost always resolves spontaneously and rarely is associated with any significant urologic pathology.

---

## 3 Physical Examination

A complete and thorough physical examination is an essential component of the evaluation of patients who present with urologic disease. The physical examination often simplifies the process and allows the urologist to select the most appropriate diagnostic studies.

In a first step, the mammary glands should be always evaluated in all patients, since gynecomastia may be a sign of several pathologies such as endocrinologic disease, alcoholism, or previous hormonal therapy for prostate cancer. The following step is the evaluation of the scrotum. Because the scrotum contains both hair and sweat glands, it is a frequent site of local infection and sebaceous cysts. Small sebaceous cysts are occasionally seen while malignant tumors

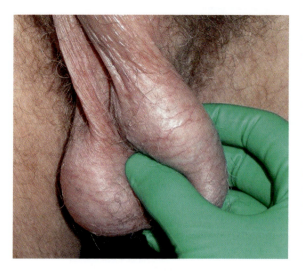

**Fig. 1** Palpation of the testes. The testes should be palpated gently between the finger tips of both hands, sliding over the surface to evaluate volume, consistence, focal masses or other pathological findings

are rare (Dogra et al. 2003). Hair follicles can become infected and may present as small pustules on the surface of the scrotum. These usually resolve spontaneously, but they can give rise to more significant infection, particularly in patients with reduced immunity and in those with diabetes. Patients often become concerned about these lesions, mistaking them for testicular tumors. Edema of the scrotum is frequently observed, it can be caused by radical resection of the lymph nodes of the inguinal and femoral areas, in which case the skin of the penis is involved. Moreover, scrotal edema could be observed in patients with cardiac decompensation, renal failure, nephrotic syndrome, or ascitis. Small hemangiomas of the skin are common and may bleed spontaneously.

A rare but severe disease associating the scrotum is Fournier's gangrene (Rosenstein and McAninch 2004), which is a synergistic polymicrobial necrotizing fasciitis of the perineum, perirectal and genital area and frequently extends to involve the lower abdominal wall. Fournier's gangrene is characterized by cutaneous and subcutaneous necrosis. The scrotal palpation of patients with Fournier's gangrene produce pain and crackles are appreciable.

The following step is the examination of the testes, which should be palpated gently between the finger tips of both hands (Fig. 1). The testes normally have a firm, rubbery consistency with a smooth surface. Volume and symmetry must be considered. The average size is

12–25 cc. The Prader's orchidometer, which consists of a string of twelve numbered wooden or plastic beads of increasing size from about 1 to 25 milliliters, can be used to accurately determine the size.

Discrepancy of testicular size with other parameters of maturation can be an important clue to various diseases. Small testes can indicate either primary or secondary hypogonadism. Testicular size can help distinguish between different types of precocious puberty. Since testicular growth is typically the first physical sign of true puberty, one of the most common uses is for confirmation that puberty is beginning in a boy with delay. Large testes (macroorchidysm) can be a clue to one of the most common causes of mental retardation, fragile X syndrome. Abnormally small testes suggest hypogonadism or an endocrinopathy such as Klinefelter's disease.

It's important also to evaluate the presence of asymmetry between the testes. The atrophic testis (postoperative orchiopexy, mumps, orchitis, or torsion of the spermatic cord) may be flabby and at times hypersensitive, but is is usually firm and hyposensitive. Although spermatogenesis may be absent, androgen function is occasionally maintained.

The most frequent cause of asymmetry between the testes is varicocele, which is an abnormal dilatation of the veins of the pampiniform plexus. The diagnosis is clinical, and upon palpation of the scrotum, a non-tender, twisted mass along the spermatic cord is felt. Palpating a varicocele can be likened to feeling a bag of worms. Varicocele becomes more obvious as the patient performs a Valsalva maneuver. Patients with varicocele should be always evaluated with ultrasonography to determine the presence and the severity of reflux and testicular hypotrophy.

The testis may be absent from the scrotum, and this may be transient (physiologic retractile testis) or true cryptorchidism, which is one of the most common birth defect of male genitalia (Leissner et al. 1999). Undescended testes are associated with reduced fertility and increased risk of testicular germ cell tumors. For this reason, the clinical evaluation of patients who underwent orchiopexy for chryptorchidism is fundamental (Wolf et al. 2001). Palpation of the groins may reveal the presence of the organ. During the examination of the testes, care must be paid for evaluation of the testicular surface. The finding of a firm or hard area within the testis should be considered a malignant tumor until proved otherwise. Tumors are often smooth but may be nodular and the testes may seem abnormally heavy. A testis replaced by tumor or damaged by a gumma is insensitive to pressure, and the usual sickening sensation is absent.

About 10% of tumors are associated with a secondary hydrocele. Transillumination should be done routinely and is helpful in determining whether scrotal masses are solid (tumor) or cystic (hydrocele, spermatocele). With the patient in a dark room, a light is placed against the scrotal sac posteriorly. A hydrocele will cause the intrascrotal mass to glow red, while light is not transmitted through a solid tumor (Galejs 1999). Subsequently, the following step is the evaluation of the epididymis, which is sometimes rather losely attached to the posterior surface of the testis, and at other times, it is quite free of it. The epididymis should be carefully palpated for size and induration, which implies infection since primary tumors are exceedingly rare (Hanson et al. 1993).The testicle and epididymis may be adherent to the scrotum, which is usually quite red and exquisitely tender.

Chronic painless induration suggests tuberculosis or schistosomiasis, although nonspecific chronic epididymitis is also possible. Epididymitis is the most frequent cause of acute scrotal pain. It can be hard to distinguish from testicular torsion. For this reason color Doppler interrogation of the scrotum is mandatory.

On physical examination, the testicle is usually found to be in its normal vertical position, of equal size compared to its counterpart, and not high-riding. Typical findings are redness, warmth, and swelling of the scrotum, with tenderness behind the testicle, away from the middle (this is the normal position of the epididymis relative to the testicle). Epididymis and testis during acute epididymitis are not distinguishable (Horstman 1997). The cremasteric reflex (if it was normal before) remains normal. This is a useful sign to distinguish it from testicular torsion. Pain relief by elevation of the testicle (positive Prehn's sign) suggests epididymitis, but is non-specific. In patients with an acute scrotum, the diagnosis of appendiceal torsion should be considered. Torsion of appendages produces pain similar to that experienced with testicular torsion, but the onset is more gradual (Lavoipierre 2000). The classic finding on physical examination is a small, firm nodule that is palpable on the superior aspect of the testis and exhibits a bluish discoloration through the overlying skin. This is called the "blue dot" sign. Careful palpation of the vas deferens may reveal

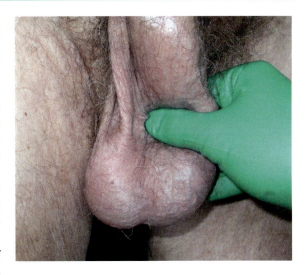

**Fig. 2** Palpation of the vas deferens, which should be researched between the finger tips of both hands. The right spot to perform this maneuver is above the upper pole of the testis

thickening (e.g., chronic infection), fusiform enlargements ("beading" caused by tuberculosis), or even absence of the vas (Lavoipierre 2000).

In patients with a diagnosis of azoospermia, it is mandatory to seek for vas deferent (Fig. 2). The latter finding is of importance in infertile males and may be associated with cystic fibrosis or ipsilateral Wolffian duct abnormality, such as renal agenesis (Kolettis and Sandlow 2002). A swelling in the spermatic cord may be cystic (e.g., hydrocele or hernia) or solid (e.g., connective tissue tumor) although the latter is rare. Lipoma in the investing fascia of the cord may simulate a hernia. Diffuse swelling and induration of the cord are seen with filarial funiculitis (Marcozzi and Suner 2001). Finally, it is necessary to seek for the presence of a hernia. To examine for a hernia, the physician's index finger should be inserted gently into the scrotum and invaginated into the external inguinal ring (Fig. 3). Hernia diagnosis is clinical. Howewer, ultrasonography is helpful for patients with equivocal physical findings and for patients who present with acute inguino-scrotal swelling (Cuckow and Frank 2000). The scrotum should be invaginated in front of the testis, and care should be taken not to elevate the testis itself, which is quite painful. Once the external ring has been located, the physician should place the fingertips of his or her other hand, over the internal inguinal ring and ask the patient to bear down (Valsalva's maneuver). A hernia will be felt as a distinct bulge that descends

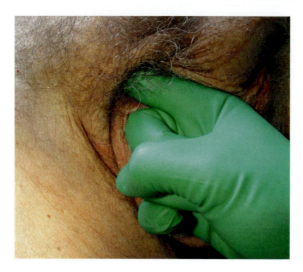

**Fig. 3** Examination of the inguinal canal. The physician's index finger should be inserted gently into the scrotum and invaginated into the external inguinal ring. While performing the procedure, the patient should be asked to perform the Valsalva maneuver to assess the presence of hernias

against the tip of the index finger in the external inguinal ring as the patient bears down. Although it may be possible to distinguish a direct inguinal hernia arising through the floor of the inguinal canal from an indirect inguinal hernia prolapsing through the internal inguinal ring, this is seldom possible and of little clinical significance because the surgical approach is essentially identical for both conditions.

# References

Abul F, Al-Sayer H, Arun N (2005) The acute scrotum: a review of 40 cases. Med Princ Pract 14:177–181

Arver S, Lehtihet M (2009) Current guidelines for the diagnosis of testosterone deficiency. Front Horm Res 37:5–20

Bemelmans BL, Meuleman EJ, Anten BW et al (1991) Penile sensory disorders in erectile dysfunction: results of a comprehensive neuro-urophysiological diagnostic evaluation in 123 patients. J Urol 146:777–782

Ciftci AO, Senocak ME, Tanyel FC et al (2004) Clinical predictors for differential diagnosis of acute scrotum. Eur J Pediatr Surg 14:333–338

Cuckow PM, Frank JD (2000) Torsion of the testis. BJU Int 86:349–353

Dogra V, Bhatt S (2004) Acute painful scrotum. Radiol Clin North Am 42:349–363

Dogra VS, Gottlieb RH, Oka M et al (2003) Sonography of the scrotum. Radiology 227:18–36

Galejs LE (1999) Diagnosis and treatment of the acute scrotum. Am Fam Physician 59:817–824

Hanson P, Rigaux P, Gilliard C et al (1993) Sacral reflex latencies in tethered cord syndrome. Am J Phys Med Rehabil 72:39–43

Horstman WG (1997) Scrotal imaging. Urol Clin North Am 24:653–671

Kolettis PN, Sandlow JI (2002) Clinical and genetic features of patients with congenital unilateral absence of the vas deferens. Urology 60:1073–1076

Lavoipierre AM (2000) Ultrasound of the prostate and testicles. World J Surg 24:198–207

Leissner J, Filipas D, Wolf HK et al (1999) The undescended testis: considerations and impact on fertility. BJU Int 83:885–891 quiz 891–882

Leocadio DE, Stein BS (2009) Hematospermia: etiological and management considerations. Int Urol Nephrol 41:77–83

Lutz MC, Roberts RO, Jacobson DJ et al (2005) Cross-sectional associations of urogenital pain and sexual function in a community based cohort of older men: olmsted county, Minnesota. J Urol 174:624–628 discussion 628

Marcozzi D, Suner S (2001) The nontraumatic, acute scrotum. Emerg Med Clin North Am 19:547–568

Nickel JC, Siemens DR, Nickel KR et al (2002) The patient with chronic epididymitis: characterization of an enigmatic syndrome. J Urol 167:1701–1704

Rosenstein D, McAninch JW (2004) Urologic emergencies. Med Clin North Am 88:495–518

Rowland D, McMahon CG, Abdo C et al (2010) Disorders of orgasm and ejaculation in men. J Sex Med 7:1668–1686

Wolf CK, Maizels M, Furness PD 3rd (2001) The undescended testicle. Compr Ther 27:11–17

# Sonographic Scrotal Anatomy

Vincenzo Migaleddu, Giuseppe Virgilio, Alberto Del Prato, and Michele Bertolotto

## Contents

V. Migaleddu (✉) · G. Virgilio
SMIRG Foundation-Sardinian Mediterranean Imaging
Research Group, Via Gorizia No. 11, 07100 Sassari, Italy
e-mail: migaleddu@smirg.org

A. Del Prato
S.C. Radiodiagnostica, Ospedale S. Bartolomeo,
Via Cisa Loc. Santa Caterina, 19038 Sarzana, Italy

M. Bertolotto
Department of Radiology, University of Trieste,
Ospedale di Cattinara, Strada di Fiume 447,
34124 Trieste, Italy

**Abstract**

High resolution ultrasound allows an excellent evaluation of the different organs contained in the scrotal sac. The testes are paired organs with smooth surface homogeneous echotexture. The epididymis is usually set on the upper and posterior-lateral aspect of the testis, but anatomical variations exist. The epididymal head is almost isoechoic to testis, while the remaining portions are usually less echogenic. The vas deferens and vessels are identified in the spermatic cord in virtually all subjects. Appendages of the testis and of the epididymis are often recognized. Doppler interrogation allows evaluation of flow characteristics of intratesticular and funicular vessels. This chapter describes the normal appearance of the scrotal content at color doppler ultrasound. Specific topics discussed are ultrasound appearance of anatomical variations of the testis and epididymis and color doppler features of the testicular and extratesticular vessels.

## 1    Introduction

High-resolution ultrasound is the imaging modality of choice for the superficially located scrotal sac and its contents. Gray-scale ultrasonography in combination with color or power doppler imaging is a well accepted technique for assessing scrotal lesions and testicular perfusion. In this chapter, the gray-scale and color doppler appearance of the different structures contained in the scrotum are described, with emphasis on anatomical variation which can be identified

M. Bertolotto and C. Trombetta (eds.), *Scrotal Pathology*, Medical Radiology. Diagnostic Imaging,
DOI: 10.1007/174_2011_172, © Springer-Verlag Berlin Heidelberg 2012

at ultrasound, and that can predispose to scrotal disease, or may be misinterpreted as pathological features.

## 2    Ultrasound and Doppler Appearance of the Spermatic Cord

Ultrasound evaluation of the normal spermatic cord is commonly considered difficult because contrast resolution with the surrounding echogenic fat is poor (Gooding 1988; Sudakoff et al. 2002). Using modern high frequency broadband probes, however, the spermatic cord can be identified in virtually all subjects. It appears as an echogenic ribbon-like structure whose echotexture is different from the surrounding fat by presence of the vas deferens and spermatic arteries and veins (Fig. 1).

The three fascial layers surrounding the cord, internal spermatic fascia, cremasteric fascia and muscle, and external spermatic fascia, cannot be discriminated at ultrasound (Sudakoff et al. 2002), but are depicted as a linear interface with slightly different echogenicity.

### 2.1    Sonographic Appearance of the Vas Deferens

According to Middleton et al. (2009), the extrapelvic portion of the normal vas deferens is reliably visualized at ultrasound in virtually all fertile men as a noncompressible, markedly hypoechoic structure, lacking vascularization at color doppler interrogation. The intrascrotal portion of the vas can be found in a variety of locations with respect to the testis and epididymis (Puttemans et al. 2006). It has a convoluted, tortuous appearance at its origin and gradually straighten distally. The suprascrotal segment presents upon longitudinal view, as a straight cordlike structure with central parallel linear reflectors, representing the anterior and posterior walls of the lumen. The cross-sectional view typically shows a "target" appearance, with the lumen appearing as central paired reflectors. In the prepubic area, the parallel

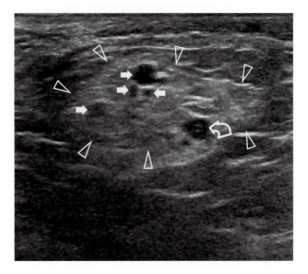

**Fig. 1** Ultrasound appearance of the spermatic cord. Cross-sectional view showing a circumscribed oval structure with slighly different echogenicity compared to the surrounding fat. Vessels (*arrows*) appear as hypo-anechoic rounded dots. The deferens (*curved arrow*) shows a target appearance, with the lumen appearing as central paired reflectors. The fascial layers surrounding the cord are stuck together, appearing as a thin linear interface (*arrowheads*)

linear reflectors representing the lumen walls are depicted inconstantly (Middleton et al. 2009). The terminal portion of the vas is depicted at transrectal ultrasound (Fig. 2).

The vas deferens has a higher ratio of muscle to lumen than any other hollow viscus in the body. This predominant muscular component explains the hypoechoic to anechoic appearance at ultrasound (Middleton et al. 2009). The mucosa is composed of pseudostratified columnar epithelium forming longitudinal folds that may act as strong reflectors (Middleton et al. 2009).

### 2.2    Ultrasound and Doppler Appearance of Spermatic Vessels

Besides the vas deferens, arteries, and veins can be identified at ultrasound, appearing as small, tubular hypoechoic structures within the echogenic connective tissue of the cord, showing color signals at color doppler interrogation (Fig. 3). Arteries are not

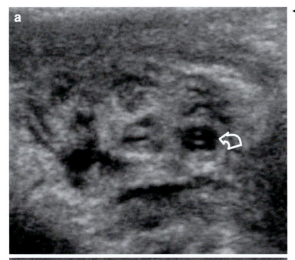

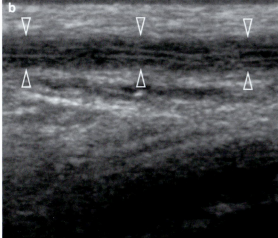

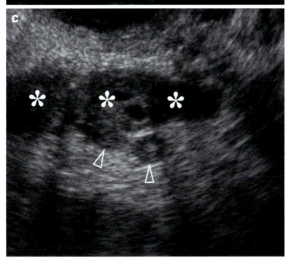

◄ **Fig. 2** Appearance of vas deferens at grey-scale ultrasound. **a** Axial view of the spermatic cord showing a markedly hypoecoic rounded structure (*curved arrow*) with target appearance by presence of central paired reflectors. **b** Longitudinal view of the spermatic cord showing a straight, markedly hypoechoic cordlike structure (*arrowheads*) with central parallel linear reflectors representing the anterior and posterior walls of the lumen. **c** Trasrectal view showing the terminal portion of the deferens (*arrowheads*) entering the seminal vesicle (*asterisks*)

compressible, and are characterized by pulsatile flows, while veins can be compressed by the probe (Middleton et al. 2009), and present transient flow, typically lasting <1 s, during the Valsalva's maneuver (Fig. 4). A prolonged venous reflux is recognized in patients with varicocele.

In the most common anatomical arrangement, three arterial vessels are identified: the larger testicular artery, and the smaller cremasteric and deferential arteries. Cases have been described, however, where one or more of these vessels are duplicated (Mostafa et al. 2008; Raman and Goldstein 2004).

The deferential artery runs parallel to the vas deferens (Raman and Goldstein 2004), which is the landmark for its identification. The cremasteric artery travels within the external fascia of the spermatic cord (Raman and Goldstein 2004). Multiple anastomotic channels among the testicular, cremasteric, and deferential arteries have been demonstrated in the human testis (Mostafa et al. 2008). Despite this fact, arteries of the spermatic cord display different flow characteristics (Aziz et al. 2005). At color doppler interrogation, testicular artery is less pulsatile than deferential and the cremasteric arteries. Lower impedance pattern with higher levels of diastolic flows are recorded in the testicular artery on duplex doppler interrogation, compared to deferential and cremasteric arteries, reflecting the low vascular resistance of the testis.

## 3 Gray-Scale Appearance of the Testis

The normal postpubertal testis presents at gray-scale ultrasound as a symmetric ovoid organs with medium level homogeneous echoes. Testis is surrounded by the

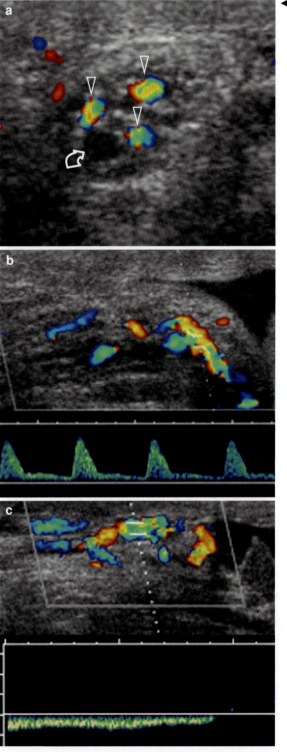

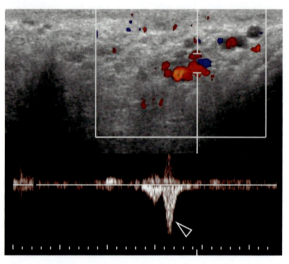

◀ **Fig. 3** Color Doppler and pulsed Doppler interrogation of the spermatic cord. **a** Axial color Doppler view of the spermatic cord obtained while standing during Valsalva's maneuver. Vessels (*arrowheads*) present with color signal, while the deferens (*curved arrow*) does not display flow. **b**, **c** Color Doppler interrogation of the vessels show arterial (**b**) and venous flows (**c**). Presence of veins with prolonged reflux (>2 s) within the inguinal channel is only consistent with grade 1 varicocele (following the classification of Sarteschi, see Imaging the Infertile Male: Varicocele for detail)

**Fig. 4** Pulsed doppler interrogation of a spermatic vein in a normal subject while standing and during Valsalva's maneuver showing only transient flow (*arrowhead*), lasting less than 1 s

fibrous tunica albuginea and by the visceral layer or the tunica vaginalis, which are stuck together appearing as a thin echogenic lines (Fig. 5). Along its posterior border, the tunica albuginea penetrates the testicular parenchyma to form the mediastinum testis, seen as an elongated hyperechoic structure of variable thickness, parallel to the testis' long axis. Conspicuity of the mediastinum testis is variable, depending on the amount of fibrous and fatty tissue, and degree of dilatation of the rete testis. The mediastinum testis is the origin of approximately 250 fine septa that form the lobules of the testis and through which radiate, testicular vessels and lymphatics. Convergence of these structures toward the mediastinum testis may cause a subtle focal striated appearance at ultrasound (Loberant et al. 2010) (Fig. 6).

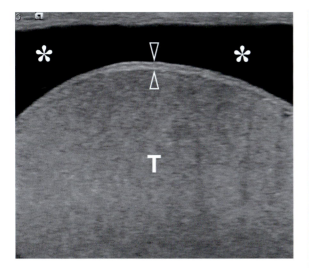

**Fig. 5** Gray-scale appearance of the scrotal content in a patient with hydrocele (*asterisks*). The testis (*T*) presents with medium level homogeneous echoes, surrounded by the tunica albuginea and by the visceral layer of the tunica vaginalis (*arrowheads*), which are stuck together and appear as parallel echogenic lines

In older subjects, atrophy of the glandular elements accompanied by an increase in interstitium may change the appearance of the testicular parenchyma, producing a more pronounced striated pattern. The combination of a striated appearance with small testicular size supports the diagnosis of testicular fibrosis. While it is normal in elderly, a similar appearance is recognized also in a variety of pathological conditions (Loberant et al. 2010).

In most of the patients, the testis is fixed to the scrotal wall by apposition of the parietal and of the visceral layers of the tunica vaginalis, which form the mesentery. The lower pole of the testis is also fixed by the scrotal ligament, also called gubernaculum testis, which is a remnant of the gubernaculum that during the fetal life drives the testis from the abdomen within the scrotum (Heyns 1987). In most of subjects, the scrotal ligament is very short, and cannot be visualized directly at ultrasound. Occasionally, however, a loose, longer ligament is present, which can be identified at grey scale ultrasound, especially if hydrocele is present, as an elongated structure connecting the lower pole of the testis to the scrotal wall (Fig. 7). The scrotal ligament may contain small vessels. A long, loose

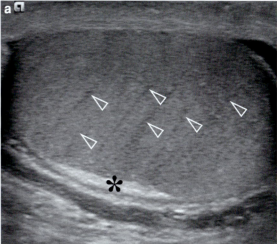

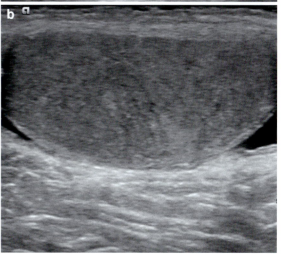

**Fig. 6** Striated appearance of the normal testis. **a** Young man. thin hypoechoic streaks (*arrowheads*) originating from the mediastinum (*asterisks*) cross the parenchyma. **b** Old man showing a more prominent and irregular striated pattern, due to age-related hypotrophy

scrotal ligament causes excessive mobility of the testis and may predispose to torsion.

The superb resolution of modern high-frequency transducers often reveals anechoic blood vessels, either arterial or venous, their nature confirmed on color doppler interrogation.

A single or double larger vascular structure representing the transtesticular vessels can be seen. A low reflective area may be produced by this oblique

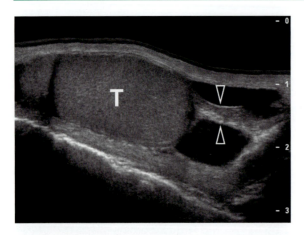

**Fig. 7** Scrotal ligament. Remnant of the gubernaculum (*arrowheads*) connecting the testis (*T*) to the inferior portion of the scrotum

interface within the lower aspect of the testis, an artifact described as the "two-tone" testis (Bushby et al. 2007).

## 4 Color-Doppler and Pulsed Doppler Appearance of the Testis

With the use of modern equipment, normal intratesticular vascularity is readily and consistently visualized at color doppler interrogation (Middleton et al. 1989). The arterial supply is given by two sets of arteries, the superficial and the transmediastinal arteries, branches of the main testicular artery.

The capsular arteries have superficial course in the tunica vasculosa located beneath the tunica albuginea; centripetal branches rising from the capsular arteries carry blood toward the mediastinum, then divide and form the recurrent rami carrying blood away from the mediastinum into the testis (Fig. 8).

The centrifugal transmediastinal arteries cross the mediastinum testis and parenchyma with straight course, and near the anterior border of the testis, divide into a limited number of terminal branches (Pais et al. 2004). These vessels are identified at color doppler ultrasound in up to 52% of patients (Middleton and Bell 1993), isolated, or accompanied by a satellite vein, also transmediastinal but of

opposite orientation (Fig. 9). Transmediastinal vessels are usually found in the superior half of the testis, but their course is variable.

Usually only one centrifugal transmediastinal artery is recognized, but occasionally two or three arteries may be present (Pais et al. 2004).

Rarely, a transmediastinal artery with centripetal course can be observed. An anatomical study has clarified that this vessel is likely an unusual type of origin of the main epididymal artery (Pais et al. 2004). As they are branches of the testicular artery, both the vessels of the capsular and of the transmediastinal group present with low impedance pattern on duplex doppler interrogation with high levels of diastolic flow. Resistance index and peak systolic velocity reduce from the central towards the peripheral branches (Martinoli et al. 1992) (Fig. 10).

## 5 Sonographic Appearance of the Epididymis

The epididymis is a curved tubular structure consisting of a head, body, and tail best evaluated in a longitudinal view. It is usually situated posterolateral to the testis and courses in a craniocaudal direction. The epididymal head is homogeneous and almost isoechoic to testis. Its maximal size is less than 10–12 mm. The body measures 2–5 mm in diameter, and is usually less echogenic than the head and testis. The tail is usually close to the inferior and posterior aspects of the testis and measures 2–5 mm. It is usually hypoechoic to the testes (Puttemans et al. 2006) (Fig. 11). The epididymal tail curves acutely, where it becomes the proximal portion of the ductus deferens which is hypo- to anechoic.

According to Hricak (1995), higher echogenicity of the epididymal head may be due to the greater number of interfaces in that portion of the epididymis. Puttermans et al. (2006), however, suggests that this feature could also be due to the little muscular component of the thin wall of the efferent tubes in the epididymal head. As the wall becomes gradually

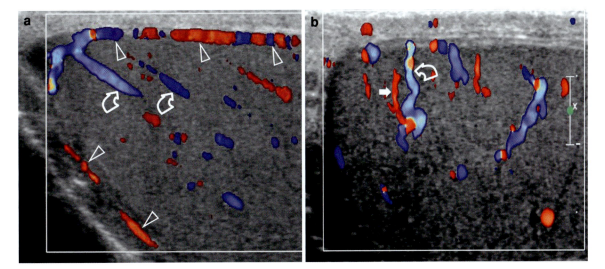

**Fig. 8** Normal appearance of testicular vessels at color doppler interrogation. **a** Capsular vessels (*arrowheads*) forming the tunica vasculosa giving origin to centripetal branches (*curved arrows*) with flow directed towards the mediastinum. **b** Recurrent artery (*arrow*) branching from a centripetal artery (*curved arrow*)

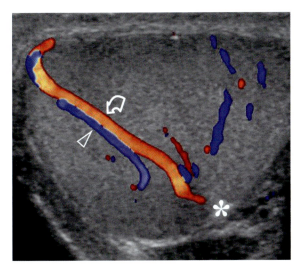

**Fig. 9** Transmediastinal testicular vessels. Longitudinal color doppler image shows an artery (*curved arrow*) branching from the mediastinum testis (*asterisks*) and running within the parenchyma with straight course towards the tunica albuginea. A satellite vein with parallel course but opposite flow orientation is recognized

thickened by smooth muscle fibers in the epididymal body and tail, wall's echogenicity decreases.

Using modern equipment and high frequency probes, color doppler ultrasound can reliably demonstrate flow within the normal epididymis. Similar to the testicular artery, the epididymal artery characteristically displays low-resistance flows.

## 6 Sonographic Appearance of Appendages

The testicular and epididymal appendages are commonly identified on ultrasound. they can be seen normally but are more easily identified in the presence of hydrocele or other scrotal fluid collections. Appendages may present no or little vascularization at color doppler interrogation (Sellars and Sidhu 2003). Occasionally both, an epididymal and testicular appendage may be seen in the same patient.

### 6.1 Appendix Testis

The appendix testis is a remnant of the Müllerian duct. It may be present in up to 92% of autopsy specimens

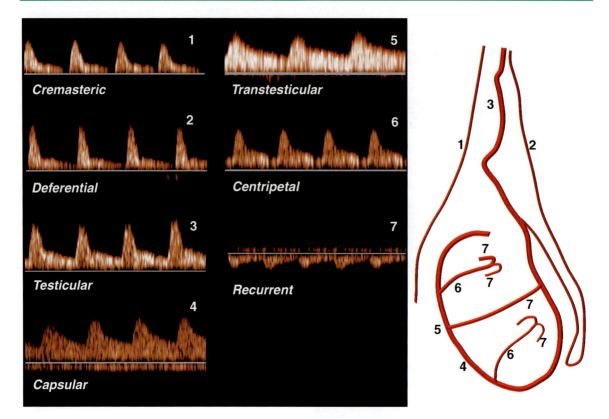

**Fig. 10** Flow characteristics of the different scrotal arteries at pulse doppler analysis in a normal subject. Compared to cremasteric and deferential arteries, the testicular artery shows low resistance flow. A progressive reduction of the peak systolic velocity and vascular resistances is appreciably progressing from the main testicular artery towards the peripheral branches

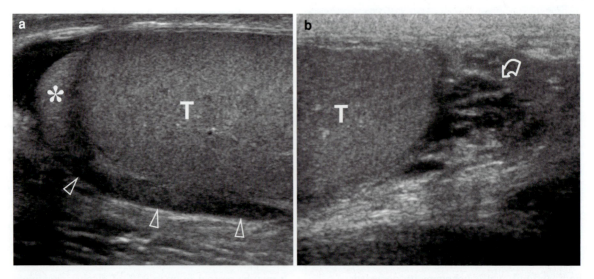

**Fig. 11** Appearance of the epididymis at gray-scale ultrasound. Longitudinal views. **a** The epididymal head (*asterisks*) is isoechoic to the testis (*T*), while the body (*arrowheads*) is relatively hypoechoic. **b** The epididymal tail (*curved arrow*) is hypoechoic to testis (*T*)

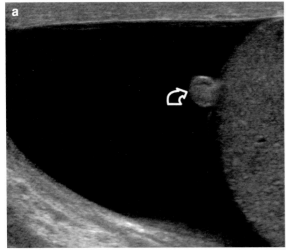

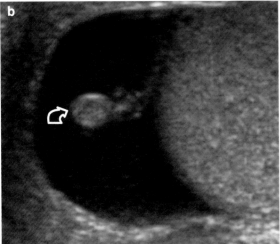

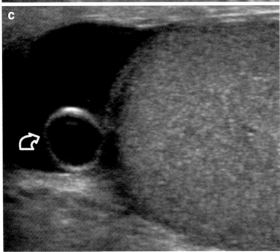

**Fig. 12** Variable appearance of appendix testis (*curved arrow*) at gray-scale ultrasound. **a** Rounded and sessile appearance. **b** Peduncolated with solid appearance. **c** Cystic appearance

and in approximately 44% of ultrasound examinations (Kantarci et al. 2005). It is usually seen as an echogenic structure of a few millimeters diameter at the angle between the epididymal head and the testis. Morphology is variable; in most cases it is oval shaped and sessile, but it may appear pedunculated, cystic, or calcified (Sellars and Sidhu 2003) (Fig. 12).

## 6.2 Appendix Epididymis

The appendix epididymis is a remnant of the Wolffian duct. It may be present in up to 34% of autopsy specimens and in approximtately 18% of ultrasound examinations (Kantarci et al. 2005). On histopathological examination it is almost invariably cystic, composed of multiple converging ducts. The lumen is filled with secretions derived from the columnar epithelial cells lining the cyst. At ultrasound, however, appendix epididymis presents with cystic appearance in only about 36% of cases (Kantarci et al. 2005) (Fig. 13). The most common morphology is a pedunculated and large nonseptated cysts. According to Kantarci et al. (2005) since the appendix epididymis is composed of thin fluid-filled ducts, solid appearance at ultrasound may be explained by presence of many interfaces between the ducts and the ultrasound beam.

## 7 Anatomical Variations of the Testis

Polyorchidism, testicular lobulations, and bell-clapper deformity can be incidentally recognized at ultrasound. Bozgeyik et al. (2008) described a patient in whom polyorchidism and lobulation of the supernumerary testis were associated.

## 7.1 Polyorchidism

Polyorchidism, or supernumerary testes, is a rare congenital abnormality where more than two testes are present. Although three testes is the most common form, as many as five have been reported. This anatomical variation is believed to result embryologically from an abnormal division of the genital ridge (Woodward et al. 2003; Amodio et al. 2004). Till 2002, approximately 75 cases had been documented (Chung and Yao 2002). The patients most

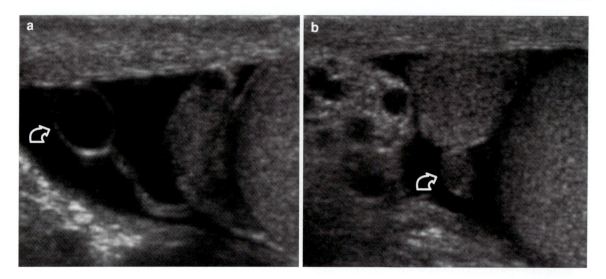

**Fig. 13** Variable appearance of appendix epidiymis (*curved arrow*) at gray-scale ultrasound. **a** Peduncolated with cystic appearance. **b** Isoechoic to testis, sessile, apparently solid

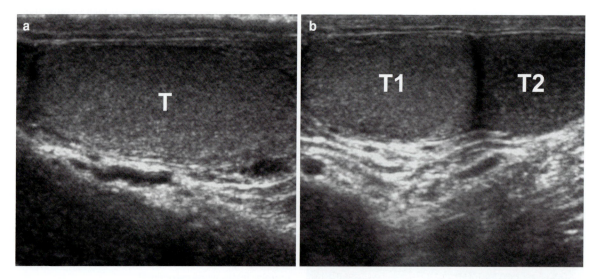

**Fig. 14** Triorchidism. Sagittal ultrasound images showing one testis (*T*) in the right hemiscrotum (**a**) and two testes (*T1* and *T2*) in the left hemiscrotum (**b**)

often present with a painless scrotal mass. In approximately 75% of cases, the supernumerary testes are intrascrotal. In the remaining cases 20% of the testes are inguinal and 5% retroperitoneal (Woodward et al. 2003). The testes may have separate or common spermatic cords, epididymis and tunica albuginea (Amodio et al. 2004; Berger et al. 2002). Color doppler ultrasound shows a normal flow pattern and vascular architecture of the supernumerary testis.

The presence of an accessory testis may be associated to various anomalies, such as criptorchidism and inguinal hernia (Chung and Yao 2002). An increased risk or torsion has also been reported (Chung and Yao 2002). In patients with polyorchidism, the accessory testis usually presents at ultrasound with the same

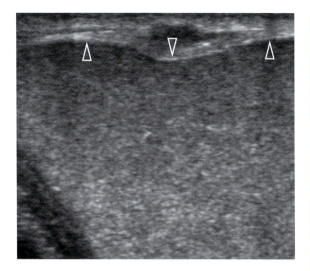

**Fig. 15** Gray-scale sagittal view revealing a lobulated appearance of the surface of the testis (*arrowheads*)

echogenicity, echotexture, and vascular pattern than the normal testes (Chung and Yao 2002; Stewart and Sidhu 2007) (Fig. 14). The epididymis, particularly when duplicated, may be difficult to evaluate. In cases with equivocal ultrasound findings, MR imaging can be helpful for making a definitive diagnosis showing the supernumerary testes with the same characteristics as normal testes (Woodward et al. 2003; Chung and Yao 2002).

## 7.2 Testicular Lobulation

This very rare anatomical variation may be an idiopathic embryologic variant (Kao and Gerscovich 2003) or may be a consequence of postoperative fibrotic changes (Kantarci et al. 2003; Mihmanli and Kantarci 2009). It may present clinically as a palpable testicular mass. Ultrasound reveals the lobulated appearance of the testis, and rules-out testicular malignancy (Fig. 15).

## 7.3 Bell-Clapper Deformity

Bell-clapper deformity is a common condition, with a 12% incidence in an autopsy series (Caesar and Kaplan

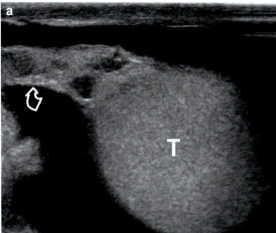

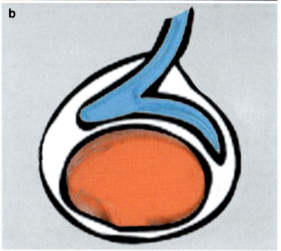

**Fig. 16** Bell-clapper deformity. **a** Gray-scale ultrasound view showing the testis (*T*) completely surrounded by hydrocele, hanging the extremity of the spermatic cord (*curved arrow*). **b** Diagram showing the deformity. The tunica vaginalis surrounds completely the testis and epididymis which are not fixed to the posterior aspect of the scrotal wall

1994), in which the tunica vaginalis completely encircles the epididymis, distal spermatic cord, and the testis rather than attaching to the posterolateral aspect of the testis (Dogra 2003). As a consequence, the testis is able to rotate freely within the tunica vaginalis. This anatomic abnormality predisposes to spermatic cord torsion.

Bell-clapper deformity is hard to be detected at ultrasound, and only a few cases have been described. In most patients, it is easier to palpate clinically than

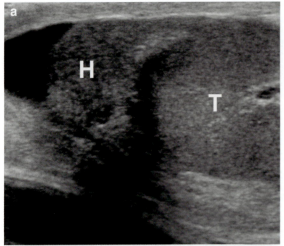

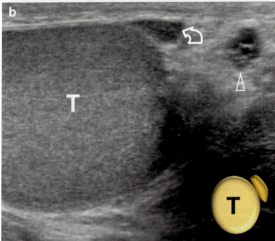

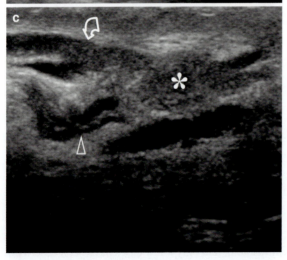

◀ **Fig. 17** Normal epididymal anatomy. **a** Longitudinal gray-scale view of the left testis showing the head of the epididymis (*H*) above the upper pole of the testis (*T*). **b** Transverse view showing the body or the epididymis (*curved arrow*) lateral to the testis (*T*) and slighly anterior to the vas deferens (*arrowhead*) The diagram shows the relationship between the testis (*T*) and the epididymis. **c** Longitudinal view showing the body of the epididymis (*curved arrow*), the tail (*asterisks*), and the vas deferens (*arrowhead*) posterior to the epididymal tail

to be visualized by an ultrasound examination (Cochlin 2005). Abnormal direction of the long axis of the testis and abnormal pattern of fluid distribution around the testis may suggest the diagnosis (Cochlin 2005). In fact, the long axis of the testis normally lies in the head-to-foot direction, while in the bell-clapper deformity, the testis is mobile and often lies in the right-to-left direction. Hydrocele makes diagnosis easier. Fluid surrounds the anterior surface of the testis and not the posterior aspect, while in the bell-clapper deformity, fluid surrounds the entire testis and epididymis (Coley 2006) (Fig. 16).

## 8 Anatomical Variations of the Epididymis

In the commonest anatomic position, the epididymal head is above the upper pole of the testis, the epididymal body lateral to the testis, and the epididymal tail anterior to the vas deferens (Fig. 17). According to Puttermans et al. (2006), this anatomical position occurs in approximately 98% of normal subjects and in 88% of infertile patients. Variations in the anatomic position of the epididymal body and tail can occur, and can be evaluated at ultrasound. In a variation occurring in approximately 6% of normal subjects and in 9% of infertile patients, the epididymal body is posterior to the testis, with the epididymal head remains above the upper pole of the testis and the epididymo-deferential loop is inverted with the vas deferens anterior to the epididymal tail (Fig. 18). Occasionally, there is an epididymal rotation in the longitudinal axis; the epididymis is inverted, with the epididymal head located below the lower pole of the testis, and the epididymal body posterior to the

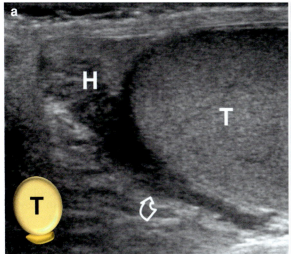
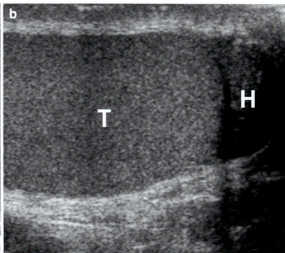

**Fig. 18** Anatomical variations of the epididymis. **a** Gray-scale longitudinal view showing the head of the epididymis (*H*) above the upper pole of the testis (*T*) and the epididymal body (curved arrow) posterior to the testis. The diagram shows the relationships between the testis (*T*) and the epididymis. **b** Uncommon anatomical variation in which the head of the epididymis (*H*) is below the lower pole of the testis (T)

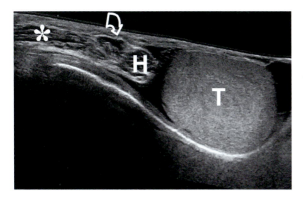

**Fig. 19** Disjunction of the epididymal tail. Longitudunal view showing the epididymis (*curved arrow*) presenting as an elongated hypoechoic formation above the testis (*T*). The head of the epididymis (*H*) is connected to the upper pole of the testis, while the tail (*asterisks*) is displaced into the inguinal canal

testis (Fig. 18). According to Puttermans et al. (2006), this anatomical variation occur in approximately 2–3% of normal subjects and 12% of infertile men.

In most of cases, the epididymo-deferential loop is below the lower pole of the testis. In some men, however, the epididymal tail reaches only up to the mid-portion of the testis before turning cephalad into the vas deferens or rarely, in case of fusion abnormalities

between the testis and the epididymis, the body and tail of the epididymis may be seen superiorly to the epididymal head (Black and Patel 1996).

# 9 Fusion Abnormalities Between the Testis and the Epididymis

Most commonly, the normal anatomy of the epididymis demonstrates the epididymal head to be firmly attached to the upper pole of the testis by the efferent ductules. The tail of the epididymis is closely opposed to the lower pole of the testis with a fibrous attachment. Variations of the relationship between the testis and the epididymis, however, has been described (Favorito et al. 2004).

Favorito et al. (2004) classified epididymal anatomy in six groups: Type I, corresponding to the commonest anatomical arrangement, in which epididymis is connected to the testis by its head and tail; type II, in which epididymis is totally connected to the testis; type III, characterized by disjunction of epididymal tail; type IV, characterized by disjunction of epididymal head; Type V, in which there is total disjunction between testis and epididymis, and Type VI, epididymal atresia.

Absence of portions of the epididymis can be identified at ultrasound in patients with obstructive azoospermia (Moon et al. 2006). Complete separation of the testis and epididymis has been described in a 21 month-old boy. The epididymis appeared as an oval structure in the inguinal region, with the same echotexture of the testis, mimicking polyorchidism (Zuppa et al. 2006).

Type III abnormality can be identified at ultrasound when the mobile epididymis moves in the inguinal canal as an elongated hypoechoic formation connected to the mediastinum testis (Fig. 19).

Although also the other fusion abnormalities between the testis and the epididymis may be clinically relevant, because they may predispose to testicular and epididymal torsion (Favorito et al. 2004; Dibilio et al. 2006; Brisson et al. 2005), their ultrasound appearance has not been described.

# References

Amodio JB, Maybody M, Slowotsky C et al (2004) Polyorchidism: report of three cases and review of the literature. J Ultrasound Med 23:951–957

Aziz ZA, Satchithananda K, Khan M et al (2005) High-frequency color doppler ultrasonography of the spermatic cord arteries: Resistive index variation in a cohort of 51 healthy men. J Ultrasound Med 24:905–909

Berger AP, Steiner H, Hoeltl L et al (2002) Occurrence of polyorchidism in a young man. Urology 60:911

Black JA, Patel A (1996) Sonography of the normal extratesticular space. Am J Roentgenol 167:503–506

Bozgeyik Z, Kocakoc E, Ozturk T (2008) Polyorchidism with lobulation and septa in supernumerary testis. Diagn Interv Radiol 14:100–102

Brisson P, Feins N, Patel H (2005) Torsion of the epididymis. J Pediatr Surg 40:1795–1797

Bushby LH, Sellars ME, Sidhu PS (2007) The "two-tone" testis: spectrum of ultrasound appearances. Clin Radiol 62:1119–1123

Caesar RE, Kaplan GW (1994) Incidence of the bell-clapper deformity in an autopsy series. Urology 44:114–116

Chung TJ, Yao WJ (2002) Sonographic features of polyorchidism. J Clin Ultrasound 30:106–108

Cochlin D (2005) Acute testicular pain. Imaging 17:91–100

Coley BD (2006) The acute paediatric scrotum. Ultrasound Clin 1:485–496

Dibilio D, Serafini G, Gandolfo NG et al (2006) Ultrasonographic findings of isolated torsion of the epididymis. J Ultrasound Med 25:417–419

Dogra V (2003) Bell-clapper deformity. Am J Roentgenol 180:1176; author reply 1176–1177

Favorito LA, Cavalcante AG, Costa WS (2004) Anatomic aspects of epididymis and tunica vaginalis in patients with testicular torsion. Int Braz J Urol 30:420–424

Gooding GA (1988) Sonography of the spermatic cord. Am J Roentgenol 151:721–724

Heyns CF (1987) The gubernaculum during testicular descent in the human fetus. J Anat 153:93–112

Hricak H (1995) Imaging techniques, anatomy, artifacts, and bioeffects. In: Hricak H, Hamm B, Kim B (eds) Imaging of the scrotum. Raven Press, New York, p 11

Kantarci F, Mihmanli I, Yilmaz MH et al (2003) Orchiopexy: a cause of benign testicular lobulation. J Ultrasound Med 22:1417–1419

Kantarci F, Ozer H, Adaletli I et al (2005) Cystic appendix epididymis: a sonomorphologic study. Surg Radiol Anat 27:557–561

Kao EY, Gerscovich EO (2003) Benign testicular lobulation: sonographic findings. J Ultrasound Med 22:299–301

Loberant N, Bhatt S, McLennan GT et al (2010) Striated appearance of the testes. Ultrasound Q 26:37–44

Martinoli C, Pastorino C, Bertolotto M et al (1992) Color-doppler echography of the testis. Study technique and vascular anatomy. Radiol Med 84:785–791

Middleton WD, Bell MW (1993) Analysis of intratesticular arterial anatomy with emphasis on transmediastinal arteries. Radiology 189:157–160

Middleton WD, Thorne DA, Melson GL (1989) Color doppler ultrasound of the normal testis. Am J Roentgenol 152:293–297

Middleton WD, Dahiya N, Naughton CK et al (2009) High-resolution sonography of the normal extrapelvic vas deferens. J Ultrasound Med 28:839–846

Mihmanli I, Kantarci F (2009) Sonography of scrotal abnormalities in adults: an update. Diagn Interv Radiol 15:64–73

Moon MH, Kim SH, Cho JY et al (2006) Scrotal US for evaluation of infertile men with azoospermia. Radiology 239:168–173

Mostafa T, Labib I, El-Khayat Y et al (2008) Human testicular arterial supply: gross anatomy, corrosion cast, and radiologic study. Fertil Steril 90:2226–2230

Pais D, Fontoura P, Esperanca-Pina JA (2004) The transmediastinal arteries of the human testis: an anatomical study. Surg Radiol Anat 26:379–383

Puttemans T, Delvigne A, Murillo D (2006) Normal and variant appearances of the adult epididymis and vas deferens on high-resolution sonography. J Clin Ultrasound 34:385–392

Raman JD, Goldstein M (2004) Intraoperative characterization of arterial vasculature in spermatic cord. Urology 64:561–564

Sellars ME, Sidhu PS (2003) Ultrasound appearances of the testicular appendages: pictorial review. Eur Radiol 13:127–135

Stewart VR, Sidhu PS (2007) The testis: the unusual, the rare and the bizarre. Clin Radiol 62:289–302

Sudakoff GS, Quiroz F, Karcaaltincaba M et al (2002) Scrotal ultrasonography with emphasis on the extratesticular space: anatomy, embryology, and pathology. Ultrasound Q 18:255–273

Woodward PJ, Schwab CM, Sesterhenn IA (2003) From the archives of the AFIP: extratesticular scrotal masses: radiologic-pathologic correlation. Radiographics 23:215–240

Zuppa AA, Nanni L, Di Gregorio F et al (2006) Complete epididymal separation presenting as polyorchidism. J Clin Ultrasound 34:258–260

# Scrotal Anatomy at MRI

Yuji Watanabe

## Contents

Y. Watanabe (✉)
Department of Radiology, Kurashiki Central Hospital,
1-1-1-Miwa, Kurashiki 710-8602, Japan
e-mail: yw5904@kchnet.or.jp

**Abstract**

This section of the chapter provides comprehensive description of MR features for normal anatomy, developmental growth, and related anomalies of the scrotum. The normal scrotum is divided by a midline septum called raphe, and each half of the scrotum contains a testis, the epididymis, and the scrotal portion of the spermatic cord. A normal testis has homogeneous texture of high signal intensity on fat-suppressed T2-weighted image, and covered with the tunica albuginea and the visceral layer of tunica vaginalis which are seen as a thin stripe of low signal intensity. The epididymis, which overlies the superolateral aspect of the testis, shows intermediate signal intensity lower than that of the testis on FST2-weighted image. Fibrous septa dividing seminiferous lobules are seen as low signal intensity and prominent on heavily T2-weighted image, especially in patients with infertility. Also described are other MR features found in abnormal anatomy such as cryptorchidism, inguinoscrotal hernia, hydrocele, bell clapper deformity, varicocele, etc.

## 1   Normal Anatomy

The scrotum is divided by a midline septum called raphe, and each half of the scrotum contains a testis, the epididymis, and the scrotal portion of the spermatic cord (Fig. 1).

A normal testis measures $5 \times 3 \times 2$ cm in size and has homogeneous texture of intermediate and high signal intensity on T1- and fat-suppressed (FS) T2-weighted images, respectively (Baker et al. 1987; Rholl et al. 1987). The tunica albuginea and the

M. Bertolotto and C. Trombetta (eds.), *Scrotal Pathology,* Medical Radiology. Diagnostic Imaging,
DOI: 10.1007/174_2011_173, © Springer-Verlag Berlin Heidelberg 2012

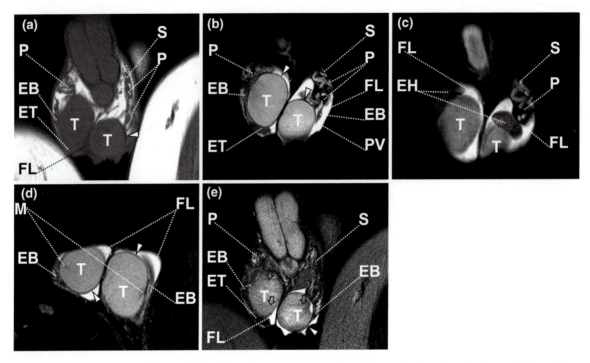

**Fig. 1** Normal anatomy in a 23 year-old healthy volunteer. **a** T1-weighted coronal image. **b** Fat-suppressed (FS) T2-weighted coronal image. **c** FST2-weighted coronal image at the anterior level to the image-b. **d** FST2-weighted transaxial image. **e** Heavily T2-weighted coronal image. T: testis, EH: epididymal head, EB: epididymal body, ET: epididymal tail, S: spermatic cord, *arrowheads*: tunica albuginea and visceral layer of tunica vaginalis, PV: parietal layer of tunica vaginalis, M: mediastinum of testis, *arrows*: fibrous septa between the numerous lobules, P: pampiniform plexus of vein, FL: fluid in the tunica vaginalis cavity

visceral layer of tunica vaginalis are fibrous coverings that protect the testis from external injuries and are seen as a thin stripe (less than 1 mm in thickness) of low signal intensity on both T1- and FST2-weighted images (Baker et al. 1987; Rholl et al. 1987; Kim et al. 2007). The epididymi Baker et al., which overlies the superolateral aspect of the testis, comprises a head, body, and tail (Aso et al. 2005; Bhatt and Dogra 2008; Hricak et al. 1995). The tail of the epididymis continues as the vas deferens in the spermatic cord. The signal intensity of the epididymis is similar to that of the testis on T1-weighted images, and shows intermediate signal intensity lower than that of the testis on FST2-weighted images (Baker et al. 1987; Rholl et al. 1987; Hricak et al. 1995).

The tunica vaginalis consists of visceral and parietal layers, normally separated by small amounts of fluid. The layer, lining the scrotal wall is termed the parietal layer, and the layer extending over the testis and epididymis is referred to as the visceral layer (Aso et al. 2005; Dogra et al. 2003). The tunica vaginalis is seen as a thin lining of low signal intensity on FST2-weighted images (Baker et al. 1987; Rholl et al. 1987; Hricak et al. 1995). The fluid in the tunica vaginalis cavity is delineated as high and very high signal intensity on FST2- and heavily T2-weighted images, respectively (Baker et al. 1987; Rholl et al. 1987).

## 2 Testis

Magnetic resonance (MR) imaging allows evaluation of different anatomical features of the testis. Among them, the mediastinum and parenchymal features should be evaluated, as well as growth characteristic and changes in infertile patients.

### 2.1 Mediastinum

The tunica albuginea covers the entire testis. The posterior surface of the tunica albuginea projects into

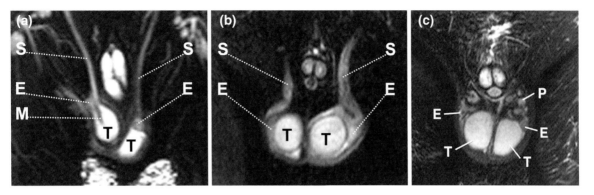

**Fig. 2** Developmental growth of testis, **a** FST2-weighted image in 1 year-old baby. **b** FST2-weighted image in 11 year-old boy. **c** FST2-weighted image in 26 year-old adult. Testicular size increases with the age. Signal intensity of the testis minimally decreases with the age. The Spermatic cord appears as a straight tubular structure in infant. In peripuberty and adolescence, the pampiniform plexus of veins becomes prominent and demonstrates the spermatic cord as tortuous tubular structures. T: testis, E: epididymis, S: spermatic cord, M: mediastinum of testis, P: pampiniform plexus of vein

the interior of the testis, forming the incomplete septum known as the mediastinum of the testis. The mediastinum appears as a low signal intensity band (1–2 cm long) along the long axis of the testis invaginating into the testis of high signal intensity on FST2-weighted and heavily T2-weighted images (Baker et al. 1987; Hricak et al. 1995), and may be mistaken for an intratesticular lesion (Dogra et al. 2003) (Fig. 1d, e).

## 2.2 Parenchyma

The testicular parenchyma consists of multiple lobules, each of which is composed of many seminiferous tubules. From the mediastinum, numerous fibrous septa extend into the testis, dividing it into 250–400 lobules, each of which consists of one to three seminiferous tubules supporting the sertoli cells and spermatocytes that give rise to sperm (Dogra et al. 2003). The seminiferous tubules lead via the tubuli recti into dilated spaces called the rete testis within the mediastinum. The rete testis, a network of epithelium-lined spaces embedded in the fibrous stroma of the mediastinum, drains into the epididymis through 10–15 efferent ductules. A normal testis shows homogeneous high signal intensity on FST2-weighted images and intermediate signal intensity on heavily T2-weighted images (Fig. 1b, d, e). Fine fibrous septa dividing the lobules are often seen as thin linear structures of low signal intensity extending from the mediastinum testis on heavily T2-weighted images (Cramer et al. 1991) (Fig. 1e).

## 2.3 Developmental Growth

Testicular size depends on age and stage of sexual development (Dogra et al. 2003). In neonates, the testis measures approximately $1.5 \times 1$ cm in length and width. Testicular volume is approximately $1–2$ cm$^3$ before puberty and reaches 4 cm$^3$ in puberty (Aso et al. 2005) (Fig. 2). The testes measures approximately $5 \times 3 \times 2$ cm in the postpubertal male (Doherty 1991). In the peripubertal period, a difference of 3 mm in anteroposterior diameter is significant (Baud et al. 1998). Although these measurements of the testes are not acquired routinely, they should be obtained in patients with cryptorchidism, varicocele, and infertility to assess changes in testicular size (Sijstermans et al. 2009).

Testicular signal intensity also varies depending on age and sexual development on FST2-weighted and heavily T2-weighted images, but does not change on T1-weighted images. In neonates and infants, the testis is visualized as an ovoid structure of very high signal intensity on FST2-weighted images. In adolescence, testicular signal intensity slightly decreases with the development of germ cell elements and tubular maturation on FST2-weighted and heavily T2-weighted images.

## 2.4 Infertility

In patients with infertility, the testes show atrophy (Simpson et al. 2009) and inhomogeneous low signal

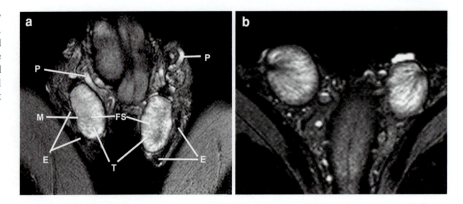

**Fig. 3** Infertility. **a** Heavily T2-weighted coronal image. **b** Heavily T2-weighted transaxial image. Testes are small and atrophic, and show inhomogeneous signal intensity with the prominent fibrous septa

intensity on FST2-weighted and heavily T2-weighted images. Fibrous septa of low signal intensity are prominent on heavily T2-weighted images, reflecting atrophy of seminiferous tubules (Fig. 3).

## 3 Processus Vaginalis

The processus vaginalis appears at about 13 weeks of fetal development as an outpouching of the parietal peritoneum, through which the testis descends from the abdomen to the scrotum between the 7th and 9th months of fetal life. After testicular descent, the processus vaginalis is obliterated and the scrotal portion of this processus remains as a peritoneum-lined cavity, the tunica vaginalis, surrounding the anterior surface of the testis (Langman 1975).

Failure of the testis to descend into the scrotum and patency or anomalous closure of the processus vaginalis result in the following conditions: cryptorchidism, inguinoscrotal hernia, and hydrocele (Aso et al. 2005).

### 3.1 Cryptorchidism

Failure of the intra-abdominal testes to descend into the scrotal sac is known as cryptorchidism (Dogra et al. 2003). The cryptorchid testis may be located at any point along the descent route from the retroperitoneum to the external inguinal ring (Nguyen et al. 1999).

MR imaging is very useful for identifying testes and is highly accurate for locating testes in the inguinal canal (Fritzsche et al. 1987; Kier et al. 1988; Shadbolt et al. 2001; Tripathi et al. 1992) (Figs. 4, 5). However, when the testis is located in the abdomen,

MR imaging may not allow detection of abdominal testes (Nguyen et al. 1999; Muglia et al. 2002). The cryptorchid testis is usually smaller relative to the normally located testis because of testicular dystrophy and degeneration (Sijstermans et al. 2009) (Fig. 4). The signal intensity change related with the degree of dystrophy and degeneration might be smaller on FST2-weighted image than on heavily T2-weighted image. The undescended testis with dystrophy and degeneration may appear as low signal intensity on diffusion-weighted imaging and high on ADC map (Kaipia et al. 2005) (Fig. 4). The undescended testis tends to twist, where dynamic subtraction contrast-enhanced imaging is necessary for evaluating testicular perfusion (Watanabe 2002; Watanabe et al. 2000, 2007) (Fig. 5).

### 3.2 Inguinal-Scrotal Hernia

Inguinal-scrotal hernia is defined as the passage of intestinal loops and/or omentum into the scrotal cavity (Garriga et al. 2009). The prevalence of inguinal hernia is higher in preterm neonates, especially at 32 weeks gestation (Shipp and Benacerraf 1995). The hernia is more frequently located on the right side, because the right processus vaginalis closes later than the left (Siegel 1997).

Though physical examination allows for accurate diagnosis in most cases, MR examination can be indicated in patients with inconclusive physical findings. Fat tissues such as omentum and mesentery, protruding through the inguinal canal, usually shows high signal intensity on T1-weighted images and very low signal intensity on FST2-weighted images. Vessels of the omentum and/or mesentery appear as curvilinear structures of T1-low and FST2-high signal

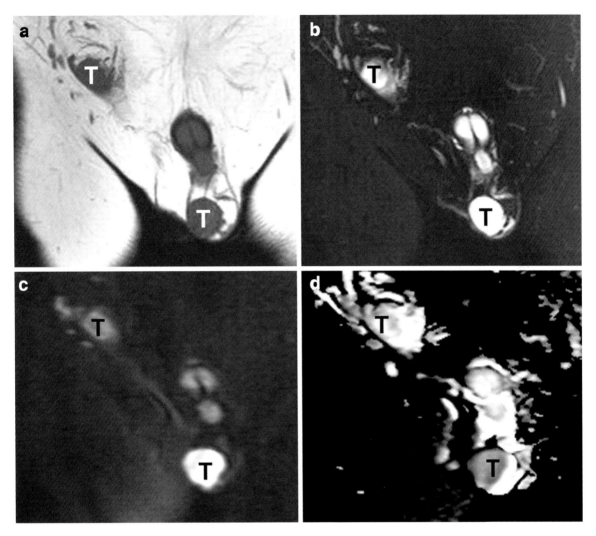

**Fig. 4** Cryptorchidism. **a** T1-weighted coronal image. **b** FST2-weighted coronal image. **c** Diffusion-weighted image at b = 800 s/mm². **d** ADC map. The right testis is located in the inguinal canal. The undescended testis is smaller than the left normal testis. The signal intensity of the undescended testis appeared similar with the left normal testis on FST2-weighted image. In contrast, the diffusion-weighted image and ADC map demonstrate the difference in the signal intensity between the undescended and normal testes. T: testis

intensity (Fig. 6). When bowel loops protrude through the inguinal canal, it is also easy to identify inguinal hernia by detecting tubular structures on T1-weighted images (Shadbolt et al. 2001).

## 4 Tunica Vaginalis

The tunica albuginea and the visceral layer of the tunica vaginalis can be seen as a thin T2-hypointensity line around the testis (Baker et al. 1987; Rholl et al. 1987). The parietal layer of the tunica vaginalis lines the scrotal wall. The space between the two leaves of the tunica vaginalis normally contains a few milliliters of fluid, seen as a thin T2-hyperintensity rim, partly surrounding the testes (Hricak et al. 1995).

The parietal and visceral layers of the tunica vaginalis join at the posterolateral aspect of the testis, where the tunica attaches to the scrotal wall (Baker et al. 1987; Garriga et al. 2009). The tunica vaginalis covers the testis and epididymis except for a small posterior area (Dogra et al. 2003).

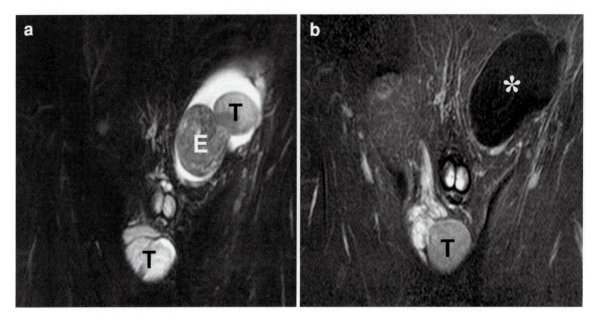

**Fig. 5** Testicular torsion of the undescended testis. **a** FST2-weighted coronal image. **b** Dynamic subtraction contrast-enhanced image. The left testis with the enlarged epididymis is located in the external inguinal ring. The left undescended testis and the left epididymis show low signal intensity with the prominent fine septa on FST2-weighted image and no contrast enhancement on the dynamic subtraction contrast-enhanced image. Subsequently, the undescended testis surgically proved to be twisted. T: testis, E: epididymis

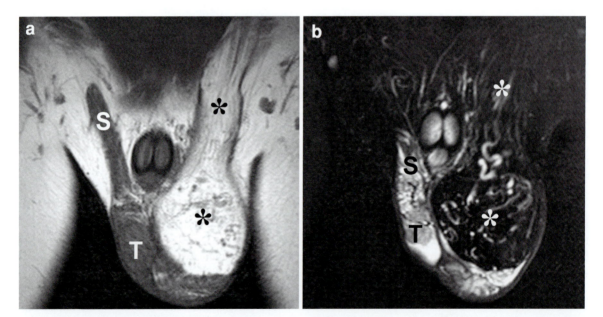

**Fig. 6** Left inguinoscrotal hernia. **a** T1-weighted coronal image. **b** FST2-weighted coronal image. The omentum (*astrisks*) protrude through the left inguinal canal and is located in the scrotum. Fat tissue of the herniated omentum shows very high signal intensity on T1-weighted image and very low signal intensity on FST2-weighted images. Vessels of the omentum appear as curvilinear structures of T1-low and FST2-high signal intensity. T: testis, S: spermatic cord

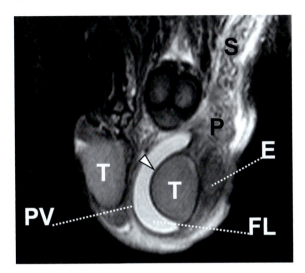

**Fig. 7** Hydrocele associated with acute epididymitis. On FST2-weighted images, hydrocele (FL) appears as a fluid collection of high signal intensity surrounding the anterior and medial aspects of the testis and extending to the inguinal canal. The swollen epididymis and spermatic cord are caused by acute epididymitis. T: testis, E: epididymis, S: spermatic cord, *arrowhead*: tunica albuginea and visceral layer of tunica vaginalis, PV: parietal layer of tunica vaginalis, P: pampiniform plexus of vein, FL: fluid in the tunica vaginalis cavity

## 4.1 Hydrocele

Hydrocele is an abnormal collection of fluid between the visceral and parietal layers of the tunica vaginalis and/or along the spermatic cord. In neonates and infants, hydroceles are congenital and associated with a patent processus vaginalis, which allows peritoneal fluid to enter the scrotal sac (Garriga et al. 2009; Martin et al. 1996). In older children and adolescents, hydroceles are usually acquired and are associated with an inflammatory process, testicular torsion, trauma, appendiceal torsion, etc. (Fig. 7).

On FST2-weighted and heavily T2-weighted images, hydrocele appears as a fluid collection of high signal intensity surrounding the anterior and medial aspects of the testis and sometimes extending to the inguinal canal (Baker et al. 1987; Rholl et al. 1987; Hricak et al. 1995) (Fig. 7).

Closure of the processus vaginalis above the testis and below the internal inguinal ring leads to a less common type of hydrocele, known as spermatic cord cyst, which appear as a fluid collection in the spermatic cord (Martin et al. 1996).

## 4.2 Bell Clapper Deformity

Failure of normal posterior anchoring of the epididymis and testis is called a bell clapper deformity because it leaves the testis free to swing and rotate within the tunica vaginalis of the scrotum like the clapper inside of a bell. This is a precondition for twisting of the testis on the axis of the spermatic cord, called spermatic cord torsion.

The deformity itself is hard to be detected by imaging. However, there are some specific MR features suggestive of bell-clapper deformity: abnormal direction of the long axis of the testis and abnormal pattern of fluid collection in the tunica vaginalis cavity. The long axis normally lies in the head-to-foot direction with mild superior-lateral to inferior-medial slope (Baker et al. 1987; Rholl et al. 1987) (Figs. 1, 2, 7). In the bell-clapper deformity where the testes are very high in mobility, the long axis sometimes appears to lie in the right-to-left direction with the epididymis right upon the testis, which can be observed on FST2-weighted and heavily T2-weighted images (Fig. 8). The fluid collection in the tunica vaginalis cavity is normally seen surrounding the anterior surface of the testis and not in the posterior aspect of the testis (Fig. 7). In the bell-clapper deformity, the fluid collection is sometimes found even in the posterior aspect of the testis and surrounding the entire testis and epididymis, which can be observed on the FST2-weighted and heavily T2-weighted images (Fig. 8).

## 5 Appendages

There are four testicular appendages, which are the remnants of the mesonephric and paramesonephric ducts (Aso et al. 2005; Dogra et al. 2003; Sellars and Sidhu 2003; Trainer 1992). One of the four, the appendix testis, can be usually identified on MR imaging as intermediate signal intensity on FST2-weighted images. The appendix testis, known as hydatid of Morgagni, is a Mullerian duct remnant, and consists of fibrous tissue and blood vessels within an envelope of columnar epithelium and is attached to the anterior surface of the upper pole of the testis.

The size is normally 5 mm in length and appears swollen particularly in cases of appendiceal torsion.

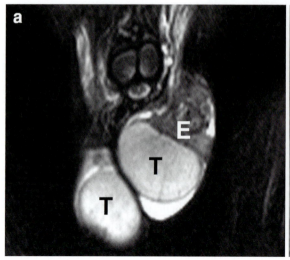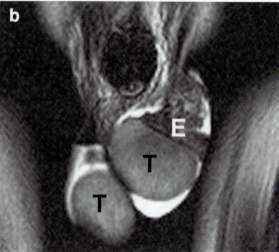

**Fig. 8** Bell-clapper deformity. **a** FST2-weighted coronal image. **b** heavily T2-weighted coronal image. On FST2-weighted coronal image, the left testis with the bell clapper deformity shows the abnormal long axis lying in the right-to-left direction. The fluid collection in the tunica vaginalis cavity is clearly seen surrounding the testis on heavily T2-weighted image. T: testis, E: epididymis

The appendix epididymis, found at the head of the epididymis, is the similar size with the appendix testis, but is less commonly identified on MR imaging. The normal appendix testis and the appendix epididymis are typically seen only when a hydrocele is present (Aso et al. 2005; Dogra et al. 2003; Hricak and Filly 1983).

## 5.1 Torsion of Appendages

In appendiceal torsion, twisted and swollen appendage is usually seen as hyperintensity oval structure with dark rim in the anterior surface of the testis on FST2-weighted images and no central contrast enhancement with ring-like enhancement on the dynamic subtraction contrast-enhanced images (Watanabe 2002; Watanabe et al. 2000) (Fig. 9).

## 6 Epididymis

The epididymis is best evaluated in a coronal plane. The epididymal head is a 5–12 mm pyramidal structure situated on the superior pole of the testis (Bree and Hoang 1996; Dambro 1998). The epididymal body is seen as a narrow tubular structure of 2–4 mm thickness. The tail of the epididymis is approximately 2–5 mm in diameter and can be seen as a curved structure at the inferior pole of the testis (Kim et al. 2007; Dogra et al. 2003).

The signal intensity of the epididymis is similar to that of the testis on T1-weighted images, intermediate signal intensity lower than that of the testis on FST2-weighted images, and low signal intensity on heavily T2-weighted images (Baker et al. 1987; Shadbolt et al. 2001; Hricak and Filly 1983; Frush and Sheldon 1998) (Fig. 1). The vas deferens can be traced from the tail of the epididymis to the spermatic cord on FST2-weighted images.

## 6.1 Acute Epididymitis

In the inflammatory process such as acute epididymitis, the entire epididymis is swollen and appears as large as the testis (Figs. 7, 10). The enlarged epididymis minimally increases the signal intensity relative to the normal side on FST2-weighted images and clearly shows intense contrast enhancement on the dynamic subtraction contrast-enhanced images, reflecting hyperemic condition (Rholl et al. 1987; Watanabe 2002; Watanabe et al. 2000) (Fig. 10).

## 7 Spermatic Cord

The spermatic cord contains the vas deferens, testicular artery, deferential artery, cremasteric artery, the pampiniform plexus of veins, and lymphatic vessels,

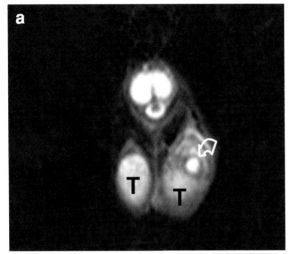

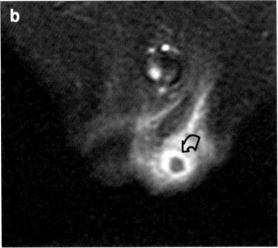

**Fig. 9** Torsion of testicular appendage. **a** FST2-weighted coronal image. **b** Dynamic subtraction contrast-enhanced image. The appendix testis (*curved arrow*) is twisted and swollen. FST2-weighted image demonstrates a hyperintense oval structure with dark rim in the anterior surface of the testis. The dynamic subtraction contrast-enhanced image shows ring-like enhancement with no central contrast enhancement. T: testis

and begins at the deep inguinal ring and descends vertically into the scrotum (Dogra et al. 2003; Krone and Carroll 1985; Langer 1993).

In infants, the spermatic cord appears as a straight tubular structure of intermediate signal intensity similar to the epididymis and lower than that of the testis on coronal FST2-weighted images (Baker et al. 1987; Shadbolt et al. 2001) (Fig. 2a). From prepuberty to adolescence, with the development of

pampiniform plexus of veins, the spermatic cord mainly demonstrates tortuous tubular structures of high signal intensity on FST2-weighted images (Baker et al. 1987; Hricak et al. 1995; Shadbolt et al. 2001) (Figs. 2b, c, 7). On transaxial images, the spermatic cord appears ovoid with a hyperintensity on FST2-weighted and contrast-enhanced images (Fig. 11a).

## 7.1 Spermatic Cord Torsion

In spermatic cord torsion, the twisted spermatic cord appears swollen and demonstrates the whirlpool appearance on transaxial FST2-weighted and contrast-enhanced images (Baud et al. 1998) (Fig. 11a). In addition, the twisted testis shows no contrast enhancement on contrast-enhanced images (Watanabe 2002; Watanabe et al. 2000, 2007) (Fig. 11b).

## 8 Vascular Supply

The right and left testicular arteries branch from the abdominal aorta, arise just distal to the renal arteries and provide the primary vascular supply to the testes (Dogra et al. 2003). They enter the spermatic cord at the deep inguinal ring and course along the posterior surface of the testis, penetrating the tunica albuginea to carry blood to the parenchyma through the mediastinum. A transmediastinal arterial branch of the testicular artery is present in approximately one-half of normal testes (Middleton and Bell 1993), and it courses through the mediastinum to supply the capsular arteries. These arteries are usually too small in diameter to be demonstrated on FST2-weighted images.

Venous blood from the testes is drained through the pampiniform plexus of draining veins, which is formed around the upper half of the epididymis in a variable fashion and continues as the testicular vein through the deep inguinal ring. Pampiniform plexus of veins appears as tortuous, tubular structures of high signal intensity on FST2-weighted and contrast-enhanced FST1-weighted images, which is more prominent in adolesence than in prepuberty (Baker et al. 1987; Rholl et al. 1987) (Figs. 1, 2, 12).

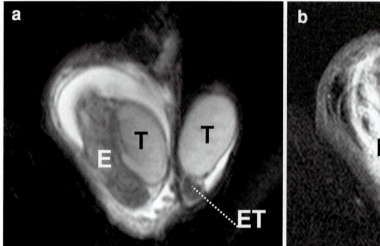
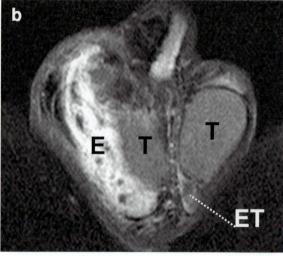

**Fig. 10** Acute epididymitis. **a** FST2-weighted coronal image. **b** Dynamic subtraction contrast-enhanced image. The right epididymis is enlarged and demonstrates slightly higher signal intensity than that of the left epididymal tail on FST2-weighted image. On the dynamic subtraction contrast-enhanced image, the right epididymis shows remarkable contrast enhancement relative to that of the left epididymal tail. T: testis, E: epididymis, ET: epididymal tail

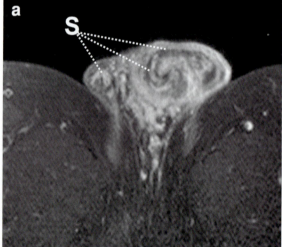
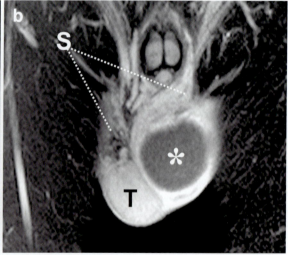

**Fig. 11** Spermatic cord torsion. **a** Contrast-enhanced FST1-weighted transaxial image. **b** Dynamic subtraction contrast-enhanced coronal image. The twisted spermatic cord appears swollen and demonstrates the whirlpool appearance on the contrast-enhanced images. The twisted testis shows no contrast enhancement on dynamic subtraction contrast-enhanced image. T: testis, S: spermatic cord

## 8.1    Varicocele

A varicocele is relatively common in adolescents, accounting for approximately 15% of adult men (Meacham et al. 1994). Varicocele involves abnormal dilatation of veins in the pampiniform plexus of the spermatic cord and is usually caused by incompetent valves in the internal spermatic vein (Aso et al. 2005; Dogra et al. 2003). The pampiniform plexus of veins, which normally range from 0.5 to 1.5 mm in diameter, can become 2 mm or larger in diameter, which can be observed on FST2-weighted and heavily T2-weighted images. The MR appearance of varicocele consists of multiple, serpiginous, tubular

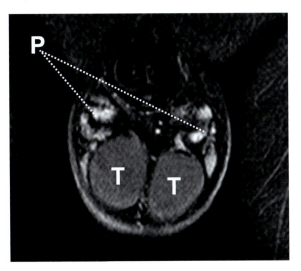

**Fig. 12** Perfusion of the normal testes. The dynamic subtraction contrast-enhanced image demonstrates symmetric and homogeneous contrast enhancement of the normal testes. Pampiniform plexus of veins shows intense contrast enhancement. T: testis, P: pampiniform plexus of vein

**Table 1** Perfusion pattern in various scrotal disorders based on contrast enhancement

| | Perfusion (contrast enhancement) | | |
|---|---|---|---|
| | Testis | Epididymis | Spermatic cord |
| Testicular torsion | None or decreased | None | Increased |
| Testicular trauma | None or partial defect | Normal | Increased |
| Testicular infarction | Partial defect | Normal | Normal |
| Acute epididymitis | Normal | Increased | Increased |
| Acute (epididymo) orchitis | Increased | Increased | Increased |
| Appendiceal torsion | Normal | Normal or Increased | Normal or Increased |
| Malignant neoplasm | Increased | Normal or Increased | Normal or Increased |

structures of T2-hyperintensity in varying sizes larger than 2 mm in diameter that are usually best visualized superior and lateral to the testis.

Varicoceles are more frequent on the left side (Niedzielski et al. 1997). Varicocele may affect testicular growth (Thomas and Elder 2002). Therefore, testicular volumes should be systematically measured and testicular parenchyma should be assessed with MR (Fig. 3).

## 8.2 Testicular Perfusion

Testicular perfusion also varies depending on age and sexual development. Before puberty, color or power doppler ultrasound is not always accurate in the detection of testicular blood flow (Atkinson et al. 1992; Bader et al. 1997; Luker and Siegel 1996). With the dynamic subtraction contrast-enhanced MR imaging, testicular perfusion is constantly detected in infant and prepubertal males as well as adolescent males (Watanabe et al. 2000). The normal testes show a gradual and steady increase of contrast enhancement (Fig. 12). The peak and upslope of contrast enhancement is more prominent in adolescence than in prepuberty. Comparison of contrast enhancement between the right and left testes,

facilitates the evaluation of contrast enhancement of the affected-side testis with the unaffected-side testis serving as a normal control (Watanabe 2002; Watanabe et al. 2000, 2007). Impaired testicular perfusion can be seen in testicular torsion, trauma, and infarction, and appears as no or a little contrast enhancement of the affected testis (Figs. 5b, 11b). Increased testicular perfusion can be seen in malignant testicular neoplasm and acute orchitis. In combination with the assessment of contrast enhancement of the epididymis and spermatic cord, the scrotal disorders can be classified as shown in Table 1 (Watanabe et al. 2000).

## References

Aso C, Enriquez G, Fite M et al (2005) Gray-scale and color doppler sonography of scrotal disorders in children: an update. Radiographics 25:1197–1214

Atkinson GO Jr, Patrick LE, Ball TI Jr et al (1992) The normal and abnormal scrotum in children: evaluation with color doppler sonography. Am J Roentgenol 158:613–617

Bader TR, Kammerhuber F, Herneth AM (1997) Testicular blood flow in boys as assessed at color doppler and power doppler sonography. Radiology 202:559–564

Baker LL, Hajek PC, Burkhard TK et al (1987) MR imaging of the scrotum: normal anatomy. Radiology 163: 89–92

Baud C, Veyrac C, Couture A et al (1998) Spiral twist of the spermatic cord: a reliable sign of testicular torsion. Pediatr Radiol 28:950–954

Bhatt S, Dogra VS (2008) Role of US in testicular and scrotal trauma. Radiographics 28:1617–1629

Bree RL, Hoang DT (1996) Scrotal ultrasound. Radiol Clin North Am 34:1183–1205

Cramer BM, Schlegel EA, Thueroff JW (1991) MR imaging in the differential diagnosis of scrotal and testicular disease. Radiographics 11:9–21

Dambro T (1998) The scrotum. Mosby, St Louis

Dogra VS, Gottlieb RH, Oka M et al (2003) Sonography of the scrotum. Radiology 227:18–36

Doherty FJ (1991) Ultrasound of the nonacute scrotum. Semin Ultrasound CT MR 12:131–156

Fritzsche PJ, Hricak H, Kogan BA et al (1987) Undescended testis: value of MR imaging. Radiology 164:169–173

Frush DP, Sheldon CA (1998) Diagnostic imaging for pediatric scrotal disorders. Radiographics 18:969–985

Garriga V, Serrano A, Marin A et al (2009) US of the tunica vaginalis testis: anatomic relationships and pathologic conditions. Radiographics 29:2017–2032

Hricak H, Filly RA (1983) Sonography of the scrotum. Invest Radiol 18:112–121

Hricak H, Hamm B, Kim B (1995) Imaging techniques, anatomy, artifacts and bioeffects: magnetic resonance imaging. Raven Press, New York

Kaipia A, Ryymin P, Makela E et al (2005) Magnetic resonance imaging of experimental testicular torsion. Int J Androl 28:355–359

Kier R, McCarthy S, Rosenfield AT et al (1988) Nonpalpable testes in young boys: evaluation with MR imaging. Radiology 169:429–433

Kim W, Rosen MA, Langer JE et al (2007) US MR imaging correlation in pathologic conditions of the scrotum. Radiographics 27:1239–1253

Krone KD, Carroll BA (1985) Scrotal ultrasound. Radiol Clin North Am 23:121–139

Langer JE (1993) Ultrasound of the scrotum. Semin Roentgenol 28:5–18

Langman J (1975) Medical embryology: Human development– normal and abnormal. 3rd edn. Williams & Wilkins, Baltimore

Luker GD, Siegel MJ (1996) Scrotal US in pediatric patients: comparison of power and standard color doppler US. Radiology 198:381–385

Martin LC, Share JC, Peters C et al (1996) Hydrocele of the spermatic cord: embryology and ultrasonographic appearance. Pediatr Radiol 26:528–530

Meacham RB, Townsend RR, Rademacher D et al (1994) The incidence of varicoceles in the general population when evaluated by physical examination, gray scale sonography and color doppler sonography. J Urol 151:1535–1538

Middleton WD, Bell MW (1993) Analysis of intratesticular arterial anatomy with emphasis on transmediastinal arteries. Radiology 189:157–160

Muglia V, Tucci S Jr, Elias J Jr et al (2002) Magnetic resonance imaging of scrotal diseases: when it makes the difference. Urology 59:419–423

Nguyen HT, Coakley F, Hricak H (1999) Cryptorchidism: strategies in detection. Eur Radiol 9:336–343

Niedzielski J, Paduch D, Raczynski P (1997) Assessment of adolescent varicocele. Pediatr Surg Int 12:410–413

Rholl KS, Lee JK, Ling D et al (1987) MR imaging of the scrotum with a high-resolution surface coil. Radiology 163:99–103

Sellars ME, Sidhu PS (2003) Ultrasound appearances of the testicular appendages: pictorial review. Eur Radiol 13:127–135

Shadbolt CL, Heinze SB, Dietrich RB (2001) Imaging of groin masses: inguinal anatomy and pathologic conditions revisited. Radiographics 21:S261–271

Shipp TD, Benacerraf BR (1995) Scrotal inguinal hernia in a fetus: sonographic diagnosis. Am J Roentgenol 165:1494–1495

Siegel MJ (1997) The acute scrotum. Radiol Clin North Am 35:959–976

Sijstermans K, Hack WW, van der Voort-Doedens LM et al (2009) Long-term testicular growth and position after orchidopexy for congenital undescended testis. Urol Int 83:438–445

Simpson WL Jr, Rausch DR (2009) Imaging of male infertility: pictorial review. Am J Roentgenol, 192:S98–107 (Quiz S108–111)

Thomas JC, Elder JS (2002) Testicular growth arrest and adolescent varicocele: does varicocele size make a difference? J Urol 168:1689–1691; discussion 1691

Trainer T (1992) Testis and the excretory duct system. Raven, New York

Tripathi RP, Jena AN, Gulati P et al (1992) Undescended testis: evaluation by magnetic resonance imaging. Indian Pediatr 29:433–438

Watanabe Y (2002) Scrotal imaging. Curr Opin Urol 12:149–153

Watanabe Y, Dohke M, Ohkubo K et al (2000) Scrotal disorders: evaluation of testicular enhancement patterns at dynamic contrast-enhanced subtraction MR imaging. Radiology 217:219–227

Watanabe Y, Nagayama M, Okumura A et al (2007) MR imaging of testicular torsion: features of testicular hemorrhagic necrosis and clinical outcomes. J Magn Reson Imaging 26:100–108

# Scrotal Trauma: Mechanisms, Presentation and Management

Giulio Garaffa and David J. Ralph

## Contents

**Abstract**

Genital injuries are rare, tend to affect relatively young people, and usually derive from blunt trauma, machinery accidents, stab wounds, firearm injury and fragmentation devices. Genital traumas require prompt assessment and treatment to minimize the potential severe impact on patients' quality of life that they may produce.

## 1 Introduction

Genital injuries are significant, since they are frequently associated with injuries to major pelvic and vascular organs and result from both blunt and penetrating mechanisms.

Since trauma is predominantly a condition that occurs in relatively young people, genital injuries may profoundly affect health related quality of life. This chapter will concentrate only on scrotal trauma and will focus on the mechanisms, evaluation and operative management of injuries.

## 2 Prevalence

The real incidence of scrotal injuries has not been determined, however, in civilian centers is expected to be low and that is the reason why most case series span many years and include relatively small numbers of patients. The scenario changes completely in the battlefield; this is consequence of the massive destruction caused by fragmentation devices combined with the use of protective torso armour, that has

G. Garaffa (✉) · D. J. Ralph
St Peter's Andrology Centre,
The London Clinic Consulting Rooms,
145 Harley Street,
W1G 6 BJ London, UK
e-mail: giuliogaraffa@googlemail.com

M. Bertolotto and C. Trombetta (eds.), *Scrotal Pathology*, Medical Radiology. Diagnostic Imaging,
DOI: 10.1007/174_2011_174, © Springer-Verlag Berlin Heidelberg 2012

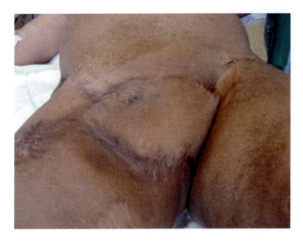

**Fig. 1** Example of the massive destruction that can be caused by a landmine explosion. The penile shaft and all scrotal content have been completely destroyed leaving a large defect in the pelvic region. The patient has been managed with a perineal urethrostomy and the pubic defect has been covered with an antero-lateral thigh flap harvested from the right thigh

led to the survival of soldiers with increasingly severe pelvic and genital organ injuries (Wessells and Long 2006) (Fig. 1).

# 3    Mechanisms

The scrotum in general has a tremendous capacity to resist injury. This is because of the laxity and looseness of the scrotal structures that allow the transfer of kinetic energy during trauma.

The laxity of scrotal tissue usually plays a protective role, allowing the skin to deform and slide away from a potential point of contact. However, in machinery injuries, rotating or suction devices can grab hold of a portion of the scrotal skin and in this situation the laxity of the skin becomes a liability because the entire genital skin can be trapped and avulsed.

Blunt scrotal trauma is the most common cause of hydrocele, intra and extra testicular haematomas, haematocele and testicular rupture.

Lacerations and avulsions of the scrotum may occur because of blunt trauma, machinery accidents, stab wounds and occasional firearm injury. Complete avulsion of the scrotum is rare and is usually the result of power takeoff, auger, or devastating motor vehicles crashes involving widespread skin avulsion and degloving.

**Table 1** AAST organ injury scale for scrotal injury

| AAST grade | Scrotal injury |
| --- | --- |
| I | Contusion |
| II | Laceration <25% of scrotal diamater |
| III | Laceration >25% of scrotal diameter |
| IV | Avulsion <50% |
| V | Avulsion >50% |

Scrotal injuries can be also consequence of chemical, electric and fire burns, although a genital involvement is present in less than 5% of burn victims.

Finally, extremely rare causes of scrotal injury are animal or human bites and self amputation.

# 4    Presentation and Initial Evaluation

Penetrating injuries to the scrotum require special consideration due to the high likelihood of associated injuries to the spermatic cord and the testis, urethra and pelvic organs. In particular, urethral injuries may occur in up to 38% of genital traumas (Cline et al. 1998).

The American Association for Surgery and Trauma (AAST) has proposed a classification of scrotal injuries according to its severity (Table 1).

The evaluation and initial management of scrotal injuries involves recognition of associated injuries, control of bleeding and mechanism-specific interventions. In particular, penetrating injuries to the genitalia may have associated injuries in up to 83% of cases.

The mechanism of injury is important when planning the treatment. Burns should be covered with appropriate dressings depending on the mechanism responsible. In general, in chemical and thermic burns, the likelihood of damage to deeper structures, the testis and spermatic cord, is directly related to the extent of the damage of the skin and dartos, with the more superficial the injury the less chance of involvement of deeper structures. The scenario is completely different in electric burns since there is no correlation between the degree of skin damage and involvement of deep structures, and therefore, these patients have to be fully investigated searching for deep structures involvement even if the superficial damage is minimal (Fig. 2).

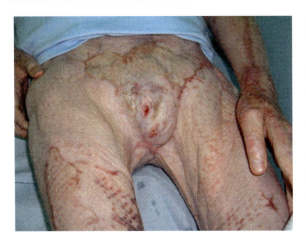

**Fig. 2** Electric burn involving the lower abdomen, the thighs and the genitalia. The skin defects in patient, who has also lost the right testicle and the distal third of the shaft penis, have been covered with meshed split thickness skin grafts harvested from the lower back

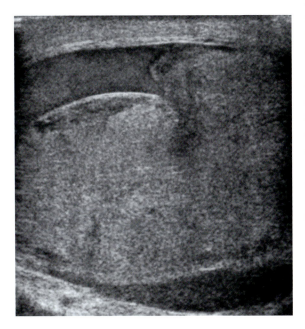

**Fig. 3** Ultrasound image demonstrating a testicular rupture. It is evident an interruption of the tunica albuginea and an extravasation of blood inside the tunica vaginalis

Bite injuries require appropriate broad spectrum antibiotic coverage and tetanous toxoid administration. In case of animal bites, the possibility of rabies transmission must be considered.

All patients with penetrative scrotal trauma should undergo immediate surgical exploration; this will allow immediate recognition and management of associated injuries to the testes, cord, corpora and urethra.

The management of non penetrative scrotal trauma is different. Immediate surgical exploration is necessary only in presence of a hematocele or when sonographic findings are suggestive of the presence of a testicular rupture (Fig. 3). In fact, testicular rupture, defined as a rupture of the tunica albuginea with protrusion of the seminiferous tubules, if not immediately identified and treated, is associated with high rates of testicular atrophy; prompt surgical intervention instead leads to salvage rates between 80 and 90% (Buckley and McAninch 2006; Altarac 1994) (Fig. 4).

## 5 Management

Scrotal skin lacerations can be closed primarily in the absence of gross infection or heavy contamination. Meticulous hemostasis is important because the scrotum accepts a large capacity of bleeding without tamponade.

In order to prevent haematomas it is advisable to carry out a layered closure of the deep fascia, of the dartos and of the skin and to leave a Penrose drain in the most dependent position. Ideally the sutures should be interrupted to reduce the risk of ischemia and to allow further drainage between the sutures. Absorbable monofilament should be the suture of choice unless the wound is contaminated or necrotic.

In cases of complete scrotal avulsion it is sometimes possible to preserve the avulsed skin and use it as a graft, however, frequently the avulsed scrotal tissue is so severely damaged that is unsuitable for grafting, as with burns or machinery injuries with rotating mechanisms.

Various authors do not advocate immediate repair following scrotal avulsion and rather favour an interval of local care in order to allow the bed to granulate and eventual necrotic areas to demarcate in order to be successfully removed (Wessells 1999).

Once the bed is granulating, scrotal reconstruction can be achieved successfully with the use of skin grafts.

Otherwise scrotal reconstruction can be successfully achieved using craniodorsal scrotal flaps as already described following total scrotectomy in the management of genital lymphoedema (Garaffa et al. 2008).

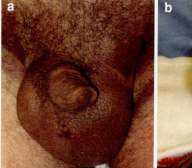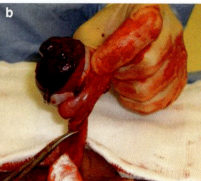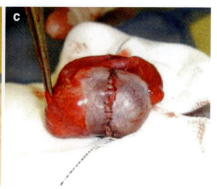

**Fig. 4** Scrotal haematoma with testicular rupture, consequence of a blunt trauma. **a** The examination of the scrotum does not allow excluding the presence of testicular rupture. **b** The exploration demonstrates the testicular rupture along the equator of the testicle. The presence of testicular rupture must always be excluded in presence of blunt scrotal trauma. **c** The rupture is repaired with reapproximation of the edges of the tunica albuginea with the use of resorbable sutures

In complete scrotal avulsion, testicular transposition into subcutaneous thigh pouches may be required. It can be a temporary or permanent measure, depending on patient's age and concomitant conditions.

Testicular contusions are by far more common than scrotal lacerations. If there is no tear of the tunica albuginea and haematocele, testicular traumas with or without intra testicular haematomas and hydroceles should be managed conservatively with administration of anti-inflammatory drugs and elevation of the scrotum. Testicular ruptures with or without haematoceles instead require prompt recognition and immediate surgical treatment to minimize the risk of testicular loss.

Although before 1968 blunt scrotal trauma was managed conservatively, non-operative management of testicular rupture is now considered obsolete since it almost invariably leads to testicular atrophy.

Most testicular ruptures can be reconstructed primarily and if an extensive loss of tunica albuginea is present, the defect can be successfully covered with a tunica vaginalis graft.

Once the associated haematocele has been evacuated and the rupture site identified, the necrotic tissue is excised with sharp dissection until healthy bleeding edges are encountered. The remaining tunica albuginea is then closed with a small absorbable suture in a continuous fashion. The testis is then placed back into the scrotal sack in its natural position and a two layer closure of the scrotum performed with absorbable sutures (Lee et al. 2008).

Usually a penrose drain is left in situ to prevent hematoma formation.

Orchidectomy is reserved to critically ill patients with complex traumatic injuries where testicular reconstruction is not a life-saving priority or if the cord is irreparably damaged.

## 6 Conclusions

Genital anatomy has evolved to maximize protection of reproductive function from blunt trauma. However, when weapons or excessive shear forces exceed the elasticity of the tissues trauma is unavoidable. The ultimate goal of reconstructive surgery is to preserve the scrotum with normal function and appearance. Primary closure of most wounds including uncomplicated bites and penetrating injuries is possible with adequate antibiotic administration. In case of severe loss of substance, good cosmetic results can be achieved with delayed closure and with the use of skin grafting.

## References

Altarac S (1994) Management of 53 cases of testicular trauma. Eur Urol 25:119–123

Buckley JC, McAninch JW (2006) Use of ultrasonography for the diagnosis of testicular injuries in blunt scrotal trauma. J Urol 175:175–178

Cline KJ, Mata JA, Venable DD et al (1998) Penetrating trauma to the male external genitalia. J Trauma 44:492–494

Garaffa G, Christopher N, Ralph DJ (2008) The management of genital lymphoedema. BJU Int 102:480–484

Lee SH, Bak CW, Choi MH et al (2008) Trauma to male genital organs: a 10 year review of 156 patients, including 118 treated by surgery. BJU Int 101:211–215

Wessells H (1999) Genital skin loss: Ussnified reconstructive approach to a heterogeneous entity. World J Urol 17:107–114

Wessells H, Long L (2006) Penile and genital injuries. Urol Clin North Am 33:117–126, vii

# Imaging Scrotal Trauma

Michele Bertolotto, Marco M. Cavallaro, Paola Martingano,
Massimo Valentino, Ciro Acampora, and Maria A. Cova

## Contents

M. Bertolotto (✉) · M. M. Cavallaro · P. Martingano ·
M. A. Cova
Department of Radiology, University of Trieste,
Ospedale di Cattinara, Strada di Fiume 447,
34124 Trieste, Italy
e-mail: bertolot@units.it

M. Valentino
S.S.D. Radiologia d'Urgenza, Dipartimento di Radiologia e
Diagnostica per Immagini Azienda Ospedaliera,
Universitaria di Parma Ospedale Maggiore,
Via Gramsci 14, 43100 Parma, Italy

C. Acampora
Radiologia Generale e Pronto Soccorso,
Azienda Ospedaliera A. Cardarelli,
Via Cardarelli 9, 80131 Naples, Italy

**Abstract**

Scrotal injuries may result from either blunt or penetrating traumas. The former usually require immediate surgical exploration, while management of the latter is more complex. If the tunica albuginea is intact the lesion can be usually managed conservatively, while immediate operation is necessary if albugineal disruption is suspected. Ultrasound is the first-line imaging modality to assess testis integrity. Contour irregularity and discontinuity of the tunica albuginea are signs of testicular rupture. Color Doppler interrogation allows direct evaluation of testicular perfusion and detection of ischemic changes following contusion, or posttraumatic torsion. Besides post-traumatic epididymitis, which is assessed effectively at color Doppler interrogation, sensitivity of ultrasound in assessment of epididymal injuries is poor. Hematomas and other fluid collections present different echotexture with time. They are hyperechoic first, and then isoechoic, with mixed echogenicity, and eventually hypoechoic. Other traumatic lesions to the scrotum in which imaging has a role are testicular dislocation, vascular lesions, and hematoceles. Due to its excellent contrast resolution, wider panoramicity, and possibility to characterize blood products, MR imaging is an accurate diagnostic adjunct in those patients for whom the findings from clinical and ultrasound evaluations are inconclusive.

M. Bertolotto and C. Trombetta (eds.), *Scrotal Pathology*, Medical Radiology. Diagnostic Imaging,
DOI: 10.1007/174_2011_175, © Springer-Verlag Berlin Heidelberg 2012

# 1    Introduction

Scrotal injuries most commonly occur in young men between 15 and 40 years, and may result from either penetrating or blunt traumas. Penetrating injuries include wounds from sharp objects and missiles as well as animal bites and self-mutilation (Haas et al. 1999). Blunt injuries are caused by crush of the scrotum against the symphysis pubis or between the thighs.

Penetrating injuries to the scrotum often undergo immediate surgical exploration. Although it is useful, especially in severe traumas, imaging is not routinely performed. Management of blunt traumas is more complex. Immediate operation often is not mandatory, and the risks associated with anesthesia, surgery, and infections have to be carefully evaluated and weighted against the possible advantages for the patient. Assessment of the tunica albuginea integrity, in particular, is essential because if it is intact the lesion can be usually managed conservatively, while immediate operation is necessary if albugineal disruption is suspected (Buckley and McAninch 2006a).

Today's approach of early operative exploration and repair in case of albugineal disruption is based on evidence that early diagnosis and intervention results in salvage of the testis in a high percent of cases. Cass (1983) and Gross (1969) compared primary conservative management with early surgical exploration and repair and found a 45% orchiectomy rate in the delayed surgical intervention group, versus a 9% orchiectomy rate in the early surgical exploration group.

Imaging helps urologists improve patient management in many patients with scrotal traumas (Buckley and McAninch 2006a). In fact, clinical examination is difficult because scrotal swelling and pain could prevent evaluation of the scrotal content. Ultrasonography is the first-line imaging modality, MR imaging has a role when ultrasound is inconclusive, while CT is indicated in polytrauma patients.

# 2    Blunt Scrotal Traumas

Blunt scrotal traumas are often associated with severe injuries of the scrotal content including rupture or avulsion of the testis, testicular fracture, hematoma, hematocele, and epididymal injury. The most important differential diagnosis is between injuries with

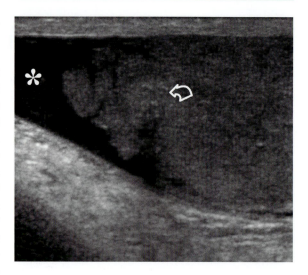

**Fig. 1** Testicular rupture. Longitudinal ultrasound scan shows contour irregularity of the upper pole of the testis (*curved arrow*) consistent with extrusion of the parenchyma. A surrounding hematocele (*asterisk*) is also shown. Surgery confirmed testicular rupture

rupture of the tunica albuginea and whose in which the albuginea is intact, because the former require immediate surgical exploration, while the latter can be managed conservatively.

## 2.1    Testicular Rupture

This severe scrotal injury is characterized by traumatic disruption of the tunica albuginea and extrusion of the testicular parenchyma into the scrotal sac.

Ultrasound is the imaging modality of choice in identification of testicular rupture. While early investigation reported low accuracy, recent series in which modern equipment and high frequency probes are used, report high sensitivity and specificity (Buckley and McAninch 2006a, b; Kim et al. 2007a; Guichard et al. 2008).

Following Kim et al. contour irregularity of the testis is the most significant predictor for diagnosis of testicular rupture (Fig. 1), with sensitivity, specificity, and accuracy of 90% (Kim et al. 2007a).

In patients with testicular rupture, as well as those with other testicular parenchymal injuries in which the tunica albuginea is not interrupted, testicular echotexture may appear heterogeneous, with focal hyperechoic or hypoechoic regions corresponding to hemorrhagic or ischemic areas.

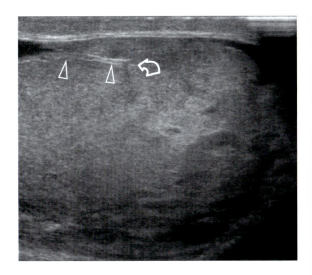

**Fig. 2** Testicular rupture. Longitudinal ultrasound scan shows interruption (*curved arrow*) of the echogenic line of the tunica albuginea (*arrowheads*) at the lower pole of the testis. Surgery confirmed testicular rupture

When high frequency probes are used on modern ultrasound equipment, an excellent depiction of the tunica albuginea and of its changes is possible (Bhatt and Dogra 2008). On ultrasound, the normal tunica albuginea appears as a hyperechoic line outlining the testis. Demonstration of its discontinuity supports a straightforward diagnosis of testicular disruption (Fig. 2). The reported accuracy of ultrasound for direct identification of the albugineal tear, however, is lower than the accuracy for recognition of contour irregularity, with a reported sensitivity of 50% and specificity of 76% (Guichard et al. 2008).

Color Doppler interrogation is useful to determine viability of the injured testis. Tunica albuginea rupture is almost always associated with a disruption of the tunica vasculosa. As a result, testicular rupture results in ischemia at a portion of parenchyma of variable extention (Fig. 3), which must be removed during surgical repair. CEUS may be performed in equivocal cases to confirm partial or complete testicular ischemia (Moschouris et al. 2009).

Limitations have been described for ultrasound in assessing patients with testicular rupture (Kim et al. 2007a; Buckley and McAninch 2006b; Chandra et al. 2007). False negative assessment may result from lack of contour irregularity in patients with small albugineal disruption. Conversely, intratesticular and extratesticular hematomas may be isoechoic to testis,

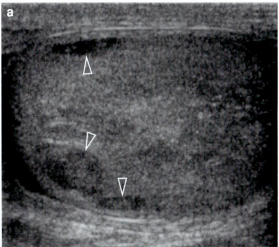

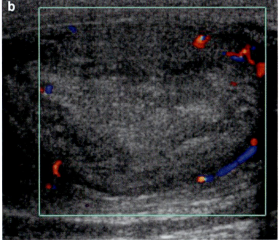

**Fig. 3** Post-traumatic testicular ischemia. **a** Grey-scale ultrasound shows multiple small subalbugineal peripheral hematomas (*arrowheads*). **b** Color Doppler interrogation shows that large portions of the testis are ischemic, consistent with extensive disruption of the tunica vasculosa

and mimic contour irregularity, leading to a false positive diagnosis of rupture.

MR imaging provides additional clinically useful information in patients with scrotal traumas and equivocal findings for albugineal disruption at ultrasound. The tunica albuginea is well visualized as a low signal intensity line which is interrupted in testicular rupture (Kim et al. 2007b). In a series of 7 patients with blunt scrotal traumas evaluated with MR imaging before exploratory surgery, presence or absence of albugineal rupture was identified correctly in all cases (Kim et al. 2009). Associated parenchymal necrosis and hemorrhage are identified as areas of mixed signal

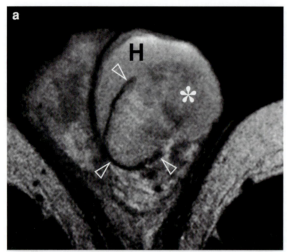

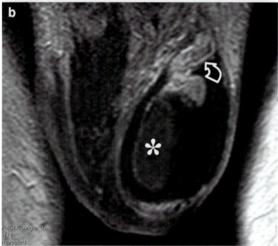

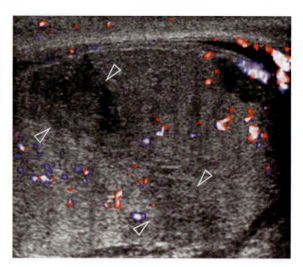

**Fig. 5** Testicular fracture. Sagittal color Doppler scan demonstrates a linear hypoechoic area (*arrowheads*) that runs obliquely across the testis and represents the testicular fracture line [reprinted with permission from Dogra and Bhatt (2004)]

**Fig. 4** Efficacy of MR imaging in assessment of testicular rupture. **a** Axial T2-weighted image shows extensive rupture of the tunica albuginea (*arrowheads*) of the right testis, with extrusion of the parenchyma (*asterisk*). The torn albuginea is identified as a low signal intensity line. Hematocele (*H*) is associated. **b** Coronal T1-weighted contrast enhanced dynamic scan shows enhancement of the spermatic cord (*curved arrow*) and of the medial portion of the left testis (*asterisk*) while the remaining portions of the parenchyma are avascular. Viability of a portion of the parenchyma was confirmed at surgery

liver, kidney, and spleen fracture lines in the testis are often difficult to identify at gray-scale ultrasound. Only about 17% of cases are seen. When visible (Fig. 5), fractures appear as linear hypoechoic avascular bands extending across the testis (Deurdulian et al. 2007). Testicular shape and ultrasound appearance of the tunica albuginea are normal. Color Doppler interrogation of the injured testis plays a significant role in guiding patient management. Testicular fractures are treated conservatively if normal flow is identified, while emergent surgery is recommended if flow is absent (Deurdulian et al. 2007).

Visibility of the fracture lines and of the integrity of the tunica albuginea markedly improves using MR imaging, as well as the presence of associated hematomas, hematoceles, and lesion extension to the spermatic cord. Parenchymal viability is assessed after gadolinium contrast administration (Kim et al. 2009).

intensity. Ischemic changes are identified after contrast medium administration (Fig. 4).

## 2.2 Testicular Fracture

In this injury, the testicular parenchyma is broken by one or more fracture lines, but the tunica albuginea is intact. Similar to injuries of other parenchymas, such as

## 2.3 Post-traumatic Testicular Torsion

Testicular torsion is a rare manifestation of scrotal trauma which requires immediate operation. It especially occurs if predisposing factors, such as a "Bell clapper deformity", are present (Bhatt and Dogra 2008). Clinical manifestations and ultrasound appearance are similar to those of non-trauma-related torsion (Bhatt and Dogra 2008). Findings vary according to the

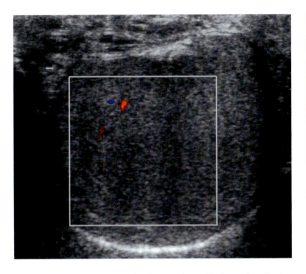

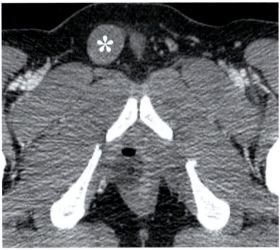

**Fig. 6** Post-traumatic testicular torsion. Patient developing severe acute left scrotal pain following trauma. Color Doppler ultrasound shows an intact left testis, which is markedly hypovascular at color Doppler interrogation. Post-traumatic torsion was found at operation

**Fig. 7** Traumatic testicular dislocation. The right testis (*asterisk*) is found in the inguinal channel. Fractures of the pelvic bones are associated (By courtesy of L.E. Derchi, Genova, Italy)

duration and degree of rotation of the spermatic cord. Early after torsion testis can appear normal at gray-scale ultrasound, with markedly reduced or absent flows, at color Doppler interrogation (Fig. 6). Absence of alterations at gray-scale ultrasound is indicative of salvageability of the testis.

## 2.4 Testicular Dislocation

Testicular dislocation is a traumatic translocation of the testis outside its normal position in the scrotum. This injury is rare, with only about 80 cases reported till 2008 (Ezra et al. 2009). Most commonly it results from impact against the fuel tank in motorcycle accidents. Abdominal organ and pelvic bone injuries are often associated (Ko et al. 2004).

Testicular dislocation is bilateral in approximately 33% of cases (Ezra et al. 2009). The possible sites of dislocation include superficial and internal regions. In order of decreasing frequency of occurrence, superficial dislocation may be inguinal, pubic, penile, preputial, crural, perineal or acetabular; internal dislocation is canalicular or intraabdominal (Ko et al. 2004; Schwartz and Faerber 1994).

Once dislocation is diagnosed, treatment by early reduction is recommended to avoid a possible spermatogenesis loss, and predisposition to malignant degeneration (Bhatt and Dogra 2008). When manual reduction is not possible, surgical intervention is necessary.

Diagnosis of testicular dislocation can be made by physical examination when a well-developed but empty scrotal sac is found or an abnormally located testis is palpated (Kochakarn et al. 2000). When a clinical suspicion exists, dislocation can be readily identified at ultrasound and MR imaging (Bedir et al. 2005). In the clinical practice, however, the dislocated testis is often identified incidentally during a CT scan, performed for evaluation of abdominal organs (Fig. 7).

In polytrauma patients, testicular dislocation is often missed because the perineum is not routinely enclosed into the scan volume, or overlooked when examining the CT images (Bedir et al. 2005). In a series of 9 trauma patients in whom testicular dislocation was retrospectively recognized, prompt diagnosis at the time of CT examination was achieved in 3 patients only (Ko et al. 2004).

## 2.5 Intratesticular Hematoma

Single or multiple intratesticular hematomas are commonly encountered in patients with scrotal traumas. Hematomas, with no direct or indirect evidence of a testicular rupture, are treated conservatively.

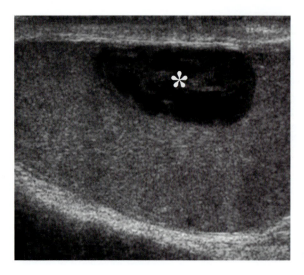

**Fig. 8** Intratesticular hematoma. Longitudinal ultrasound image showing a complex cystic intratesticular lesion (*asterisk*) which was completely avascular at color Doppler interrogation (not shown)

There is, however, a high incidence rate of infection and necrosis, which may necessitate orchiectomy (Dogra and Bhatt 2004).

Ultrasound is the imaging modality of choice for evaluation and follow-up of intratesticular hematomas. MR imaging is indicated in selected cases only.

The sonographic appearance of intratesticular hematomas varies with time (Bhatt and Dogra 2008). Hyperacute and acute hematoma may appear hyperechoic, isoechoic to the surrounding testicular parenchyma, or have a diffusely heterogeneous echotexture. Chronic hematoma is usually hypoechoic. Intralesional flows are lacking at color Doppler interrogation (Fig. 8).

Differential diagnosis between hematomas and testicular tumors is important (Yagil et al. 2010). Although they are usually incidental findings, or present as palpable masses, testicular tumors may be identified in as much as 10–15% of patients with scrotal traumas (Dogra and Bhatt 2004). Both tumors and intratesticular hematomas may have similar appearance at gray-scale ultrasound, but most tumors display vascularization at color Doppler interrogation, while hematomas do not (Yagil et al. 2010). Tumor can be excluded if the lesion shows progressive resolution during the follow-up (Fig. 9).

MR imaging is not routinely recommended in imaging testicular hematoma since enough information is usually obtained with color Doppler ultrasound. It can be used, however, when findings at ultrasound are equivocal (Muglia et al. 2002; Parenti et al. 2009). Characteristic signal changes are appreciated with time on T1- and T2-weighted images (Fig. 10), as methemoglobin within subacute blood is hyperintense on T1-weighted images, while hemosiderin deposition produces a low-signal-intensity rim on T2-weighted images (Kim et al. 2007b). Lack of internal enhancement eases differential diagnosis with hypovascular tumors, which display contrast enhancement after administration of gadolinium contrast material in virtually all cases.

## 3 Extratesticular Injuries

In patients with scrotal traumas, extratesticular injuries are more common that testicular lesions and are usually managed conservatively. Among them, epididymal injuries, lesions of the spermatic cord, fluid collections, and lesions of the scrotal wall should be considered.

### 3.1 Post-traumatic Epididymitis

Hyperemia and swelling are the most common epididymal changes in patients with scrotal trauma. Post-traumatic epididymitis has a similar appearance at ultrasound than the infectious ones (Bhatt and Dogra 2008). Epididymis is enlarged. Heterogeneous echotexture with hypoechoic and hyperechoic areas may be secondary to small hematomas and contusions. Reactive hydrocele or hematocele, and scrotal wall thickening are usually associated. At color Doppler evaluation epididymis is hyperemic (Fig. 11), with high velocity, low resistance flows. The history of scrotal trauma allows differential diagnosis with infectious epididymitis (Bhatt and Dogra 2008).

### 3.2 Other Epididymal Injuries

Post-traumatic epididymal injuries are not uncommon, but their preoperative identification is difficult (Learch et al. 1995). These conditions are usually identified incidentally during surgical exploration performed for suspicious testicular rupture. In a series

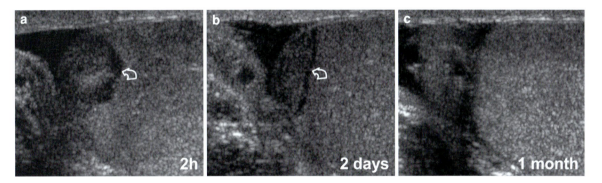

**Fig. 9** Time changes of intratesticular hematoma. Patients presenting at ultrasound complaining for testicular pain after a minor scrotal trauma. **a** Sagittal scan performed within 2 h after the trauma shows rounded lesions at the upper pole of the testis (*curved arrow*). **b** Follow-up examination performed 2 days after the trauma shows a crescent lesion in the upper pole of the testis (*curved arrow*). **c** One month ultrasound follow-up shows complete disappearance of the lesion

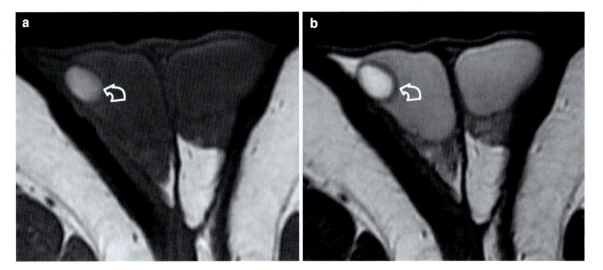

**Fig. 10** Appearance of intratesticular hematoma at MR imaging. Axial T1-weighted (**a**) and T2-weighted (**b**) images show a predominantly hyperintense lesion (*curved arrow*) on both sequences with a low-signal-intensity hemosiderin rim with T2-weighted images

of 33 patients who underwent surgical exploration for blunt scrotal traumas, epididymal lesions were identified in seven. At ultrasound, there were four false-positive and three false-negative results (Guichard et al. 2008).

Despite poor sensitivity and specificity, in trauma patients, epididymis should be investigated to seek traumatic lesions. Hematomas are depicted as heterogeneous, well-defined avascular masses (Fig. 12). Rupture presents with ill-defined epididymis, heterogeneous echotexture, and absence of blood flow (Bhatt and Dogra 2008). These findings, however, are nonspecific and do not allow a confident diagnosis.

MR imaging has been seen more sensitive than ultrasound in characterization of epidydimal hematoma (Kim et al. 2009).

## 3.3 Injury of the Scrotal Wall

This common traumatic lesion usually undergoes spontaneous resolution. Blood extravasation within the scrotal wall may appear at ultrasound as a thickened,

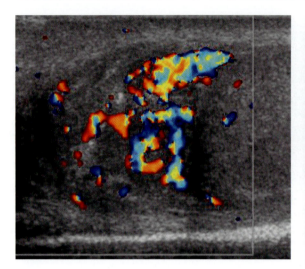

**Fig. 11** Post-traumatic epididymitis. Longitudinal color Doppler view showing enlarged hyperemic epididymis with heterogeneous echotexture

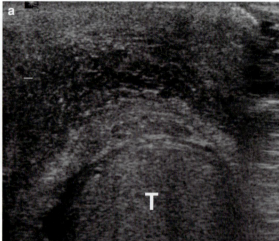

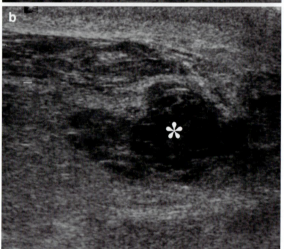

**Fig. 13** Injury of the scrotal wall. Patient developing severe scrotal swelling following blunt trauma. **a** Axial ultrasound image showing diffuse, inhomeogeneous thickening of the scrotal wall, consistent with blood extravasation. The testis (*T*) is intact. **b** Longitudinal ultrasound view showing a circumscribed hematoma within the scrotal wall (*asterisk*), presenting as a heterogeneous fluid collection

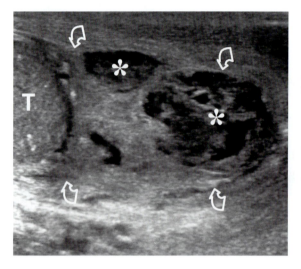

**Fig. 12** Hematomas of the epididymal tail. Longitudinal ultrasound view of the scrotal content in a trauma patient showing an enlarged and inhomogeneous epididymal tail (*curved arrows*) containing fluid-filled heterogeneous lesions (*asterisk*) avascular at color Doppler interrogation (not shown) consistent with hematomas (T = testis)

## 3.4 Spermatic Cord Hematoma

This lesion may follow blunt scrotal trauma, or may be a complication of hernia repair. Occasionally, it can also result from the rupture of a varicocele (Gordon et al. 1993), or may represent an extension of a retroperitoneal hemorrhage (McKenney et al. 1996).

Spermatic cord hematoma may be identified incidentally during an abdominal CT scan performed to evaluate a polytrauma patient. Iodinated contrast administration may allow recognition of associated

inhomogeneous area, or as a circumscribed fluid collection (Fig. 13) whose appearance changes with time (Bhatt and Dogra 2008; Deurdulian et al. 2007). MRI shows an avascular lesion in the scrotal wall whose signal intensity characteristically changes with time on T1- and T2-weighted images (Kim et al. 2009).

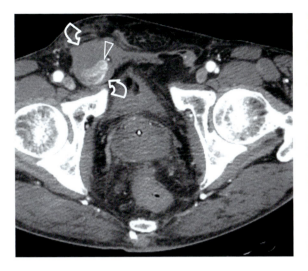

**Fig. 14** Hematoma of the spermatic cord. Abdominal contrast-enhanced CT in a polytrauma patient showing hematoma of the right spermatic cord (*curved arrow*) with active extravasation of contrast by an injured spermatic vessel (*arrowhead*)

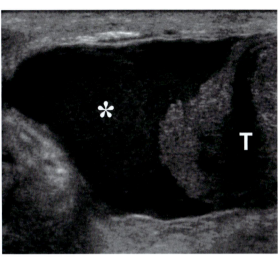

**Fig. 16** Hematocele due to testicular rupture after blunt scrotal trauma. Longitudinal ultrasound image shows uniformly echogenic fluid (*asterisk*). The testis (*T*) presents contour irregularity, with extrusion of the parenchyma

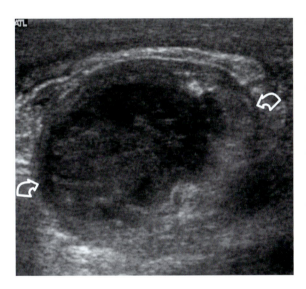

**Fig. 15** Hematoma of the spermatic cord. Transversal ultrasound scan of the spermatic cord showing an avascular heterogeneous mass (*curved arrows*) lacking color flows (not shown)

rupture of the spermatic vessels with active bleeding (Fig. 14). In most patients, however, spermatic cord hematoma is evaluated at ultrasound (Fig. 15) which shows a heterogeneous, well-defined, avascular mass located superior to the testis (Bhatt and Dogra 2008). Associated rupture of the spermatic vessels and

testicular ischemia may be recognized at color Doppler interrogation.

MR imaging typically shows an avascular mass related to the spermatic cord showing the characteristic behavior of blood products on the T1- and the T2-weighted images (Kim et al. 2009; Cassidy et al. 2010).

Management of spermatic cord hematoma is usually conservative. Operation is necessary only in patients with associated testicular ischemia secondary to spermatic vessel disruption.

## 4 Hydrocele and Hematocele

Reactive hydrocele is often identified in patients with acute or chronic scrotal traumatism. Blood extravasation within the parietal and visceral layers of the tunica vaginalis is also commonly encountered, and surgery is not indicated except in the rare cases of ischemia caused by compression of the testis (Pavlica and Barozzi 2001).

Like hematomas and other blood collections, the ultrasound appearance of hematoceles varies with its age, being echogenic acutely, and becoming more complex and hypoechoic later (Figs. 16 and 17). Chronic hematoceles may develop septa and loculations, internal fluid–fluid levels, and eventually calcifications (Pavlica and Barozzi 2001; Dogra et al. 2003).

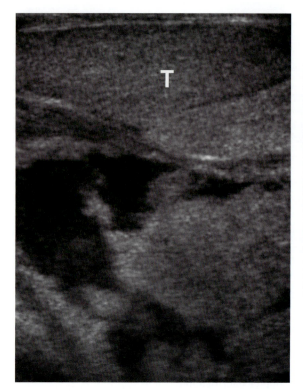

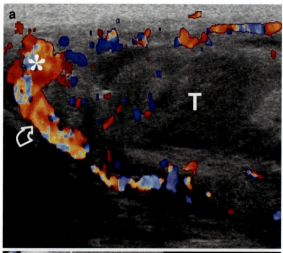

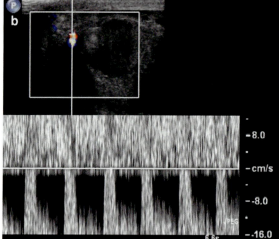

**Fig. 17** Chronic hematocele. Longitudinal ultrasound image of the scrotum obtained 2 weeks after a blunt trauma showing an heterogeneous fluid collection surrounding the testis (*T*)

When isoechoic, hematoceles can prevent accurate delineation of testicular margins. As a consequence, it may be difficult to differentiate hematoma from extruded testicular content (Deurdulian et al. 2007) and, on the countrary, small albugineal tears may be missed. MR imaging may have a role in these patients, thanks to high tissue contrast and excellent depiction of the tunica albuginea (Muglia et al. 2002; Parenti et al. 2009).

On MR imaging, hematoceles display the characteristic signal changes with time already described for the other blood collections (Muglia et al. 2002).

## 5    Post-traumatic Pseudoaneurysm and Arteriovenous Fistula

These extremely rare vascular lesions may be intratesticular or extratesticular, and may result from either blunt and penetrating traumas.

**Fig. 18** Post-traumatic arteriovenous fistula in a patient with testicular rupture. **a** Color Doppler image showing enlarged capsular vessels (*curved arrow*) and a focal area with a mosaic of colors (*asterisk*). **b** Duplex Doppler interrogation of the area showing high-velocity, turbulent flows consistent with post-traumatic arteriovenous communication. The testis (*T*) is inhomogenous with irregular contours, poorly vascularized at color Doppler interrogation

The typical sonographic appearance of pseudoaneurysm, as elsewere in the body, is that of an anechoic mass containing variably turbulent flow. The neck can be identified, with flow entering the aneurysm during systole and exiting during diastole, producing a characteristic to-and-from pattern (Dee et al. 2000).

Arteriovenous fistulas are identified at Doppler interrogation as a color blush displaying aliasing and high velocity, turbulent flow (Fig. 18).

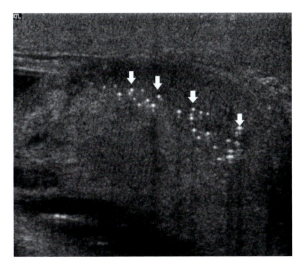

**Fig. 19** Gunshot wound of the testis. Longitudinal ultrasound image showing air bubbles inside the testis (*arrows*) indicating the track of the bullet fragment [reprinted with permission from Secil (2005)]

## 6 Penetrating Injuries

Gunshot and other missile wounds are the most common penetrating scrotal injuries. Ultrasound helps to assess preoperatively the severity of injuries, in order to allow their appropriate management. In a study of 19 patients with gunshot wounds to the scrotum, 9 were managed conservatively (Learch et al. 1995). Other authors, however, recommend surgical exploration for all penetrating scrotal injuries that are not obviously superficial (Bandi and Santucci 2004). Pathologic findings range from a small hematocele to testicular rupture. Air can be identified either in extratesticular or intratesticular location (Fig. 19), appearing as echogenic foci with a reverberation artifact (Secil 2005). Pellets, bullets, and other foreign bodies are identified (Bhatt and Dogra 2008). Color Doppler imaging is useful to identify vascular injury, such as transection of the spermatic cord, which may result in testicular ischemia.

Other isolated penetrating injuries to the scrotum can be the result of knife wounds and animal bites, or may be self-inflicted. Immediate surgical intervention is usually necessary and imaging is not routinely required.

Penetrating scrotal injuries may also be encountered in polytrauma patients. CT and ultrasound are indicated in these cases, to assess the extension of the lesion and associated injuries to the pelvic organs and bones.

Degloving injuries, also referred to as avulsion injuries, may result in exposure of the scrotal contents (Wessells and Long 2006). Thermal, electrical, or chemical burn injuries are rare. They present with skin loss associated to varying damage to the scrotal contents (Bhatt and Dogra 2008). Color Doppler ultrasound may be indicated to assess whether the testes are viable or not, demonstrating presence or absence of blood flow.

## References

Bandi G, Santucci RA (2004) Controversies in the management of male external genitourinary trauma. J Trauma 56:1362–1370

Bedir S, Yildirim I, Sumer F et al (2005) Testicular dislocation as a delayed presentation of scrotal trauma. J Trauma 58:404–405

Bhatt S, Dogra VS (2008) Role of US in testicular and scrotal trauma. Radiographics 28:1617–1629

Buckley JC, McAninch JW (2006a) Diagnosis and management of testicular ruptures. Urol Clin North Am 33:111–116, vii

Buckley JC, McAninch JW (2006b) Use of ultrasonography for the diagnosis of testicular injuries in blunt scrotal trauma. J Urol 175:175–178

Cass AS (1983) Testicular trauma. J Urol 129:299–300

Cassidy FH, Ishioka KM, McMahon CJ et al (2010) MR imaging of scrotal tumors and pseudotumors. Radiographics 30:665–683

Chandra RV, Dowling RJ, Ulubasoglu M et al (2007) Rational approach to diagnosis and management of blunt scrotal trauma. Urology 70:230–234

Dee KE, Deck AJ, Waitches GM (2000) Intratesticular pseudoaneurysm after blunt trauma. AJR Am J Roentgenol 174:1136

Deurdulian C, Mittelstaedt CA, Chong WK et al (2007) US of acute scrotal trauma: optimal technique, imaging findings, and management. Radiographics 27:357–369

Dogra V, Bhatt S (2004) Acute painful scrotum. Radiol Clin North Am 42:349–363

Dogra VS, Gottlieb RH, Oka M et al (2003) Sonography of the scrotum. Radiology 227:18–36

Ezra N, Afari A, Wong J (2009) Pelvic and scrotal trauma: CT and triage of patients. Abdom Imaging 34:541–544

Gordon JN, Aldoroty RA, Stone NN (1993) A spermatic cord hematoma secondary to varicocele rupture from blunt abdominal trauma: a case report and review. J Urol 149:602–603

Gross M (1969) Rupture of the testicle: the importance of early surgical treatment. J Urol 101:196–197

Guichard G, El Ammari J, Del Coro C et al (2008) Accuracy of ultrasonography in diagnosis of testicular rupture after blunt scrotal trauma. Urology 71:52–56

Haas CA, Brown SL, Spirnak JP (1999) Penile fracture and testicular rupture. World J Urol 17:101–106

Kim SH, Park S, Choi SH et al (2007a) Significant predictors for determination of testicular rupture on sonography: a prospective study. J Ultrasound Med 26:1649–1655

Kim W, Rosen MA, Langer JE et al (2007b) US MR imaging correlation in pathologic conditions of the scrotum. Radiographics 27:1239–1253

Kim SH, Park S, Choi SH et al (2009) The efficacy of magnetic resonance imaging for the diagnosis of testicular rupture: a prospective preliminary study. J Trauma 66:239–242

Ko SF, Ng SH, Wan YL et al (2004) Testicular dislocation: an uncommon and easily overlooked complication of blunt abdominal trauma. Ann Emerg Med 43:371–375

Kochakarn W, Choonhaklai V, Hotrapawanond P et al (2000) Traumatic testicular dislocation a review of 36 cases. J Med Assoc Thai 83:208–212

Learch TJ, Hansch LP, Ralls PW (1995) Sonography in patients with gunshot wounds of the scrotum: imaging findings and their value. AJR Am J Roentgenol 165:879–883

McKenney MG, Fietsam R Jr, Glover JL et al (1996) Spermatic cord hematoma: case report and literature review. Am Surg 62:768–769

Moschouris H, Stamatiou K, Lampropoulou E et al (2009) Imaging of the acute scrotum: is there a place for contrast-enhanced ultrasonography? Int Braz J Urol 35:692–702 discussion 702–695

Muglia V, Tucci S Jr, Elias J Jr et al (2002) Magnetic resonance imaging of scrotal diseases: when it makes the difference. Urology 59:419–423

Parenti GC, Feletti F, Brandini F et al (2009) Imaging of the scrotum: role of MRI. Radiol Med 114:414–424

Pavlica P, Barozzi L (2001) Imaging of the acute scrotum. Eur Radiol 11:220–228

Schwartz SL, Faerber GJ (1994) Dislocation of the testis as a delayed presentation of scrotal trauma. Urology 43:743–745

Secil M (2005) Medical Image. Lothario's scrotum. N Z Med J 118:U1691

Wessells H, Long L (2006) Penile and genital injuries. Urol Clin North Am 33:117–126, vii

Yagil Y, Naroditsky I, Milhem J et al (2010) Role of Doppler ultrasonography in the triage of acute scrotum in the emergency department. J Ultrasound Med 29:11–21

# Acute Scrotal Pain: Clinical Features

Vincenzo Mirone, Paolo Verze, and Davide Arcaniolo

## Contents

**Abstract**

Acute scrotum is defined as an acute painful swelling of the scrotum or its contents, and is accompanied by local signs and general symptoms. Acute scrotal pain with or without swelling and erythema in child or adolescent male should always be treated as an emergency condition. The most frequent differential diagnosis of an acute scrotum includes spermatic cord torsion, torsion of testicular appendages, epididymo-orchitis, and trauma. The cause of an acute scrotum can usually be established based on careful history, physical examination, and appropriate diagnostic tests. The onset, character, and severity of symptoms should be clearly established to determine the appropriate and timely management. A correct diagnosis is mandatory as treatment options could differ dramatically depending on the disease process. Among these conditions, the spermatic cord torsion is of major concern because it requires immediate surgical intervention to avoid testicular loss.

## 1 Introduction

Acute scrotal pain with or without swelling and erythema should always be treated as an emergency condition (Burgher 1998). The presence of acute testicular pain or swelling is often referred to as "acute scrotum" and can be determined by many different causes. There are a number of differential diagnoses to consider (Jefferson et al. 1997; Brandes et al. 1994) (Table 1). In fact, emergencies that involve the scrotum may be confined to the scrotal

V. Mirone (✉) · P. Verze · D. Arcaniolo
Urologic Clinic, University Federico II of Naples,
Via S. Pansini 5, 80132, Naples, Italy
e-mail: mirone@unina.it

M. Bertolotto and C. Trombetta (eds.), *Scrotal Pathology*, Medical Radiology. Diagnostic Imaging,
DOI: 10.1007/174_2011_176, © Springer-Verlag Berlin Heidelberg 2012

**Table 1** Differential diagnosis for acute scrotal pain and swelling

| Pain and swelling | Pain alone | Swelling Alone |
| --- | --- | --- |
| Testicular torsion | Acute or Chronic epididymitis | Hydrocele/Varicocele |
| Torsion of appendages | Torsion of appendages | Hernia |
| Acute epididimitis | Adductor tendinitis | Idiopatic scrotal oedema |
| Hernia | Hematocele | Cyst of epididymis |
| Fournier's gangrene | Dermatological lesions | Neoplasia |
| Trauma | Vasculitis (Henoch-Schönlein purpura) | Spermatocele |
| Vasculitis (Henoch-Schönlein purpura) | | |

structures or referred from other sources. It must also be taken into account that the scrotum itself contains numerous structures: the testicles, epididymis, spermatic cord, and the scrotal tissue itself, comprised of several muscular and fascial layers. A correct diagnosis is mandatory as treatment options (observation, surgery, antibiotics, etc.) could differ dramatically depending on the disease process. Testicular torsion, epididymo-orchitis, and torsion of the testicular appendages are the most common etiologies of acute scrotum, especially in younger men.

Amongst emergencies involving the scrotum, those involving the testis certainly take on greater importance as the loss of a testicle due to a disregarded torsion, or a missed diagnosis of testicular cancer, can bring disastrous consequences.

## 2 Torsion

Torsion of the spermatic cord (testicular torsion) is defined as the process whereby there is cessation of blood flow to the testicle because of an occlusion of arterial blood supply resulting from the twisting of the artery and associated structures. When not treated timely, this condition can lead to testicular loss.

The incidence of torsion is about one in 125 males per year in Europe and it occurs most commonly in boys aged 13–17 years old. It is considered the most common cause of acute scrotal pain and swelling in boys from birth to 18 years of age. Testicular torsion must be considered a surgical emergency because the cord occlusion can lead to an irreversible ischaemic injury to the testicular parenchyma, depending on the

degree and duration of the torsion (McAndrew et al. 2002).

From the anatomical point of view, testicular torsion can be classified as either intravaginal or as extravaginal.

## 2.1 Extravaginal Torsion

This type of torsion can be either prenatal (in utero) or postnatal (in newborns). It is characterized by a lack of fixation of the gubernaculum testis and testicular tunica to the scrotal wall, which determines the torsion of the entire testis, spermatic cord, and tunica vaginalis, often to the level of the internal inguinal ring. Cryptorchidism is considered the most important risk factor for extravaginal torsion (Benjamin 2002).

## 2.2 Intravaginal Torsion

This is the more common type of testicular torsion. In intravaginal torsion, the spermatic cord twist occurs within the tunica vaginalis. This is probably due to a failure of normal posterior anchoring of the gubernaculum, epididymis, and testis, which leaves the testis free to swing and rotate within the tunica vaginalis of the scrotum (Kapoor 2008).

This anatomic relationship, in which the testicle has a transverse lie, is termed the bell-clapper deformity. This horizontal lie becomes a risk factor for torsion and after puberty the testis' added weight increases its likelihood of twisting on its vascular stalk. An abrupt contraction of the cremaster muscle can cause an initial rotation of the testis. This contortion is caused by the spiral configuration of the muscle's insertion onto the cord, twisting it in such a way that each testis' anterior surface rotates toward the midline.

## 2.3 Clinical Presentation

The most common age for the development of torsion is early puberty, while the newborn period is the second most common. The vascular compromise results in the rapid onset of swelling because of venous outflow obstruction in the face of continued arterial inflow.

Patients are usually presented with a sudden acute testicular pain, often being awakened from sleep, but sometimes the onset is more gradual and the pain less severe. In many cases, there is a history of previous episodes of severe, self-limiting scrotal pain and swelling. In testicular torsion, pain may be accompanied by nausea and vomiting and ipsilateral lower abdomen pain. Patients usually do not refer a history of associated lower urinary tract symptoms (Kapoor 2008).

If the patient has mild pain, which has increased over few days' time, a torsion of the testicular appendage should be suspected, rather than testicular torsion itself. If the patient complains of intermittent acute pain, which completely resolves, a diagnosis of intermittent testicular torsion should be suspected (Eaton et al. 2005).

Typically, a patient with testicular torsion lies relatively still on the exam table, but feels a sharp pain upon walking.

When palpating the scrotum the normal testicle, which should be in a vertical position, must be palpated first. Next, the spermatic cord of the affected testis is palpated. If painful and swollen, the suspicion of torsion is raised. Finally, the affected testis is palpated. Careful palpation of the scrotum will assess the asymmetric positioning of the testis within the scrotal sac. Examination will almost always detect an acutely sore and tender scrotum. The testis may be high-riding in the scrotum in an abnormal transverse position (Kapoor 2008).

Pain at the lower pole of the testis is more likely to signify torsion than pain at the upper pole of the testis, which is where many of the testicular appendages

are located. Hydrocele and scrotal oedema can be detected in established cases. A cremasteric reflex should be elicited next, before palpation, as absence of a cremasteric reflex is frequently associated with torsion. This finding is usually difficult to assess due to the presence of pain and swelling (Nelson et al. 2003).

While scrotal ultrasound with a color doppler is commonly used, some clinics have the capacity to use rapid nuclear medicine imaging with technetium-99 m radionuclide scanning which can detect blood flow to the testicle and is equally efficient (Nussbaum Blask et al. 2002). MR imaging can also be used to detect torsion. However, further intraoperative exploration may be required if a timely accurate image modality is obtained and index suspicion is high. In fact, the testicle can be completely salvaged with up to 6 h of torsion, but is unlikely to be salvaged beyond 12 h, so expedient diagnosis and surgical detorsion should be pursued (Mushtaq et al. 2003; Whitaker 1982).

## 2.4 Intermittent Torsion of the Spermatic Cord

There are cases of some adolescents reporting episodic bouts of severe, acute scrotal pain, and swelling, accompanied by nausea and vomiting, that can resolve themselves without treatment. In these cases, physical examination following such episodes results normal, but most of these individuals are found to have a bell-clapper deformity. It is assumed that they must be experiencing spontaneous torsion and detorsion (Eaton et al. 2005).

Misdiagnosis may create a cohort of boys with intermittent spermatic cord torsion who are at risk for acute unresolved torsion and potential testicular loss. Elective scrotal exploration and bilateral testicular fixation is strongly recommended when intermittent spermatic cord torsion is a likely diagnosis (Hayn et al. 2008).

## 3 Torsion of Testicular Appendages

Four types of testicular appendages are recognized: the appendix testis (hydatid of Morgagni, remnant of the Müllerian duct); the appendix of epididymis (remnant of Wolffian ducts); the paradydimis (organ of Giraldes, remnant of mesonephric duct); and the vas aberrans of Haller.

Testicular appendages become important clinically once they undergo torsion. The peak incidence of this event occurs in young teenagers due to the ensuing hormonal stimulation brought on by adolescence which increases testicular mass causing a propensity for the testes to twist on the vascular pedicle (Gatti and Murphy 2007).

The onset of the pain in appendage torsions can be either insidious, with mild scrotal discomfort, or acute, making it indistinguishable from a torsion of the cord. Physical examination of the scrotum may reveal a small (3–5 mm) tender nodule at the upper pole of the testis or epididymis or even a bluish change in the skin color of the affected side. This feature is due to visualization of the infarcted appendage through the skin ('blue dot sign'). The blue dot is strongly specific for torsion, even though it is detectable in only about 21% of patients (McCombe and Scobie 1988).

These findings are characteristic of the early stage, while as time passes, a massive edema develops, making physical examination really difficult. At this stage an ultrasound examination could be useful to evaluate whether testicular torsion is present. The presence of the cremasteric reflex should help to distinguish testicular torsion from torsion of the appendages.

The appendix testis is the testicular appendage most susceptible to torsion and often presents the same symptoms as those for testicular torsion. Torsion afflicts most often adolescents who report a sudden onset of testicular pain. If diagnosis is uncertain, meaning that testicular torsion is suspected, then surgical exploration is mandatory (Gatti and Murphy 2007).

# 4       Acute Epididymitis

Epididymitis is an inflammation of the epididymis that causes pain and swelling. It is classified as acute or chronic according to the onset and clinical course (Grabe et al. 2010). In some cases, the testis is involved in the inflammatory process (epididymo-orchitis). Acute epididymitis is a pain and swelling of the epididymis lasting for a short period of less than 6 weeks representing the main differential diagnosis of testicular torsion.

## 4.1      Acute Infective Epididymitis

In bacterial epididymitis, the infection usually spreads from the urethra, prostate, or bladder. Chlamydia trachomatis, Neisseria gonorrhoeae and the coliforms, and less frequently mycobacteria, brucella, and cryptococcus are the main pathogens. In the case of young children and older men, it is the coliforms that are responsible for infection and the epididymitis is almost always associated with bacteriuria or structural and/or functional abnormalities of the urinary tract. On the contrary, gonococcal and chlamydial infections are most likely to be found in men less than 35 years of age. Such infections are more commonly associated with urethritis, rather than bacteriuria. Coliform infection can also be found in young homosexuals who practice anal intercourse (Naber and Weidner 1999).

## 4.2      Non-Infective Inflammatory Epididymitis

This is a rare pathological entity that has been reported in association with Behçet's disease and Henoch-Schönlein purpura. Iatrogenic epididymitis has also been observed after administration of amiodarone (Nikolaou et al. 2007).

## 4.3      Clinical Presentation

Typically, the scrotal pain and swelling of epididymitis have a gradual onset, but in many cases pain can be described as sharp and acute. Fever or other non-specific signs of infection can be associated. Pain may radiate along the spermatic cord and reach the abdomen. Other presenting symptoms include urethral discharge, dysuria, and other irritative lower urinary tract symptoms. These could also be signs of developing erythema, which is usually unilateral and found primarily in the posterior part of the scrotum, causing the epididymis to double in size in as little as 3–4 h.

Physical examination findings range from inflammation and swelling of the tail of the epididymis to a massively inflamed erythematous hemiscrotum such that anatomical landmarks become unrecognizable. The spermatic cord is usually tender and swollen. A reactive hydrocele can be found which is caused by the secretion of inflammatory fluid between the layers of the tunica vaginalis. The most important differential diagnosis is torsion of the spermatic cord which is more probable if the onset of pain is sudden and severe in a patient younger than 20 years of age. When these symptoms are present, further scrotal exploration should be carried out if any pending doubt remain.

## 5    Testicular Trauma

While the scrotum's mobility provides protection from serious injury, its exposure and dependent position can make it susceptible to traumatic injury. The testicles are further protected by the tough surrounding tunica albuginea and by the cremasteric reflex (Deurdulian et al. 2007).

Blunt trauma, most often caused by athletic activity, is the cause of up to 85% of testicular injury and can result in local haematoma, ecchymosis of the scrotum, or injury to the testicle, epididymis, or spermatic cord. When blunt trauma occurs, patients usually suffer from immediate post-traumatic scrotal pain, nausea, vomiting and, at times, fainting. Most often they present a tender, swollen scrotum, and an impalpable testis (Munter and Faleski 1989).

In testicular rupture a disruption to the tunica albuginea is found, whereas in intratesticular haematoma, the tunica albuginea remains intact.

Trauma can result in haematoceles, which is an accumulation of blood in the space between the tunica albuginea and the tunica vaginalis. Hydrocele is a result of the accumulation of serum liquid in the space between the tunica albuginea and the tunica vaginalis.

Penetrating injuries caused by knives, gunshot or missiles include lacerations, haematomas, and delayed blast-type injuries while projectile trauma can damage all of the scrotal contents. Injury caused by animal and human bites can involve the scrotum including the scrotal contents. Apart from externally-inflicted trauma, scrotal injury can also be caused by self-mutilation or assault (Deurdulian et al. 2007).

## References

Benjamin K (2002) Scrotal and inguinal masses in the newborn period. Adv Neonatal Care 2:140–148

Brandes SB, Chelsky MJ, Hanno PM (1994) Adult acute idiopathic scrotal edema. Urology 44:602–605

Burgher SW (1998) Acute scrotal pain. Emerg Med Clin North Am 16:781–809, vi

Deurdulian C, Mittelstaedt CA, Chong WK et al (2007) US of acute scrotal trauma: optimal technique, imaging findings, and management. Radiographics 27:357–369

Eaton SH, Cendron MA, Estrada CR et al (2005) Intermittent testicular torsion: diagnostic features and management outcomes. J Urol 174:1532–1535; discussion 1535

Gatti JM, Murphy JP (2007) Current management of the acute scrotum. Semin Pediatr Surg 16:58–63

Grabe M, Bjerklund-Johansen TE, Botto H et al (2010) Guidelines on Urinary tract infection. European Association of Urology (EAU) pp 79–81

Hayn MH, Herz DB, Bellinger MF et al (2008) Intermittent torsion of the spermatic cord portends an increased risk of acute testicular infarction. J Urol 180:1729–1732

Jefferson RH, Perez LM, Joseph DB (1997) Critical analysis of the clinical presentation of acute scrotum: a 9 year experience at a single institution. J Urol 158:1198–1200

Kapoor S (2008) Testicular torsion: a race against time. Int J Clin Pract 62:821–827

McAndrew HF, Pemberton R, Kikiros CS et al (2002) The incidence and investigation of acute scrotal problems in children. Pediatr Surg Int 18:435–437

McCombe AW, Scobie WG (1988) Torsion of scrotal contents in children. Br J Urol 61:148–150

Munter DW, Faleski EJ (1989) Blunt scrotal trauma: Emergency department evaluation and management. Am J Emerg Med 7:227–234

Mushtaq I, Fung M, Glasson MJ (2003) Retrospective review of paediatric patients with acute scrotum. ANZ J Surg 73:55–58

Naber KG, Weidner W (1999) Prostatitis, epididymitis, orchitis. In: Armstrong D, Cohen J (eds) Infectious diseases. Mosby. Harcourt Publishers Ltd, London, pp 1–58

Nelson CP, Williams JF, Bloom DA (2003) The cremasteric reflex: a useful but imperfect sign in testicular torsion. J Pediatr Surg 38:1248–1249

Nikolaou M, Ikonomidis I, Lekakis I et al (2007) Amiodarone-induced epididymitis: a case report and review of the literature. Int J Cardiol 121:e15–e16

Nussbaum Blask AR, Bulas D, Shalaby-Rana E et al (2002) Color Doppler sonography and scintigraphy of the testis: a prospective, comparative analysis in children with acute scrotal pain. Pediatr Emerg Care 18:67–71

Whitaker RH (1982) Diagnoses not to be missed. Torsion of the testis. Br J Hosp Med 27:66–69

# Acute Scrotal Pain: Management

Giuseppe Ocello, Andrea Lissiani, and Carlo Trombetta

## Contents

**Abstract**

A variety of scrotal and non-scrotal pathologies may present with acute scrotal pain. Differential diagnosis is important, since management is different. When history and physical examination strongly suggest the presence of testicular torsion and the duration of pain is less than 12 h, urgent surgical exploration is mandatory. When pain is present for more than 12 h or the diagnosis is unclear, color Doppler ultrasound can be helpful in decision making. It is important to remember that most patients with an acute scrotum do not have testicular torsion. In case of epididymo-orchitis, pathogen-directed antibiotic therapy is required. Furthermore, bed rest, scrotal elevation and the use of non-steroidal anti-inflammatory agents are useful in reducing the duration of the symptoms.

## 1   Introduction

Testicular pain may have many causes, some of which are emergencies that require immediate medical attention. Besides traumas, however, the most important differential diagnosis is between testicular torsion, which requires immediate surgery, and inflammatory disorders, that are usually treated conservatively.

The three most important details to obtain from the patient in order to reach a confident differential diagnosis include the patient's age, the description of the pain and sexual history. History, in particular, in conjunction with the physical examination, can provide important clues as to the exact cause for the pain. Age is a key factor, since many conditions most often

G. Ocello · A. Lissiani · C. Trombetta (✉)
Department of Urology, Ospedale di Cattinara, University of Trieste, Strada di Fiume 447, 34124 Trieste, Italy
e-mail: trombcar@units.it

M. Bertolotto and C. Trombetta (eds.), *Scrotal Pathology,* Medical Radiology. Diagnostic Imaging,
DOI: 10.1007/174_2011_177, © Springer-Verlag Berlin Heidelberg 2012

**Table 1** Disorders presenting with acute scrotal pain

| Testicular | Intra/extravaginal torsion |
| --- | --- |
| | Torsion of the appendages |
| | Segmental testicular infarction |
| | Orchitis |
| | Tumors |
| Paratesticular | Epididymitis |
| | Incarcerated hernia |
| Scrotal wall | Fournier's Gangrene |
| | Idiopatic/secondary edema |
| | Trauma |
| | vasculitis |
| | Thrombophlebitis of the pampiniform plexus |
| | Filariasis |

occur in certain age groups. Testicular torsion, for instance, has a peak incidence in the neonatal and postpuberal stages while torsion of the appendices most often occurs during early adolescence. The description of the pain can provide important clues to the underlying etiology. Testicular and appendiceal torsion, for instance, present with sudden onset of the pain while epididymitis usually presents with a gradual onset of pain that increases in severity and extends over a period of hours to days. If concomitant urethritis is present, patients will also give a history of dysuria. Fever is also present in the inflammatory conditions while is typically absent in torsion.

The urologist should be aware that symptoms may occasionally be misleading. While conditions affecting the scrotum can secondarily cause referred pain to the abdomen and inguinal canal, a spectrum of abdominal pathologies may present clinically with acute scrotal pain.

In this chapter, the most clinically significant conditions that present with acute scrotal pain are presented (Table 1), with emphasis to clinical presentation, diagnosis and management.

## 2 Testicular Torsion

Intravaginal testicular torsion is due to anatomical variations that allow excessive testicular mobility inside the scrotum. The testis can present rotation that ranges from 360° to 720° in its own axis, causing

reduction or interruption of vascularization (Favorito et al. 2004). Extravaginal torsion could occur in uterus and in neonates and involves the gubernaculum testis that is not fixed to the scrotal wall and allows the testis to twist with its spermatic cord and tunica vaginalis around its axis inside the scrotum (Eifinger et al. 2010).

Intravaginal torsion most often occur in adolescents. The testis will present irreversible damage if the torsion is not resolved within up to 6 h (Turgut et al. 2008).

## 2.1 Management of Testicular Torsion

In suspected testicular torsion and/or scrotal pain, a complete abdominal, genitourinary, and prostate examination is important. Scrotal examination should include inspection, palpation, elicitation of the cremasteric reflex and, in selected case transillumination. In classic testicular torsion, the patient presents with severe pain and usually cannot deambulate easily. At close examination, the torsed testicle occupies a high position in the scrotal bag, just underneath the external inguinal ring. The cremasteric reflex is elicited next by pinching or lightly stroking from caudally to cranially the superior-medial aspect of the thigh. The presence of the reflex is indicated by elevation of the ipsilateral testicle. In patients with testicular torsion cremasteric reflex is absent. The palpation is often painful: when possible, the spermatic cord is found swollen and sometimes the epididymis faces anteriorly.

Color Doppler ultrasound allows differential diagnosis between testicular torsion and other causes of acute scrotal pain with excellent sensitivity of up to 90% and specificity of up to 99% (Kalfa et al. 2007).

In patients with testicular torsion the treatment of choice is to attempt manual and then surgical detorsion. After surgical detorsion the testis is placed in a weave gauze pad for a few minutes. If appropriate color and turgor returns, the orchidopexis should be performed with the fixation of the testis to the scrotal wall. Fixation of the controlateral testis is recommended as well (Venugopal et al. 2010). In the presence of necrosis, the testicle must be removed (Fig. 1) in order to avoid the risk of antisperm antibodies formation (Anderson and Williamson 1988).

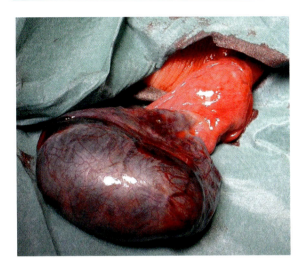

**Fig. 1** Intraoperative photo of intravaginal testicular torsion

## 3    Torsion of Appendages

Patients are most often adolescents presenting with sudden onset of scrotal pain. Clinical presentation is almost the same as that for testicular torsion even if clinical examination reveal a normal positioned testicle. In the early-stage, the twisted appendage can be palpated as a small tender mass close to the upper pole of the testis. Ultrasound allows diagnosis confirmation. Twisted solid appendages usually appear as rounded structures of variable echogenicity, often with inhomogeneous echotexture, lacking vascularization at color Doppler interrogation. Perilesional enhancement can occasionally be present.

In case of established diagnosis of appendiceal torsion, analgesic and anti-inflammatory medications are the therapy of choice. Surgical exploration, however, is mandatory if testicular torsion can't be completely excluded.

## 4    Inflammation

Epididymitis is an inflammatory reaction of the epididymis due to several infection agents or to local trauma. It is associated with fever, lower urinary tract symptoms and sensation of mass in the scrotum. It may present at any age. Epididymitis has a 2–3 day period of progressive increase in scrotal discomfort, and the pain is localized to the scrotum but sometime extends along the spermatic cord to reach the ipsilateral flank. A hot, erythematous scrotum is found at physical examination. Fever is also quite often present.

Inflammation involves the spermatic cord first, and then proceeds cephalad to the tail, to the head of the epididymis, and eventually to the testis. It can present in a sexually transmitted form but usually is associated with urinary tract infections and prostatitis. It can also be caused by reflux of sterile urine into the epididymis, causing local chemical inflammation. The most common sexually transmitted infections are caused by Neisseria gonorrhoeae or Chlamydia trachomatis. Those non-sexually transmitted are usually enterobacteriaceae or Pseudomonas. Complications of epididymo-orchitis include abscess, testicular ischemia, and pyocele formation. Post-inflammatory testicular ischemia is rare.

The most common manifestation of genitourinary tuberculosis in males is epididymo-orchitis. Local symptoms of the disease are usually insidious and progressive, and can be confused with other infections, cysts, and tumors. Tuberculous Epididymoorchitis can also complicate intravesical BCG therapy for superficial bladder carcinoma (Salvador et al. 2007).

Although characteristic features have been described (Muttarak and Peh 2006), Tuberculous epididymoorchitis may be indistinguishable from conventional bacterial infection both clinically and at imaging. The diagnosis is based on clinical suspicion arising from history of tuberculosis. Typical ultrasound features, when present, help in differential diagnosis with conventional bacterial epididymo-orchitis.

### 4.1    Management

Clinical examination and palpation is usually easy and the diagnosis is quite clear even if sometimes testicular torsion cannot be ruled out. Urinalysis or urethral smear help to evaluate the presence of infection. Color Doppler ultrasound is the imaging modality of choice revealing the pathognomic increased blood flow.

The appropriate therapy for scrotal inflammation is usually instituted empirically, giving broad-spectrum intravenous antibiotics, typically quinolones when possible, along with anti-inflammatory medications, bed rest, and scrotal elevation. When the testis is extensively involved in the inflammatory process, with ischemic changes or abscess formation, surgical removal may be necessary. Screening urinalysis is an important adjunct to the physical examination and radiological exams to rule out urinary tract infection or epididymo-orchitis.

Patients with tuberculous epididymitis or epididymo-orchitis usually respond to antituberculous therapy. Surgery, however, may be required in severe cases.

## 5    Trauma

A variety of traumatic mechanisms have been reported to result in scrotal trauma, with a common endpoint of blunt and/or penetrating trauma to the scrotal area. The aetiology includes avulsions after motor vehicle accidents, self-mutilation, work accident machinery-related, blunt injury, assaults (sharp or high-velocity missiles) and penetrating injury.

Two factors protect the testes from minor external trauma. First, a thin layer of physiologic hydrocele separates the tunica albuginea from the tunica vaginalis, and allows the testis to slide freely within the scrotal sac. Secondly, the testes are suspended within the scrotum by the spermatic cord, allowing them to move freely. In cases of penetrating trauma or severe blunt trauma, these protective features are not sufficient to prevent damage to the testis.

Testicular injuries can be divided into three categories based on the mechanism of injury including blunt, penetrating, and deglooving traumas. Blunt traumas account for approximately 85% of cases (Morey et al. 2004). Most common events are characterized by the testis that crushes against the pubic bone as a result of car or motorcycle accidents. Right testis is injured more often than the left. The testicular insult from blunt trauma can range from contusion to complete rupture, the latter happening approximately in 50% of all blunt scrotal traumas (Cass and Luxenberg 1988). It has been calculated that approximately 50 kg of force is required to rupture the testicle. A tear in the tunica albuginea leads to extrusion of the seminiferous tubules and allows an intratesticular hemorrhage to escape into the tunica vaginalis. Disruption of the tunica vaginalis or extension to the epididymis leads to bleeding into the scrotal wall, resulting in a scrotal hematoma.

Penetrating traumas account for 15% as a result from a variety of accidents associated with complex injuries or self-mutilation, which is relatively frequent in drug addicts or psychiatric patients. In children the most common penetrating traumas to the scrotum are caused by straddle-type falls or falls on sharp objects (Monga and Hellstrom 1996) while adults are generally involved in stab or gunshots injuries.

Even in isolated scrotal injuries, abdominal pain, nausea, emesis, and difficulty with voiding may occur. Embarrassment associated with the site, mechanism, or circumstance of injury often result in delayed presentation and may complicate diagnostic evaluation.

### 5.1    Management

Scrotal ultrasonography with Doppler studies is valuable for diagnosing and staging testicular injuries (Bhatt and Dogra 2008). The presence of contour irregularities or direct visualization of the interruption of the tunica albuginea are pathognomonic signs for testicular rupture. The absence of blood flow on ultrasonography may represent spermatic cord torsion, avulsion, or infarction. Other imaging studies, such as MR imaging, may be used to obtain additional information in equivocal cases (Parenti et al. 2009). Surgical exploration is mandatory in case of doubtful diagnosis after appropriate clinical and radiographic evaluations, clinical findings consistent with testicular injury, disruption of the tunica albuginea, absence of blood flow on color Doppler examination. Clinical hematoceles which are expanding or large ($\geq 5$ cm) should be explored as well. If the testis is fractured, testicular debridement and surgical closure of the tunica albuginea are necessary. Early surgical intervention for blunt trauma is associated with higher salvage rates (94 vs. 79%). Inappropriately protracted expectant management promotes testicular infection, atrophy, and necrosis. Delay in repair may result in loss of spermatogenesis.

Penetrating scrotal traumas usually require exploration to determine the severity of the injury and to identify, and control intratesticular bleeding.

Scrotal or perineal burns may be caused by electrical or chemical agents and are more common in children. For superficial burns (I–II degrees), a conservative treatment is prefered, while for deep lesions the main problem is to control the infection and repair tissue damage, for example, with eschar excision and allograft.

## 6 Fournier's Gangrene

Fournier gangrene is a necrotizing infection that involves the soft tissues of the male genitalia. Men are ten times more likely than women to develop it. Men aged 60–80 with a predisposing condition are most susceptible, as well as women who have had a bacterial infection in the vaginal area, episiotomy, septic abortion, hysterectomy. Rarely, children may develop Fournier's gangrene as a complication from a burn, circumcision, or an insect bite.

The necrotizing process commonly originates from an infection in the anorectum, urogenital tract, or skin of the genitalia. Anorectal causes include infection in the perianal glands, manifesting as a consequence of colorectal injury or as a complication of colorectal malignancy, inflammatory bowel disease, colonic diverticulitis, or appendicitis. Urogenital tract causes, include infection in the bulbourethral glands, urethral injury, iatrogenic injury secondary to urethral stricture manipulation, or lower urinary tract infection. Dermatologic causes include hidradenitis suppurativa, ulceration due to scrotal pressure, trauma, intentional trauma (skin popping or piercing), or complications of surgery. Other causes of Fournier gangrene, although less common, include bone marrow malignancy, systemic lupus erythematosus, Crohn disease, and HIV infection. Additionally, Fournier gangrene may result from iatrogenic or traumatic perineal injury (Gamagami et al. 1998; Gould et al. 1997; Brings et al. 1997).

Comorbid diseases that compromise the immune system have been implicated as necessary predisposing factors for the development of Fournier gangrene. The following are common predisposing comorbidities or risk factors: diabetes mellitus, morbid obesity, cirrhosis, vascular disease of the pelvis, malignancies, high-risk behaviors (alcoholism, intravenous drug abuse), immunodeficiency, trauma, or surgery to the external genitalia, perirectal and perianal abscesses, urethral injury following endoscopic surgery with extravasation of urine (Gould et al. 1997). Bacterial infection leads to obliterative endarteritis and thrombosis of the subcutaneous vessels that in turn causes ischemic necrosis of the subcutaneous fat and overlying skin. The infection rapidly spreads along the Dartos fascia of the scrotum and penis, Colles' fascia of the perineum, and Scarpa's fascia of abdomen.

### 6.1 Diagnosis

Diagnosis of Fournier gangrene is most commonly made clinically. Imaging is useful when clinical findings are unclear or the extent of disease is difficult to discern. On abdominal radiographs, subcutaneous emphysema and soft-tissue edema may be seen (Levenson et al. 2008; Rajan and Scharer 1998; Uppot et al. 2003). On ultrasound the scrotal wall is thickened and contains hyperechoic foci with reverberation artifacts and dirty shadowing, revealing presence of gas. Reactive hydroceles may be present (Uppot et al. 2003). The testes and epididymides are usually normal. CT can often show the cause of Fournier gangrene, such as perianal abscesses, incarcerated inguinal hernias, or fistulous tracts. Moreover, it plays an important role in the evaluation of disease extent for appropriate surgical treatment and is the imaging modality of choice in the postoperative follow-up to monitor the therapeutic response (Levenson et al. 2008). Compared with other imaging modalities, CT can better depict the extent of soft-tissue gas, and presence of any fluid collection or abscess (Levenson et al. 2008). CT is also important in differentiating Fournier gangrene from other less aggressive inflammatory entities such as soft-tissue edema or cellulitis, which may appear similar to Fournier gangrene at physical examination.

### 6.2 Management

Even though properly treated, Fournier's gangrene is a potentially lethal disease, with a mortality rate ranging from 15 to 50%. Advanced age, severity of comorbidities, renal insufficiency, hepatic dysfunction, and necrosis extension before the debridement are negative predictors against survival (Erol et al. 2010).

The management of Fournier's gangrene is surgical debridement of necrotic tissue and broad-spectrum antibiotics, intravenous fluid administration, and hyperbaric oxygen therapy, which stimulates leukocytes, improves tissue neovascolarization, and inhibits toxin formation from anaerobic bacteria. The first cycle of hyperbaric oxygen therapy should start 24 h after the debridement, and end a week after the surgical closure of the wound, which can heal by secondary intention, or require skin grafting or flap reconstruction.

## 7    Tumors

Any solid mass arising from the testis must be considered as a testicular tumor unless otherwise proven. Tumors most often occur between 20 and 40 years of age and present as incidental findings with a painless, hard nodule. About 95% of all testis tumors are represented by germ cell neoplasms (seminoma, choriocarcinoma, yolk sac tumor, teratoma, and embrional carcinoma). Stromal testis tumors are rare and show benign behavior. Men over 50 years are more likely to have a testicular lymphoma. Benign testicular tumors are very rare and include: testicular cyst, tunica cyst, dermo-epidermoid cyst and epidermoid tumor of the epididymis.

### 7.1    Management

Scrotal ultrasound confirms the diagnosis of a heterogeneous vascularized testicular mass. CT scan of the thorax and abdomen are necessary to rule out the presence of lymphadenopathy. Dosage of tumoral markers (alpha fetoprotein, beta human chorionic gonadotropin, and lactate dehydrogenase) completes the diagnostic pattern. Treatment is always a radical inguinal orchifunicolectomy as a first step.

## 8    Other Causes of Acute Scrotal Pain

A variety of scrotal and non-scrotal disorders may present clinically with acute scrotal pain. Among scrotal diseases, testicular and paratesticular tumors, segmental testicular infarction (Bilagi et al. 2007), isolated torsion of the epididymis (Dibilio et al. 2006), isolated torsion of a spermatocele (Takimoto et al. 2002), idiopathic and secondary acute scrotal edema (Aso et al. 2005), vasculitis (Sudakoff et al. 1992; Ben-Sira and Laor 2000; Dayanir et al. 2001), filariasis of the spermatic cord (Chaubal et al. 2003),

thrombophlebitis of the pampiniform plexus (Vincent and Bokinsky 1981) are treated elsewhere in this book. Among non-scrotal causes of acute scrotal pain renal colic, strangulated hernia, acute appendicitis, acute pancreatitis, adrenal hemorrhage and splenic fracture have been reported (Pavlica and Barozzi 2001; Dogra et al. 2003; Tillett et al. 2006; Worden 1996). Clinical history and physical examination are usually sufficient to reach diagnosis. Ultrasound or other imaging modalities are helpful in patients with equivocal physical findings.

## References

Anderson JB, Williamson RC (1988) Testicular torsion in Bristol: a 25-year review. Br J Surg 75:988–992

Aso C, Enriquez G, Fite M et al (2005) Gray-scale and color Doppler sonography of scrotal disorders in children: an update. Radiographics 25:1197–1214

Ben-Sira L, Laor T (2000) Severe scrotal pain in boys with Henoch-Schonlein purpura: incidence and sonography. Pediatr Radiol 30:125–128

Bhatt S, Dogra VS (2008) Role of US in testicular and scrotal trauma. Radiographics 28:1617–1629

Bilagi P, Sriprasad S, Clarke JL et al (2007) Clinical and ultrasound features of segmental testicular infarction: six-year experience from a single centre. Eur Radiol 17:2810–2818

Brings HA, Matthews R, Brinkman J et al (1997) Crohn's disease presenting with Fournier's gangrene and enterovesical fistula. Am Surg 63:401–405

Cass AS, Luxenberg M (1988) Value of early operation in blunt testicular contusion with hematocele. J Urol 139:746–747

Chaubal NG, Pradhan GM, Chaubal JN et al (2003) Dance of live adult filarial worms is a reliable sign of scrotal filarial infection. J Ultrasound Med 22:765–769 quiz 770-762

Dayanir YO, Akdilli A, Karaman CZ et al (2001) Epididymoorchitis mimicking testicular torsion in Henoch-Schonlein purpura. Eur Radiol 11:2267–2269

Dibilio D, Serafini G, Gandolfo NG et al (2006) Ultrasonographic findings of isolated torsion of the epididymis. J Ultrasound Med 25:417–419 quiz 420-411

Dogra VS, Gottlieb RH, Oka M et al (2003) Sonography of the scrotum. Radiology 227:18–36

Eifinger F, Ahrens U, Wille S et al (2010) Neonatal testicular infarction–possibly due to compression of the umbilical cord? Urology 75:1482–1484

Erol B, Tuncel A, Hanci V et al (2010) Fournier's gangrene: overview of prognostic factors and definition of new prognostic parameter. Urology 75:1193–1198

Favorito LA, Cavalcante AG, Costa WS (2004) Anatomic aspects of epididymis and tunica vaginalis in patients with testicular torsion. Int Braz J Urol 30:420–424

Gamagami RA, Mostafavi M, Gamagami A et al (1998) Fournier's gangrene: an unusual presentation for rectal carcinoma. Am J Gastroenterol 93:657–658

Gould SW, Banwell P, Glazer G (1997) Perforated colonic carcinoma presenting as epididymo-orchitis and Fournier's gangrene. Eur J Surg Oncol 23:367–368

Kalfa N, Veyrac C, Lopez M et al (2007) Multicenter assessment of ultrasound of the spermatic cord in children with acute scrotum. J Urol 177:297–301 discussion 301

Levenson RB, Singh AK, Novelline RA (2008) Fournier gangrene: role of imaging. Radiographics 28:519–528

Monga M, Hellstrom WJ (1996) Testicular trauma. Adolesc Med 7:141–148

Morey AF, Metro MJ, Carney KJ et al (2004) Consensus on genitourinary trauma: external genitalia. BJU Int 94:507–515

Muttarak M, Peh WC (2006) Case 91: tuberculous epididymo-orchitis. Radiology 238:748–751

Parenti GC, Feletti F, Brandini F et al (2009) Imaging of the scrotum: role of MRI. Radiol Med 114:414–424

Pavlica P, Barozzi L (2001) Imaging of the acute scrotum. Eur Radiol 11:220–228

Rajan DK, Scharer KA (1998) Radiology of Fournier's gangrene. AJR Am J Roentgenol 170:163–168

Salvador R, Vilana R, Bargallo X et al (2007) Tuberculous epididymo-orchitis after intravesical BCG therapy for superficial bladder carcinoma: sonographic findings. J Ultrasound Med 26:671–674

Sudakoff GS, Burke M, Rifkin MD (1992) Ultrasonographic and color Doppler imaging of hemorrhagic epididymitis in Henoch-Schonlein purpura. J Ultrasound Med 11:619–621

Takimoto K, Okamoto K, Wakabayashi Y et al (2002) Torsion of spermatocele: a rare manifestation. Urol Int 69:164–165

Tillett JW, Elmore J, Smith EA (2006) Torsion of an indirect hernia sac within a hydrocele causing acute scrotum: case report and review of the literature. Pediatr Surg Int 22:1025–1027

Turgut AT, Bhatt S, Dogra VS (2008) Acute painful scrotum. Ultrasound Clin 3:93–107

Uppot RN, Levy HM, Patel PH (2003) Case 54: Fournier gangrene. Radiology 226:115–117

Venugopal S, Schoeman D, Damola A et al (2010) Acute scrotal pain with a twist. Ann R Coll Surg Engl 92:W24–W26

Vincent MP, Bokinsky G (1981) Spontaneous thrombosis of pampiniform plexus. Urology 17:175–176

Worden AC (1996) Acute ureteral colic manifested by scrotal pain. Am Fam Physician 54:1896

# Imaging Acute Scrotal Pain in Adults: Torsion of the Testis and Appendages

Ahmet T. Turgut and Vikram S. Dogra

## Contents

A. T. Turgut (✉)
Department of Radiology
Ankara Training and Research Hospital,
06590 Ankara, Turkey
e-mail: ahmettuncayturgut@yahoo.com

V. S. Dogra
Department of Imaging Sciences,
University of Rochester School of Medicine,
601 Elmwood Ave, Box 648,
Rochester, NY 14642, USA

**Abstract**

Torsion of the spermatic cord is a common cause of acute scrotal pain and a delay in intervention may cause irreversible testicular damage. Intravaginal testicular torsion, which is associated either with a long mesorchium or bell-clapper deformity, accounts for most of the cases. Gray-scale US combined with color and pulsed Doppler modes is the method of choice for patients with the clinical presentation of testicular torsion, where the findings depend on the duration of torsion and the degree of twisting of the spermatic cord. The absence of testicular blood flow on color or power Doppler US is considered diagnostic of ischemia. On the other hand, the presence of color or power Doppler flow in a patient with a typical clinical presentation for torsion may be consistent with partial testicular torsion. The main role of ultrasound in the torsion of testicular appendix is to rule out testicular torsion or epididymo-orchitis. Optimization of the color and pulsed Doppler parameters is crucial for increasing the diagnostic yield.

## 1 Clinical Background

Torsion of testis and testicular appendages is among the major causes of acute scrotal pain, which is the most commonly encountered urological emergency. The entity involves the twisting of the spermatic cord which may result in the strangulation of the testicular blood flow and rotation of the testis in the longitudinal axis of the spermatic cord. The ability to differentiate torsion properly from other common causes of acute scrotal pain like epididymo-orchitis and trauma is crucial, as

M. Bertolotto and C. Trombetta (eds.), *Scrotal Pathology*, Medical Radiology. Diagnostic Imaging,
DOI: 10.1007/174_2011_178, © Springer-Verlag Berlin Heidelberg 2012

testicular ischemia is associated with significant morbidity which necessitates proper patient management.
Testicular salvage rate is closely associated with prolonged ischemia. Despite its propensity to effect
patients of any age, testicular torsion, with a prevalence
of 1 in 4,000 under the age of 25, mainly effects pediatric patients and young males (Barada et al. 1989).

## 2 Anatomical Considerations and Mechanism

Apart from the extravaginal torsion which is a rare
phenomenon occurring in the newborns when the
scrotum is not securely attached to the tunica vaginalis,
intravaginal torsion, accounting for 65–80% of the
cases, is the most common type (Favorito et al. 2004). It
is associated either with a long mesorchium, which is a
long intrascrotal portion of the spermatic cord or with
bell-clapper deformity, involving a tunica vaginalis
completely encircling the epididymis, distal spermatic
cord, and testis rather than attaching to the posterolateral aspect of the testis. The increased incidence of
torsion in cryptorchidism is attributable to its association with the aforementioned long mesorchium. On the
other hand, bell-clapper deformity with a reported
prevalence of 12% in one autopsy series (Dogra et al.
2001), is usually bilateral and refers to a testis which is
free to swing and rotate within the tunica vaginalis,
resembling a clapper inside a bell (Dogra 2003). Bell
clapper deformity, which predisposes to the rotation of
the testis and spermatic cord, can be diagnosed with
greater accuracy by ultrasound (US) in the presence of
moderate degree of hydrocele surrounding the distal
portion of the spermatic cord and testis (Fig. 1). As this
deformity predisposes to testicular torsion, orchiopexy
involving surgical anchoring of both testes should be
considered as this will prevent future twisting. Furthermore, sexual activity and physical exercise are associated with increased incidence of intravaginal torsion
(Lin et al. 2007).

## 3 Clinical Evaluation

Testicular torsion was first described in 1776 by
Hunter (Noske et al. 1998). By the age of 25 years,
the chance of torsion of the testis or its appendages is
approximately 1 in 160 (Williamson 1976). The

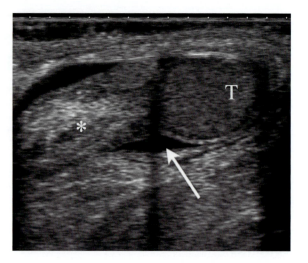

**Fig. 1** Bell-clapper deformity. Ultrasound image showing
hydrocele (*arrow*) encircling the distal third of the spermatic
cord (*asterisk*). The child underwent a bilateral orchiopexy
(Reprinted from Dogra et al. 2006 with permission)

clinical evaluation of these patients is usually a
diagnostic challenge even for an experienced urologist due to the associated pain and swelling. Clinically, patients with torsion mostly present with
sudden onset of severe scrotal pain particularly at
night, followed by nausea, vomiting, and a low grade
fever (Dogra et al. 2006). The symptoms may be
intermittent or variable in partial and intermittent
varieties of the entity. The entity can be classified
according to the duration of the symptoms. In this
regard, acute torsion refers to the symptoms beginning in less than 24 h, whereas subacute torsion
implies spanning of the duration of the pain to
6–10 days. The symptoms with a history of longer
duration, on the other hand, is consistent with chronic
torsion. The intensity of the symptoms and the degree
of testicular ischemia are closely associated with the
duration of the torsion, the number of twists in the
spermatic cord and the degree to which the spermatic
cord vessels are compressed.

A swollen, tender, and erythematous hemiscrotum is
the predominant physical examination finding. Inability
to distinguish the testis from the epididymis due to
localized swelling may result in a diagnostic dilemma
and the condition can be misdiagnosed as epididymitis,
as both entities have similar presentations (Dogra et al.
2006). The cremasteric reflex is usually absent, which is
the most sensitive physical examination finding

(Kadish and Bolfe 1998; Kass and Lundak 1997). Additionally, pain is not relieved by elevating the scrotum above the symphisis pubis, which is called as Prehn's sign. A high-riding testicle refers to the shortening of the torsed spermatic cord causing elevation of the testis toward the inguinal canal (Dogra et al. 2006). In the standing position, the normal testis of an adult hangs in a near-vertical position, whereas the torsion will result in near-horizontal lie of the testis (Angell 1963).

Testicular salvage rate is closely associated with prolonged ischemia. If surgical treatment is started within 4–6 h after the onset of the symptoms the chance of testicular salvage is quite high, whereas the salvage rate drops to 70% within 6–12 h and most testes which are not detorsed by 10–12 h will be unsalvagable because of irreversible damage (Oyen 2002). In this regard, it is of utmost importance to utilize a diagnostic tool which is specific enough to enable the urologist to make a choice properly between surgical intervention and conservative management so that testicular infarct and unnecessary surgical exploration can be avoided as much as possible. Nevertheless, prompt surgical exploration is recommended in case the torsion cannot be ruled out.

Notably, unilateral testicular injury may have an insult on the uninvolved testis through an ischemia–reperfusion mechanism (Dogra et al. 2006). Recently, the treatment of torsion by detorsion alone has been reported not to prevent testicular damage, which may result in infertility (Adivarekar et al. 2005). If a necrotic testis, a sequela of the testicular torsion, is not removed surgically, the contralateral testis may also be damaged through an autoimmune response (Donohue and Utley 1978).

# 4 US Evaluation

Apart from clinical history and physical examination, US is helpful as it can usually suggest a more specific diagnosis in the management of patients with acute scrotal pain. Broadband high-frequency gray-scale US combined with color and pulsed Doppler modes is the modality of choice, as it can, not only reveal anatomical details but also characterize testicular perfusion. US findings depend on the duration of torsion and the degree of twisting of the spermatic cord. In this regard, awareness for the typical and atypical US features as well as pitfalls of testicular torsion is critical.

## 4.1 Technical Considerations

In addition to the grayscale images revealing the size and the echogenicity of each testis, color, power, and spectral Doppler evaluation is a requirement for the direct assessment of testicular perfusion. Importantly, comparison of the findings of the aforementioned evaluation for one side with those of the opposite side may be helpful to establish a diagnosis, which necessitates transverse scanning depicting portions of each testis on the same field of view. Accordingly, bilateral spectral Doppler tracings should be obtained.

If the blood flow cannot be detected properly, color and pulsed Doppler parameters should be optimized for revealing the flow signals in the testis and paratesticular structures and for demonstrating low-flow velocities with the highest sensitivity. This optimization involves increasing the frequency of the transducer probe used, increasing the gain up to just below the noise level, decreasing the wall filter and decreasing the pulse repetition frequency (Wilbert et al. 1993). Naturally, the focal zone where the image optimization is performed should be set to the expected location of the vessels. Additionally, the color box should be kept small enough to increase the frame rate and improve color resolution. As a technical prerequisite, the sample volume should be set to a correct size, which is about two-thirds of the vessel lumen (Lin et al. 2007). On the other hand, care should be taken to examine the asymptomatic side initially so that the gray-scale and color Doppler gain settings can be set optimally allowing a baseline for comparison with the structures on the affected side (Dogra et al. 2006). Despite being prone to motion artifacts, power Doppler is the most sensitive mode in the evaluation of tissues with decreased blood flow thanks to its higher power gain and independence from angle correction (Lin et al. 2007). Notably, the application of additional techniques like Valsalva maneuver and upright positioning may be helpful for better evaluation of venous return. Despite the fact that an asymmetry in the findings of the aforementioned evaluation may be a clue for the diagnosis of torsion, it should be kept in mind that bilateral involvement may occur in about 2% of the cases.

# 5    Testicular Torsion

## 5.1    Intravaginal Torsion

### 5.1.1    Gray-Scale US

In general, grayscale US findings for testicular torsion which depend on the length of time passed from the beginning of the symptoms are nonspecific. In the early period immediately after the onset of the torsion, grayscale US evaluation of the testis reveals no abnormality, though a progressive hypoechogenecity develops secondary to edema. Hence, a normal US appearance of testis and epididymis becomes an occasional finding in 2–4 h. Importantly, an apparently normal testis in the setting of an acute torsion warrants further evaluation with color and spectral Doppler US to improve the diagnostic yield. Importantly, a normal testicular echogenecity is a strong indicator for the viability of the testicular tissue (Middleton et al. 1997). After 4–6 h, the appearance of a swollen and enlarged testis with a more spherical morphology and decreased echogenecity, being mostly diffuse in distribution, predominates (Fig. 2). It should be kept in mind that a partial infarct may result in an focal or partially hypoechoic pattern (Fig. 3). A heterogenous testicular echotexture or diffuse, focal, or multifocal hyperechogenecity due to vascular congestion, hemorrhage and infarction can be detected after 24 h, referring to a phase of torsion labeled as late or missed torsion (Fig. 4). Besides, an enlarged and more spherical epididymal head with decreased echogenecity can be detected, as the arterial blood supply of the epididymis is derived from the testicular artery. If the epididymis is also effected by the hemorrhagic infarction, a hyperechoic appearance due to parenchymal bleeding predominates (Schulsinger et al. 1991).

On gray-scale US, care should be taken to compare the positions of affected testis with the normal one and also to assess the positional relationship of the mediastinum testis and epididymis. In this regard the long axis of the testis converts to an oblique or even horizontal position in relation to the long axis of the thigh (Kass and Lundak 1997). The abnormal position of mediastinum can be a clue for the diagnosis of torsion (Prando 2009). Testicular torsion can also be inferred by the traction of the epididymis and mediastinum testis to the inguinal canal (Prando 2002).

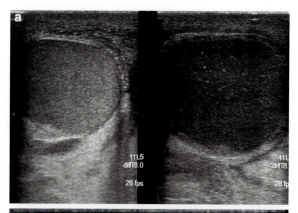
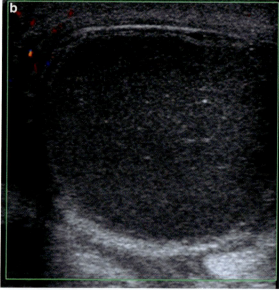

**Fig. 2** Testicular torsion. **a** Transverse gray-scale ultrasound image of the scrotum revealing an enlarged and edematous appearence of the symptomatic left testis with diffuse hypoechogenecity compared to the asymptomatic right testis. **b** Color Doppler ultrasound demonstrates complete absence of blood flow within the left testis

On transverse scanning, the enlarged and heterogenous epididymis followed by the mediastinum can be seen immediately distal to the inguinal canal (Prando 2002). The visibility of the lobar architecture of the affected testis is enhanced due to interstitial and septal edema (Prando 2009). Likewise, a well-identified and thickened mediastinum which is less echogenic than the uninvolved testis can be detected (Prando 2002).

As a consequence of the efforts aiming to identify the exact site of torsion, the sonographic real time "whirlpool sign" referring to the detection of a mass with concentric layers formed by coiling of the cord

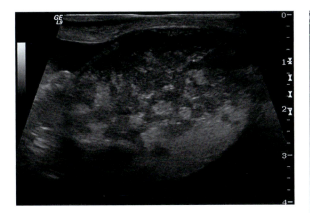

**Fig. 3** Longitudinal gray-scale US image showing focal hypoechoic areas with patchy distribution throughout the testicular parenchyma interspersed with normal testicular parenchyma and scarce, hyperechoic foci representing hemorrhage implying partial torsion in the subacute stage

vessels secondary to the twisting of the spermatic cord has been reported to be the most definitive sign of torsion, with a reported rate of 100% for sensitivity and specificity, respectively (Figs. 4b , 5b) (Vijayaraghavan 2006). The whirlpool mass, produced by moving the transducer in a downward direction along the inguinal canal perpendicular to the axis of the cord resembles a doughnut or a target. The author noted that the whirlpool mass can be located just distal to the external ring, above or posterior to the testis or in the inguinal canal in case of an undescended testis (Vijayaraghavan 2006). However, in several other studies, the sensitivity of this sign was found to be lower, despite having a satisfactory specificity (Baud et al. 1998; Kalfa et al. 2004). Additionally, a prominent increase in the thickness of the peritesticular soft tissues (>5 mm) and scrotal skin due to edema, which can partially involve the contralateral hemiscrotum can be detected (Fig. 6) (Prando 2009). Another finding of the entity which is a reactive hydrocele usually located posterior to the testis can be detected after 6 h and may contain internal echoes and scattered fine septations in time (Prando 2002; van Dijk and Karthaus 1994). Chronic torsion, on the other hand, is characterized by a small, hard, and diffusely hypoechoic testis with an accompanying hyperechoic mass representing the extratesticular components of the torsion (Prando 2002). Notably, the thickness of the scrotal wall and skin turns to normal and hydrocele disappears at this stage (Prando 2009).

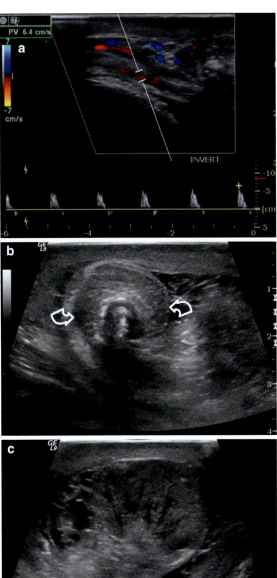

**Fig. 4** Testicular torsion. **a** Spectral Doppler waveform showing high resistance blood flow pattern with reversal of diastolic flow in the spermatic cord suggesting loss of tissue perfusion consistent with acute complete torsion or impending testicular infarction. Longitudinal **b** ultrasound image shows whirlpool sign (*curved arrows*) resembling a snail shell, revealing spiral aspect of the twisted spermatic cord which is highly specific for torsion. **c** Markedly heterogenous parenchymal echotexture with interspersed areas of cystic degeneration in the symptomatic testis implies testicular infarction. On color Doppler ultrasound, no flow is detected within the symptomatic testis (*not shown here*)

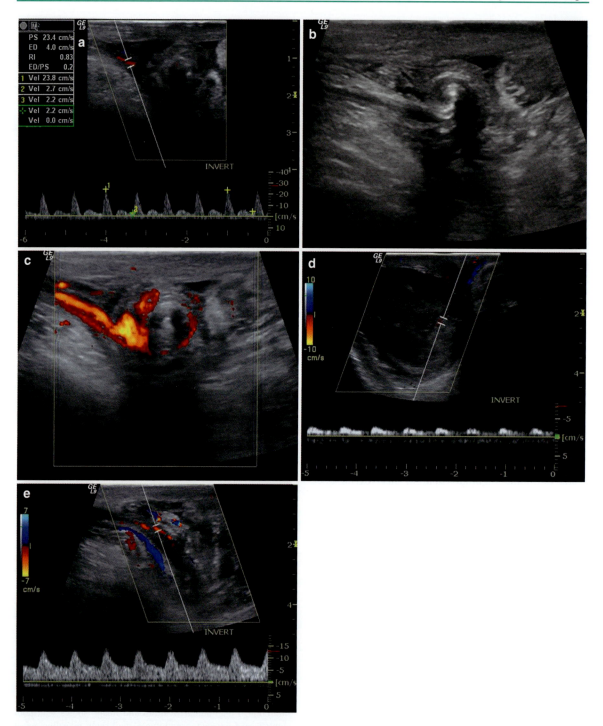

**Fig. 5** Partial testicular torsion. **a** Spectral Doppler waveform showing high resistance blood flow pattern with decreased amplitude of diastolic flow in the spermatic cord. **b** Longitudinal gray-scale ultrasound image demonstrating buckling of the spermatic cord resulting in the formation of whirlpool mass. **c** On power Doppler ultrasound, flow can be detected in the vessels of the whirlpool mass suggesting incomplete nature of the torsion. **d** Color Doppler ultrasound image showing no substantial flow throughout most of the testicular parenchyma with only a small amount of blood flow where the spectral Doppler analysis revealed relatively decreased arterial flow. The patient was found to have partial torsion when he was operated on. Thereby, detorsion and orchiopexy were performed. **e** Spectral Doppler waveform obtained in the immediate post-operative period demonstrating a normal low-resistance flow pattern

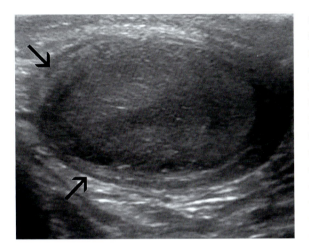

**Fig. 6** Testicular torsion. Longitudinal gray-scale ultrasound image shows the heterogenous echotexture of the torsed testis and the hyperechoic ring consistent with concentric layers of thickened tunica albuginea (*arrows*)

### 5.1.2 Color Flow Doppler US

Testicular perfusion can be assessed best by color, power, and spectral Doppler US. The relevant evaluation typically begins with color Doppler US, which can demonstrate the presence of blood flow and early perfusion changes reliably. In several reports focusing on the value of color Doppler US, the sensitivity of the technique ranged from 79 to 89%, whereas its specificity was between 77 and 100% (Nussbaum-Blask and Rushton 2006; Wilbert et al. 1993). On the other hand, power Doppler US using the integrated power of the Doppler signal to depict the presence of blood flow yields higher power gains and enables better assessment of the diminished testicular blood (Dogra et al. 2006). In this regard, inability to detect any blood flow in the involved testis implying ischemia is the cardinal finding for the diagnosis of testicular torsion and can easily be distinguished from the normal flow in the contralateral testis (Fig. 2b). In early torsion, color flow Doppler evaluation is strongly recommended owing to the fact that gray-scale US evaluation reveals no abnormality at this phase. On the other hand, hypervascularity in the extratesticular soft tissues is associated with testicular infarction (Dogra et al. 2006).

Hemodynamically, testicular torsion first causes compromise of the venous flow, followed by obstruction of the arterial flow and testicular ischemia, the severity of which is related to the degree of torsion. Sonographically, no blood flow can be detected in a spermatic cord with a twisting degree exceeding 450°. Nevertheless, high resistance blood flow pattern characterized by a decrease or reversal of diastolic flow in the spermatic cord suggesting an impending testicular infarction can also be detected (Fig. 4a). In general, the presence of testicular blood flow should always be confirmed by quantitative spectral Doppler evaluation using the time-velocity spectrum. As the normal testis is a low impedance organ, the spectral waveform of the intratesticular arteries show a low-resistance pattern with high levels of diastolic flow. The mean resistive index (RI) value obtained in normal intratesticular arteries is 0.62 (range, 0.48–0.75) (Siegel 1997). In cases with an apparently diminished testicular blood flow, which can be best visualized in close proximity to the mediastinum testis, spectral Doppler analysis of the remaining testicular blood flow should be performed (Prando 2002). In a similar fashion, the spectral Doppler analysis of patients with a small amount of residual arterial flow detected in the torsed testis after an incomplete torsion, will yield a high resistance waveform pattern with an elevated RI and diminished or reversed diastolic flow (Dogra and Bhatt 2004).

Infrequently, only a small arterial signal can be detected in the testis, which should not preclude the diagnosis of torsion, particularly in the appropriate clinical setting (Fig. 5d) (Dogra et al. 2006). In this regard, arterial flow may not necessarily be absent for torsion to be present (Dogra et al. 2006). In early torsion, diminished arterial velocity and a decreased or absent diastolic flow resulting in an increased RI representing severe venous obstruction or occlusion can be detected (Dogra et al. 2004). Nevertheless, increased RI and absent or reversed diastolic flow can also be a complication of severe epididymo-orchitis, where the venous outflow obstruction is secondary to swelling and edema rather than cord obstruction caused by torsion (Dogra et al. 2004). Contrary to decreased flow in torsion, the overall blood flow to the involved side is increased in epididymitis, which may be a clue for an appropriate diagnosis.

### 5.2 Partial (Incomplete) Testicular Torsion

Torsion of the spermatic cord is not necessarily an all-or-nothing phenomenon as the vascular pedicle can twist in different degrees, ranging from one-quarter (90°) twist up to three complete turns (Prando 2009). Partial torsion occurs usually when the degree of twisting is less than 360°, whereas complete torsion refers to a rotation with more than 360° (Hörmann et al. 2004). The true incidence of the entity is unknown, because detorsion may automatically occur in some cases, whereas others may undergo surgery immediately without any ultrasound evaluation as they may be presumed to be complete torsion and some others may be classified as torsion/detorsion (Cassar et al. 2008). The arterial blood supply, which is not necessarily absent, can be detected as far as the mediastinum testis and the venous flow can be partially or totally obstructed (Hörmann et al. 2004). Nevertheless, the clinical and sonographic diagnosis of partial testicular torsion, also called as incomplete torsion or transient torsion, may be problematic and the cases may present a diagnostic challenge. Despite the current progress in US technology, false-negative findings in the evaluation of partial testicular torsion, still cannot be avoided.

In general, US findings for the entity vary depending on the duration and the degree of rotation. A grayscale US usually yields no abnormality in patients with partial torsion (Cassar et al. 2008). The value of color and power Doppler US and spectral Doppler analysis for a definite diagnosis of partial testicular torsion has not been established yet, though the findings have proved to be useful. In this regard, a consistently present intratesticular flow on color Doppler US can be detected, though asymmetry of the color flow Doppler findings revealing decreased intratesticular flow compared to the uninvolved testis can be helpful for the diagnosis (Fig. 5d). On the other hand, spectral Doppler analysis has also been considered to be useful and is particularly more reliable in detecting subtle asymmetry (Sanelli et al. 1999). In this regard, subtle spectral Doppler variations should be regarded as an indirect clue for testicular torsion, particularly in the setting of a typical clinical history.

In an earlier report, color Doppler imaging with spectral analysis was noted to be useful in a canine model, where diastolic component of the arterial

signal was found to be enhanced at 180° torsion (Mevorach et al. 1991). Besides, the effectiveness of the technique was emphasized by several other authors (Cassar et al. 2008; Dogra et al. 2001; Sanelli et al. 1999). Variability of the amplitude of the spectral Doppler waveform and relative to the uninvolved testis or within the same testis has been reported to be the most common abnormality, followed by the reversal of diastolic flow implying total obstruction of the venous flow (Cassar et al. 2008). Besides, increased resistance to arterial flow due to the decrease in the diastolic flow velocities can be detected. Nevertheless, a cut-off value for RI above or below which a diagnosis could be made confidently has not been determined yet (Cassar et al. 2008).

It is noteworthy that a reliable spectral Doppler analysis should include evaluation of the upper, mid, and lower poles of each testis, so that the operator can be aware of the aforementioned variability in the spectral Doppler findings. Additionally, the specificity of ultrasound for incomplete torsion can further be enhanced with the demonstration of "whirlpool sign" where flow can be detected in the vessels of the whirlpool mass, distal to it, and in the testis, contrary to complete torsion (Fig. 5c) (Vijayaraghavan 2006). Finally, the presence of color or power Doppler signal in a patient with a typical clinical presentation for torsion should not exclude torsion and the possibility for partial testicular torsion should be considered.

## 5.3 Intermittent Torsion (Torsion-Detorsion Syndrome)

Intermittent torsion is characterized by recurrent episodes of acute and sharp unilateral testicular pain and scrotal swelling, interspersed with long symptom-free intervals. Physical examination findings include a very mobile or horizontally positioned testis, an anteriorly located epididymis and bulky spermatic cord due to partial twisting. When examined in the asymptomatic period or immediately after the regression of the symptoms, color Doppler US may reveal paradoxically increased blood flow in the affected testis with a decreased arterial resistance

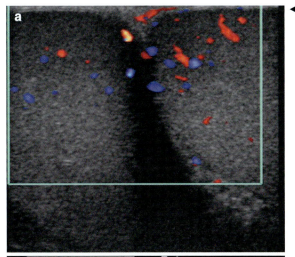

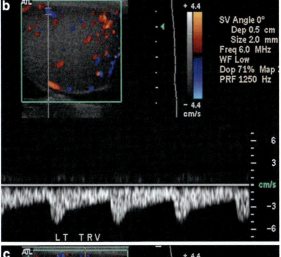

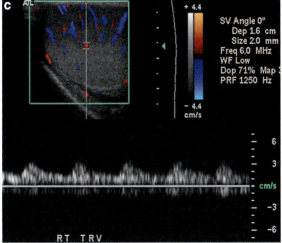

◀ **Fig. 7** Torsion-detorsion syndrome. The patient presenting with a history of intermittent left testicular pain was asymptomatic at the time of examination. **a** Color flow Doppler on transverse plane demonstrates increased blood flow to the left testis. Comparing spectral Doppler waveform of the left testis **b** with that of the right testis **c**, the blood flow to the left testis is apparently increased. (Reprinted from Dogra et al. 2006 with permission)

(Fig. 7) (Dogra et al. 2006). This intratesticular hypervascularization can be confused with mumps orchitis, which is the most common cause of orchitis without associated epididymitis (Dogra et al. 2003). Apart from the clinical history of parotitis within 1–6 weeks, US finding of enlarged and hyperemic testis with increased venous flow may be clue for the diagnosis (Dogra et al. 2003). Notably, the testis may be normal in size or enlarged and focal or segmental hypoechoic testicular infarcts may or may not be present in patients with intermittent torsion (Dogra et al. 2006, 2004). Surgical exploration and orchiopexy is the choice of management for the patients with intermittent torsion. If the clinical suspicion for intermittent torsion is high, exploration may reveal a bell-clapper deformity, which may necessitate bilateral orchiopexy (Ameur et al. 2003; Kamaledeen and Surana 2003). Likewise, a horizontal testicular position is a strong indication for surgical exploration and testicular fixation (Schulsinger et al. 1991).

## 5.4 Mimics of Testicular Torsion

Several other conditions resulting in the ultrasound findings consistent with decreased testicular perfusion and high resistance blood flow can mimic testicular torsion. Among these are poor technical parameters, scrotal skin thickening, marked scrotal edema (Dogra et al. 2006), inguinal hernia (Turgut et al. 2007), external compression by large hydroceles or extratesticular hematomas (Dogra et al. 2006; Turgut et al. 2006), severe epididymitis or vasculitis causing venous occlusion (Dogra et al. 2004), and protein S and antitrombin III deficiency (Ameur et al. 2003). Despite being rare, testicular infarction without torsion of the spermatic cord can occur spontaneously. The entity is usually idiopathic and characterized by a

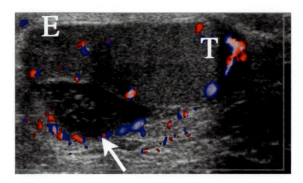

**Fig. 8** Testicular appendigeal torsion. A 10 year-old boy presented with testicular pain. Color flow Doppler demonstrates a hypoechoic mass with peripheral hyperemia (*arrow*) separate from epididymis (*E*). This hypoechoic mass resolved on follow-up. *T*, Testis. (Reprinted from Dogra et al. 2006 with permission)

focal area of decreased echogenecity which is usually located anteriorly near the upper pole of the testis (Fukuhara et al. 2005).

## 6 Torsion of Epididymis

Isolated torsion of the epididymis, which has been rarely reported in the literature (Dibilio et al. 2006; Elert et al. 2002; Ravichandran et al. 2003), may also cause acute scrotal pain. Anatomically, anomalous attachment of the epididymis to the testis or the presence of a long and tortuous epididymis with a long mesorchium may be the predisposing factors (Dibilio et al. 2006). In a recent case report by Dibilio et al. (2006) epididymis which was found attached to the testis at the level of the head only was surgically found to be twisted on its pedicle. On US, a normal testis with a normal vascular flow, a markedly enlarged, heterogeneous epididymis with only a few or no vascular signals and a highly vascularized epididymal head with whirling appearence of the vessels can be detected (Dibilio et al. 2006). Notably, the aforementioned predisposing anomalies are more common in patients with undescended testes compared to the normal population.

## 7 Torsion of Appendages

Torsion of appendix testis and appendix epididymis can also cause acute scrotal pain and the clinical presentation may be similar to that of testicular

torsion. The classical physical examination finding is "blue dot" sign referring to a small, firm, and palpable nodule on the superior aspect of the testis with a bluish discoloration through the overlying skin (Skoglund et al. 1970). More than 90% of twisted appendices involve the appendix testis (Dogra et al. 2006).

On US, an appendix testis with spherical shape and size larger than 5 mm with no internal blood flow and increased periapendiceal vascular signals is suggestive of a torsion of appendix testis (Fig. 8) (Oyen 2002; Yang et al. 2005). The identification of an appendix testis larger than 5.6 mm strongly suggests torsion (Dogra et al. 2006). A torsed appendix may be either hypoechoic or hyperechoic relative to the testis or epididymis. The torsion of appendix testis or appendix epididymis is frequently accompanied by reactive hydrocele and skin thickening. Finally the main role of ultrasound in the torsion of testicular appendix is to rule out testicular torsion or epididymo-orchitis.

## 8 Conclusion

Ultrasound is the first step for the evaluation of patients with the clinical presentation of torsion of spermatic cord. Optimization of scan parameters for gray-scale, color and power Doppler ultrasound and pulsed Doppler US with spectral analysis is crucial for accuracy in making or success in excluding the diagnosis of the entity. Apart from the classical clinical and imaging features associated with complete torsion, various ultrasound findings implying atypical forms of the entity as partial (incomplete) testicular torsion or intermittent torsion should be considered during the management of the patients.

## References

Adivarekar PK, Bhagwat SS, Raghavan V et al (2005) Effect of Lomodex-MgSO(4) in the prevention of reperfusion injury following unilateral testicular torsion: an experimental study in rats. Pediatr Surg Int 21:184–190

Ameur A, Zarzur J, Albouzidi A et al (2003) Testicular infarction without torsion in cryptorchism. Prog Urol 13:321–323

Angell JC (1963) Torsion of the testicle. A plea for diagnosis. Lancet 1:19–21

Barada JH, Weingarten JL, Cromie WJ (1989) Testicular salvage and age-related delay in the presentation of testicular torsion. J Urol 142:746–748

Baud C, Veyrac C, Couture A et al (1998) Spiral twists of the spermatic cord: a reliable sign of testicular torsion. Pediatr Radiol 28:950–954

Cassar S, Bhatt S, Paltiel HJ et al (2008) Role of spectral Doppler sonography in the evaluation of partial testicular torsion. J Ultrasound Med 27:1629–1638

Dibilio D, Serafini G, Gandolofo N et al (2006) Ultrasonographic findings in isolated torsion of the epididymis. J Ultrasound Med 25:417–419

Dogra V (2003) Bell-clapper deformity. Am J Roentgenol 180:1176–1177

Dogra VS, Bhatt S (2004) Acute painful scrotum. Radiol Clin North Am 42:349–363

Dogra VS, Sessions A, Mevorach RA et al (2001) Reversal of diastolic plateau in partial testicular torsion. J Clin Ultrasound 29:105–108

Dogra VS, Bhatt S, Rubens DJ (2006) Sonographic evaluation of testicular torsion. Ultrasound Clin 1:55–66

Dogra VS, Gottlieb RH, Oka M et al (2003) Sonography of the scrotum. Radiology 227:18–36

Dogra VS, Rubens DJ, Gottlieb RH et al (2004) Torsion and beyond: new twists in spectral Doppler evaluation of the scrotum. J Ultrasound Med 23:1077–1085

Donohue RE, Utley WL (1978) Torsion of spermatic cord. Urology 11:184–190

Elert A, Hegele A, Olbert P et al (2002) Isolated epididymal torsion in dissociation of testis-epididymis. Urologe A 41:364–365

Favorito LA, Cavalcante AG, Costa WS (2004) Anatomic aspects of epididymis and tunica vaginalis in patients with testicular torsion. Int Braz J Urol 30:420–424

Fukuhara Y, Shiga Y, Omori Y et al (2005) Idiopathic testicular infarction: a case report. Hinyokika Kiyo 51:129–131

Hörmann M, Balassy C, Philipp MO et al (2004) Imaging of the scrotum in children. Eur Radiol 14:974–983

Kadish HA, Bolfe RG (1998) A retrospective review of pediatric patients with epididymitis, testicular torsion, and torsion of testicular appendages. Pediatrics 102:73–76

Kalfa N, Veyrac C, Baud C et al (2004) Ultrasonography of the spermatic cord in children with testicular torsion: impact on the surgical strategy. J Urol 172:1692–1695

Kamaledeen S, Surana R (2003) Intermittent testicular pain: fix the testes. BJU Int 91:406–408

Kass EJ, Lundak B (1997) The acute scrotum. Pediatr Clin North Am 44:1251–1266

Lin EP, Bhatt S, Rubens DJ et al (2007) Testicular torsion: twists and turns. Semin Ultrasound CT MRI 28:317–328

Mevorach RA, Lerner RM, Greenspan BS et al (1991) Color Doppler ultrasound compared to a radionuclide scanning of spermatic cord torsion in a canine model. J Urol 145:428–433

Middleton WD, Middleton MA, Dierks M et al (1997) Sonographic prediction of viability in testicular torsion: preliminary observations. J Ultrasound Med 16:23–27

Noske HD, Kraus SW, Altinkilic BM et al (1998) Historical milestones regarding torsion of the scrotal organs. J Urol 159:13–16

Nussbaum-Blask AR, Rushton HG (2006) Sonographic appearance of the epididymis in pediatric testicular torsion. Am J Roentgenol 187:1627–1635

Oyen RH (2002) Scrotal ultrasound. Eur Radiol 12:19–34

Prando D (2002) Torsion of the spermatic cord: sonographic diagnosis. Ultrasound Quart 18:41–57

Prando D (2009) Torsion of the spermatic cord: the main grayscale and Doppler sonographic signs. Abdom Imaging 34:648–661

Ravichandran A, Blades RA, Watson ME (2003) Torsion of the epididymis: a rare cause of acute scrotum. Int J Urol 10:556–557

Sanelli PC, Burke BJ, Lee L (1999) Color and spectral Doppler sonography of partial torsion of the spermatic cord. Am J Roentgenol 172:49–51

Schulsinger D, Glassberg K, Strashun A (1991) Intermittent torsion: association with horizontal lie of the testicle. J Urol 145:1053–1055

Siegel MJ (1997) The acute scrotum. Radiol Clin North Am 35:959–976

Skoglund RW, McRoberts JW, Ragde H (1970) Torsion of the spermatic cord: a review of the literature and an analysis of 70 new cases. J Urol 104:604–607

Turgut AT, Unsal A, Ozden E et al (2006) Unilateral idiopathic hydrocele has a substantial effect on the ipsilateral testicular geometry and resistivity indices. J Ultrasound Med 25:837–843

Turgut AT, Olçücüoğlu E, Turan C et al (2007) Preoperative ultrasonographic evaluation of testicular volume and blood flow in patients with inguinal hernias. J Ultrasound Med 26:1657–1666

van Dijk R, Karthaus HFM (1994) Ultrasonography of the spermatic cord in testicular torsion. Eur J Radiol 18:220–223

Vijayaraghavan SB (2006) Sonographic differential diagnosis of acute scrotum: real-time whirlpool sign, a key sign of torsion. J Ultrasound Med 25:563–574

Wilbert DM, Schaerfe CW, Stern WD et al (1993) Evaluation of the acute scrotum by color-coded Doppler ultrasonography. J Urol 149:1475–1477

Williamson RC (1976) Torsion of the testis and allied conditions. Br J Surg 63:465–476

Yang DM, Lim JW, Kim JE et al (2005) Torsed appendix testis: gray scale and color Doppler sonographic findings compared with normal appendix testis. J Ultrasound Med 24:87–91

# Imaging Acute Scrotal Pain in Adults-2: Inflammation and Other Disorders

Aarti Shah, Gordon G. Kooiman, and Paul S. Sidhu

## Contents

A. Shah · P. S. Sidhu (✉)
Department of Radiology, King's College Hospital, Denmark Hill, London, SE5 9RS, UK
e-mail: paulsidhu@nhs.net

G. G. Kooiman
Department of Surgery, King's College Hospital, Denmark Hill, London, SE5 9RS, UK

## Abstract

The commonest cause for acute scrotal pain in the adult patient is bacterial epididymitis, normally managed successfully with antibiotics, with complete resolution of symptoms. Ultrasonography in acute scrotal disorders provides a comprehensive and diagnostic overview, without recourse to any other imaging modalities. In acute epididymo-orchitis, inflammation of the epididymis is readily apparent as thickening and an increase in colour Doppler flow representing increased blood flow. The involvement of the testis with inflammation, orchitis, is also normally well identified with ultrasonography and atypical features identified with the addition of colour Doppler techniques. Complications arising from severe inflammatory change such as abscess formation, segmental infarction or pyocele may be seen with the addition of contrast, a useful technique. Other causes of acute scrotal pain such as tuberculosis, vasculitis and other rare conditions may be identified with ultrasonography, and the appropriate clinical management instituted. Conditions that arise outside the scrotum causing scrotal pain such as acute appendicitis, inguinal hernia and Fournier's gangrene have features that allow for a diagnosis using ultrasonography. This article describes all the features seen on ultrasonography that allow for a confident diagnosis.

## 1 Introduction

An acutely painful scrotum is a common presenting complaint for men of all ages. It is important to distinguish the surgical versus non-surgical causes of

M. Bertolotto and C. Trombetta (eds.), *Scrotal Pathology*, Medical Radiology. Diagnostic Imaging,
DOI: 10.1007/174_2011_179, © Springer-Verlag Berlin Heidelberg 2012

acute scrotal pain as the viability of the testis depends on timely clinical evaluation and imaging. Clinical evaluation can be limited by pain preventing palpation of the scrotum. Ultrasonography remains the imaging modality of choice for accurate imaging of acute scrotal pain as it is readily available and can be performed rapidly without any preparation of the patient. The commonest cause of acute scrotal pain in adults is epididymo-orchitis. The peak incidence of acute spermatic cord torsion lies between the ages of 14–16 years and gradually decreases with age but is uncommon beyond the fourth decade. Most episodes of epididymo-orchitis are managed by community based physicians and in clinics dealing with sexually transmitted diseases without recourse to imaging. Nevertheless, imaging is needed when there is uncertainty as to the cause of the scrotal pain—infection may be responsible, but other more unusual causes may be present. The present chapter examines inflammatory and less common causes of acute scrotal pain, excluding spermatic cord torsion, in the adult patient and details the imaging features.

## 2 What does the Urologist Require from Imaging?

Urologists are regularly called upon for advice or clinical assessment of patients with acute scrotal pain. In the clinical history, the age of the patient is relevant as well as details regarding the onset, severity and duration of symptoms. Sudden, severe pain, often waking the patient at night with associated nausea and vomiting, is more suggestive of spermatic cord torsion whereas a more gradual onset of pain, with rigors points towards infection. A recent history of mumps, urethritis, urinary tract infection, or scrotal trauma may prove relevant. Diabetes mellitus, granulomatous disease, immune compromise and rarely, a history of vasculitis or sarcoidosis are important conditions to be considered. A clinical history of chronic urinary retention, bladder outflow surgery or urethral catheterisation may also indicate an inflammatory aetiology of the scrotal pain. Physical examination of the abdomen and scrotum is often difficult in patients with acute scrotal pain but nevertheless, this must be carefully performed. The tail of the epididymis may be swollen in early epididymitis but this may also be present with early spermatic cord torsion.

Considerable scrotal swelling is usually present in epididymo-orchitis but is also seen with spermatic cord torsion due to oedema of the spermatic cord and testis. Ultrasonography is a useful extension of the physical examination and offers the Urologist a rapid and reliable tool in the differential diagnosis of epididymitis and spermatic cord torsion. The results of other investigations including a leucocytosis and raised C-reactive protein may help formulate a diagnosis as might urine microscopy and culture.

If spermatic cord torsion is suspected, the correct management is immediate surgical exploration. However, colour Doppler ultrasonography in experienced hands may confirm or refute the diagnosis, as long as it does not delay surgical management. When epididymo-orchitis is suspected, scrotal ultrasonography will usually confirm the diagnosis and provide reassurance for the patient. Baseline and repeat ultrasonography may be useful in monitoring the response of severe infections to antibiotic therapy and rule out abscess formation. A painful testicular lump or indeed a painful hydrocele suggestive of testicular malignancy with acute haemorrhage will, of course, warrant careful ultrasonography.

## 3 Epididymo-Orchitis

### 3.1 Clinical Aetiology

Epididymitis refers to the acute inflammation of the epididymis, usually secondary to ascending infection from the prostatic urethra and seminal vesicles, but can also occur from haematogenous spread. Epididymitis is the commonest cause of scrotal pain in adolescent boys and men over the age of 35 years. Involvement of the testis, orchitis, can occur in 20–40% of patients with epididymitis. Primary orchitis without involvement of the epididymis is rare but can be seen in mumps and HIV infection. In the patient with acute scrotal pain, it is useful to consider epididymitis and orchitis together under the umbrella term 'epididymo-orchitis' as most cases of orchitis occur secondary to local spread of an ipsilateral epididymitis. Furthermore, the clinical management does not rely upon differentiation between the two entities. The causative organism in epididymitis is usually bacterial and varies according to the age of the patient. In young sexually active males, sexually

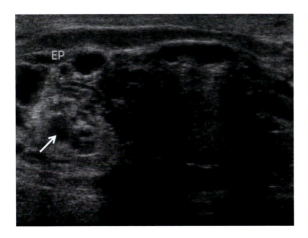

**Fig. 1** Scrotal infestation with *Wuchereria bancrofti*, causing epididymitis in filariasis, with dilated areas (*arrow*) infested with the parasite (*EP* epididymis) (courtesy of Dr. Mukund Joshi, Mumbai, India)

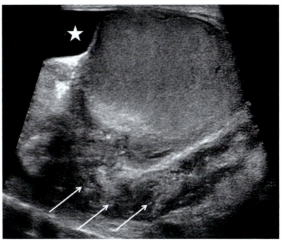

**Fig. 2** Acute epididymo-orchitis on gray-scale imaging mainly affecting the epididymal tail (*arrows*) which is thickened and heterogenous in appearance, with a small underlying hydrocele (*star*)

transmitted bacterial infection such as *Neisseria gonorrhoae* and *Chlamydia trachomatis* are most commonly responsible. Urinary tract infections caused by *Escherichia coli* and *Proteus mirabilis* are the underlying cause in young boys and elderly men. Less common causes of inflammatory change include brucellosis, tuberculosis and cryptococcosis (Bayram and Kervancioglu 1997; Muttarak et al. 2001). Parasitic infections that may lead to epididymitis such as filariasis are only seen in the endemic areas of Africa, Asia and South America, with the causative organism usually *Wuchereria bancrofti* (Fig. 1). Non-infectious causes include sarcoidosis, trauma, autoimmune conditions (e.g. Behcet's disease) and inflammation secondary to the administration of pharmaceutical drugs (e.g. amiodarone) (Toyoshima et al. 2000).

## 3.2 Clinical Presentation and Sonographic Technique

Classically, patients present with fever, dysuria and a tender, sometimes enlarged scrotum. On clinical examination, scrotal elevation can relieve the pain caused by acute epididymo-orchitis but not pain caused by testicular torsion, a finding called Prehn's sign. In most cases however, differentiation between torsion and epididymo-orchitis is clinically difficult. The classical finding in acute spermatic cord torsion is to palpate the affected testis lying in an elevated

horizontal position, a difficult sign to elicit in the presence of acute pain.

Ultrasonography is the primary imaging modality used to resolve this clinical dilemma in the acute setting. Routine examination involves imaging both testes in at least two planes using a broadband high frequency linear transducer (ideally up to 10 MHz). It is best practice to image the asymptomatic side first in order to familiarise the patient with the process, obtain an impression of the normal appearances for the patient and then proceed to the symptomatic side. In acute epididymitis, initial imaging will indicate that the testis on the affected side lies in its normal position in distinction with acute spermatic cord torsion, where the testis may be high riding with a more transverse orientation.

## 3.3 Gray-Scale Sonographic Appearances

On gray-scale ultrasonography imaging of acute epididymitis, the epididymis is enlarged with the tail usually affected first (Fig. 2). The epididymis may appear focally or diffusely affected and a spectrum of echogenicity is seen depending upon the timing of evolution of symptoms. There may be a separation of the layers of the scrotal wall by oedema. A reactive hydrocele may be initially present with thickening of the overlying skin. Over time, a complex septation within a hydrocele can develop (Fig. 3).

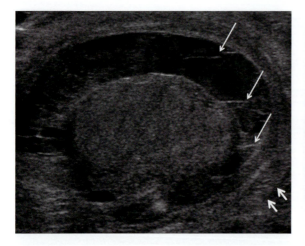

**Fig. 3** Severe acute epididymo-orchitis with thickening of the scrotal skin (*short arrows*) and a septated hydrocele (*long arrows*)

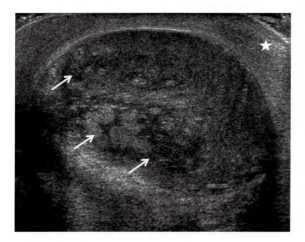

**Fig. 4** Severe acute epididymo-orchitis with thickening of the scrotal skin (*star*) and focal areas mixed reflectivity (*arrows*) indicating areas of infection and orchitis

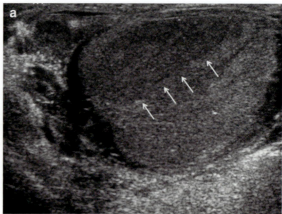

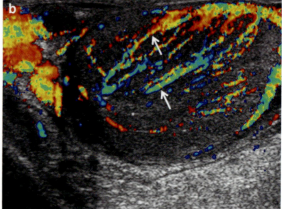

**Fig. 5** Patient with acute epididymo-orchitis mimicking a focal tumour. **a** A focal area of low reflectivity (*arrows*) at the upper aspect of the right testis. **b** The pattern of vascular distribution on colour Doppler ultrasound demonstrates a linear pattern (*arrows*) in keeping with the hyperaemia associated with inflammation

Similarly, within the testis, there is swelling and diffuse low reflectivity which may later evolve to increasingly well defined, patchy areas of low reflectivity (Cook and Dewbury 2000) (Fig. 4). The testicular hilum is the predominant site of infective change with focal hypoechoic areas which may mimic a testicular tumour (Fig. 5). Follow up is important in these patients with focal orchitis to ensure resolution.

## 3.4 Colour Doppler Sonographic Appearances

The gray-scale sonographic findings of acute epididymo-orchitis can be rather non-specific and may even appear normal, despite the presence of inflammation. The ability to demonstrate the presence or absence of blood flow within the testes using colour Doppler ultrasound is probably the single most useful factor in distinguishing the pathologies that cause acute scrotal pain (Fig. 6). Modern ultrasound machines have made demonstration of colour Doppler flow much more technically feasible. A study of 155 patients presenting with an acute scrotum showed that the sensitivity and specificity of physical examination in association with colour Doppler ultrasound was equal to 100% (Pepe et al. 2006). The use of colour Doppler ultrasound remains highly dependent on the expertise and technique of the operator. There are several Doppler parameters that an operator must bear in mind to achieve high quality Doppler examinations. In order

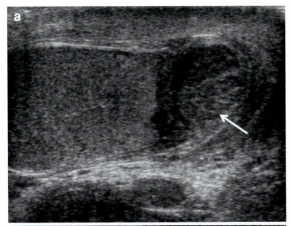

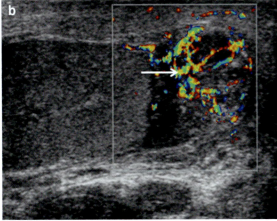

**Fig. 6** Patient with acute epididymal-orchitis. **a** Minimal changes on gray scale imaging of the epididymal tail (*arrow*). **b** There is increase in colour Doppler flow in the epididymal tail (*arrow*)

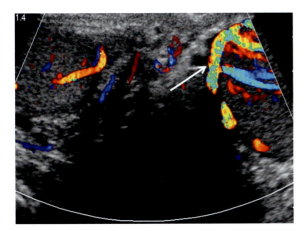

**Fig. 7** A 'spectacle' view of both testes in a transverse direction demonstrating increased colour Doppler flow to the left testis (*arrow*) affected by acute epididymo-orchitis

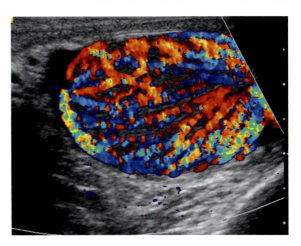

**Fig. 8** An exaggerated colour Doppler image of a patient with acute epididymo-orchitis demonstrating increased flow within the tunica vasculosa seen as lines of colour flow radiating from the mediastinum testis out to the periphery

to optimise detection of low velocity flow, the pulse repetition frequency (PRF) and filtration must be set low and a small colour sampling box should be used. The gain is increased until noise is seen and then reduced slightly. Comparison of the contralateral, asymptomatic side is essential to exclude technical reasons as the cause of absent flow and to allow the diagnosis of unilateral increased flow to be made. This is achieved by including both testes on the screen at the same time, with the Doppler box covering part of each of the testis in cross-section (Figs. 6, 7).

Once the identification of spermatic cord torsion has been excluded by the presence of intra-testicular blood flow, then a subjective assessment must be made as to whether there is hyperaemia of the testis or epididymis. Increased number and concentration of vessels on colour Doppler when compared with the normal side, indicate increased blood flow to the area of inflammation. Demonstration of increased blood flow on colour Doppler examination is an established method of diagnosing epididymo-orchitis (Horstman et al. 1991). Additionally, in the acute phase, increased flow within the tunica vasculosa can be seen as lines of colour flow radiating from the mediastinum testis out to the periphery (Fig. 8). It has been suggested that this can persist after resolution of the orchitis as linear low reflectivity lines that are referred to as 'septal accentuation' (Cook and Dewbury 2000). Whilst this appearance could be explained by chronic

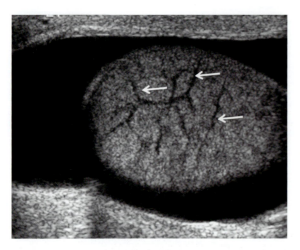

**Fig. 9** Resolution of the orchitis has left a hydrocele and linear low reflectivity lines (*arrows*) that are referred to as 'septal accentuation', and may also be a manifestation of an infiltrative process such as lymphoma or leukaemia

fibrosis secondary to an inflammatory process, in the absence of a relevant clinical history, a differential for a striated testicular pattern should include an infiltrative process such as lymphoma or leukaemia (Casalino and Kim 2002) (Fig. 9).

## 3.5 Limitations of Colour Doppler Ultrasonography

Increased colour flow does not always indicate a diagnosis of epididymo-orchitis. Firstly, reactive changes such as epididymal head enlargement and increased colour Doppler flow from torsion of a testicular appendix can mimic epididymitis. Although rare, this should be considered and excluded before the diagnosis of primary epididymitis can be made (Karmazyn et al. 2006). Secondly, testicular malignancies can also show increased colour Doppler flow (Horstman et al. 1992). The use of spectral Doppler ultrasonography with measurement of peak systolic and end-diastolic velocities before and after antibiotic treatment may be useful to differentiate orchitis from tumour, but is a cumbersome technique (Varsamidis et al. 2001). Thirdly, when the testis regains its blood supply following spontaneous detorsion, there is increased colour Doppler flow which could be misdiagnosed as orchitis (Oyen 2002). This is especially important to recognise as there is a risk of retorsion unless surgical fixation is performed. Similarly, a lack

of colour Doppler flow may not always represent torsion. For example, a very severe epididymo-orchitis can rarely cause inflammatory swelling of the spermatic cord that is sufficiently severe as to compress the vascular supply to the testis and lead to ischaemia (Eisner et al. 1991). These appearances can mistakenly be interpreted as suggestive of testicular torsion. Appearances similar to those of epididymo-orchitis can occasionally be seen with leukaemia, lymphoma, scrotal trauma and testicular metastases. It is important to correlate with the clinical context and follow up to resolution especially if the diagnosis is uncertain. In the younger patient with recurrent episodes of epididymitis, further evaluation with renal ultrasonography and voiding cystourethrography for associated anomalies of the urogenital tract is recommended. These include ectopic ureter to the seminal vesicles and lower urinary tract anomalies, such as recto-ureteral fistula and strictures of the urethra (Cappele et al. 2000).

## 3.6 Additional Imaging Techniques

### 3.6.1 Power Doppler Ultrasonography
Occasionally, epididymo-orchitis will have no grayscale sonographic abnormalities; hyperaemia may be the only positive finding. Power Doppler can be used to make detection of this easier. A study by Farriol et al. demonstrated a subjective increase in the number and length of vessels with power Doppler compared to colour Doppler (Farriol et al. 2000). Power Doppler is up to five times more sensitive for detection of blood flow than colour Doppler and is particularly good at registering relatively slow moving flow such as seen in the testes. Power Doppler is however susceptible to motion artefact and this must be considered to avoid false positive results.

### 3.6.2 Magnetic Resonance Imaging
With epididymo-orchitis, T2 weighted images show heterogeneous areas of low signal intensity. On T1 weighted images, the epididymis can appear enlarged and hyper-enhancing with administration of contrast. Orchitis may appear as heterogeneous testicular enhancement with hypo-intense bands (Kim et al. 2007).

### 3.6.3 Nuclear Medicine
Radionuclide imaging of the scrotum has been used accurately for differentiating ischaemia from infection

(Lutzker and Zuckier 1990). With increasing use of ultrasonography, experience with radionuclide imaging is decreasing and currently this examination is rarely performed in the acute setting.

## 3.7 Imaging Complications of Epididymo-Orchitis

Complications from untreated epididymo-orchitis include chronic hydrocele, abscess formation, haematoma, testicular infarction, chronic pain and infertility. Follow up ultrasonography is recommended to exclude these, especially where there is gray-scale change within the testis (Dogra et al. 2003).

### 3.7.1 Hydrocele

A hydrocele is defined as accumulation of fluid within the parietal and visceral layers of the tunica vaginalis. A small amount of 'physiological' fluid can be visualised in this space in over 80% of normal patients (Leung et al. 1984). A hydrocele is an uncommon cause of acute scrotal pain in isolation but reactive hydroceles are commonly seen with epididymo-orchitis and are sometimes painful, simply due to their mass effect. A hydrocele with internal echogenicity or septation implies that this may be long-standing, raising the possibility of an atypical infective aetiology such as tuberculosis (Muttarak et al. 2001), brucellosis (Ozturk et al. 2005) or a chronic granulomatous disorder such as sarcoidosis (Astudillo et al. 2004).

### 3.7.2 Abscess

An intra-testicular abscess can develop as a consequence of epididymo-orchitis and must be considered as a differential for epididymo-orchitis that is refractory to therapy. The ultrasonographic features of an intra-testicular abscess include a heterogeneous, usually hypoechoic, focal lesion with irregular margins (Fig. 10). An abscess may rupture into the scrotal sac and form a pyocele. Occasionally, it may be difficult to distinguish an abscess from a tumour. An abscess may also form in the epididymis (Fig. 11). An abscess, wherever it forms, requires careful clinical management and follow-up ultrasonography. Overlying skin changes with swelling is indicative of an infectious process rather than a malignant one.

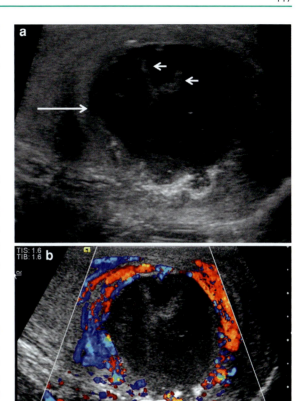

**Fig. 10** Patient with acute epididymo-orchitis not responding to therapy. **a** A focal low reflective lesion (*long arrow*) in the testis with evidence of septations (*short arrows*). **b** The colour Doppler image demonstrates absence of vascularity within the lesion and surrounding increased vascularity; hyperaemia surrounding an intra-testicular abscess

### 3.7.3 Infarction

Testicular infarction can be seen as a consequence of epididymo-orchitis due to severe inflammation resulting in obstruction to venous out-flow. This may be responsible for severe pain with sonographic appearances that may be difficult to interpret without a relevant clinical history (see Sect. 4).

## 3.8 Tuberculous Epididymo-Orchitis

Due to its indolent course, granulomatous disease presents very occasionally with symptoms of acute pain or a scrotal mass. Infectious causes include tuberculosis, syphilis, fungi and parasites. Approximately 30% of cases of extra-pulmonary tuberculosis

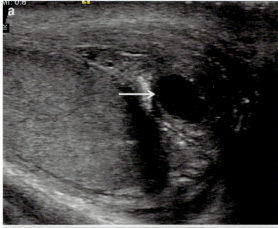

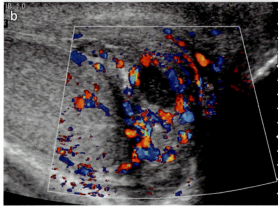

**Fig. 11** Hyperaemia surrounding an epididymal abscess. **a** A focal low reflective area (*arrow*) in the epididymis of a patient with acute epididymo-orchitis. **b** The colour Doppler image demonstrates absence of vascularity within the lesion and surrounding increased vascularity

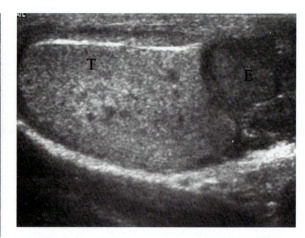

**Fig. 12** A 32-year-old man with a history of chest and renal tuberculosis presented with left scrotal enlargement. Sagittal image demonstrates nodular enlargement of the tail of epididymis (E) and multiple hypoechoic nodules in the testis (T); tuberculous epididymo-orchitis (courtesy of Dr. Malai Muttarak, Bangkok, Thailand)

involve the urogenital tract (Kim 2000). The kidney is the commonest site of involvement, and spread to the genitalia occurs in a small subset of patients. The disease usually develops in young males with initial involvement of the epididymis via haematogenous spread or direct extension from the prostate and seminal vesicles. The pathologic findings in tuberculous epididymo-orchitis are caseating necrosis, fibrosis and formation of granulation tissue. Over time, this may lead to abscess formation. Acute epididymo-orchitis secondary to tuberculosis is well recognised, but is more likely to present as a chronic disease. Clinically, unless there is a previous history of tuberculosis, it can be difficult to distinguish tuberculous epididymitis from bacterial epididymitis. The diagnosis may be suspected clinically when there is a failure to respond to conventional antibiotic therapy.

The following sonographic patterns of tuberculous epididymitis have been described (Muttarak et al. 2001) (Figs. 12, 13):

a. Diffusely enlarged heterogeneously hypoechoic tuberculous epididymitis,
b. Diffusely enlarged homogeneously hypoechoic tuberculous epididymitis,
c. Nodular, enlarged heterogeneously hypoechoic tuberculous epididymitis.

Orchitis, as with pyogenic epididymo-orchitis, occurs as a result of direct extension from the epididymis, and isolated involvement of the testis is rare. Similar descriptions to the ones used for epididymitis can be applied to the changes seen within the testis. Additionally, multiple small hypoechoic nodules have been described as the 'miliary appearance' and are characteristic of tuberculous orchitis (Drudi et al. 1997).

It has been suggested that certain gray-scale and colour Doppler findings may favour a diagnosis of tuberculous epididymo-orchitis, over that of bacterial epididymo-orchitis. Gray scale imaging, showing a heterogeneously hypoechoic pattern of epididymal enlargement with concomitant hypoechoic lesions in the testis is likely to represent tuberculous disease (Chung et al. 1997). Diffusely increased colour Doppler flow is seen in bacterial epididymitis whereas with tuberculous disease, the colour Doppler flow increase is more focal in nature and is usually located peripherally within the epididymis (Yang et al. 2000).

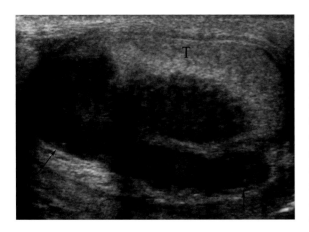

**Fig. 13** A 59-year-old man presented with right scrotal pain and enlargement. Sagittal image shows nodular enlargement of the head and body of epididymis (*arrows*) and a hypoechoic mass in the testis (T); tuberculous epididymo-orchitis (courtesy of Dr. Malai Muttarak, Bangkok, Thailand)

Other features that support the diagnosis of scrotal tuberculosis include scrotal skin thickening, abscesses, sinus tracts and calcifications. Abscess formation as a consequence of tuberculous infection has similar gray-scale appearances to pyogenic abscesses in that both are heterogeneously hypoechoic with an absence of blood flow on colour Doppler (Yang et al. 2000). Differentiation between the two types of abscess is clinically relevant because a pyogenic abscess will resolve with antibacterial therapy, whereas a tuberculous one may require surgical management. Studies have shown the size of the abscess and pattern of blood flow as being useful, in making this distinction (Yang et al. 2001). The tuberculous epididymal abscess is larger than pyogenic epididymal abscess and a possible explanation for this finding could be the more chronic duration in the former. Also, colour Doppler reveals a subjective decrease in peripheral flow of a tuberculous abscess, when compared with pyogenic.

## 4 Testicular Infarction

Global testicular infarction can be seen as a result of torsion of the spermatic cord, severe epididymo-orchitis or trauma (Sidhu 1999). On gray-scale ultrasonography, in the acute stage, the testis appears enlarged and hypoechoic. Over time, there is a decrease in size and increase in reflectivity. Colour Doppler ultrasound reveals poor or absent flow.

Segmental testicular infarction is an uncommon cause of acute scrotal pain in adult men. It is usually diagnosed following full (Costa et al. 1999) or partial (Ruibal et al. 2003) orchidectomy. Factors associated with this entity include epididymo-orchitis (Bird and Rosenfield 1984), trauma, haematological disorders such as polycythemia and sickle cell disease (Gofrit et al. 1998), vasculitides such as hypersensitivity angiitis (Baer et al. 1989) and polyarteritis nodosa (Braeckman et al. 2002) as well as previous scrotal or inguinal surgery. Segmental testicular infarction has also been described secondary to the bell-clapper deformity, an anatomical anomaly that allows excessive testicular mobility, thus making the testis vulnerable to torsion (Ledwidge et al. 2002). In most cases however, the aetiology is described as idiopathic, with no underlying cause found. Most patients present with acute scrotal pain but there may be a history of recurrent pain. In severe epididymo-orchitis, the mechanism for an area of infarction in the testis, often segmental in distribution, is compromise to the venous drainage of the testis caused by the oedema of inflammatory change.

The gray-scale ultrasound appearances of segmental infarction are variable – a focal area of low reflectivity is the usual finding but high reflectivity areas have also been documented (Bilagi et al. 2007). These differences may reflect whether the infarction is ischaemic (low reflectivity) or haemorrhagic (high reflectivity) in nature. Studies differ on the commonest location of the infarction within the testis. Some report a predilection for the upper or middle (Fernandez-Perez et al. 2005) whilst others show an equal distribution (Bilagi et al. 2007). Infarctions are usually wedge-shaped with the vertex orientated at the testicular mediastinum (Fig. 14). A similar pattern of wedge-shaped infarction can be seen in the spleen and kidney (Balcar et al. 1984). Rounded lesions, however, were not uncommon (Fig. 15). It is suggested that the shape of the infarcted lesion may be a feature of the type of ischaemic insult. In a round lesion, the venous drainage to the testis is compromised and in a wedge shaped lesion, the arterial (Bilagi et al. 2007). The appearance may resemble a focal testicular tumour (Sriprasad et al. 2001).

The most significant and universal finding is that of absent vascularity within the lesion on colour Doppler ultrasound based on comparison with both the vascularity of the surrounding testicular parenchyma of the

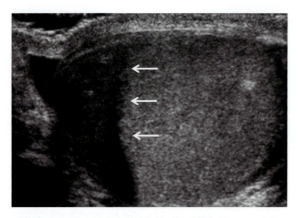

**Fig. 14** A wedge shaped area of low reflectivity (*arrows*) at the upper aspect of the testis in a patient with segmental infarction

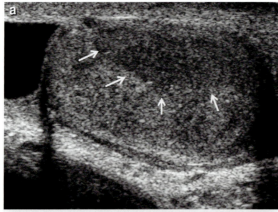

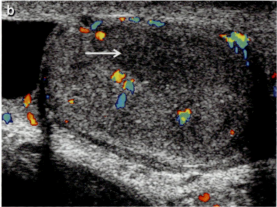

**Fig. 15** Segmental infarction. **a** The gray-scale image demonstrates a rounded low reflective area (*arrows*) at the upper aspect of the testis representing a segmental infarction. **b** The colour Doppler image demonstrates the absence of colour Doppler flow (*arrow*)

affected testis as well as the unaffected testis (Fig. 15). Making the differential diagnosis between segmental testicular infarction and testicular tumour is difficult (Kim et al. 2007). On gray-scale images, often, testicular tumours cannot be distinguished from benign aetiologies. This is especially the case with rounded, hypoechoic lesions that can occur as a result of infarction. Previously, the use of colour Doppler in tumours less than 1.6 cm was shown to have a limited role because they did not always demonstrate increased vascularity (Horstman et al. 1992). However, with improvements in colour Doppler sensitivity, flow can be identified in focal testicular lesions up to 5 mm in size (Sidhu et al. 2004). Certain patterns of colour Doppler flow are thought to be more suggestive of malignant disease for example, a 'criss–cross' pattern within a lesion (Bushby et al. 2001). Additional imaging such as MR may be used as an adjunct to ultrasonography when diagnostic uncertainty remains.

## 4.1 Other Imaging Modalities

### 4.1.1 MR Imaging

Segmental infarction is isointense to the testicular parenchyma on T1 weighted images and has variable signal intensity on T2 weighted images. Following administration of intravenous gadolinium chelate as contrast, an area of infarction appears as a focal avascular area with a bright rim. Haemorrhage within the lesion is seen as high signal intensity foci on T1 weighted images. Retraction of the tunica albuginea adjacent to the lesion can be seen and is thought to represent a more chronic picture (Fernandez-Perez et al. 2005).

### 4.1.2 Contrast-Enhanced Ultrasound

There is growing interest in the use of contrast-enhanced ultrasound (CEUS) in demonstrating areas of increased or decreased flow within the scrotum. A recent study failed to demonstrate any additional diagnostic benefit of CEUS over conventional studies using colour Doppler in the acute setting (Moschouris et al. 2009) but investigations by other groups shows promise (Shah et al. 2010). A possible role for CEUS could be when colour Doppler findings are equivocal, and to clearly demonstrate an area of non-perfusion (Fig. 16). The finding of a focal intra-testicular lesion that is avascular on colour Doppler should raise the possibility of segmental testicular infarction or an area

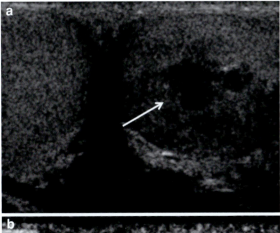

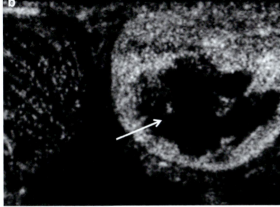

Fig. 16 Patient with severe pain and acute epididymo-ochitis. **a** Gray-scale ultrasound shows an irregular shaped, low reflective area (*arrow*) in the testis. **b** Following the administration of microbubble contrast, the focal area of low reflectivity demonstrates no enhancement (*arrow*) in keeping with an area of infarction secondary to venous impairment

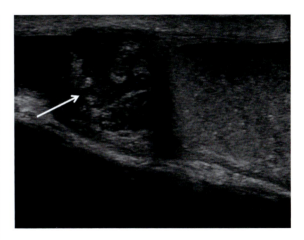

Fig. 17 A heterogeneous mainly low reflective epididymal head (*arrow*) in a patient with sarcoidoisis

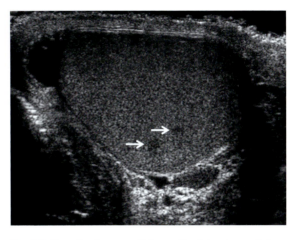

Fig. 18 Two focal areas of low reflectivity (*arrows*) in a patient with known sarcoidosis

of venous infarction for although this is thought to be a rare entity, its prevalence may be underestimated. Patients with negative tumour markers can be closely followed up. If the findings on ultrasonography remain static or are reduced, then a conservative approach to management, which spares the patient unnecessary surgery, can be safely adopted (Madaan et al. 2008).

# 5 Other Inflammatory Conditions

## 5.1 Testicular Sarcoidosis

Sarcoidosis is a chronic granulomatous disorder that may rarely involve the genital tract. It is usually asymptomatic but may present with acute scrotal pain

when the epididymis becomes enlarged. The sonographic findings are those of an enlarged, heterogeneous epididymis (Fig. 17) with multiple, usually bilateral, hypoechoic nodules (Woodward et al. 2003) (Fig. 18). MR imaging shows low signal intensity intra-testicular lesions on T2 weighted imaging that enhance after contrast administration (Kim et al. 2007).

## 5.2 Acute Appendicitis

The processes vaginalis represents an embryonic conduit between the abdomen and scrotum that would normally close in the first few years of life. If this remains patent then rarely, appendicitis can present as a scrotal mass (Satchithananda et al. 2000). The finding of an acute scrotum has been documented with ruptured and non-ruptured appendicitis. It can be detected as testicular inflammatory change or an abscess along with inflammatory change in the appendix on ultrasonography. Rarely, inguino-scrotal abscesses and epididymo-orchitis can develop following appendicectomy as an extra-abdominal postoperative complication (Bingol-Kologlu et al. 2006).

## 5.3 Strangulated Hernia

Incarcerated inguinal hernias can present as an acutely painful scrotum. The hernia is typically firm and tender, and is usually not reducible clinically. By definition, a strangulated hernia is one where the vascular supply to the herniated bowel is compromised leading to ischaemia and subsequent necrosis. Sonographic signs of incarcerated hernias include free fluid in the hernial sac, thickening of the wall of the herniated loop, fluid within the lumen of the herniated bowel and dilated bowel loops in the abdomen. Lack of peristalsis and absence of blood flow, if present, are clues to the potential diagnosis, but are not specific signs. This is because non-incarcerated bowel can show lack of peristalsis and the absence of blood flow seems to be a late sign indicating bowel necrosis (Rettenbacher et al. 2001). The sensitivity of CT for the detection of small bowel obstruction and in determining the location and cause of obstruction is well established (Frager et al. 1994).

## 5.4 Fournier's Gangrene

Fournier's gangrene is defined as a polymicrobial necrotising fasciitis of the scrotal wall and represents a surgical emergency due to the high associated mortality. Most cases have a perianal or colorectal focus and less often the spread originates from the urogenital tract (Rajan and Scharer 1998). The pathogens involved are usually anaerobic *Streptococci* in association with other bacteria such as *Proteus spp.*, *Escherichia coli, Staphylococcus aureus*, beta-haemolytic *Streptococci* and occasionally *Pseudomonas spp.*

The process begins as a localised cellulitis and progresses rapidly to involve deeper fascial planes.

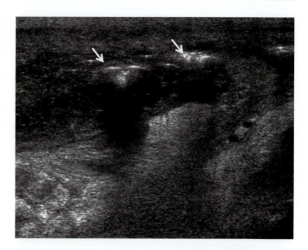

**Fig. 19** A patient with Fournier's gangrene demonstrates focal areas of high reflectivity (*arrows*) in the subcutaneous tissue representing gas formation

The spread of the organisms causes an obliterative endarteritis which eventually results in tissue necrosis. Plain radiographs may demonstrate the presence of soft tissue gas tracking along the involved tissue planes before it becomes clinically evident. The sonographic findings include a thickened, oedematous scrotal wall usually with the underlying testis spared. The hallmark on ultrasonography is the finding of subcutaneous gas which is the by-product of anaerobic metabolism of the organisms involved. This is demonstrated as numerous discrete, hyperechoic foci with posterior acoustic shadowing (Fig. 19). This can be differentiated from bowel gas within a scrotal hernia by the more superficial location of the locules of gas in necrotising fasciitis (Dogra et al. 1994).

Imaging with CT is useful for delineating the extent of involvement of the anterior abdominal wall, perineum and pelvis. It can locate the presence of abdominal, pelvic and retroperitoneal collections which may be secondary to the necrotising process or causing it. This allows the surgical management to be planned accordingly. CT appearances are those of soft-tissue thickening, stranding of fat around the areas of inflammation and low attenuation corresponding to area of subcutaneous gas (Rettenbacher et al. 2001).

## 5.5 Vasculitis

Very rarely, vasculitic disorders such as polyarteritis nodosa (PAN) and systemic lupus erythematosus

(SLE) can involve the testis (Fries et al. 1990). Testicular pain or tenderness is included in the American College of Rheumatology diagnostic criteria for PAN (Fries et al. 1990). The inflammatory reaction within the testicular arteries may lead to the absence of testicular blood flow on colour Doppler, mimicking torsion. It is in these patients with vasculitis, where blood flow is so slow that it is beyond the resolution of the Doppler to detect it, that CEUS could play a role in establishing perfusion of the testis (Moschouris et al. 2009). Henoch-Schonlein purpura is one of the most common systemic vasculitis in children and the reported incidence of scrotal involvement is between 2% and 38% (Clark and Kramer 1986). The clinical signs include swelling, discolouration and tenderness of the scrotum. As is the case of adult patients, the confirmation of testicular blood flow within the testis using colour Doppler sonography is essential to support the diagnosis of vasculitis and avoid surgical exploration for torsion.

## 5.6 Spontaneous Venous Thrombosis

Spontaneous thrombosis of the testicular vein can present as an acutely painful inguino-scrotal mass (Roach et al. 1985). Reports on this rare entity reveal that it can occur spontaneously or secondary to exercise, pampiniform ectasia or Henoch-Schonlein purpura. Sonographically it appears as a hypoechoic non-compressible mass with no blood flow and can mimic an incarcerated hernia.

## 5.7 Intra-Testicular Tumours

Although rare, testicular neoplasm should be considered in patients presenting with testicular pain (Wilson and Cooksey 2004). The pain may be secondary to haemorrhage into the tumour which is spontaneous or secondary to even minor trauma.

## 6 Conclusion

Ultrasonography with the use of colour Doppler, when performed sufficiently rapidly as to avoid delay in surgery, is vital to provide diagnostic information in the patient with acute scrotal pain. This assessment needs to be performed with good quality ultrasound equipment by an operator trained in optimising Doppler parameters to obtain high quality imaging. Diagnostic information obtained from urgent ultrasonography is invaluable for determining whether the management of the patient is surgical or conservative. Where there remains diagnostic uncertainty, MR imaging may have a limited role. Contrast-enhanced ultrasound is one of the newer techniques currently being evaluated.

## References

Astudillo L, Payoux P, Game X et al (2004) Bilateral testicular and epididymal involvement in sarcoidosis. Am J Med 116:646–647

Baer HM, Gerber WL, Kendall AR et al (1989) Segmental infarct of the testis due to hypersensitivity angiitis. J Urol 142:125–127

Balcar I, Seltzer SE, Davis S et al (1984) CT patterns of splenic infarction: a clinical and experimental study. Radiology 151:723–729

Bayram MM, Kervancioglu R (1997) Scrotal gray-scale and color Doppler sonographic findings in genitourinary brucellosis. J Clin Ultrasound 25:443–447

Bilagi P, Sriprasad S, Clarke JL et al (2007) Clinical and ultrasound features of segmental testicular infarction: six-year experience from a single centre. Eur Radiol 17: 2810–2818

Bingol-Kologlu M, Fedakar M, Yagmurlu A et al (2006) An exceptional complication following appendectomy: acute inguinal and scrotal suppuration. Int Urol Nephrol 38: 663–665

Bird K, Rosenfield AT (1984) Testicular infarction secondary to acute inflammatory disease: demonstration by B-scan ultrasound. Radiology 152:785–788

Braeckman P, Joniau S, Oyen R et al (2002) Polyarteritis nodosa mimicking a testis tumour: a case report and review of the literature. Cancer Imaging 2:96–98

Bushby L, Sriprasad SI, Sidhu PS (2001) Focal testicular abnormalities: evaluation of lesion vascularity using high frequency colour Doppler ultrasound. Eur J Ultrasound 13:S30

Cappele O, Liard A, Barret E et al (2000) Epididymitis in children: is further investigation necessary after the first episode? Eur Urol 38:627–630

Casalino DD, Kim R (2002) Clinical importance of a unilateral striated pattern seen on sonography of the testicle. AJR Am J Roentgenol 178:927–930

Chung JJ, Kim MJ, Lee T et al (1997) Sonographic findings in tuberculous epididymitis and epididymo-orchitis. J Clin Ultrasound 25:390–394

Clark WR, Kramer SA (1986) Henoch-Schonlein purpura and the acute scrotum. J Pediatr Surg 21:991–992

Cook JL, Dewbury K (2000) The changes seen on high-resolution ultrasound in orchitis. Clin Radiol 55:13–18

Costa M, Calleja R, Ball RY et al (1999) Segmental testicular infarction. BJU Int 83:525

Dogra VS, Smeltzer JS, Poblette J (1994) Sonographic diagnosis of Fournier's gangrene. J Clin Ultrasound 22:571–572

Dogra VS, Gottlieb RH, Oka M et al (2003) Sonography of the scrotum. Radiology 227:18–36

Drudi FM, Laghi A, Iannicelli E et al (1997) Tubercular epididymitis and orchitis: US patterns. Eur Radiol 7:1076–1078

Eisner DJ, Goldman SM, Petronis J et al (1991) Bilateral testicular infarction caused by epididymitis. AJR Am J Roentgenol 157:517–519

Farriol VG, Comella XP, Agromayor EG et al (2000) Gray-scale and power Doppler sonographic appearances of acute inflammatory diseases of the scrotum. J Clin Ultrasound 28:67–72

Fernandez-Perez GC, Tardaguila FM, Velasco M et al (2005) Radiologic findings of segmental testicular infarction. AJR Am J Roentgenol 184:1587–1593

Frager D, Medwid SW, Baer JW et al (1994) CT of small-bowel obstruction: value in establishing the diagnosis and determining the degree and cause. AJR Am J Roentgenol 162:37–41

Fries JF, Hunder GG, Bloch DA et al (1990) The American College of Rheumatology 1990 criteria for the classification of vasculitis. Summary. Arthritis Rheum 33:1135–1136

Gofrit ON, Rund D, Shapiro A et al (1998) Segmental testicular infarction due to sickle cell disease. J Urol 160:835–836

Horstman WG, Middleton WD, Melson GL et al (1991) Color Doppler US of the scrotum. Radiographics 11:941–957 discussion 958

Horstman WG, Melson GL, Middleton WD et al (1992) Testicular tumors: findings with color Doppler US. Radiology 185:733–737

Karmazyn B, Steinberg R, Livne P et al (2006) Duplex sonographic findings in children with torsion of the testicular appendages: overlap with epididymitis and epididymoorchitis. J Pediatr Surg 41:500–504

Kim SH (2000) Urogenital tuberculosis. In: Pollack HM, McClennan BL, Dyer R et al (eds) Clinical Urography, 1 edn. Saunders, Philadelphia, pp 1193–1228

Kim W, Rosen MA, Langer JE et al (2007) US MR imaging correlation in pathologic conditions of the scrotum. Radiographics 27:1239–1253

Ledwidge ME, Lee DK, Winter TC 3rd et al (2002) Sonographic diagnosis of superior hemispheric testicular infarction. AJR Am J Roentgenol 179:775–776

Leung ML, Gooding GA, Williams RD (1984) High-resolution sonography of scrotal contents in asymptomatic subjects. AJR Am J Roentgenol 143:161–164

Lutzker LG, Zuckier LS (1990) Testicular scanning and other applications of radionuclide imaging of the genital tract. Semin Nucl Med 20:159–188

Madaan S, Joniau S, Klockaerts K et al (2008) Segmental testicular infarction. Conservative management is feasible and safe: part 2. Eur Urol 53:656–658

Moschouris H, Stamatiou K, Lampropoulou E et al (2009) Imaging of the acute scrotum: is there a place for contrast-enhanced ultrasonography? Int Braz J Urol 35:692–702 discussion 695–702

Muttarak M, Peh WC, Lojanapiwat B et al (2001) Tuberculous epididymitis and epididymo-orchitis: sonographic appearances. AJR Am J Roentgenol 176:1459–1466

Oyen RH (2002) Scrotal ultrasound. Eur Radiol 12:19–34

Ozturk A, Ozturk E, Zeyrek F et al (2005) Comparison of brucella and non-specific epididymorchitis: gray scale and color Doppler ultrasonographic features. Eur J Radiol 56:256–262

Pepe P, Panella P, Pennisi M et al (2006) Does color Doppler sonography improve the clinical assessment of patients with acute scrotum? Eur J Radiol 60:120–124

Rajan DK, Scharer KA (1998) Radiology of Fournier's gangrene. AJR Am J Roentgenol 170:163–168

Rettenbacher T, Hollerweger A, Macheiner P et al (2001) Abdominal wall hernias: cross-sectional imaging signs of incarceration determined with sonography. AJR Am J Roentgenol 177:1061–1066

Roach R, Messing E, Starling J (1985) Spontaneous thrombosis of left spermatic vein: report of 2 cases. J Urol 134:369–370

Ruibal M, Quintana JL, Fernandez G et al (2003) Segmental testicular infarction. J Urol 170:187–188

Satchithananda K, Beese RC, Sidhu PS (2000) Acute appendicitis presenting with a testicular mass: ultrasound appearances. Br J Radiol 73:780–782

Shah A, Lung PF, Clarke JL et al (2010) Re: new ultrasound techniques for imaging of the indeterminate testicular lesion may avoid surgery completely. Clin Radiol 65:496–497

Sidhu PS (1999) Clinical and imaging features of testicular torsion: role of ultrasound. Clin Radiol 54:343–352

Sidhu PS, Sriprasad S, Bushby LH et al (2004) Impalpable testis cancer. BJU Int 93:888

Sriprasad S, Kooiman GG, Muir GH et al (2001) Acute segmental testicular infarction: differentiation from tumour using high frequency colour Doppler ultrasound. Br J Radiol 74:965–967

Toyoshima M, Chida K, Masuda M et al (2000) Testicular sarcoidosis. Nihon Kokyuki Gakkai Zasshi 38:63–66

Varsamidis K, Varsamidou E, Mavropoulos G (2001) Doppler ultrasonography in testicular tumors presenting with acute scrotal pain. Acta Radiol 42:230–233

Wilson JP, Cooksey G (2004) Testicular pain as the initial presentation of testicular neoplasms. Ann R Coll Surg Engl 86:284–288

Woodward PJ, Schwab CM, Sesterhenn IA (2003) From the archives of the AFIP: extratesticular scrotal masses: radiologic-pathologic correlation. Radiographics 23:215–240

Yang DM, Chang MS, Oh YH et al (2000) Chronic tuberculous epididymitis: color Doppler US findings with histopathologic correlation. Abdom Imaging 25:559–562

Yang DM, Yoon MH, Kim HS et al (2001) Comparison of tuberculous and pyogenic epididymal abscesses: clinical, gray-scale sonographic, and color Doppler sonographic features. AJR Am J Roentgenol 177:1131–1135

# Imaging Acute Scrotal Pain in Children

Brian D. Coley and Venkata R. Jayanthi

## Contents

**Abstract**

Acute scrotal pain in a child requires prompt clinical evaluation. When the etiology is unclear, ultrasound is the imaging modality of choice for further evaluation. Documenting testicular perfusion is essential, as this largely determines whether or not emergent surgery is needed. While many etiologies of acute scrotal pain are the same in children and adults, knowledge of entities unique to the pediatric population will help make more rapid and certain diagnoses.

## 1   Introduction

Acute scrotal pain requires prompt clinical evaluation and diagnosis to differentiate between surgical and non-surgical conditions. The differential diagnostic possibilities of scrotal pain in children depend upon the patient's age. In the neonate, the principle diagnoses are testicular torsion (pre- or post-natal), hernias, and hydroceles. In the older child, common diagnoses include testicular torsion, appendage testis or epididymis torsion, and epididymitis; less common conditions include hernias and hydroceles, vasculitis, idiopathic scrotal edema, trauma, and peritonitis. Testicular torsion is always the primary concern, as testicular salvage is related to the duration of torsion making prompt diagnosis crucial. Testicular torsion requires immediate surgical intervention, whereas the other causes of acute scrotal pain are typically managed medically.

While the rapidity of symptom onset, associated symptoms, and physical exam findings may suggest the diagnosis, imaging is often required (Kass and

B. D. Coley (✉)
Department of Radiology,
Nationwide Children's Hospital,
700 Children's Drive,
Columbus, OH 43205, USA
e-mail: brian.coley@nationwidechildrens.org

V. R. Jayanthi
Department of Pediatric Urology,
Nationwide Children's Hospital,
700 Children's Drive,
Columbus, OH 43205, USA

M. Bertolotto and C. Trombetta (eds.), *Scrotal Pathology*, Medical Radiology. Diagnostic Imaging,
DOI: 10.1007/174_2011_180, © Springer-Verlag Berlin Heidelberg 2012

Lundak 1997). Ultrasound with color Doppler has proven to be highly sensitive and specific in determining the causes of acute scrotal pain, and is the imaging modality of choice (Aso et al. 2005; Bhatt et al. 2006; Deurdulian et al. 2007; Dogra et al. 2003; Gronski and Hollman 1998; Karmazyn et al. 2005; Paltiel 2000; Prando 2002; Sung et al. 2006; Traubici et al. 2003; Weber et al. 2000; Coley and Siegel 2002; Karmazyn 2010; Baker et al. 2000; Kalfa et al. 2004; Lam et al. 2005; Pepe et al. 2006; Schalamon et al. 2006; Siegel 1997; Coley 2006).

## 2 Testicular Torsion and Infarction

### 2.1 Intravaginal Torsion

Testicular torsion (also referred to as spermatic cord torsion) has two incidence peaks, one perinatal and one peripubertal. Intravaginal torsion can occur at any age, but is most common in adolescents and young adults (Prando 2002; Arce et al. 2002; McAndrew et al. 2002). Intravaginal torsion can occur when the tunica vaginalis completely surrounds the testis and inserts high on the spermatic cord, preventing normal fixation of the testis to the scrotum. This is referred to the "bell and clapper" anomaly and allows the testis to rotate freely on its vascular pedicle (Prando 2002). Spermatic cord twisting results first in compromised venous outflow, and then arterial inflow, resulting in testicular ischemia and eventual infarction.

Patients present with abrupt onset of scrotal pain, often accompanied by nausea, vomiting, anorexia, and low-grade fever. Among children and adolescents presenting with acute scrotal pain, spermatic cord torsion is present in 5–31% (Karmazyn et al. 2005; Baker et al. 2000; Lam et al. 2005; Pepe et al. 2006; Schalamon et al. 2006; McAndrew et al. 2002). Nausea and vomiting are more common in testicular torsion than in other causes of acute pain, with a positive predictive value of over 96% (Jefferson et al. 1997).

If the history and physical exam strongly indicate testicular torsion, then surgery should be performed without the delay to perform imaging studies. However, the history may be unclear and the physical exam may be difficult to perform in an ill child. Physical exam findings include a tender testis, swelling, an abnormal transverse lie of the testis within the scrotum, erythema, and loss of the

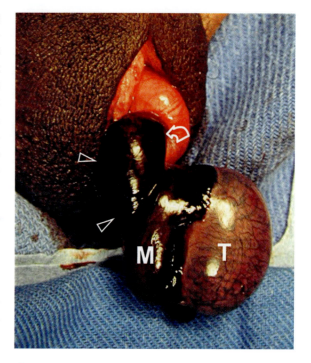

**Fig. 1** Testicular torsion. Intraoperative photograph of a teenager with over 12 h of left scrotal pain shows a twist of the spermatic cord (*curved arrow*) with infarction of the inferior cord (*arrowheads*). Note the paratesticular mass (*M*) comprised of infracted cord and epididymis, and the discolored and congestions testis (*T*). There was no improvement after untwisting the cord, and histology showed testicular hemorrhagic infarction

cremasteric reflex. The twisted spermatic cord may be felt posterior to the testis and may be confused for a congested, inflamed epididymis. Imaging should be used for those patients with unclear diagnoses, in whom torsion is unlikely and another diagnosis needs to be addressed, and in those with symptoms longer than 24 h when the chance of testicular salvage is remote and emergency surgery unwarranted.

The treatment for testicular torsion is immediate detorsion, fixation of the testis to the scrotal wall, and contralateral orchidopexy (Bolln et al. 2006). Manual detorsion can be performed and can restore testicular perfusion; however, this is only a temporizing measure since the underlying anatomic defect predisposing to torsion persists (Garel et al. 2000). Testicular salvage is directly related to the time from onset of symptoms with only 20% salvage after 12 h and virtually no salvage after 24 h (Fig. 1) (Siegel 1997). Non-viable testes are removed to prevent immune-mediated injury to the contralateral testis.

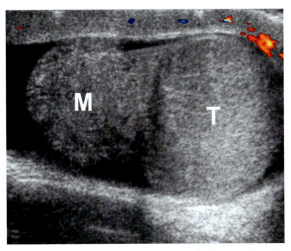

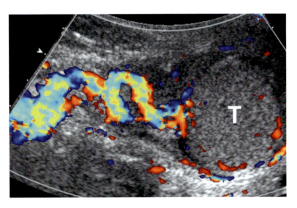

**Fig. 3** Testicular torsion and cord twist. Longitudinal color Doppler sonogram of the testis and cord in a teenager with acute pain shows flow within a tortuous and twisted spermatic cord, with no flow entering the testis (*T*)

**Fig. 2** Acute testicular torsion. Longitudinal color Doppler sonogram of the right scrotum in a 14-year-old with acute pain shows an abnormal orientation of the testis (*T*), a paratesticular mass of swollen epididymis and cord (*M*), and a small hydrocele. There is a flow seen in the scrotal soft tissues, but none in the testis. The testis was still viable at surgery

The sonographic appearance of testicular torsion depends upon the duration of ischemia. Acutely the testis may appear normal, but the testis is typically enlarged and hypoechoic due to edema; rarely will the torsed testis be hyperechoic (Paltiel 2000). As ischemia progresses and infarction begins to occur, the testis becomes progressively heterogeneous, which generally indicates non-viability (Dogra et al. 2003; Akin et al. 2004; Kaye et al. 2008; Middleton et al. 1997). The gray scale findings with testicular torsion are rarely normal. Common findings are an abnormal transverse position of the testis, a paratesticular "mass" from swollen spermatic cord and epididymis, a hydrocele, and sometimes scrotal skin thickening (Fig. 2) (Dogra et al. 2003; Karmazyn et al. 2005; Prando 2002; Karmazyn 2010; Kalfa et al. 2004; Arce et al. 2002; Baud et al. 1998; Dogra et al. 2004; Vijayaraghavan 2006; Blask and Rushton 2006). The actual twist of the spermatic cord may be visible (Fig. 3), and transverse imaging along the spermatic cord shows better the twist of the cord and spermatic vessels improving detection (Arce et al. 2002; Vijayaraghavan 2006).

While the gray scale findings in torsion are rarely normal, the diagnosis of acute testicular torsion requires demonstrating arterial blood flow to the asymptomatic testis, and absent or reduced arterial flow to the symptomatic testis (Fig. 4). The sensitivity

of color Doppler with current ultrasound equipment in the diagnosis of testicular torsion in most studies is over 95%, with technically adequate studies having a sensitivity of nearly 100% (Karmazyn et al. 2005; Paltiel 2000; Weber et al. 2000; Baker et al. 2000; Lam et al. 2005; Pepe et al. 2006). The negative predictive value of a normal ultrasound examination is from 97.5–100% (Weber et al. 2000; Lam et al. 2005). It must be remembered that the presence of Doppler flow in a painful testis does not exclude the diagnosis of torsion, and it is critical to compare the symmetry of flow between the two testes. Early, incomplete, or partial testicular torsion is not uncommon, and these testes may demonstrate arterial flow, although quantitatively diminished from the asymptomatic testis (Fig. 5) and often with diminished diastolic flow due to vascular congestion and increased impedance (Aso et al. 2005; Gronski and Hollman 1998; Prando 2002; Lam et al. 2005; Dogra et al. 2001).

A non-surgical painful testis must show hyperemia relative to the asymptomatic side; otherwise testicular torsion must still be considered. An exception to this is spontaneous detorsion, which results in increased blood flow to the testis and peritesticular tissues and can give the appearance of an inflammatory or infectious condition (Siegel 1997; Burks et al. 1990). Spontaneous detorsion is accompanied by a dramatic and marked relief of pain, which allows distinction between detorsion and inflammatory conditions. While a child with spontaneous detorsion does not require emergent surgery, patients are at risk for

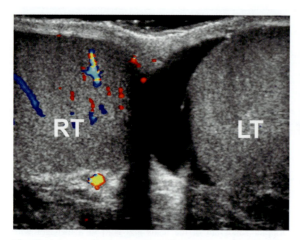

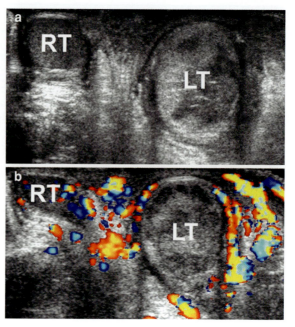

**Fig. 4** Acute testicular torsion. Transverse color Doppler sonogram of the scrotum in a 15-year-old with acute left sided pain shows an enlarged and slightly hypoechoic left testis (*LT*) with a small hydrocele. There is no blood flow to the left testis, with blood flow readily seen to the normal and asymptomatic right testis (*RT*)

**Fig. 6** Late testicular torsion. **a** Transverse sonogram of the scrotum in a 3-year-old with 5 days of left scrotal pain shows an enlarged and very heterogeneous left testis (*LT*) with surrounding soft tissue swelling. The right testis (*RT*) is normal. **b** Corresponding color Doppler sonogram shows flow to the normal right testis (*RT*). There is hyperemia around the infarcted left testis (*LT*), which shows no internal flow

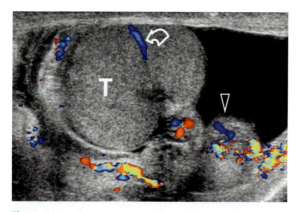

**Fig. 5** Incomplete testicular torsion. Longitudinal color Doppler sonogram of the left scrotum in a 12-year-old with acute pain shows an abnormal orientation of the testis (*T*) that lies superior to the epididymal head and cord (*arrowhead*). There is still arterial perfusion to the testis (*curved arrow*), which was viable at surgery

## 2.2 Extravaginal Torsion

Extravaginal torsion occurs in neonates because the tunica vaginalis is not yet fused to the overlying dartos muscle. This allows the testicle along with its surrounding hydrocele sac to twist spontaneously. Extravaginal torsion may occur post-natally, but is usually a pre-natal event, with the newborn presenting with a firm and discolored scrotum (Brown et al. 1990; Devesa et al. 1998; Groisman et al. 1996; Youssef et al. 2000; Chiang et al. 2007). While most commonly unilateral, bilateral extravaginal perinatal torsion does occur (Zinn et al. 1998), the testis is usually necrotic at birth; surgical salvage is rare. In utero extravaginal torsion is generally not considered a surgical emergency and it is not clear if surgery is required at all. Contralateral torsion is relatively rare, and it is controversial whether elective contralateral orchidopexy is necessary (Snyder and Diamond 2010). In the rare case where extravaginal torsion occurs post-natally or produces only partial ischemia, the testis may be viable and thus surgery warranted

recurrent torsion and should undergo orchidopexy (Siegel 1997; Burks et al. 1990).

Ultrasound findings become more marked in cases of late torsion (>24 h). The testis becomes more heterogeneous secondary to infarction, and color Doppler typically shows marked hyperemia of the scrotal wall and paratesticular soft tissues, but no flow within the testis (Fig. 6). If not removed, the torsed and infarcted testis will atrophy, usually becoming hyperechoic due to fibrosis or calcification.

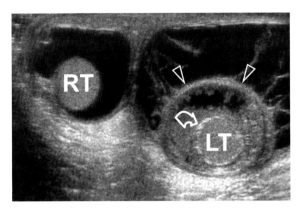

**Fig. 7** Perinatal torsion. Transverse sonogram of the scrotum in a newborn with left scrotal swelling shows a normal right testis (*RT*) with a small hydrocele. The left testis (*LT*) shows peripheral calcification in the tunica albuginea (*curved arrow*) indicating a more chronic torsion. The tunica vaginalis is seen (*arrowheads*) with edema and hemorrhage between it and the wall of the scrotum. There was normal color Doppler flow to the right testis and none to the left testis

(Zinn et al. 1998; Ahmed et al. 2008). Other diagnostic considerations of a swollen scrotum in a neonate include hydrocele, hernia, meconium periorchitis, intraperitoneal bleeding, and tumor.

Sonographic findings of extravaginal torsion vary depending on the duration of torsion. Recent torsion results in enlarged heterogeneous testis (Traubici et al. 2003; van der Sluijs et al. 2004). More chronically torsed testis may be normal sized, but are hypoechoic and begin to develop peripheral calcifications in the tunica albuginea (Traubici et al. 2003; van der Sluijs et al. 2004). Associated scrotal skin thickening and hydroceles are common (Fig. 7) (Traubici et al. 2003). Doppler signals are absent in the affected testis and in the spermatic cord. If not recognized at birth, the natural history of these testes is to atrophy and often calcify (Traubici et al. 2003). The contralateral testis may demonstrate compensatory hypertrophy, a finding seen in other cases of congenital monorchism (Koff 1991).

## 2.3 Other Causes of Infarction

### 2.3.1 Segmental Testicular Infarction

Infarction of only a portion of the testis is uncommon. Segmental infarction has been seen in association with spermatic cord torsion, sickle cell disease, vasculitis, polycythemia, and secondary to surgical complications (Fernandez-Perez et al. 2005). Patients may present with acute scrotal pain. Sonography shows a solid wedge-shaped avascular lesion that frequently has a vertex directed toward the mediastinum testis. Most segmental infarction occurs in the upper and middle thirds of the testis (Fernandez-Perez et al. 2005).

### 2.3.2 Miscellaneous Causes

In addition to torsion of the spermatic cord, other etiologies that may lead to complete or partial testicular infarction include epididymitis, orchitis, trauma, arteritis, and endocarditis. The appearance is similar to that seen in other causes of testicular torsion or ischemia.

Testicular ischemia can also result from extrinsic compression of the testis or spermatic cord, and has been reported with hernias (Turgut et al. 2007), hydroceles (Mihmanli et al. 2004; Turgut et al. 2006), and epididymitis (Akin et al. 2004).

## 3 Appendiceal torsion

Torsion of epididymal or testicular appendage is the most common cause of prepubertal acute scrotal pain, with an incidence of 26–67% in patients presenting to the emergency department, and a peak age incidence of 7–14 years (Aso et al. 2005; Lam et al. 2005; McAndrew et al. 2002; Campobasso et al. 1996; Sidler et al. 1997; Baldisserotto et al. 2005; Corbett and Simpson 2002). Most cases of prepubertal "epididymitis" are probably due to appendiceal torsion, as the imaging findings are similar and most children have no anatomic, functional, or infectious predisposition for true epididymitis. The appendages are embryologic remnants which tend to be pedunculated thus allowing them to twist (Aso et al. 2005; Yang et al. 2005). The appendix epididymis is present in about 25% of males, and the appendix testis is present in 92% (Coley 2006) and is thus the one more prone to torsion.

Patients with appendiceal torsion present with acute pain, but it is often of more gradual onset than patients with testicular torsion, and systemic symptoms are usually absent (Jefferson et al. 1997). On physical exam, tenderness may be diffuse, but is more often located to the superior aspect of the scrotum. The torsed appendage may be palpable as a firm

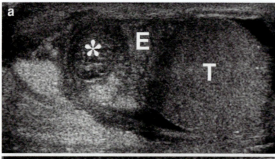

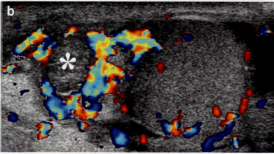

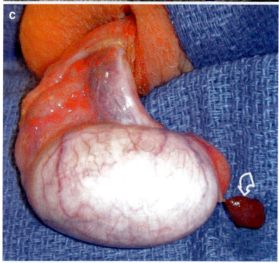

**Fig. 8** Appendiceal torsion. **a** Longitudinal sonogram in a 10-year-old boy shows an enlarged and echogenic epididymis (*E*) with a heterogeneous ovoid mass (*) representing a torsed appendage. The testis (*T*) is normal. **b** Corresponding color Doppler image shows tremendous hyperemia within the epididymis and normal testicular flow. The torsed appendage (*) is avascular. **c** Intraoperative photo in a different patient shows a torsed necrotic appendage (*curved arrow*) with hyperemia and swelling of the epididymis and testis

most cases resolving with conservative management (e.g. analgesics and scrotal support). The natural history is for the torsed appendage to atrophy and occasionally calcify and become a scrotal loose body; rarely will surgical resection be required for persistent pain.

Sonographic findings of appendiceal torsion are a small variably echogenic mass next to the superior testis or epididymal head (Baldisserotto et al. 2005; Yang et al. 2005). Normal appendages are small ovoid or triangular structures 3 mm or less in size, and are difficult to visualize in the absence of hydrocele fluid. Torsed appendages are usually 5 mm or larger in size, and often spherical (Baldisserotto et al. 2005; Yang et al. 2005). With careful examination, the detection of torsed appendages with ultrasound is nearly 90%. There is concomitant scrotal skin thickening, epididymal enlargement and heterogeneity, and often a reactive hydrocele (Baldisserotto et al. 2005; Yang et al. 2005; Monga et al. 1999). Color Doppler shows the torsed appendage to be avascular, but inciting tremendous hyperemia in the surrounding paratesticular soft tissues and epididymis (Fig. 8), and sometimes increased testicular blood flow as well (Baldisserotto et al. 2005; Yang et al. 2005). Later ultrasound findings will show a shrinking and increasingly echogenic appendage that may go on to calcify.

# 4 Epididymitis and Orchitis

## 4.1 Acute Epididymitis

The true incidence of acute epididymitis in children is uncertain due to studies employing varied diagnostic criteria, but probably accounts for between 6 and 47% of cases of acute scrotal pain (Lam et al. 2005; McAndrew et al. 2002; Campobasso et al. 1996; Sidler et al. 1997; Corbett and Simpson 2002). Epididymitis is most common after puberty. Many if not most prepubertal patients diagnosed with epididymitis (especially with negative urine cultures) actually represent cases of appendiceal torsion, as discussed above (Kass and Lundak 1997; Kadish and Bolte 1998).

Sexually transmitted organisms such as *Neisseria gonorrhoeae* and *Chlamydia trachomatis* are commonly present in older patients with epididymitis

paratesticular nodule, and a bluish discoloration through the scrotal skin seen ("blue dot sign"). This, however, is relatively rare; most boys will have a diffusely swollen and erythematous hemiscrotum. Appendiceal torsion is not a surgical emergency with

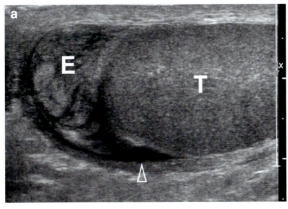

**Fig. 9** Epididymitis. **a** Longitudinal sonogram of the right scrotum in a teenager with pain and scrotal erythema shows an enlarged heterogeneous epididymis (*E*) and a normal testis (*T*). There is a small reactive hydrocele (*arrowhead*). **b** Corresponding color Doppler image shows increased epididymal flow without testicular hyperemia

(Akin et al. 2004). In younger boys urinary tract infections (especially with *Escherichia coli*) are more common, although urine cultures are positive in only 10–25% of cases of epididymitis (Lau et al. 1997). In younger patients non-infectious epididymitis may be secondary to anatomic congenital anomalies like an ectopic ureter draining into the vas deferens or seminal vesicles. Bladder outlet obstruction, whether functional or anatomic, can cause reflux of urine into the ejaculatory ducts and produce epididymitis even in the setting of sterile urine (Aso et al. 2005; Bukowski et al. 1995; Hudnall and Meservy 2004; Karmazyn et al. 2009). Epididymitis may also be secondary to trauma, and can be idiopathic (Gordon et al. 1996).

Clinically, patients with epididymitis typically have a more gradual onset of pain than other causes of the acute scrotum, and constitutional symptoms are less (Kass and Lundak 1997). Tenderness is often localized. Severe cases may have more diffuse tenderness and scrotal edema, and fever and pyuria may be present.

Sonography shows an enlarged epididymis that may be diffuse or focal, with the epididymal head most commonly involved (Aso et al. 2005; Akin et al. 2004). More diffuse and severe swelling is seen in children with anatomic abnormalities and in cases of recurrent epididymitis (Karmazyn et al. 2009). Epididymal echogenicity is usually decreased, but can be variable due to edema or hemorrhage (Fig. 9a) (Siegel 1997; Akin et al. 2004). Scrotal skin thickening and a reactive hydrocele are common associated findings (Aso et al. 2005; Sudakoff et al. 2002).

Color Doppler shows increased blood flow in the involved epididymis (Fig. 9b) compared with the asymptomatic side (Aso et al. 2005; Karmazyn et al. 2009), and provides confirmatory evidence of the gray scale findings. In 20% of patients with epididymitis, however, the gray scale appearance of the epididymis will be normal and the inflammatory process only revealed by color Doppler (Dogra et al. 2003). As with examination of the testes, comparison of the symptomatic to the asymptomatic side can be useful in determining whether abnormal flow is present.

## 4.2 Orchitis

### 4.2.1 Primary Orchitis

Primary orchitis is less common than that associated with secondary epididymo-orchitis; it is usually viral in origin. Orchitis secondary to mumps occurs in about 30% of infected postpubertal males, and is more common in underdeveloped countries with decreased immunization rates. Both testes are usually involved. Sonographically, the testes are enlarged, usually hypoechoic (although sometimes heterogeneous), and are hyperemic with color Doppler (Dogra et al. 2003; Tarantino et al. 2001). In one-third of patients, the epididymis is also enlarged and hyperemic (Tarantino et al. 2001). Testicular atrophy may result and later fertility is probably reduced (Masarani et al. 2006).

### 4.2.2 Secondary Orchitis

The most common cause of orchitis is secondary spread of inflammation from epididymitis, which occurs in approximately 20–40% of postpubertal cases (Dogra et al. 2003; Gronski and Hollman 1998; Kim et al. 2007). The testis is usually enlarged and tender, and is usually diffusely hypoechoic on sonography (Cook and Dewbury 2000). Focal lesions are less common, but may occur next to the inflamed epididymis. Color Doppler shows increased flow. Like with epididymitis, gray scale imaging is normal in up to 40% of patients, and the testicular inflammation is only detected with color Doppler (Dogra et al. 2003).

### 4.3 Complications of Epididymitis and Orchitis

Complications of epididymo-orchitis include testicular ischemia and infarction, scrotal and testicular abscess, and testicular atrophy (Cook and Dewbury 2000). Testicular ischemia occurs when an enlarged epididymis or edematous spermatic cord compresses spermatic vessels. The testicular artery may be directly compressed, but compression and compromise of the draining pampiniform venous plexus and lymphatics is probably more important in producing testicular ischemia (Sue et al. 1998). The sonographic findings are the same as those described for testicular torsion, including an enlarged, heterogeneous testis with decreased or absent color flow. Infarction may involve the entire testis, or be focal or multifocal, appearing as hyperechoic or hypoechoic lesions (Dogra et al. 2003; Cook and Dewbury 2000). With testicular abscess formation, ultrasound shows a hypoechoic or complex collection with low-level echoes. Color Doppler shows an avascular complex intratesticular mass with peripheral hypervascularity (Sudakoff et al. 2002). A pyocele can occur if the abscess breaks through the tunica vaginalis (Kim et al. 2007).

Scrotal abscess can result from spread from epididymitis or a testicular abscess, but can also result from secondary infection of hydroceles or hematoceles, or from extension of intraperitoneal infection into the scrotal sac via a patent process vaginalis (Dogra et al. 2003). Appendicitis is the most common cause (Bingol-Kologlu et al. 2006), but necrotizing enterocolitis and other intraabdominal infections can also be causes. Sonography shows a complex scrotal fluid collection with scrotal skin thickening and hyperemic soft tissues(Chung et al. 1999; Srinivasan and Darge 2009). The testis and epididymis may be difficult to see if displaced, but when imaged are often swollen and hyperemic (Chung et al. 1999; Srinivasan and Darge 2009).

## 5 Edema and Vasculitis

### 5.1 Idiopathic Scrotal Edema

Idiopathic scrotal edema produces unilateral or bilateral marked scrotal swelling, typically in patients less than 10 years of age (Klin et al. 2002). The cause is unknown, but it probably is a result of some kind of allergic reaction (Klin et al. 2002). On physical examination the affected scrotum is painful and diffusely edematous and erythematous (Klin et al. 2002). The scrotal contents are normal to palpation. Clinically the condition may resemble cellulitis or a reaction to an insect bite, but there is no skin break and no other sign of infection. At sonography, there is thickening and edema of the scrotal soft tissues with a mean wall thickness of over 11 mm (Fig. 10) (Klin et al. 2002; Lee et al. 2009). The testes and epididymes are normal (Grainger et al. 1998). Color Doppler shows increased flow along the echogenic striations in the edematous scrotum (Lee et al. 2009). Idiopathic scrotal edema resolves spontaneously over several days with symptomatic treatment and without consequence, although it may recur in up to 21% of patients (Klin et al. 2002).

### 5.2 Henoch-Schönlein Purpura

While polyarteritis nodosa is the most common vasculitis to involve the adult scrotum and testis, in children Henoch-Schönlein purpura is the most common, usually afflicting children less than ten years of age. Henoch-Schönlein purpura is a small vessel vasculitis that involves the skin, gastrointestinal tract and kidneys, and is generally preceded by an

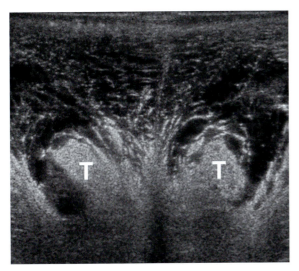

**Fig. 10** Idiopathic scrotal edema. Transverse sonogram of the scrotum in a 7-year-old with scrotal pain and swelling shows tremendous edema of the scrotal skin and soft tissues. The testes (*T*) were normal

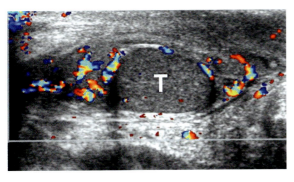

**Fig. 11** Henoch-Schönlein Purpura. Longitudinal color Doppler sonogram of the left scrotum in a 5-year-old with scrotal swelling and known Henoch-Schönlein purpura shows a normal testis (*T*) with hyperemia of the epididymal head and tail along with scrotal skin thickening

infection, especially Group A beta hemolytic streptococcus (Tizard and Hamilton-Ayres 2008). The scrotum is be involved in 15–38% of cases, and the clinical scenario is usually enough for diagnosis. Occasionally, scrotal disease may present before the disease is clinically apparent elsewhere, or scrotal pain may be sufficiently severe that imaging is warranted (Tizard and Hamilton-Ayres 2008; Ben-Sira and Laor 2000). At ultrasound, the testes are usually normal. The epididymes, however, are enlarged and heterogeneous and usually associated with scrotal skin thickening and a reactive hydrocele. Color Doppler imaging shows epididymal hyperemia with normal testicular flow (Fig. 11) (Ben-Sira and Laor 2000).

## 6  Trauma

Scrotal trauma is common in childhood, especially in adolescents. While there are many causes, approximately 50% of scrotal injuries are from athletic activity (Deurdulian et al. 2007; Dogra et al. 2003). Since the physical examination of the scrotum can be limited by pain and swelling, ultrasound is important to evaluate for hematocele, testicular hematoma, and the more serious testicular fracture and rupture.

A hematocele is a collection of blood between the layers of the tunica vaginalis, and is common after trauma to the scrotum. At ultrasound, acute hematoceles appear as complex fluid collections. As the hemorrhage organizes, septations form and the intervening fluid become less echogenic (See in Chapter Imaging scrotal lumps in children) (Deurdulian et al. 2007). Most hematoceles resorb, but chronic hematoceles can show scrotal wall thickening and internal calcifications (Sudakoff et al. 2002). Hematomas of the scrotal wall or peritasticular soft tissues can also occur, and will appear variably echogenic depending upon their age.

With sufficient force to the scrotum, a testicular hematoma may result. The importance of imaging is to document perfusion within the testis. Acutely, ultrasound shows an enlarged testis with the hematoma being heterogeneous but usually hyperechoic to surrounding testicular parenchyma (Deurdulian et al. 2007; Megremis et al. 2005). Like hematomas elsewhere, as the blood liquefies, the hematoma becomes septated and complex with more anechoic areas (Deurdulian et al. 2007; Megremis et al. 2005). Color Doppler should show a normally perfused testis except for focal areas of absent vascularity in the hematoma (Deurdulian et al. 2007; Megremis et al. 2005). Later imaging may reveal focal atrophy from resorption of injured non-viable parenchyma, or diffuse testicular atrophy from intra-tunica swelling and secondary ischemia (Cross et al. 1999).

With increasing force, a testicular fracture may occur. At sonography, testicular fracture appears as a hypoechoic band crossing the testicular parenchyma. The testicular contour remains smooth and well defined and the thin echogenic line of the tunica albuginea is intact. An associated hematocele is common. Doppler evaluation of the testis is essential. If perfusion to all

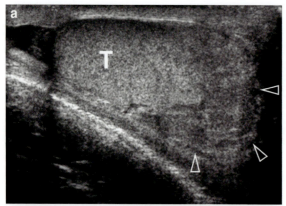

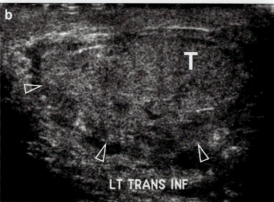

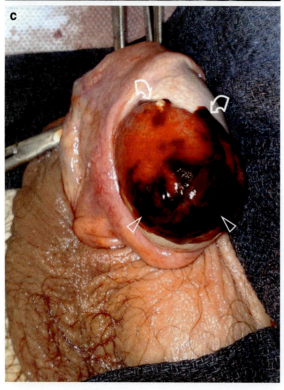

◀**Fig. 12** Testicular rupture. **a** Longitudinal sonogram of the left testis in a 14-year-old after a bicycle accident shows a normal superior testis (*T*), but inferiorly the parenchyma appears disorganized and the margins of the testis is ill defined (*arrowheads*). **b** Transverse sonogram inferiorly shows the lower portion of the testis (*T*), but without sharp borders. There is solid amorphous material appearing around the lower pole of the testis (*arrowheads*) indicating extrusion of testicular contents. **c** Intraoperative photograph shows the tear of the tunica albuginea (*curved arrows*) and the extruded intratesticular contents (*arrowheads*)

portions of the testis can be documented, then the testis should be viable and conservative treatment carried out. Areas without identifiable flow indicate ischemia and non-viability, which is an indication for emergent surgical exploration (Deurdulian et al. 2007; Buckley and McAninch 2006).

The most serious injury is testicular rupture, resulting from disruption of the tunica albuginea allowing extrusion of testicular contents into the scrotal sac. At ultrasound, the testicular parenchyma is often heterogeneous due to hemorrhage, the borders of the testis my be irregular and ill-defined, and the thin white line of the tunica albuginea is interrupted (Fig. 12) (Deurdulian et al. 2007; Buckley and McAninch 2006). Actual visualization of extruded intra-testicular contents may be difficult in the presence of a hematocele and scrotal wall hematoma. The accuracy of sonographic diagnosis ranges between 56 and 94% (Buckley and McAninch 2006; Bhatt and Dogra 2008; Herbener 1996). Doppler rarely demonstrates flow, but emergent surgery is indicated because more than 80% of ruptured testes can be saved with immediate surgery (Buckley and McAninch 2006; Bhatt and Dogra 2008), but less than 50% are salvaged if treatment is delayed (Deurdulian et al. 2007). Complications of delayed diagnosis include testicular necrosis, abscess, and loss of spermatogenesis (Siegel 1997; Buckley and McAninch 2006).

Penetrating scrotal trauma is uncommon in pediatrics. The role of sonography is the same as in blunt trauma: to identify the nature and extent of injury, to determine if the tunica albuginea is intact, and assess if there is blood flow to the testis (Deurdulian et al. 2007; Bhatt and Dogra 2008). Testicular rupture is not uncommon with penetrating injuries, and the salvage rate is much less (approximately 35%) (Cline et al. 1998) compared with blunt trauma.

# 7    Conclusion

When the history and physical exam findings do not allow a specific diagnosis in a boy with acute scrotal pain, ultrasound is the imaging modality of choice for further evaluation. Many of the entities causing scrotal pain in children are the same as adults, but some such as appendiceal torsion and idiopathic scrotal edema are generally limited to pediatric ages. Evaluating the relative flow to each testis, as well as correlating the imaging findings to the patient's current level of pain is essential to accurately determine surgical problems (complete torsion, incomplete torsion, detorsion) from non-surgical conditions (appendiceal torsion and inflammatory conditions).

# References

Ahmed SJ, Kaplan GW, DeCambre ME (2008) Perinatal testicular torsion: preoperative radiological findings and the argument for urgent surgical exploration. J Pediatr Surg 43:1563–1565

Akin EA, Khati NJ, Hill MC (2004) Ultrasound of the scrotum. Ultrasound Q 20:181–200

Arce JD, Cortes M, Vargas JC (2002) Sonographic diagnosis of acute spermatic cord torsion: rotation of the cord, a key to the diagnosis. Pediatr Radiol 32:485–491

Aso C, Enriquez G, Fite M et al (2005) Gray-scale and color Doppler sonography of scrotal disorders in children: an update. RadioGraphics 25:1197–1214

Baker L, Sigman D, Mathews R et al (2000) An analysis of clinical outcomes using color Doppler testicular ultrasound for testicular torsion. Pediatrics 105:604–607

Baldisserotto M, de Souza L, Pertence A et al (2005) Color Doppler sonography of normal and torsed testicular appendages in children. AJR 184:1287–1292

Baud C, Veyrac C, Couture A et al (1998) Spiral twist of the spermatic cord: a reliable sign of testicular torsion. Pediatr Radiol 28:950–954

Ben-Sira L, Laor T (2000) Severe scrotal pain in boys with Henoch-Schonlein purpura: incidence and sonography. Pediatr Radiol 30:125–128

Bhatt S, Dogra VS (2008) Role of US in testicular and scrotal trauma. RadioGraphics 28:1617–1629

Bhatt S, Rubens DJ, Dogra VS (2006) Sonography of benign intrascrotal lesions. Ultrasound Q 22:121–136

Bingol-Kologlu M, Fedakar M, Yagmurlu A et al (2006) An exceptional complication following appendectomy: acute inguinal and scrotal suppuration. Int Urol Nephrol 38:663–665

Blask ARN, Rushton HG (2006) Sonographic appearance of the epididymis in pediatric testicular torsion. AJR 187:1627–1635

Bolln C, Driver CP, Youngson G (2006) Operative management of testicular torsion: current practice within the UK and Ireland. J Pediatr Urol 2:190–193

Brown SM, Casillas VJ, Montalvo BM et al (1990) Intrauterine spermatic cord torsion in the newborn: sonographic and pathologic correlation. Radiology 177:755–757

Buckley JC, McAninch JW (2006) Use of ultrasonography for the diagnosis of testicular injuries in blunt scrotal trauma. J Urol 175:175–178

Bukowski TP, Lewis AG, Reeves D et al (1995) Epididymitis in older boys: dysfunctional voiding as an etiology. J Urol 154:762–765

Burks DD, Markey BJ, Burkhard TK et al (1990) Suspected testicular torsion and ischemia: evaluation with color Doppler sonography. Radiology 175:815–821

Campobasso P, Donadio P, Spata E et al (1996) Acute scrotum in pediatric age: analysis of 265 consecutive cases. Pediatr Med Chir 18:15–20

Chiang MC, Chen HW, Fu RH et al (2007) Clinical features of testicular torsion and epididymo-orchitis in infants younger than 3 months. J Pediatr Surg 42:1574–1577

Chung SE, Frush DP, Fordham LA (1999) Sonographic appearances of extratesticular fluid and fluid-containing scrotal masses in infants and children: clues to diagnosis. AJR 173:741–745

Cline KJ, Mata JA, Venable DD et al (1998) Penetrating trauma to the male external genitalia. J Trauma 44:492–494

Coley BD (2006) The acute pediatric scrotum. Ultrasound Clinics 1:485–496

Coley BD, Siegel MJ (2002) Male genital tract. In: Siegel MJ (ed) Pediatric Sonography, 3rd edn. Lippincott, Williams & Wilkins, Philadelphia, pp 579–624

Cook JL, Dewbury K (2000) The changes seen on high-resolution ultrasound in orchitis. Clin Radiol 55:13–18

Corbett HJ, Simpson ET (2002) Management of the acute scrotum in children. ANZ J Surg 72:226–228

Cross JJ, Berman LH, Elliott PG et al (1999) Scrotal trauma: a cause of testicular atrophy. Clin Radiol 54:317–320

Deurdulian C, Mittelstaedt CA, Chong WK et al (2007) US of acute scrotal trauma: optimal technique, imaging findings, and management. RadioGraphics 27:357–369

Devesa R, Munoz A, Torrents M et al (1998) Prenatal diagnosis of testicular torsion [see comments]. Ultrasound Obstet Gynecol 11:286–288

Dogra V, Sessions A, Mevorach R et al (2001) Reversal of diastolic plateau in partial testicular torsion. J Clin Ultrasound 29:105–108

Dogra V, Gottlieb R, Oka M et al (2003) Sonography of the scrotum. Radiology 227:18–36

Dogra VS, Rubens DJ, Gottlieb RH et al (2004) Torsion and beyond: new twists in spectral Doppler evaluation of the scrotumJ. J Ultrasound Med 23:107–1085

Fernandez-Perez GC, Tardaguila FM, Velasco M et al (2005) Radiological findings of segmental testicular infarction. AJR 184:1587–1593

Garel L, Dubois J, Azzie G et al (2000) Preoperative manual detorsion of the spermatic cord with Doppler ultrasound monitoring in patients with intravaginal acute testicular torsion. Pediatr Radiol 30:41–44

Gordon LM, Stein SM, Ralls PW (1996) Traumatic epididymitis: evaluation with color Doppler sonography. AJR 166:1323–1325

Grainger AJ, Hide IG, Elliott ST (1998) The ultrasound appearances of scrotal oedema. Eur J Ultrasound 8:33–37

Groisman GM, Nassrallah M, Bar-Maor JA (1996) Bilateral intra-uterine testicular torsion in a newborn. Br J Urol 78:800–801

Gronski M, Hollman AS (1998) The acute paediatric scrotum: the role of colour Doppler ultrasound. Eur J Radiol 26:183–193

Herbener TE (1996) Ultrasound in the assessment of the acute scrotum. J Clin Ultrasound 24:405–421

Hudnall TW, Meservy C (2004) Vas deferens ectopia: an uncommon finding. Pediatr Radiol 34:179

Jefferson RH, Perez LM, Joseph DB (1997) Critical analysis of the clinical presentation of acute scrotum: a 9-year experience at a single institution. J Urol 158:1198–1200

Kadish HA, Bolte RG (1998) A retrospective review of pediatric patients with epididymitis, testicular torsion, and torsion of testicular appendages. Pediatrics 102:73–76

Kalfa N, Veyrac C, Baud C et al (2004) Ultrasonography of the spermatic cord in children with testicular torsion: impact on the surgical strategy. J Urol 172:1692–1695

Karmazyn B (2010) Scrotal Ultrasound. Ultrasound Clinics 5:61–74

Karmazyn B, Steinberg R, Kornreich L et al (2005) Clinical and sonographic criteria of acute scrotum in children: a retrospective study of 172 boys. Pediatr Radiol 35:302–310

Karmazyn B, Kaefer M, Kauffman S et al. (2009) Imaging and urologic abnormalities associated with epididymitis in children. Pediatr Radiol (in press)

Kass EJ, Lundak B (1997) The acute scrotum. Pediatr Clin North Am 44:1251–1266

Kaye JD, Shapiro EY, Levitt SB et al (2008) Parenchymal echo texture predicts testicular salvage after torsion: potential impact on the need for emergent exploration. J Urol 180(4 Suppl):1733–1736

Kim W, Rosen MA, Langer JE et al (2007) US-MR imaging correlation in pathologic conditions of the scrotum. Radio-Graphics 27:1239–1253

Klin B, Lotan G, Efrati Y et al (2002) Acute idiopathic scrotal edema in children-revisited. J Pediatr Surg 37:1200–1202

Koff SA (1991) Does compensatory testicular enlargement predict monorchism? J Urol 146:632–633

Lam W, Yap T, Jacobsen A et al (2005) Colour Doppler ultrasonography replacing surgical exploration for acute scrotum: myth or reality? Pediatr Radiol 35:597–600

Lau P, Anderson PA, Giacomantonio JM et al (1997) Acute epididymitis in boys: are antibiotics indicated? Br J Urol 79:797–800

Lee A, Park SJ, Lee HK et al (2009) Acute idiopathic scrotal edema: ultrasonographic findings at an emergency unit. Eur Radiol (in press)

Masarani M, Wazait H, Dinneen M (2006) Mumps orchitis. J R Soc Med 99:573–575

McAndrew HF, Pemberton R, Kikiros CS et al (2002) The incidence and investigation of acute scrotal problems in children. Pediatr Surg Int 18:435–437

Megremis S, Michalakou M, Mattheakis M et al (2005) An unusual well-circumscribed intratesticular traumatic

hematoma: diagnosis and follow-up by sonography. J Ultrasound Med 24:547–550

Middleton WD, Middleton MA, Dierks M et al (1997) Sonographic prediction of viability in testicular torsion: preliminary observations. J Ultrasound Med 16:23–27 quiz 29–30

Mihmanli I, Kantarci F, Kulaksizoglu H et al (2004) Testicular size and vascular resistance before and after hydrocelectomy. AJR 183:1379–1385

Monga M, Scarpero HM, Ortenberg J (1999) Metachronous bilateral torsion of the testicular appendices. Int J Urol 6:589–591

Paltiel HJ (2000) Sonography of pediatric scrotal emergencies. Ultrasound Q 16:53–72

Pepe P, Panella P, Pennisi M et al (2006) Does color Doppler sonography improve the clinical assessment of patients with acute scrotum? Eur J Radiol 60:120–124

Prando D (2002) Torsion of the spermatic cord: sonographic diagnosis. Ultrasound Q 18:41–57

Schalamon J, Ainoedhofer H, Schleef J et al (2006) Management of acute scrotum in children-impact of Doppler ultrasound. J Pediatr Surg 41:1377–1380

Sidler D, Brown RA, Millar AJ et al (1997) A 25-year review of the acute scrotum in children. S Afr Med J 87:1696–1698

Siegel MJ (1997) The acute scrotum. Radiol Clin North Am 35:959–976

Snyder HM, Diamond DA (2010) In utero/neonatal torsion: obsevation versus prompt exploration. J Urol 183:1675–1677

Srinivasan AS, Darge K (2009) Neonatal scrotal abscess: a differential diagnostic challenge for the acute scrotum. Pediatr Radiol 39:91

Sudakoff G, Quiroz F, Karcaaltincaba M et al (2002) Scrotal ultrasonography with emphasis on the extratesticular space: anatomy, embryology, and pathology. Ultrasound Q 18:255–273

Sue SR, Pelucio M, Gibbs M (1998) Testicular infarction in a patient with epididymitis. Acad Emerg Med 5:1128–1130

Sung T, Riedlinger W, Diamond D et al (2006) Solid extratesticular masses in children: radiographic and pathologic correlation. AJR 186:483–490

Tarantino L, Giorgio A, de Stefano G et al (2001) Echo color Doppler findings in postpubertal mumps epididymo-orchitis. J Ultrasound Med 20:1189–1195

Tizard EJ, Hamilton-Ayres MJJ (2008) Henoch Schonlein purpura. Arch Dis Child Ed Pract 93:1–8

Traubici J, Daneman A, Navarro O et al (2003) Testicular torsion in neonates and infants: sonographic features in 30 patients. AJR 180:1143–1145

Turgut AT, Unsal A, Ozden E et al (2006) Unilateral idiopathic hydrocele has a substantial effect on the ipsilateral testicular geometry and resistivity indices. J Ultrasound Med 25:837–843

Turgut AT, Olcucuoglu E, Turan C et al (2007) Preoperative ultrasonographic evaluation of testicular volume and blood flow in patients with inguinal hernias. J Ultrasound Med 26:1657–1666

van der Sluijs JW, den Hollander JC, Lequin MH et al (2004) Prenatal testicular torsion: diagnosis and natural course. An ultrasonographic study. Eur Radiol 14:250–255

Vijayaraghavan SB (2006) Sonographic differential diagnosis of acute scrotum: real-time wirlpool sign, a key sign of torsion. J Ultrasound Med 25:563–574

Weber DM, Rosslein R, Fliegel C (2000) Color Doppler sonography in the diagnosis of acute scrotum in boys. Eur J Pediatr Surg 10:235–241

Yang DM, Lim JW, Kim JE et al (2005) Torsed appendix testis: gray scale and color Doppler sonographic findings compared with normal appendix testis. J Ultrasound Med 24:84–91

Youssef BA, Sammak BM, Al Shahed M (2000) Case Report. Pre-natally diagnosed testicular torsion ultrasonographic features. Clin Radiol 55:150–151

Zinn HL, Cohen HL, Horowitz M (1998) Testicular torsion in neonates: importance of power Doppler imaging. J Ultrasound Med 17:385–388

# Painless Scrotal Lumps: Classification and Clinics

Giacomo Novara, Massimo Iafrate, and Vincenzo Ficarra

## Contents

### Abstract

The discovery of a scrotal mass is frequently a source of great concern for patients, who usually assume that all masses are malignant. Fortunately, many palpable or suspected scrotal masses are actually benign. In this article the relevant clinical features of scrotal masses are described, with emphasis of clinical signs that allow differential diagnosis between testicular and extratesticular lesions, and aid in identifying specific pathological conditions. Prevalence, epidemiology, and management of the different pathologies will be discussed.

## 1    Introduction and Classification

All the scrotal structures (spermatic cord, epididymis, and testis) can be involved in a variety of pathologic conditions producing unilateral or bilateral scrotal swelling or masses due to the accumulation of fluids, growth of abnormal tissue, or inflammatory process of the normal contents of the scrotum.

Scrotal masses can be distinguished as painful or painless according to the different symptoms at diagnosis. The most frequent and important scrotal painful diseases are represented by post-traumatic haematoma, torsion of the spermatic cord, torsion of the appendix of epididymis, acute inflammation of the testicle and/or epididymis (acute orchitis and epididymitis) and scrotal abscess. Painful, scrotal lumps represent an emergency clinical situation defined as acute scrotum requiring a quick differential diagnosis and an appropriate treatment to preserve the testicle functions.

G. Novara · M. Iafrate · V. Ficarra (✉)
Department of Surgical and Oncological Sciences,
Urology Clinic, University of Padua,
Monoblocco Ospedaliero, IV Floor,
Via Giustiniani 2, 35128 Padua, Italy
e-mail: vincenzo.ficarra@unipd.it

M. Bertolotto and C. Trombetta (eds.), *Scrotal Pathology*, Medical Radiology. Diagnostic Imaging,
DOI: 10.1007/174_2011_181, © Springer-Verlag Berlin Heidelberg 2012

**Table 1** Painful and painless, non traumatic scrotal lumps

| Structures involved | Painful disease | Painless disease |
| --- | --- | --- |
| Testis | Orchytis | Tumor |
| | Torsion of appendix | |
| Epididymis | Epididymidis | Cystic masses |
| | Torsion of appendix | Solid masses |
| Spermatic cord | Torsion | Hydrocele |
| | | Varicocele |
| | | Lipoma |
| | | Inguinal hernia |
| | | Solid masses |

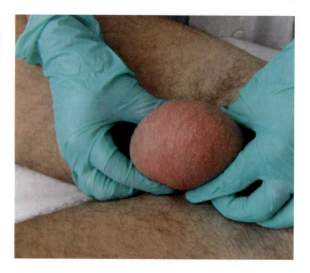

**Fig. 1** Physical examination of testis and epididymis in a patient with a left hydrocele

The most important and frequent painless scrotal lumps are represented by hydrocele, varicocele, and testicular tumors. Less frequent lesions, asymptomatic or associated with scrotal discomfort can be represented by epididymal solid tumors and cysts, spermatocele and lipoma of spermatic cord. Moreover a painless scrotal mass can be produced by non-urological disease as well as edema of the scrotal wall or inguinal hernia (Table 1).

## 2    Overall Clinical Evaluation

A combination of historical information and physical examination is helpful in differentiating some of the more confusing lesions. Usually, painless scrotal swelling may be incidentally detected by the patient while bathing or performing a self-examination or due to the presence of associated discomfort due to the mass dimension. The presence of an abnormal mass within the scrotum is best defined by careful palpation. This maneuver should be carried out in an orderly fashion starting from the testes, following with the epididymis, the cord structures and finally the external rings. Moreover, each structure should be palpated from side to side for detecting differences. All the scrotal structures should be palpated gently between the fingers tips of both hands (Fig. 1). The testes normally have a firm, rubbery consistency with a smooth surface. A firm or hard area within the testis should be considered a malignant tumor until proved otherwise. The epididymis should be palpable as a ridge posterior to each testis. Masses in the epididymis are almost always benign. For

this reason, during physical examination it is extremely important noting whether the mass arises from the testicle or from the epididymis. The spermatic cord is usually examined before with the patient in the standing position and then in supine position. This structure varies in thickness and often this depends on the presence or absence of lipoma of the cord. The physician should evaluate the presence or absence of enlarged venous structures that become more obvious as the patient performs a Valsalva maneuver (Fig. 2). Finally, the physical examination should take in consideration the palpation of the inguinal canal in standing position. Increasing intra-abdominal pressure by asking the patient to perform the Valsalva maneuver helps to define the presence of an inguinal hernia.

Independently by its origin, it is important defining the characteristics of the painless scrotal mass using a careful palpation. Specifically it is fundamental defining whether it is hard, firm, or cystic. Transillumination is helpful in determining whether scrotal masses are solid (tumor) or cystic (hydrocele, spermatocele). Any mass that radiates a reddish glow of light through the lesion represents a cystic, fluid-filled structure (Fig. 3). Occasionally also bowel in a hernia sac could result in a transilluminable mass. Vice versa, light is not transmitted through a solid tumor as well as in the presence of a hematoceles and varicoceles.

Ultrasound is an important procedure in the diagnosis of the painless scrotal lumps. This simple and inexpansive procedure offers superb imaging of

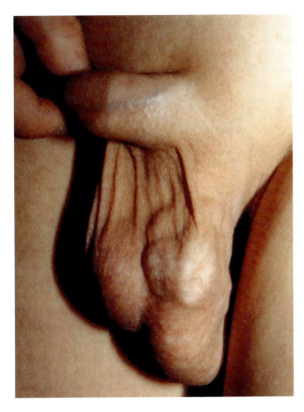

**Fig. 2** Visible (stage III) left varicocele that becomes more obvious as the patient performs a Valsalva maneuver

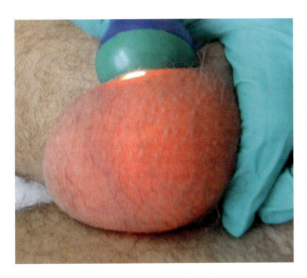

**Fig. 3** Transillumination of a left hydrocele

the scrotal contents and may be used to determine or confirm the cystic or solid aspect of the scrotal lumps and to differentiate intratesticular from extratesticular masses. Moreover, ultrasound should be considered useful above all when inflammatory or neoplasm of the testis or epididymis is associated with a secondary hydrocele that prevents an adequate scrotal palpation.

Color-flow Doppler is very helpful in the evaluation of patients with acute scrotal pain to distinguish inflammatory diseases from torsion of cord or infarction. However, this diagnostic procedure can be used also to confirm the diagnosis of varicocele in the context of painless scrotal swelling.

## 3 Hydrocele

Hydrocele is a collection of fluid between the tunica vaginalis and the testis. Although the most common form of hydrocele is localized surrounding the testis (hydrocele of the tunica vaginalis), this condition could be localized also within the spermatic cord (hydrocele of the cord). All hydroceles in infants and children result from persistence or delayed closure of the processus vaginalis. Simple hydroceles, in which the processus appears to be obliterated and fluid trapped within the tunica vaginalis of the scrotum, commonly seen at birth, are frequently bilateral, and may be quite large. They transilluminate and may appear quite tense but are not painful. No fluid is evident in the groin in most cases, but occasionally a large, simple hydrocele extends toward the internal inguinal ring. Most simple scrotal hydroceles found at birth deserve long-term observation, and most resolve during the first 2 years of life. The classic description of a communicating hydrocele is that of a hydrocele that vacillates in size, usually related to activity.

Most communicating hydroceles are smaller in the morning and become more prominent as the day progresses, enlarging in response to the upright position, activities that increase intra-abdominal pressure, and in many cases, fever. The scrotal swelling may be soft or tense, and it may change in consistency. In infants, the hydrocele sac may be thick or thin. Thin sacs frequently present a bluish hue through thin scrotal skin. Hydroceles easily transilluminate. Tense hydroceles may prohibit adequate palpation of the testis. Because most undescended testes are found at exploration to have an accompanying patent processus, it is important that a cryptorchid testis not be missed when assessing a child with a communicating hydrocele. Inguinal hernias represent the same anatomic defect that is seen in cases of communicating hydrocele. Small intestine, omentum, bladder, or genital contents may be found in the sac.

Communicating hydroceles are by definition congenital in origin. However, it is not uncommon for a communicating hydrocele to be manifested for the first time clinically in an older child or adolescent. In our experience, many of these late-onset communicating hydroceles are found to be omental hernias in which descent of a plug of omentum through the internal inguinal ring has caused a sudden increase in the amount of fluid in the scrotum. In some of these cases, a palpable thickening in the inguinal canal may suggest the presence of entrapped omentum.

One of the vagaries of closure of the processus vaginalis that may occur is segmental closure of the processus, which leaves a loculated hydrocele of the cord that may or may not communicate with the peritoneal cavity (communicating hydrocele of the cord). Hydrocele of the cord is usually manifested as a painless groin mass contiguous with the cord structures and located at any position from just above the testis to the inguinal canal. The mass is mobile and transilluminates. It may vacillate in size when communication with the peritoneal cavity is present. The differential diagnosis of inguinal masses also includes sarcomas of the cord and paratesticular tissues and inguinal hernia (especially with impacted omentum). Ultrasound may be helpful in determining the diagnosis (Fig. 4). Inguinal exploration of a hydrocele of the cord in most cases delineates a circumscribed, cystic mass connected to an obliterated or patent processus vaginalis. High ligation of a patent processus at the internal ring and excision or unroofing of the encysted hydrocele are curative.

An abdominoscrotal hydrocele is a rare clinical entity in which a large, bilobed hydrocele spans the internal inguinal ring; it consists of a large inguinoscrotal component and a large intra-abdominal component. It is thought that the abdominal component results from a large inguinoscrotal hydrocele that is separated from the peritoneal cavity by only a short obliterated segment at the internal ring. As fluid continues to accumulate, the hydrocele expands into the relatively low pressure of the abdominal cavity and forms the abdominal component (Gentile et al. 1998). The diagnosis is usually made on physical examination when a child with a large hydrocele has a

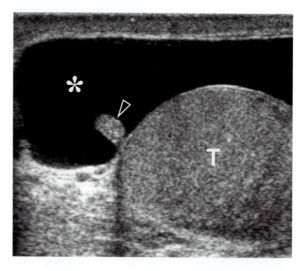

**Fig. 4** Uncomplicated hydrocele. Longitudinal ultrasound image showing a transonic collection (*) around an otherwise normally appearing testis (*T*). Arrowhead indicates an appendix testis

palpable abdominal mass. Pressure on the abdominal mass generally results in an increase in size of the scrotal hydrocele. Ultrasound examination is definitive. At inguinal exploration, it is important to remove the entire abdominal component, which is advanced into the wound as the proximal end of the sac is dissected. Failure to recognize the abdominal component is a cause of recurrence.

In adult patients, the hydrocele may develop rapidly secondary to local injury (e.g. after surgical treatment of varicocele), radiotherapy, acute nonspecific or tuberculous epididymitis, or orchitis. About 10% of testicular tumors present a reactive hydrocele. Chronic hydrocele is the most common condition, usually detected in men past the age of 40 years. This pathological condition can be bilateral. Usually, the patient presents with progressive swelling and local discomfort on the involved side of the scrotum. Pain can be referred only if hydrocele is accompanied by acute epididymal infection. The patient can require a treatment for its bulk or weight. Physical examination shows smooth, symmetrical enlargement of one side of the scrotum in which it is very difficult to feel the testis.

The diagnosis is made by finding a rounded cystic intrascrotal mass that is not tender unless underlying inflammatory disease is present. The mass transilluminates, and a tense hydrocele must be differentiated from tumor of testis, which does not transilluminate. However, in young men with idiopathic hydrocele, a careful ultrasound examination of the testes and epididymis should be done in order to rule out cancer or infection.

## 4 Varicocele

Many scrotal masses of unknown origin referred from primary care physicians are found to be varicoceles. A varicocele is a dilation of the scrotal portion of the pampiniform plexus and internal spermatic venous system primarily affecting the left side of the scrotum. It has been postulated that increased pressure in the left internal spermatic vein may result from compression of the left renal vein between the aorta and the superior mesenteric artery, which causes decreased drainage of the left internal spermatic vein (the "nutcracker effect"). This disease is found in about 10–15% of young men. The prevalence in infertile adult men reaches 30–40% of cases. More than 90% of cases are left sided. Increased venous pressure in the left renal vein, presence of collateral venous anastomoses, and incompetent valves of the internal spermatic vein were traditionally considered as the three primary factors inducing the varicocele formation (Fig. 5).

Two pathophysiological hypotheses can be drawn according to the morphological findings described in the different studies (Tilki et al. 2007; Iafrate et al. 2009; Bahren et al. 1983). The increase in the pressure within the spermatic veins would cause the mechanical distension of the venous wall and the release of endothelial mediators, which might cause the increase in the number of smooth muscle cells and the deposition of extracellular matrix, which could ultimately cause an alteration of blood flow and reflux (Tanji et al. 1999). The alterations in the complex muscle structure might be caused by hypoxia due to the reduction in the number of vasa vasorum. The presence of hypoxia within the internal spermatic veins of varicocele patients has been recently confirmed by Lee et al. (2006), who reported the overexpression of hypoxia-inducible factor-1alfa (HIF-1alfa). HIF-1alfa can stimulate the production of vascular endothelial growth factor (VEGF), platelet-derived growth factor (PDGF), and transforming growth factor-alpha (TGF-alpha) with the latter

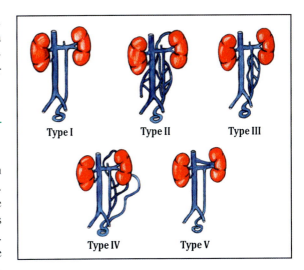

**Fig. 5** Barhen classification of varicocele (Bahren et al. 1983). *Type I*: single refluxing internal spermatic vein (40% of the cases); *Type II*: presence of several retroperitoneal veins, tributing to lumbar veins, retroaortic vein, and vena cava (22% of the cases); *Type III*: duplication of the spermatic vein into two parallel vessels with several cross-communications (21% of the cases); *Type IV*: collateral veins from renal and perirenal veins (13% of the cases); *Type V*: renal vein bifurcation, with pre- and retro-aortic branches (4% of the cases)

possibly being the main responsible for the increase in the fibrotic tissue of the venous wall in response to hypoxia. Further specific experimental studies are needed to confirm these hypotheses.

The presence of a varicocele is known to be associated with an adverse effect on spermatogenesis in a subset of men. The pathophysiology of this testicular dysfunction has been attributed to one or a combination of several mechanisms, including reflux of adrenal metabolites, hyperthermia, hypoxia, local testicular hormonal imbalance, and intratesticular hyperperfusion injury. The toxic effect of varicocele may be manifested as testicular growth failure, semen abnormalities, Leydig cell dysfunction, and histologic changes (tubular thickening, interstitial fibrosis, decreased spermatogenesis, maturation arrest).

Because adolescent varicocele is usually asymptomatic, many are discovered on routine physical examination performed for school entry, driver's license examination, or preseason sports participation. Sometimes, the varicocele may be incidentally detected by the patient while bathing or performing a self-examination or due to the presence of associated discomfort due to the mass dimensions above all after

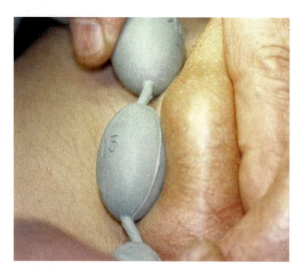

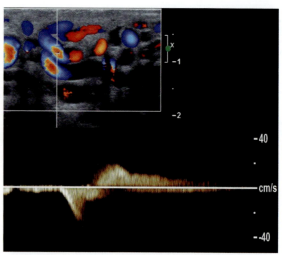

**Fig. 6** Examination of testicular volume by Prader orchidometer

**Fig. 7** Doppler interrogation of the left spermatic cord showing the presence of high grade reflux, with inversion of the blood flow

prolonged standing position or physical activity. Rarely, patients seek evaluation for a painful varicocele, usually one that is symptomatic with inguinal or scrotal aching discomfort that in many cases is relieved by assuming the supine position. The usually painless nature of this disease is explained by the fact that the majority of cases are diagnosed in adult age during the diagnostic protocol for infertility.

Physical examination should be carried out in a warm room with the patient in both the supine and standing positions and with and without a Valsalva maneuver. Failure to use the standing position or Valsalva maneuver may result in missing some cases of varicocele. A varicocele is a painless, compressible mass above and in some cases surrounding the testis. The classic description of the varices is the consistency of a "bag of worms" that decompresses when the patient is in the supine position. Varicoceles have been graded according to physical characteristics: grade I (small, palpable only with a Valsalva maneuver); grade II (moderately sized, easily palpable without a Valsalva maneuver); and grade III (large, visible through the scrotal skin) (Fig. 2). Bilateral varicoceles are palpable in less than 2% of males. If the varicocele does not decompress in supine position, the physician must suspect inferior vena cava or renal vein obstruction or retroperitoneal masses compressing the internal spermatic veins.

The physical examination must be completed above all in adolescent patient with an accurate assessment of testicular volume and consistency. The first parameter could be estimated using the Prader or disk orchidometer (Fig. 6). The volume of left testis can be compared with those of the controlateral testis with the aim to documenting the presence of hypotrophic process due to the varicocele. Clearly, a more detailed measurement of the testes can be obtained using the ultrasound examination. The evaluation of the testicular consistency is extremely subjective and less reproducible. Color-flow Doppler is a helpful examination to confirm the clinical features and to allow us the detection of subclinical, unpalpable varicocele (Fig. 7).

## 5 Testicular Tumors

Approximately 8,500 new cases related to testicular cancer are estimated to be reported in the United States in 2010 (Jemal et al. 2010). Considerable variability in the worldwide incidence of adult germ cell tumors (GCTs) does exist. The average annual age-adjusted rate is highest in Scandinavia (Denmark and Norway), Switzerland, Germany, and New Zealand; it is intermediate in the United States and Great Britain and low in Africa and Asia. Peak incidences of testicular tumors occur in late adolescence to early adulthood (20–40 years), in late adulthood (older than 60 years), and in infancy (0–10 years). Overall, the highest incidence is noted in young adult males, making these neoplasms the most common solid tumors of men aged 20–34 years and the second most common of men aged 35–40 years in the United States and Great Britain. Seminoma is rare before 10 years of age and after 60 years of age, but it is the most common histologic type overall, with a peak incidence between 35 and 39 years.

Spermatocytic seminoma (approximately 10% of all seminomas) occurs most often in patients older than 50 years. Embryonal carcinoma and teratocarcinoma occur predominantly between 25 and 35 years. Choriocarcinoma (1–2% of all GCTs) occurs more often in the 20–30-year age group. Yolk sac tumors are the predominant lesions of infancy and childhood but are frequently found in combination with other germ cell elements in young adults. Histologically benign, pure teratoma occurs most often in children but frequently appears in combination with other elements in adulthood. Malignant testicular lymphomas are predominantly tumors of men older than 50 years. 2–3% of testicular tumors are bilateral, occurring either simultaneously or successively.

The overall incidence rates of testicular tumors vary and have been tabulated as follows: seminoma, 30–60%; embryonal carcinoma in its pure form, 3–4%, although it is present in 40% of non-seminomatous GCTs; teratoma, 5–10%; and pure choriocarcinoma, 1%. Tumors of more than one histologic type are considered a separate entity and are also known as mixed GCTs; they make up approximately 60% of all GCTs (Mostofi 1973).

More recent epidemiologic studies have reported that the relative risk of testicular cancer in patients with cryptorchidism is 3–14 times the normal expected incidence (Henderson et al. 1979; Schottenfeld et al. 1980; Farrer et al. 1985). Between 5 and 10% of patients with a history of cryptorchidism develop malignancy in the contralateral, normally descended gonad.

Previous scrotal or testicle trauma, sex hormonal fluctuations and testicular atrophy are the most important acquired causes of the development of testicular tumors.

The usual presentation of a testicular tumor is a nodule or painless swelling of one gonad. This may be noted incidentally by the patient or by his sexual partner. The classic description is that of a lump, swelling, or hardness of the testis. 30–40% of patients may complain of a dull ache or a heavy sensation in the lower abdomen, anal area, or scrotum. In approximately 10% of patients, acute pain is the presenting symptom. Occasionally, patients with a previously small atrophic testis note enlargement. Acute onset of pain is rare unless there is associated epididymitis or bleeding within the tumor. In approximately 10% of patients, the presenting manifestations may be due to metastases and include a neck mass (supraclavicular lymph node metastasis); respiratory symptoms, such as cough or dyspnea (pulmonary metastasis); gastrointestinal disturbances, such as anorexia, nausea, vomiting, or hemorrhage (retroduodenal metastasis); lumbar back pain (bulky retroperitoneal disease involving the psoas muscle or nerve roots); bone pain (skeletal metastasis); central and peripheral nervous system manifestations (cerebral, spinal cord, or peripheral root involvement); or unilateral or bilateral lower-extremity swelling (iliac or caval venous obstruction or thrombosis). Gynecomastia, seen in about 5% of patients with testicular GCTs, may be regarded as a systemic endocrine manifestation of these neoplasms. Gynecomastia may or may not be associated with elevated levels of hCG, human chorionic somatomammotropin, prolactin, estrogens, or androgens. Relationships among gynecomastia, morphologic characteristics of the primary tumor, and endocrine abnormalities remain incompletely defined.

Physical examination of the testis is performed by bimanual examination of the scrotal contents, beginning with the normal contralateral testis. This provides a baseline and allows the examiner to note the relative size, contour, and consistency of the normal testis as well as the suspected gonad. Physical examination of the testis is performed by careful palpation of the testis between the thumb and the first two fingers of the examining hand. The normal testis is homogeneous in consistency, freely movable, and separable from the epididymis. Any firm, hard, or fixed area within the substance of the tunica albuginea should be considered suspicious until proved otherwise. Further examination of the suspected tumor should be directed toward possible involvement of the cord, scrotal investments, or skin. In general, seminoma tends to expand within the testis as a painless, rubbery enlargement. Embryonal carcinoma or

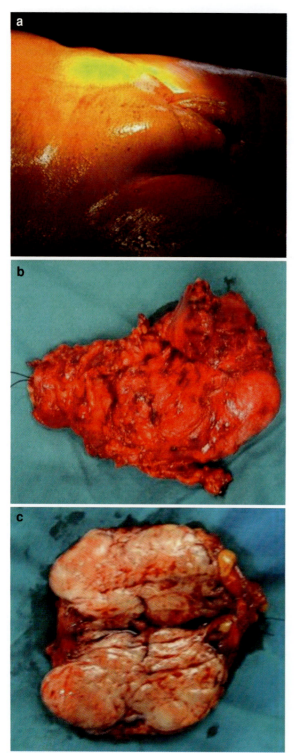

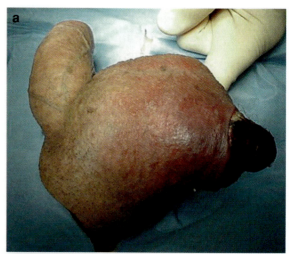

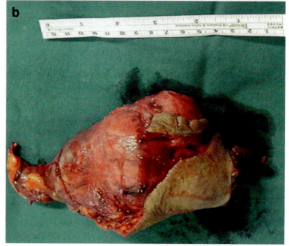

**Fig. 9** Rare case of a testicular tumor infiltrating the scrotal wall and emerging from the scrotal skin. **a** Findings at physical examination. **b** Corresponding surgical specimen

teratocarcinoma may produce an irregular, rather than discrete, mass, although this distinction is not always easily appreciated. Testicular tumors tend to remain ovoid, being limited by the tough investing tunica albuginea. In 10–15% of patients, spread to the epididymis or cord may occur. A hydrocele may be present and increase the difficulty of appreciation of a testicular neoplasm (Figs. 8 and 9).

Physical examination should also include palpation of the abdomen for evidence of nodal disease or visceral involvement. Routine assessment of the supraclavicular lymph nodes may reveal adenopathy in patients with advanced disease. Examination of the chest may disclose gynecomastia or the presence of respiratory tract involvement.

**Fig. 8** Large testis cancer presenting with an hard inguinoscrotal mass. **a** Findings at physical examination. **b, c** Macroscopic view of the intact **b** and bivalve **c** specimen

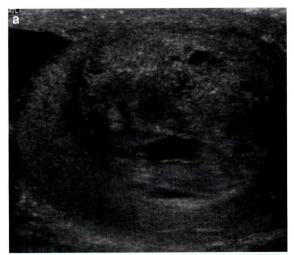

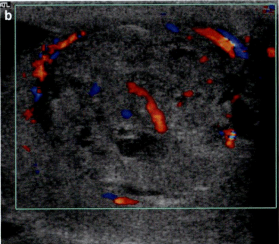

**Fig. 10** Testicular neoplasm. **a** Grey-scale longitudinal ultrasound view showing inhomogeneous, solid neoplasm. **b** Color Doppler interrogation of the testis showing intralesional blood flow

The differential diagnosis of a testicular mass includes testicular torsion, epididymitis, or epididymo-orchitis. Less common problems include hydrocele, hernia, hematoma, spermatocele, or syphilitic gumma. In any patient with a solid, firm, intratesticular mass, testicular cancer must be the considered diagnosis until proved otherwise. In patients in whom the diagnosis is unclear or in whom a hydrocele precludes adequate examination, imaging studies should be used as an important second step.

Ultrasonography of the scrotum is basically an extension of the physical examination. Any hypoechoic area within the tunica albuginea is markedly suspicious for testicular cancer (Fig. 10). Intrascrotal

fluid collection is no barrier to examination of the underlying testicular parenchyma by ultrasonography.

## 6 Epididymal Cyst and Spermatocele

Epididymal cysts are usually asymptomatic, and in adolescents they are often found on routine physical examination, in many cases a preparticipation sports-related examination. Increased awareness of the importance of testicular self-examination in adolescents has made self-discovery an important contribution to the diagnosis of spermatocele. Epididymal cysts are smooth, spherical, and in many cases located at the head of the epididymis. Although most cysts are small, on occasion a large cyst or one that has gradually enlarged is identified (Fig. 11). The cysts transilluminate.

Usually, physical examination is sufficient to differentiate an epididymal cyst from other scrotal pathology. Scrotal ultrasound has proved successful in the differential diagnosis of scrotal masses in children and adolescents (Finkelstein et al. 1986). Intervention for spermatocele is rarely indicated.

A spermatocele is a sperm-filled cyst of the epididymis. Although the cause is often unknown, it may be caused by obstruction of the epididymal ducts. It may occur anywhere in the epididymis but is more common in the caput region. It is exceedingly common, increasing in frequency with age, and identified incidentally in up to 30% of men undergoing high-resolution scrotal ultrasonography. A spermatocele is usually painless and does not obstruct the epididymal tubule from which it arises. Spermatocelectomy is indicated when the spermatocele is associated with unremitting pain or has grown to an uncomfortably large size. By definition, a spermatocele contains sperm. Puncture with a 30-gauge needle and identification of sperm in the aspirated fluid confirm the diagnosis.

## 7 Tumors of Testicular Adnexa

Most nontransilluminable epididymal masses are benign adenomatoid tumors. Malignant epididymal tumors are exceedingly rare (Siracusano et al. 1991).

Adenomatoid is the most common paratesticular tumor, accounting for approximately 30% of all paratesticular tumors. Most of these tumors occur in

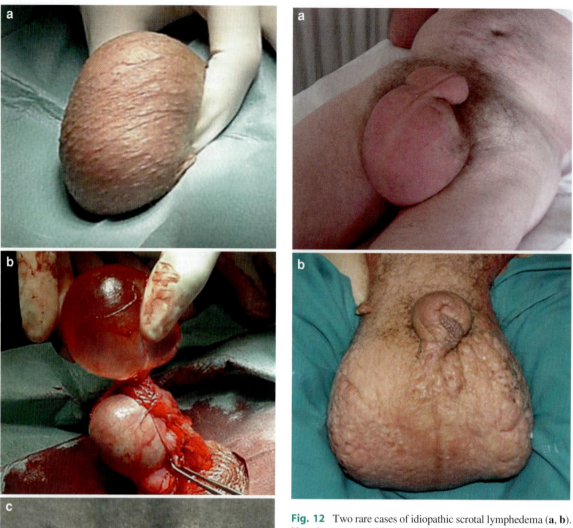

**Fig. 12** Two rare cases of idiopathic scrotal lymphedema (**a**, **b**). Note the verrucous-like growths on the penis and scrotal wall, due to lymphatic stasis

individuals in their 20's or 30's, but tumors have also been seen in patients ranging from 20 to 80 years of age. This is a benign tumor consisting of mesothelial cells which may resemble endothelium. Epididymis is the most frequent location. In the context of the epididymis, the globus minor is the most frequent site. Clinically, this tumor is an asymptomatic, well circumscribed mass ranging between 0.5 and 4 cm in size, generally found on routine examination. An occasional patient presents with mild pain or discomfort in association with the nodule.

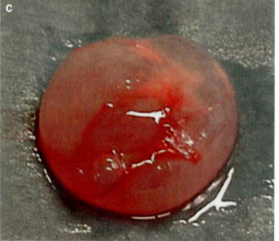

**Fig. 11** Large epididymal cyst. **a** Findings at physical examination. **b** Intraoperative view. **c** Final specimen

Paratesticular mesothelioma is more common in older individuals but may be encountered in any age group, including children. Usually, the tumor presents as a firm, painless scrotal mass in association with a hydrocele. Gradual enlargement of the hydrocele or sometimes the mass itself is seen in approximately 50% of patients.

Cystadenoma of the epididymis corresponds to benign epithelial hyperplasia. Approximately one third of the cases are bilateral and may be seen as part of von Hippel-Lindau disease. The tumor occurs most often in young adults and produces either minimal local discomfort or no symptoms. When seen in elderly patients, it is frequently an incidental finding at orchiectomy.

Paratesticular rhabdomyosarcoma occurs predominantly in children and adolescents and, with some exceptions, is most commonly seen during the first two decades of life. Clinically, this tumor usually presents as a large interscrotal mass that compresses the testis and the epididymis, sometimes reaching the external inguinal ring; the location varies somewhat, depending on the exact point of origin.

## 8    Scrotal Edema

Idiopathic edema of the scrotum is occasionally seen in children. It may involve one or both sacs and penis, perineum, or the inguinal region. The exact cause is not known; the condition may represent an allergic response or angioneurotic edema. Antihistamines may be of value, although the condition resolves spontaneously. Scrotal edema has been observed consequent to development of a fistula between the peritoneum and the subcutaneous tissue following paracentesis for cirrhosis of the liver. Even more rare is the diagnosis of scrotal lymphedema, where the alteration of the lymphatic drainage of the scrotum may be idiopathic or secondary to Wuchereria bancrofti infestation (Fig. 12).

## References

Bahren W, Lenz M, Porst H et al (1983) Side effects, complications and contraindications for percutaneous sclerotherapy of the internal spermatic vein in the treatment of idiopathic varicocele. ROFO 138:172–179

Farrer JH, Walker AH, Rajfer J (1985) Management of the postpubertal cryptorchid testis: a statistical review. J Urol 134:1071–1076

Finkelstein MS, Rosenberg HK, Snyder HM 3rd et al (1986) Ultrasound evaluation of scrotum in pediatrics. Urology 27:1–9

Gentile DP, Rabinowitz R, Hulbert WC (1998) Abdomino-scrotal hydrocele in infancy. Urology 51:20–22

Henderson BE, Benton B, Jing J et al (1979) Risk factors for cancer of the testis in young men. Int J Cancer 23:598–602

Iafrate M, Galfano A, Macchi V et al (2009) Varicocele is associated with an increase of connective tissue of the pampiniform plexus vein wall. World J Urol 27:363–369

Jemal A, Center MM, DeSantis C et al (2010) Global patterns of cancer incidence and mortality rates and trends. Cancer Epidemiol Biomarkers Prev 19:1893–1907

Lee JD, Jeng SY, Lee TH (2006) Increased expression of hypoxia-inducible factor-1alpha in the internal spermatic vein of patients with varicocele. J Urol 175:1045–1048 discussion 1048

Mostofi FK (1973) Proceedings: testicular tumors. Epidemiologic, etiologic, and pathologic features. Cancer 32:1186–1201

Schottenfeld D, Warshauer ME, Sherlock S et al (1980) The epidemiology of testicular cancer in young adults. Am J Epidemiol 112:232–246

Siracusano S, Tanda F, Trombetta C et al (1991) Melanotic neuroectodermal tumor of the epididymis in infancy. A case report and review of the literature. Eur Urol 20:49–51

Tanji N, Fujiwara T, Kaji H et al (1999) Histologic evaluation of spermatic veins in patients with varicocele. Int J Urol 6:355–360

Tilki D, Kilic E, Tauber R et al (2007) The complex structure of the smooth muscle layer of spermatic veins and its potential role in the development of varicocele testis. Eur Urol 51:1402–1409 discussion 1410

# Painless Scrotal Lumps: Current Therapeutic Approach and Follow-up

Sara Benvenuto, Stefano Bucci, Carlo Trombetta,
Paolo Umari, and Michele Rizzo

## Contents

### Abstract

Scrotal lesions can be broadly grouped by anatomical location as intratesticular or extratesticular. The clinician must consider a wide differential diagnosis based on this location, and a reliable and rapid differentiation of harmless from serious conditions such as cancer of the testis, is essential. Solid testicular masses are considered germ cell tumors until proven otherwise, but numerous other possible pathologies exist. The paratesticular region has the broadest differential diagnosis, as it contains numerous distinct structures and it is a common location for ectopic tissue and metastatic disease.

## 1   Introduction

Scrotal lesions can be broadly grouped by anatomical location in which they develop as intratesticular or extratesticular. The clinician must consider a wide differential diagnosis based on this location. Extratesticular lesions are more common than intratesticular ones. Solid testicular masses are considered tumors until proven otherwise, but numerous other possible pathologies exist (Doherty 1991). The paratesticular region has the broadest differential diagnosis, as it contains a lot of distinct structures and is a common location for ectopic tissue and metastatic disease (Krone and Carroll 1985).

In more than 95% of cases, intratesticular solid masses should be considered malignant. If the mass is extratesticular and cystic, the lesion is almost certainly benign and a specific diagnosis is often possible (Doherty 1991; Krone and Carroll 1985; Langer 1993).

S. Benvenuto · S. Bucci · C. Trombetta (✉)
P. Umari · M. Rizzo
Department of Urology, University of Trieste,
Ospedale di Cattinara, Strada di Fiume 447,
34124 Trieste, Italy
e-mail: trombcar@units.it

M. Bertolotto and C. Trombetta (eds.), *Scrotal Pathology,* Medical Radiology. Diagnostic Imaging,
DOI: 10.1007/174_2011_182, © Springer-Verlag Berlin Heidelberg 2012

Ultrasonography is the modality of choice for characterization of palpable testicular lesion (Rifkin et al. 1985). The role of imaging in the evaluation of scrotal masses is to confirm the presence of a mass, to define whether it is intratesticular or extratesticular, and to characterize it as much as possible for a specific diagnosis. For all these indications, ultrasonography is usually sufficient, since intratesticular versus extratesticular pathologic conditions can be differentiated with 98–100% sensitivity (Frates et al. 1997).

**Table 1** Intratesticular masses

| | |
|---|---|
| Tumors | Germ cell tumor |
| | Non-germ cell tumor |
| | Non primary tumors |
| Benign lesions | Cysts |
| | Epidermoid cyst |
| | Intratesticular varicocele |
| | Abscess |
| | Hemorrhage |

## 2 Intratesticular Masses

Several malignant and benign lesions may present as intratesticular masses (Table 1). The main goal of imaging is to attempt differentiation between tumors which must be removed surgically, and lesions that can be managed conservatively.

### 2.1 Testicular Tumors

Testicular neoplasms can manifest in a variety of ways. The most common manifestation is a painless scrotal mass. Testicular carcinoma is the most common malignancy in young men and boys 15–34 years of age (Luker and Siegel 1994; Ulbright et al. 1999). Overall, however, it is a relatively rare tumor, constituting only about 1% of all malignant neoplasms in men.

Every patient with a suspected testicular mass must undergo inguinal exploration with exteriorization of the testis within its tunics, and immediate orchiectomy with division of the spermatic cord at the internal inguinal ring has to be performed if a tumor is found (Weiss et al. 2001). If the diagnosis is not clear, a testicular biopsy is taken for frozen section histological examination.

The surgical technique for inguinal exploration and orchiectomy (Fig. 1) requires an incision into the skin 2 cm superior and parallel to the inguinal ligament, following the line connecting the internal and external rings, identification of the external oblique fibers and external inguinal ring, and incision along the direction of the fibers from the external inguinal ring. After having identified and mobilized the ilioinguinal nerve, and separated it so as not to resect it during the radical orchiectomy, the spermatic cord is isolated at

the pubic tubercle. Then, the point of entry of the cord into the scrotum is stretched with a finger, to deliver the testicle into the operative site. The gubernaculum is identified and then clamped, divided, and ligated. The spermatic cord is taken in two portions (a vascular portion and the vas deferens) by doubly clamping, dividing, and ligating as close as possible to the internal ring. Finally, the testis is removed from the operative field and sent for pathology. A testicular prosthesis may be placed into the hemiscrotum.

Patients who are having an orchiectomy as treatment for testicular cancer should consider banking sperm if they plan to have children following surgery. Although it is possible to father a child if only one testicle is removed, some surgeons recommend banking sperm as a precaution in case the other testicle should develop a tumor at a later date (Petersen et al. 2002, 1998).

Primary testicular neoplasms can be categorized into germ cell and non germ cell tumors (Sobin and Wittekind 2002), and several histotypes should be considered since treatment and prognosis may differ (Table 2).

### 2.1.1 Germ Cell Tumor

Intratubular germ cell neoplasia (Tin) is thought to be the precursor of most germ cell tumor (Richie 1997). The prevailing theory is that these abnormal cells develop either along a unipotential gonadal line and form seminoma or along totipotential cell lines and form non-seminomatous tumor (Table 2). The totipotential cells may remain largely undifferentiated in embryonal carcinoma, or develop toward embryonic differentiation, like in teratoma or toward extraembryonic differentiation, like in yolk sac tumor or choriocarcinoma (Ellis et al. 1984).

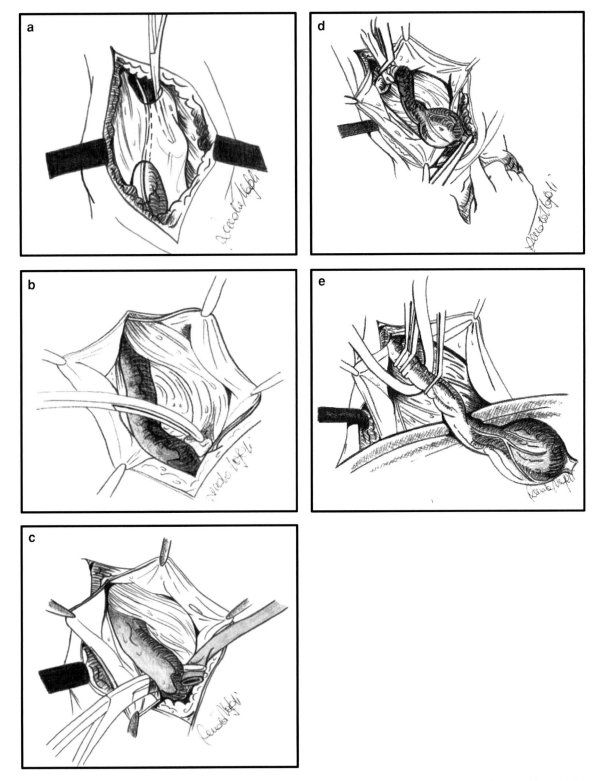

Fig. 1 Inguinal exploration and orchiectomy. **a** The external oblique fascia is entered and tented up over the length of the inguinal canal. The nerve is not injured. **b** Blunt dissection. **c** A Penrose drain is passed around the spermatic cord that is free. **d** The Penrose drain is encircled around the cord just distal to the internal ring and clamped. The gubernaculum is clamped and cut. **e** The spermatic cord is clamped and cut

**Table 2** Classification of primary testicular tumors

| Germ cell tumors | Intratubular germ cell neoplasia |
|---|---|
| | Seminoma (including cases with syncytiotrophoblastic cells) |
| | Embryonal carcinoma |
| | Yolk sac tumor |
| | Choriocarcinoma |
| | Teratoma (mature, immature, with malignant component) |
| Sex cord/gonadal stromal tumors | Leydig cell tumor |
| | Sertoli cell tumor |
| | Granulosa cell tumor |
| | Other sex cord/gonadal stromal tumors |
| Miscellaneous non-specific stromal tumors | Ovarian epithelial tumors |
| | Tumors of the collecting ducts and rete testis |
| | Tumors (benign and malignant) of non-specific stroma |

It has been demonstrated that stage and prognosis are directly related to early diagnosis.

Asymptomatic testicular tumors of small volume are often misinterpreted as germ cell tumors and inguinal orchiectomy is performed. It is highly recommended to perform an organ-sparing procedure in every small intraparenchymal lesion to gain the histological diagnosis. Abdominal and pelvic CT scanning is indicated once the diagnosis is confirmed.

#### 2.1.1.1 Seminoma

This tumor is extremely radiosensitive, and its treatment is a true success story. Radiation therapy for low-stage tumors is very effective. After modern staging procedures, about 15–20% of stage I seminoma patients have subclinical metastatic disease, usually in the retroperitoneum, and will relapse after orchiectomy alone (Richie 1997).

Patients with advanced stage disease receive chemotherapy, which may be followed by radiation therapy. Seventy percent of patients with relapse, however, are suitable for treatment with radiotherapy alone because of small volume disease at the time of recurrence. Only about 20% of these patients relapse again after salvage radiotherapy and then need salvage chemotherapy.

Adjuvant carboplatin therapy is an alternative to radiotherapy or surveillance in stage I seminoma. Adjuvant radiotherapy to a para-aortic field or to a hockey stick field (para-aortic and ipsilateral iliacal nodes), with moderate doses (total 20–24 Gy), will reduce the relapse rate to only 1–3%. Another possible site of failure is in the left renal hilum. Para-aortic irradiation should be tailored according to the site of the primary tumor. The rate of severe radiation-induced long-term toxicity is less than 2% (Zagars 1999). Moderate chronic gastrointestinal side-effects are seen in about 5% of patients and moderate acute gastrointestinal toxicity in about 60%. The main concern surrounding adjuvant radiotherapy is the potentially increased risk of radiation-induced secondary non-germ-cell malignancies. A scrotal shield can be of benefit during adjuvant radiotherapy in order to prevent scattered radiation toxicity in the contralateral testis.

Contralateral biopsy has been advocated to rule out the presence of Tin. The morbidity of Tin treatment and the fact that most of these metachronous tumors are at a low stage at presentation, make it controversial to recommend a systematic contralateral biopsy in all patients. It is still difficult to reach a consensus whether the existence of contralateral Tin has to be identified in all cases (Heidenreich and Moul 2002; Herr and Sheinfeld 1997). However, biopsy of the contralateral testis should be offered to high-risk patients for contralateral Tin with a testicular volume less than 12 ml, a history of cryptorchidism, and age under 40 years (Dieckmann et al. 2007). Because this may produce infertility, the patient must be carefully counselled before treatment commences. In addition to infertility, Leydig cell function and testosterone production may be impaired long-term following radiotherapy for Tin. Radiation treatment may be delayed in fertile patients who wish to father children.

In seminoma patients physical examination, chest radiography, and evaluation of tumor markers are recommended every 2 months for the first year and every 3 months for the second year. Moreover, patients should have CT scanning every 4 months for the first 2 years and every 6 months for a minimum of 5 years.

### 2.1.1.2  Non Seminomatous Tumors

These tumors are not radiosensitive as seminomas and the patient may receive chemotherapy as part of the treatment protocol. If retroperitoneal lymph node dissection (RPLND) is performed, about 30% of patients are found to have retroperitoneal lymph node metastases, which correspond to pathological stage II disease. A laparoscopic RPLND may become a good alternative to an open staging RPLND, but cannot currently be recommended as a standard diagnostic tool.

Choriocarcinoma is a rare germ cell tumor and it is composed of an admixture of cytotrophoblastic and syncytiotrophoblastic cells (Albers et al. 2003). Often, there is early widespread metastasis, and patients may present with symptoms referable to their metastases rather than a palpable testicular mass. Physical examination, chest radiography, and evaluation of tumor markers should be performed every month for the first year and every 2 months for the second year. The prognosis is poor, and death usually occurs within 1 year of diagnosis (Kakiashvili et al. 2007; Cullen et al. 1996).

### 2.1.2  Non-Germ Cell Tumors

Sex cord, stromal, and sex cord stromal germ cell tumors are benign lesions in the 90% of cases (Cheville et al. 1998).

Especially in patients with symptoms of gynaeco-mastia or hormonal disorders, a non-germ-cell tumor should be considered and immediate orchiectomy should be avoided. In cases of germ cell tumor in either frozen section or paraffin histology, orchiec-tomy is recommended as long as a contralateral nor-mal testicle is present (Bercovici et al. 1984).

It is highly recommended, however, to proceed with an organ-sparing approach in small intraparenchymal testicular lesions until final histology is available. This approach should be considered, in particular, for patients with gynaecomastia, hormonal disorders or suggestive features on ultrasound. Secondary orchi-ectomy can be performed if final pathology reveals a non-stromal (e.g., germ cell) tumor. Organ-sparing surgical approaches are justified as long as the remaining testicular parenchyma is sufficient for endocrine (and in stromal tumors also exocrine) function.

In stromal tumors with histological signs of malignancy, especially in patients of older age, orchiectomy and retroperitoneal lymphadenectomy are recommended to prevent metastases (Ellis et al. 1984).

In patients with non-germ cell tumors without histological signs of malignancy an individualized surveillance strategy after orchiectomy is recom-mended. CT follow-up may be most appropriate since specific tumor markers are not available.

Tumors that have metastasized to lymph nodes, lung, liver or bone respond poorly to chemotherapy or radiation and survival is poor (Chang et al. 1998).

### 2.1.3  Non-Primary Tumors

Non-primary tumors such as lymphoma, leukemia, and metastases can also manifest as testicular masses.

Lymphoma can occur in the testis in one of three ways: as the primary site of involvement, as the clinical manifestation of clinically occult disease, or as the site of recurrent disease (Doll and Weiss 1986). Testicular lymphoma is a lethal disease with a median survival of approximately 12–24 months. It is the most common testicular malignancy in men older than 60 years of age. Doxorubicin based chemother-apy with prophylactic intrathecal chemotherapy and radiation to the contralateral testis seems most promising (Verma et al. 2008).

Some patients with localized disease are cured following orchiectomy, but the majority will have evidence of disseminated disease within 6–12 months (Doll and Weiss 1986).

## 2.2  Benign Intratesticular Lesions

Benign intratesticular lesions are rare, but recognition is important to avoid unnecessary surgical interven-tion. Benign lesions include intratesticular simple cysts, epidermoid cyst, tunica albuginea cyst, intratesticular varicocele, abscess, and hemorrhage.

### 2.2.1 Epidermoid Cysts

Epidermoid cysts constitute approximately 1% of testicular lesions. They are composed of keratinizing, stratified, squamous epithelium with a well defined fibrous wall. Imaging appearance is often characteristic (Heiken 2000; Fu et al. 1996), but atypical cases are difficult to characterize. Since teratomas and other malignant tumor may occasionally have a similar appearance, orchiectomy is usually performed. However, if the lesion has been thoroughly evaluated and if there is a strong likelihood that it is an epidermoid cyst, testis sparing enucleation is indicated, rather than orchiectomy (Rushton et al. 1990).

### 2.2.2 Non Neoplastic Conditions

Non neoplastic conditions that can appear as a testicular mass include orchitis, hemorrhage and ischemia or infarction. They are more likely to manifest with an acute scrotum. Granulomatous orchitis has a more indolent course, compared with conventional bacterial orchitis, and also manifests as a testicular mass. Tuberculosis, syphilis, fungi, and parasites may be the causes.

Benign testicular cysts may be located within the tunica albuginea, or within the parenchyma. Simple testicular cysts are usually not palpable. If the cystic lesion has any solid components, it must be considered malignant until proved otherwise, and orchiectomy must be performed (Hamm et al. 1988). Imaging allows differentiation between intracistic amorphous material, such as clot and debris, and vegetations.

## 3 Extra Testicular Masses

Extratesticular solid masses are also most likely benign, with the prevalence of malignancy being approximately 3% (Beccia et al. 1976). Beyond fluid collections, varicocele, and hernia the most common benign extratesticular lesions are epididymal cysts and spermatoceles.

Lipoma and adenomatoid tumors are relatively common benign lesions as well. The remaining benign and malignant lesions are rare (Table 3).

Extratesticular masses may be classified on the basis of their composition, as cystic or solid. Several early reports suggest that extratesticular lesions

**Table 3** Extratesticular masses

| | |
|---|---|
| Tunical lesions | Hydroceles |
| | Hematoceles |
| | Mesothelioma |
| Paratesticular masses | Inguinal hernia |
| | Cysts/spermatocele |
| | Varicocele |
| | Lipoma |
| | Polyorchidism |
| | Fibrous pseudotumor |

hyperechoic relative to the testis are likely to be benign. Yet, more recently, several studies of hyperechoic extratesticular malignancies have been reported.

## 3.1 Fluid Collections

Several pathologic processes can involve the space of the tunical vaginalis. Hydroceles, accumulation of serous fluid, may be congenital or acquired as a reaction to tumor, infection, trauma or idiopathic (Doherty 1991). Surgical therapy can be divided into two approaches.

The procedure of choice for pediatric hydroceles, which is typically communicating, is an inguinal approach with ligation of the processus vaginalis high within the internal inguinal ring. A scrotal approach with excision or eversion and suturing of the tunica vaginalis is recommended for chronic non-communicating hydroceles (Sandlow 2007). Hematoceles acute or chronic may exert mass effect. Most hematoceles spontaneously resolve with conservative therapy (Cunningham 1983).

## 3.2 Varicocele

Dilatation of the pampiniform venous plexus and the internal spermatic vein, is the most frequently encountered mass of spermatic cord. Varicoceles can be treated surgically, by radiological embolization/ sclerotization with different approaches, and with coils or detachable balloons.

First described by Iaccarino (1980), embolization requires selective catheterization of the spermatic

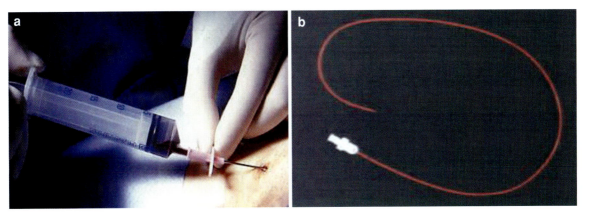

**Fig. 2** Scleroembolization technique: Femoral approach. **a** The femoral vein is entered below the inguinal ligament using the standard Seldinger technique. **b** The 6-F C3 femoral-visceral catheter used to catheterize selectively the renal vein

vein, followed by its occlusion with either a sclerosant or a solid embolization agent.

### 3.2.1 Upper Approach

In the Upper approach, the catheter is inserted in the basilic or internal jugular vein, although the latter access is poorly accepted without premedication (DD and Bonnel 1992; Gonzalez et al. 1981). The catheter is a torque 7-F (Cordis), with a distal curve suitable for both sides, and is 1.25 m long. This approach generally permits bilateral catheterization up to the deep orifice of the inguinal canal.

### 3.2.2 Anterograde Scrotal Approach

In the antegrade scrotal approach local anesthesia is induced at the level of the penile root by injecting 10 ml of 2% carbocaine into spermatic cord and under the area of planned incision. After a 2 cm long incision, a rubber band is drawn underneath the spermatic cord.

The dark yellow fat is identified and a dilated and straight vein of the spermatic cord is selected. Then, a 24 G thin-walled cannula is introduced into the largest spermatic vein (toward the renal vein). After injection of a few milliliters of saline the needle is secured with a single ligature.

### 3.2.3 Femoral Approach

In femoral approach the venography is performed through the femoral vein under local anesthesia on an outpatient basis. The femoral vein is entered below the inguinal ligament using the standard Seldinger technique. A 6-F C3 femoral-visceral catheter is commonly used to catheterize selectively the renal vein (Fig. 2). Renal phlebography is performed injecting 20 ml of contrast medium under Valsalva manoeuvre. The catheter is often changed with another, endhole one, for selective catheterization of the left spermatic vein. Once the vein has been cannulated, spermatic phlebography is obtained by injecting 5 ml 50% diluted contrast medium.

### 3.2.4 Sclerotherapy Procedure

Testicles should be shielded by a capsule to avoid excessive exposure to radiation. Before sclerotherapy 5 ml of nonionic contrast agent is injected into the vein under the fluoroscopic control. Then, 2 ml of sclerosing agent (sodium-tetra-decilsulphate 3%) is injected using an air block technique during which the patient performs a Valsalva maneuver. At the end of the procedure the cannula is removed and the vein ligated.

### 3.2.5 Scleroembolization Procedure

After selective catheterization of the spermatic vein, a guide wire is introduced deeply into the vein and the first catheter is replaced by a smaller one previously curved for this purpose that permits very distal catheterization. At the iliac level the distance between ureter and spermatic vessels is maximum making it the best site for scleroembolization. The procedure is performed by injecting a mousse of 4–8 ml sodium tetradecilsulphate 3% (Fibrovein®), which is continued until complete occlusion of the vein has been achieved, as documented by stagnation of the contrast medium (Figs. 3 and 4). The whole procedure lasts 10 min.

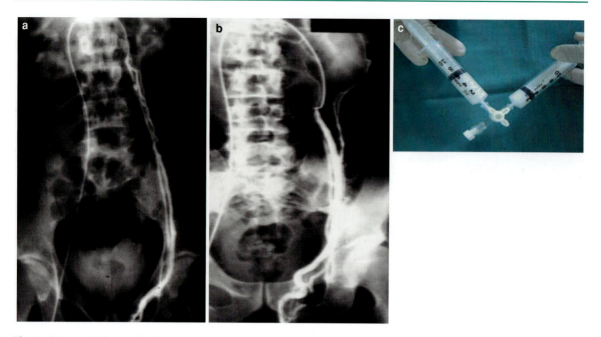

**Fig. 3** Scleroembolization Technique: femoral approach. **a**, **b** Selective spermatic phlebography. **c** The mousse of 4–8 ml sodium tetradecilsulphate 3% (Fibrovein®)

Tetradecyl sodium sulfate is more effective than hypertonic glucose solution. It is the ideal agent for small veins (collaterals or small varicoceles), but can cause moderate pain at the time of injection.

### 3.2.6 Coils or Detachable Balloons

In Europe, coils are more often used than detachable balloons, the latter in contrast are more popular in the United States (DD and Bonnel 1992). Coils are non-ferromagnetic and much cheaper than balloons. They are cost-effective and easy to use.

### 3.2.7 Complications

Coil and balloon migration are rare and always linked to excessively distal release (Gonzalez et al. 1981; Verhagen et al. 1992). All cases reported to date have been asymptomatic. This complication becomes increasingly rare as the operator's experience grows. Thrombosis of the pampiniform plexus can occur when sclerosants are used. It should be prevented by compressing the pampiniform plexus at the time of the injection. It can be prevented by beginning the embolization with coils or if tissue adhesive is used.

Thrombosis is a worrisome complication, which is observed in less than 5% of cases, and is usually painful (White 1994). It calls for prolonged antibiotic and antinflammatory treatment. When asymptomatic (1–2% of cases), it is demonstrated by palpation of an induration in the spermatic vein within the cord (White 1994). Doppler ultrasound shows an increased diameter of the veins of the pampiniform plexus which contain a hypoechogenic thrombus with little or no detectable venous flow.

### 3.2.8 Surgical Management

In the surgical treatment, high ligation of the spermatic vein by the extraperitoneal route, at the level of the anterosuperior iliac spine, is currently the most widely used treatment of varicocele. Ligation by the inguinal or subinguinal route is preferred by some authors in the case of voluminous varicocele with dilation of the cremasteric veins (GM 1990). The subinguinal route involves an incision just above the external orifice of the inguinal canal, followed by ligation of all visible veins under microscope vision; the deferential vein and lymphatic vessels must be respected, as their dissection leads to a high rate of postoperative hydrocele. The procedure can be performed under local anesthesia by infiltrating of the inguinal canal. Post operative analgesics are always required, and normal activity can be resumed a few days after the operation.

**Fig. 4** Scleroembolization technique. Femoral approach. **a, b** Complete occlusion of the internal spermatic vein (stagnation of the contrast medium) in two different patients

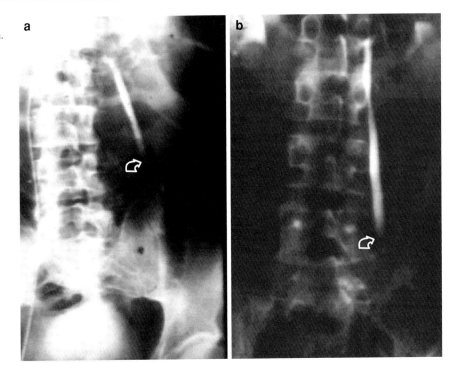

Laparoscopy has not proven superior to open surgery. It is costly and requires an experienced operator to avoid the risk of severe complications.

### 3.2.9 Choice of the Therapeutic Approach

Surgery is still the most popular treatment for varicocele (Wells 1995). It is the easiest approach and can be done by all urologists. When a trained operator is available, scleroembolization is the first-line choice, since it is the only method allowing strict outpatient treatment with resumption of daily activities the following day (Hargreave 1993). Like all operator-dependent techniques, scleroembolization has a learning curve, which can be shortened by intensive training of an interventional radiologist. After a few months of regular practice, generally it takes about 1 h.

Surgical treatment is rarely needed and generally reserved only in case of venous catheterization failure. Laparoscopy has few proponents and is criticized by many urologists (HS and Lee 1993). It requires a very experienced operator to avoid rare but potentially worrisome complications, such as injury of the vas deferens or epigastric artery (Wells 1995). Given persistent uncertainties regarding the need to treat varicoceles in subfertile men, it is generally agreed that laparoscopy is not an alternative to the other two available techniques.

## 3.3 Inguinal Hernia

Hernia is a common paratesticular mass and its ultrasound appearance depends on its content. Hernias with omentum can be more difficult to diagnose because their appearance overlap that of lipomas (Subramanyam et al. 1982).

Surgical correction of inguinal hernias, called herniorrhaphy or hernioplasty, is now often performed as outpatient surgery. There are various surgical strategies which may be considered in the planning of inguinal hernia repair. When herniotomy is combined with a reinforced repair of the posterior inguinal canal wall with autogenous (patient's own tissue) or heterogeneous (like steel or prolene mesh) material the procedure is termed hernioplasty, as opposed to herniorrhaphy, in which no autogenous or heterogeneous material is used for reinforcement (Trabucco EE and Rollino 1998; TA 1998).

## 3.4 Epididymal Cysts and Spermatoceles

The most common epididymal masses are cysts, which are lined with epithelium and contain clear fluid, or spermatoceles, which are characterized by milky fluid containing spermatozoa. Surgical intervention is not indicated for the incidental asymptomatic spermatocele. However, if discomfort, pain, or progressive enlargement is bothersome to the patient, discussion regarding excision may ensue.

Spermatocelectomy via a trans-scrotal approach is the primary operative intervention for spermatocele, and it may be offered to any reasonable surgical candidate. Sclerotherapy is an alternative to excision, but results appear to be less effective. Sclerotherapy is usually reserved for men who have no desire for future paternity, as the risk of ensuing chemical epididymitis and resultant epididymal damage may impair fertility. Aspiration alone is associated with a high recurrence rate (Walsh et al. 2007).

## 3.5 Lipoma

Lipomas are the most common extratesticular neoplasms and often originate from the spermatic cord. Simple surgical excision is the treatment of choice. The palpable borders of the mass are marked on the skin before infiltrating with anesthesia, skin is incised down to the lipoma capsule, and the lesion is dissected from the surrounding tissue.

## 3.6 Adenomatoid Tumor

Adenomatoid tumor is the most common epididymal tumor, second only to lipoma. Patients usually present with a painless scrotal mass. It is believed to be of mesothelial origin, and is benign. Surgical excision is unnecessary unless it is large enough to cause discomfort to the patient. Malignant tumors of the epididymis are rare and include sarcomas, metastases, and adenocarcinoma.

## 3.7 Fibrous Pseudotumors

This paratesticular lesion presents clinically as a mobile mass arising from the tunica vaginalis. It is not a neoplasm but a benign fibroinflammatory reaction resulting in nodular appearance. Recognizing the benign nature of this lesion should allow for a more

conservative scrotal exploration with frozen section confirmation, rather than an orchiectomy.

## 3.8 Granulomatous Masses of Epididymis

A granulomatous reaction including tuberculosis, brucellosis, syphilis, and parasitic and fungal infection, present with a painless scrotal mass. Preoperative diagnosis may be difficult, it can be obtained based on patient history combined with imaging and clinical features.

## 3.9 Mesotelioma

The tunica vaginalis is lined by mesothelial cell, which in rare cases may be involved in mesothelioma. Malignant mesothelioma of the tunica vaginalis is a rare primary tumor that occurs in a broad age range (Plas et al. 1998). Although trauma, herniorrhaphy and long term hydrocele (Gurdal and Erol 2001) have been considered as the predisposing factors for development of malignant mesothelioma, the only well established risk factor is asbestos exposure (Plas et al. 1998; Jones et al. 1995). Surgical intervention is necessary, as this is an aggressive tumor with poor prognosis (Liguori et al. 2007). The ultrasound features of mesothelioma of the tunica vaginalis testis have not been widely reported. Hydrocele, either simple or complex is present and may be associated with: (1) well organized soft tissue fronds of mixed echogenicity (a hypoechoic centre surrounded by a hyperechoic rim) which extends into the hydrocele (Fields et al. 1992); (2) multiple extratesticular nodular masses of increased echogenicity arising from the scrotal wall (Tyagi et al. 1989); and (3) focal thickening of the tunica vaginalis testis with presence of nodularity (Bruno et al. 2002).

## 3.10 Polyorchidism

This rare anatomical variation presents clinically with a painless scrotal mass (Figler et al. 1996). Differential diagnosis with other scrotal lesions is straightforward based on imaging features.

# References

Albers P, Siener R, Kliesch S et al (2003) Risk factors for relapse in clinical stage I nonseminomatous testicular germ cell tumors: results of the German Testicular Cancer Study Group Trial. J Clin Oncol 21:1505–1512

Beccia DJ, Krane RJ, Olsson CA (1976) Clinical management of non-testicular intrascrotal tumors. J Urol 116:476–479

Bercovici JP, Nahoul K, Tater D et al (1984) Hormonal profile of leydig cell tumors with gynecomastia. J Clin Endocrinol Metab 59:625–630

Bruno C, Minniti S, Procacci C (2002) Diagnosis of malignant mesothelioma of the tunica vaginalis testis by ultrasound-guided fine-needle aspiration. J Clin Ultrasound 30:181–183

Chang B, Borer JG, Tan PE et al (1998) Large-cell calcifying Sertoli cell tumor of the testis: case report and review of the literature. Urology 52:520–522, discussion 522–523

Cheville JC, Sebo TJ, Lager DJ et al (1998) Leydig cell tumor of the testis: a clinicopathologic, DNA content, and MIB-1 comparison of nonmetastasizing and metastasizing tumors. Am J Surg Pathol 22:1361–1367

Choi SHS, Lee T (1993) Adolescent varicocele. Curr Opin Urol 6:305–311

Cornud FDD, Bonnel D (1992) Traitement non chirurgical des varicocele spar embolisation des veines spermatiques et interet du Doppler couleur dans le bilan pre et post embolisation. Contracept Fertil Sex 20:1048–1053

Cullen MH, Stenning SP, Parkinson MC et al (1996) Short-course adjuvant chemotherapy in high-risk stage I nonseminomatous germ cell tumors of the testis: a Medical Research Council report. J Clin Oncol 14:1106–1113

Cunningham JJ (1983) Sonographic findings in clinically unsuspected acute and chronic scrotal hematoceles. AJR Am J Roentgenol 140:749–752

Dieckmann KP, Kulejewski M, Pichlmeier U et al (2007) Diagnosis of contralateral testicular intraepithelial neoplasia (TIN) in patients with testicular germ cell cancer: systematic two-site biopsies are more sensitive than a single random biopsy. Eur Urol 51:175–183, discussion 183–175

Doherty FJ (1991) Ultrasound of the nonacute scrotum. Semin Ultrasound CT MR 12:131–156

Doll DC, Weiss RB (1986) Malignant lymphoma of the testis. Am J Med 81:515–524

Ellis JH, Bies JR, Kopecky KK et al (1984) Comparison of NMR and CT imaging in the evaluation of metastatic retroperitoneal lymphadenopathy from testicular carcinoma. J Comput Assist Tomogr 8:709–719

Fields JM, Russell SA, Andrew SM (1992) Case report: ultrasound appearances of a malignant mesothelioma of the tunica vaginalis testis. Clin Radiol 46:128–130

Figler TJ, Olson MC, Kinzler GJ (1996) Polyorchidism and rete testis adenoma: ultrasound and MR findings. Abdom Imaging 21:470–472

Frates MC, Benson CB, DiSalvo DN et al (1997) Solid extratesticular masses evaluated with sonography: pathologic correlation. Radiology 204:43–46

Fu YT, Wang HH, Yang TH et al (1996) Epidermoid cysts of the testis: diagnosis by ultrasonography and magnetic resonance imaging resulting in organ-preserving surgery. Br J Urol 78:116–118

GM Thomas A (1990) Current management of varicocele. Urol Clin North Am 17:893–907

Gonzalez R, Narayan P, Formanek A et al (1981) Transvenous embolization of internal spermatic veins: nonoperative approach to treatment of varicocele. Urology 17:246–248

Gurdal M, Erol A (2001) Malignant mesothelioma of tunica vaginalis testis associated with long-lasting hydrocele: could hydrocele be an etiological factor? Int Urol Nephrol 32:687–689

Hamm B, Fobbe F, Loy V (1988) Testicular cysts: differentiation with US and clinical findings. Radiology 168:19–23

Hargreave TB (1993) Varicocele–a clinical enigma. Br J Urol 72:401–408

Heidenreich A, Moul JW (2002) Contralateral testicular biopsy procedure in patients with unilateral testis cancer: is it indicated? Semin Urol Oncol 20:234–238

Heiken JP (2000) Tumor of the testis and testicular adnexa. In: Pollack HM, McClennan BL (eds) Clinical urography, 2nd edn. Saunders, Philadelphia, pp 1716–1741

Herr HW, Sheinfeld J (1997) Is biopsy of the contralateral testis necessary in patients with germ cell tumors? J Urol 158:1331–1334

Iaccarino V (1980) A non surgical treatment of varicocele: transcatheter sclerotherapy of gonadal veins. Ann Radiol 23:369–371

Jones MA, Young RH, Scully RE (1995) Malignant mesothelioma of the tunica vaginalis. A clinicopathologic analysis of 11 cases with review of the literature. Am J Surg Pathol 19:815–825

Kakiashvili DA-CL, Sturgeon JF, Warde PR, Chung P, Moore M, Wang L, Azuero J, Jewett MA (2007) Non risk-adapted surveillance management for clinical stage I nonseminomatous testis tumors. J Urol 177:278

Krone KD, Carroll BA (1985) Scrotal ultrasound. Radiol Clin North Am 23:121–139

Langer JE (1993) Ultrasound of the scrotum. Semin Roentgenol 28:5–18

Liguori G, Garaffa G, Trombetta C et al (2007) Inguinal recurrence of malignant mesothelioma of the tunica vaginalis: one case report with delayed recurrence and review of the literature. Asian J Androl 9:859–860

Luker GD, Siegel MJ (1994) Pediatric testicular tumors: evaluation with gray-scale and color Doppler US. Radiology 191:561–564

Petersen PM, Giwercman A, Skakkebaek NE et al (1998) Gonadal function in men with testicular cancer. Semin Oncol 25:224–233

Petersen PM, Giwercman A, Daugaard G et al (2002) Effect of graded testicular doses of radiotherapy in patients treated for carcinoma-in situ in the testis. J Clin Oncol 20:1537–1543

Plas E, Riedl CR, Pfluger H (1998) Malignant mesothelioma of the tunica vaginalis testis: review of the literature and assessment of prognostic parameters. Cancer 83:2437–2446

Richie JP (1997) Neoplasms of the testis. In: Walsh PC (ed) Campbell's Urology, 7th edn. Saunders, Philadelphia, pp 2411–2452

Rifkin MD, Kurtz AB, Pasto ME et al (1985) Diagnostic capabilities of high-resolution scrotal ultrasonography: prospective evaluation. J Ultrasound Med 4:13–19

Rushton HG, Belman AB, Sesterhenn I et al (1990) Testicular sparing surgery for prepubertal teratoma of the testis: a clinical and pathological study. J Urol 144:726–730

Sandlow JI (2007) Surgery of the scrotum and seminal vesicles. In: Wein AJ (ed) Campbell-Walsh urology, 9th edn. Saunders Elsevier, Philadelphia

Sobin LH, Wittekind C (2002) TNM classification of malignant tumours. John Wiley and Sons, New York

Subramanyam BR, Balthazar EJ, Raghavendra BN et al (1982) Sonographic diagnosis of scrotal hernia. AJR Am J Roentgenol 139:535–538

Trabucco EETA (1998) Flat plugs and mesh hernioplasty in the inguinal box: description of the surgical technique. Hernia 2:133–138

Trabucco EE AFT, Rollino R (1998) Ernioplastlca inguinale tension-free con rete presagomata senza suture secondo trabucco. Chirurgia Minerva Medica, Torino

Tyagi G, Munn CS, Kiser LC et al (1989) Malignant mesothelioma of tunica vaginalis testis. Urology 34: 102–104

Ulbright TM, Amin MB, Young RH (1999) Tumors of the testis, adnexa spermatic cord, and scrotumAtlas of tumor pathology. Armed Forced Institute of Pathology, Washington, pp 1–290

Verhagen P, Blom JM, van Rijk PP et al (1992) Pulmonary embolism after percutaneous embolization of left spermatic vein. Eur J Radiol 15:190–192

Verma N, Lazarchick J, Gudena V et al (2008) Testicular lymphoma: an update for clinicians. Am J Med Sci 336:336–341

Walsh TJ, Seeger KT, Turek PJ (2007) Spermatoceles in adults: when does size matter? Arch Androl 53:345–348

Weiss RM, George NJR, O'Reilly PH (2001) Comprehensive urology. Mosby, London

Wells I (1995) Embolization of varicoceles. Curr Opin Urol 5:82–84

White R (1994) Radiologic management of varicoceles using embolotherapy. In: Whitehead E, Nagler H (eds) Management of impotence and infertility. Lippincott, Philadelphia, pp 228–240

Zagars GK (1999) Management of stage I seminoma: radiotherapy. In: Horwich AH (ed) Testicular cancer: investigation and management. Chapman and Hall Medical, London, p 99

# Imaging Scrotal Lumps in Adults: Tumors

Lorenzo E. Derchi and Alchiede Simonato

## Contents

**Abstract**

Ultrasound features of solid scrotal tumors are often non-specific, and most of them have no special character to help identification of their nature. Ultrasound, however, identifies the lesion in virtually all cases, allows differentiation between intratesticular and extratesticular masses, and gives an accurate estimate of its extent and relationship with adjacent tissues. A cystic extratesticular mass is usually a epididymal cyst, a relatively common finding, which is almost invariably benign. Purely cystic testicular nodules, without any mural irregularity, can be classified as benign. Careful attention, however, must be paid to identify any sign of complexity. Given the high sensitivity of ultrasound, MRI may have a role in a few clinical situations: when diffuse, non-specific testicular involvement is seen on ultrasound scanning, when fibrous lesions, lipomas, or haemorrhage are suspected, or when clinical and ultrasound findings are inconclusive.

## 1 Introduction

Radiology plays a very important role in the evaluation of patients with scrotal masses by providing highly effective informations about presence, location, and extension of the disease process and by trying to identify its nature (Woodward et al. 2002, 2003; Akbar et al. 2003; Dogra et al. 2003; Hamm 1997; Oyen 2002).

The most appropriate techniques are ultrasonography (Dogra et al. 2003; Hamm 1997; Oyen 2002) and Magnetic Resonance (MR) Imaging (Baker et al. 1987a, b; Kim et al. 2007). Plain film radiology and

L. E. Derchi (✉)
Dicmi-Radiologia, University of Genova,
Largo R. Benzi 8, 16132 Genova, Italy
e-mail: derchi@unige.it

A. Simonato
Department of Urology, Università di Genova,
Largo R. Benzi 8, 16132 Genova, Italy

M. Bertolotto and C. Trombetta (eds.), *Scrotal Pathology,* Medical Radiology. Diagnostic Imaging,
DOI: 10.1007/174_2011_183, © Springer-Verlag Berlin Heidelberg 2012

computed tomography may be useful only in rare cases to search for gas or calcifications within the scrotum.

Different mass lesions that can be encountered in the scrotum are presented in this chapter.

## 2    Lesion Detection

A scrotal mass is often identified by the patient as an abnormal lump during self-palpation. Less frequently, medical attention may be searched also after observing a change in the normal feeling of the testicle and even by presence of pain. In addition, small, non-palpable, nodules of the testis or of other scrotal structures can be identified as an incidental finding during imaging studies performed for indications other than the presence of a palpable mass.

Although testicular tumors are relatively rare and account for 1% of all malignancies in men, the primary goal of imaging is to identify whether the palpable mass is actually a cancer of the testis.

The imaging anatomy of the scrotum and the imaging techniques used to evaluate its many structures have been presented elsewhere in this book. In this chapter, it has to be stressed that an US study is a dynamic examination which entails interaction with the patient: palpation of the scrotum during scanning helps to correlate physical findings with the results of ultrasound. This is particularly useful in patients with small, mobile extratesticular masses which may be easily missed if a focused examination is not performed.

Given the high sensitivity of ultrasound, MR imaging is not frequently used to evaluate a scrotal mass. It can be indicated in a few clinical situations: when there are discrepancies between ultrasound and clinical findings, when diffuse, non specific, testicular involvement is seen on ultrasound scanning, when fibrous lesions, lipomas of hemorrhage are suspected, or when clinical and US findings are inconclusive (Woodward et al. 2002; Baker et al. 1987a, b; Kim et al. 2007). It has to be noted that this technique is used more frequently over time (Serra et al. 1998; Muglia et al. 2002; Parenti et al. 2009).

## 3    Role of Imaging

In patients with a scrotal mass, imaging is requested basically to answer five clinical questions (Woodward et al. 2002, 2003; Akbar et al. 2003). The first relates

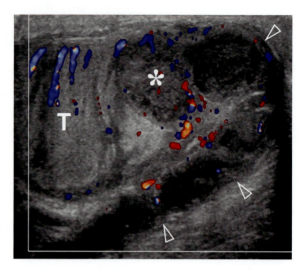

**Fig. 1** Chronic epididymitis. There is diffuse enlargement of the epididymis (*arrowheads*) and an epididymal nodule (*astrisks*) at the level of the tail mimicking an intratesticular mass. *T* = testis

to the actual presence of a mass. Enlargement of the scrotum from hernias, hydroceles, or lesions of the scrotal wall is usually easily identified by physical examination. In some cases, however, this can be difficult, and imaging has to be requested. Ultrasound is almost 100% sensitive in detecting the presence of a scrotal mass lesion. Palpation during scanning helps greatly to correlate physical findings with ultrasound images. False negative results are rarely encountered. They are mostly due to the presence of isoechogenic intratesticular lesions or diffuse testicular involvement, which may be difficult to recognize by ultrasound, or by presence of inguinal hernias containing fat and lipomas (or liposarcomas) of spermatic cord which may be isoechoic to surrounding subcutaneous tissue.

The second question is whether the mass is intra- or extratesticular. Ultrasound is 98–100% sensitive in differentiating intra- versus extra-testicular lesions, and again, simultaneous evaluation with palpation and ultrasound imaging helps to locate the mass. Also in this case, however, difficulties can be encountered since some epididymal inflammation can cause nodules which compress the testicle and may mimic a testicular mass (Fig. 1). Determining the exact location of the mass is very important, since most intratesticular masses are malignant and the greatest part of those which are extratesticular are benign.

Testicular tumors may be bilateral (up to 2% of seminomas and up to 38% of lymphomas can involve both testes, even simultaneously) and an ultrasound study has always to be performed on both sides to determine whether the mass is unilateral or bilateral.

Whether imaging can help in the identification of the nature of the scrotal mass is the fourth question, and this is probably the most important of all. It must be stated that, unfortunately, an histological diagnosis cannot be based on imaging methods alone. However, epidemiological, clinical and laboratory findings, together with the results of imaging, are important in offering helpful diagnostic criteria. As already said, localization of the lesion can be useful, since most extratesticular lesions are benign and most intratesticular masses are malignant. Furthermore, most cystic lesions are benign, while solid nodules are more often malignant. Then, combining location and structural pattern of the lesion, helps to narrow the differential diagnosis. A cystic extratesticular mass is usually an epididymal cyst, a relatively common finding, which is almost invariably benign. A cystic testicular nodule can be encountered in up to 8–10% of patients; it can be classified as benign if it is purely cystic, without any mural irregularity, and if it is localized at the tunica albuginea or near the mediastinum testis. A series of small, dilated, fluid-filled tubules with thin and regular walls, located at the mediastinum testis can be recognized as a dilated rete testis (Tartar et al. 1993). Although cystic lesions can be easily recognized by ultrasound, care must be taken before calling any intratesticular lesion as "cystic". Careful attention to the characteristics of the contents and margins of the lesion, as well as of the parenchyma surrounding it is needed. Winter has reported a patient in whom a cystic teratoma presented initially as a purely cystic lesion and solid components could be recognized within the mass, only at a follow-up study after 5 months (Winter 2009). When there is a question at US if solid components are present, MR imaging after contrast injection can help.

Solid lesions, whether intra or extratesticular, cannot be classified with certainty, and most of them have no special ultrasound or MR imaging character to help identification of their nature. Also benign lesions can present as focal intratesticular masses (Tackett et al. 1986). Color-Doppler signals can be identified in most testicular nodules. Although Horstman et al. (1992), stated that testicular nodules smaller than 1.6 cm are usually avascular, the increased sensitivity of modern ultrasound machines allows nowadays to see vessels within both benign and malignant nodules of smaller size. Some truly avascular lesions do exist, however, and this finding can be useful to lower the probability of malignancy. Tsili et al. have suggested that contrast-enhanced MR imaging can differentiate between seminoma and non-seminomatous tumors. Presence of intratesticular lesions of predominantly low signal intensity on T2-weighted images, with septa enhancing more than tumor tissue after contrast injection was more suggestive for the diagnosis of seminoma. Tumors that were markedly heterogeneous both before and after contrast injection were indicative of non-seminomatous neoplasms (Tsili et al. 2007). Furthermore, MR imaging has been found very accurate in local staging of the disease process, being able to recognize involvement of the tunica albuginea, the spermatic cord, the epididymis (Tsili et al. 2010).

Tumor markers ($\alpha$-fetoprotein, human chorionic gonadotropin and lactate dehydrogenase) can be of great help in the diagnosis of solid testicular nodules. Increased $\alpha$-fetoproteins are found in yolk-sac tumors and in mixed germ-cell tumors with yolk-sac elements; human chorionic gonadotropin is elevated in tumors containing syncytiotrophoblasts, such as choriocarcinomas. Increase of one or both of these markers is found in more than 80% of cases with nonseminomatous germ cell tumors. Lactate hydrogenase is a less specific marker which correlates with the bulk of disease and can be used in staging (Woodward et al. 2002).

## 4 Intratesticular Tumors

Testicular neoplasms can be classified into two categories: germ cell tumors and non-germ cell tumors. Germ cell tumors arise from spermatogenic cells, and are almost invariably malignant. Non germ cell tumors derive from sex cords and stroma, and are malignant in only 10% of cases.

Also non primary tumors, such as lymphomas, leukaemia, and metastases can be encountered; lymphomas are more common in the elderly (Woodward et al. 2002).

## 4.1 Germ Cell Neoplasms

These lesions are the most common testicular neoplasms. Many can present more than one histological type, and are classified as mixed lesions.

### 4.1.1 Seminoma

Seminoma are the most common germ cell tumor of the testis, accounting for 35–50% of all testicular neoplasms (considering both the pure and mixed forms). These can present as small masses or can be large, involving the whole testis. Most are homogeneously hypoechoic at ultrasound and, at MR imaging, have homogeneous hypointense pattern on T2-weighted images. Intratumoral vascular signals can be shown at color-Doppler, usually with irregularly shaped vessels, the so-called criss-cross pattern. When large, they are usually multilobulated, with many nodules continuing one into another. However, multifocal tumors may be encountered, with clearly separated nodules (Fig. 2).

### 4.1.2 Embryonal Cell Carcinoma

Embryonal cell carcinoma is a non seminomatous germ cell tumor, and is the second in frequency. It is present in 87% of mixed germ cell tumors, while it is rare as a pure lesion (2–3%). Its biological behavior is more aggressive than seminoma. Consequently, it has often a more irregular appearance at both ultrasound and MR imaging, with inner heterogeneous texture (and frequent anechoic areas) and less defined outer borders (Fig. 3).

### 4.1.3 Yolk Sac Tumors

Are the most common testicular tumors in the pediatric age group. The pure form is rare in adults, but yolk sac elements can be present in up to 44% of mixed germ cell tumors of adults. Imaging findings have been reported as non-specific. We have met cases in which testicular enlargement with diffuse and quite subtle change of the echotexture of the testicular parenchyma was the only sign of disease.

### 4.1.4 Teratoma

Teratoma are the second most common pediatric tumor. Teratomatous elements are found in about 50% of all mixed germ cell tumors of adults. They are composed of different germ layers (mesoderm, endoderm, and ectoderm), and are classified as

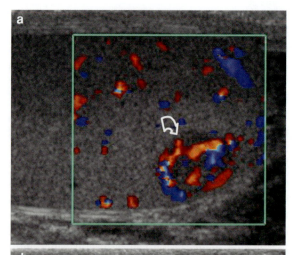
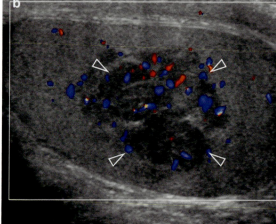
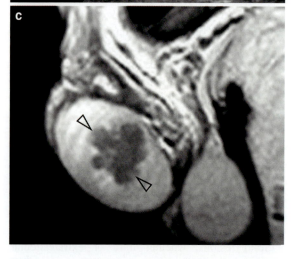

**Fig. 2** Two patients with seminoma. **a** Small tumor presenting at color Doppler ultrasound as hyoechoic homogeneous and hypervascular nodule (*curved arrow*). **b, c** Ultrasound and MR images of larger tumor. The lesion is heterogeneously hypoechoic and hypervascularized. At T2-weighted MR it is heterogeneous and hypointense (*arrowheads*)

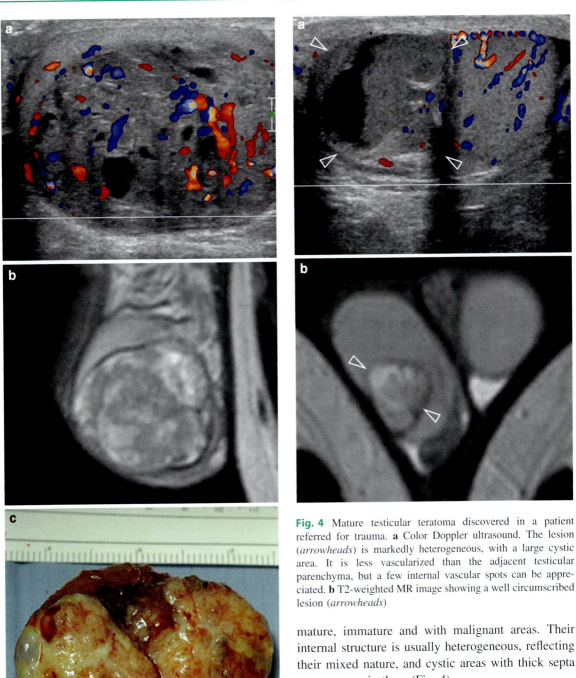

**Fig. 4** Mature testicular teratoma discovered in a patient referred for trauma. **a** Color Doppler ultrasound. The lesion (*arrowheads*) is markedly heterogeneous, with a large cystic area. It is less vascularized than the adjacent testicular parenchyma, but a few internal vascular spots can be appreciated. **b** T2-weighted MR image showing a well circumscribed lesion (*arrowheads*)

mature, immature and with malignant areas. Their internal structure is usually heterogeneous, reflecting their mixed nature, and cystic areas with thick septa are common in them (Fig. 4).

### 4.1.5 Epidermoid Cysts

Epidermoid cysts are benign testicular germ cell tumor (about 1% of testicular neoplasms). Their pathogenesis is uncertain: they may result from monodermal development of a teratoma or due to squamous metaplasia of surface mesothelium. They are true cysts, filled-in with solid, laminated, cheesy material, with no

**Fig. 3** Embryonal cell carcinoma. **a** color Doppler ultrasound image showing a large, heterogeneous, intratesticular mass. The lesion is well vascularized at color-Doppler. **b** At T2-weighted MR the lesion presents with heterogeneous signal intensity. **c** Surgical specimen of the mass

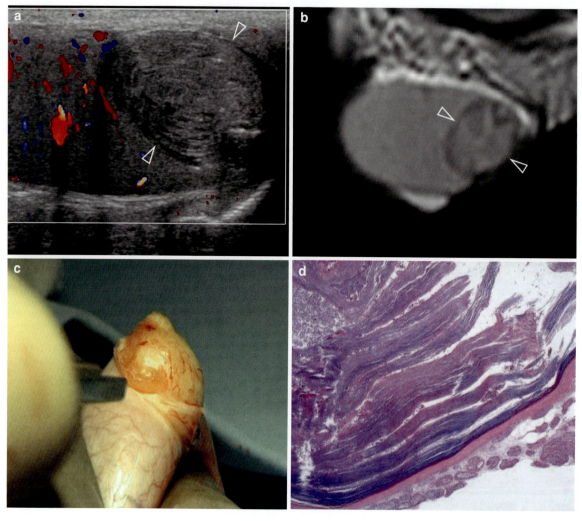

**Fig. 5** Epidermoid cyst of the testis in a 14 year boy. **a** The lesion (*arrowheads*) has a typical onion-skin echotexture, and is avascular at color-Doppler. **b** T2-weighted MR image shows a well circumscribed lesion, but without a target-like apperance. **c** Intraoperative photograph showing enucleation of the cyst. **d** Histology specimen; the multilayered internal structure of the lesion is well appreciated

malignant potential. Their nature can be often recognized, both at ultrasound and MR imaging. On ultrasound, they appear as well circumscribed, round masses, with hyperechoic wall (sometimes calcified) and laminated, onion-skin internal appearance; there are no flow signals on color-Doppler. On MR imaging, they have a target appearance, with low-signal-intensity capsule and internal content with high signal on both T1- and T2-images (Langer et al. 1999; Dogra et al. 2001; Manning et al. 2010). Multiple and bilateral lesions have been reported (Cittadini et al. 2004). Imaging findings are characteristic, but not pathognomonic. Teratoma and other tumors may mimic

epidermoid cysts, and great care in evaluating for irregular borders, as possible signs of malignancy, as well as attention to presence of irregularities within the surrounding testicular parenchima, has to be taken. When an epidermoid cyst is suspected, testis-sparing surgery rather than orchidectomy is suggested (Fig. 5).

### 4.1.6 Choriocarcinoma

Choriocarcinoma is a rare disease, seen in less than 1% of pure germinal tumors. It can be a component of mixed neoplasms in 8%. It is a very aggressive neoplasm, and patients often present with symptoms due to metastases. It has been reported with a

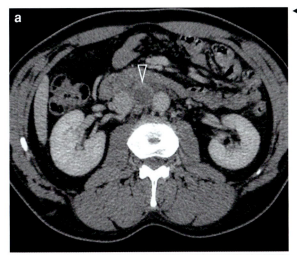

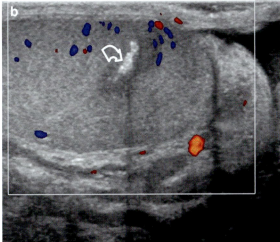

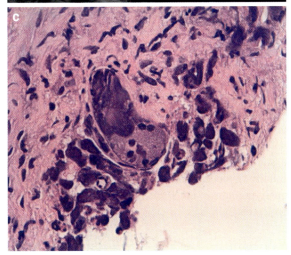

◀ **Fig. 6** "Burned-out" testicular cancer. **a** Patient with enlarged retroperitoneal lymphnodes at CT (*arrowhead*). **b** Ultrasound study of the testis shows a linear cluster of calcifications (*curved arrow*) with slight hypoechoic irregularities within the surrounding parenchyma. **c** Specimen from core-needle biopsy of lymphnodes confirmed the diagnosis of germ-cell tumor

### 4.1.7 Mixed Germ Cell Tumors

Such lesions contain more than one germ cell components. They represent 32–60% of all germ cell tumors, and virtually all combination of cell types can occur. Their imaging appearances are usually heterogeneous and variable, reflecting the many diversities of this kind of neoplasms.

### 4.1.8 Regressed or "Burned-Out" Germ Cell Tumors

This is a well-known but poorly understood phenomenon. Patients present with metastatic germ cell tumor but the primary cancer has involuted. The pathogenesis may be that the high metabolic rate of the lesion has outgrown its blood supply, leading to involution and necrosis of the primary focus of disease after it had already spread out metastases. The testes are normal or even small at palpation. Imaging is quite important in these patients and aims at recognizing a small, non palpable testicular anomaly (Shawker et al. 1983; Tasu et al. 2003; Fabre et al. 2004). At ultrasound, a small nodule of variable reflectivity, a hyperechogenic scar or a cluster of calcifications may be the only visible sign of the lesion. At histology, small amounts of residual viable tumor or only a scar with collagen and inflammatory cells can be found (Fig. 6). Patel and Patel (2007) report that, in a patient in whom ultrasound was able to identify only a cluster of calcification, contrast enhancement could be detected at that level at MR imaging, thus further suggesting the presence of neoplasm.

### 4.2 Non Germ-Cell Neoplasms

Such lesions are far less common than germ-cell tumors. Can be more frequently encountered in the pediatric age group, where they can be found in 10–30% of cases.

Only 10% of such lesions are malignant; however, there are no imaging clues which help to differentiate benign lesions from malignancies.

heterogeneous, non-specific appearance. Both the metastases and the primary tumor are often hemorrhagic.

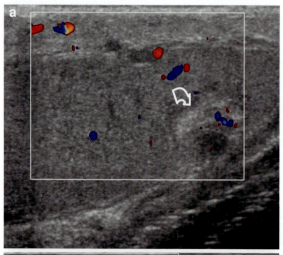

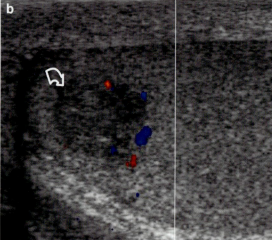

**Fig. 7** Two different patients with Leydig cell tumor. **a** Heterogeneously hyperechoic lesion (*curved arrow*) with internal vascular signals at color-Doppler. **b** Relatively homogeneous hypoechogenic lesion (*curved arrow*) displaying flow signals only at the periphery

### 4.2.1 Leydig Cell Tumors

Leydig cell tumors arise from interstitial stoma, and are the most common non germ-cell neoplasms, being encountered in up to 3% of all testicular tumors. Can be hormonally "active", with secretion of either androgen or estrogen hormones; an associated endocrinopathy, with precocious virilization, gynecomastia or decreased libido can be clinically seen. They have been reported as non-specific nodular lesions, either hyper or hypoechogenic, with possible cystic internal areas. There seems to be no possibility to differentiate them from malignant germ cell neoplasms. Vessels can be visibile at color-

Doppler (Woodward et al. 2002; Maizlin et al. 2004) (Fig. 7).

### 4.2.2 Sertoli Cell Tumors

Sertoli cell tumors arise from cells forming the sex cords, and are less than 1% of all testicular tumors. Although more rarely than Leydig cell lesions, they can cause gynecomastia. Have been described as well-defined, rounded-hypoechoic nodules. Internal vessels can be seen at color-Doppler (Fig. 8). At MR imaging they have been described as hyperintense on T2-weighted images and hypervascular. A subgroup of such lesions is the so-called large cell calcifying Sertoli cell tumors, more common in pediatric patients. They can be bilateral, with easily visible calcifications. They have been associated with Peutz-Jegher and Carney syndromes (Woodward et al. 2002; Drevelengas et al. 1999) (Fig. 9).

### 4.2.3 Other Non-Germ-Cell Neoplasms

Other, less common, stromal tumors can be seen, such as granulosa cell tumors, fibroma-thecomas, and mixed cells stromal tumors. Gonadoblastoma, a neoplasm with mixed elements of germ cell and non-germ cells can also be encountered, usually in the setting of gonadal dysgenesis and intersex syndromes.

## 4.3 Metastases

Metastases to the scrotum are rare, and generally seen in the setting of disseminated disease. A 0.68% incidence rate of metastases to the testes have been reported in an autopsy series of 738 solid malignancies (Garcia-Gonzalez et al. 2000), The most common tumors which metastasize to the scrotum are lung, prostate and melanoma; however, any malignancy can potentially give secondary involvement to scrotal tissues. Such lesions have non-specific patterns, being usually hypoechogenic at ultrasound, hyperintense or hypointense at T2-weighted MR images, and hypervascular.

## 4.4 Lymphoma

Testicular lymphoma is the most common testicular neoplasm in men over 60 years. It may occur either as

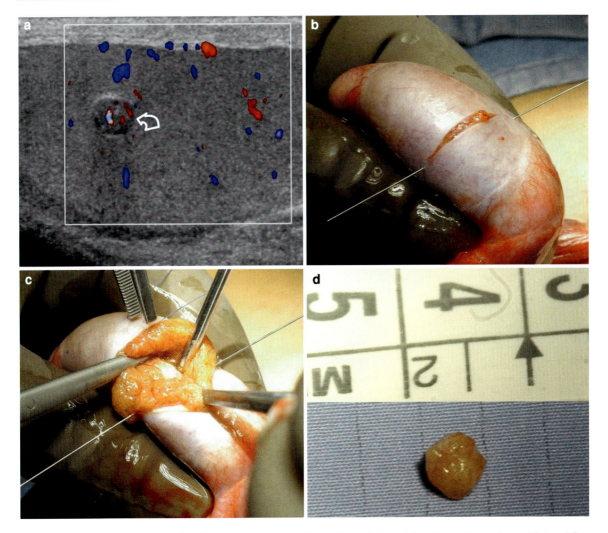

Fig. 8 **a** Ultrasound image of Sertoli cell tumor presenting as a 5 mm hypoechoic nodule with regular borders and internal flow signals. **b, c** The patient underwent enucleation of the lesion after intraoperative ultrasound localization. **d** Surgical specimen

primary involvement or as a site of recurrence. It may be bilateral in up to 40% of cases, and it may involve epididymis in 60% of cases and spermatic cord in 40%. Two different forms have been described: the nodular one, in which ultrasound shows hypoechogenic nodules (Fig. 10) which have hypointense appearance on T2-weighted MR images (Woodward et al. 2002; Mazzu et al. 1995; Eskey et al. 1997) and a diffuse one. This form presents at US as a diffuse hypoechogenic enlargement of the involved testis; there is marked hypervascularity, and the intraparenchymal vessels have a rectilinear course. These findings are quite similar to those observed in orchitis, and should not be interpreted as due to inflammation (Fig. 11).

## 4.5    Leukemia

The testis is a common site of leukemia recurrence in children, and lesions may be uni- or bilateral. Testicular leukemia has been described as either focal or diffuse involvement of the testis, more commonly with hypoecogenic structure (Woodward et al. 2002; Mazzu et al. 1995).

## 4.6    The Small, Indeterminate Testicular Mass

This is a problem which is becoming more and more frequent with the widespread use of ultrasound for

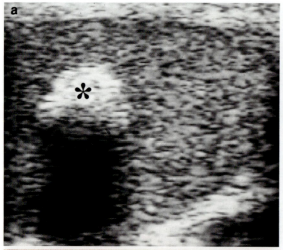

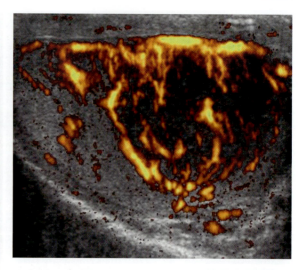

Fig. 10 Primary non Hodgkin's lymphoma of the testis. Longitudinal ultrasound view in a 74 year-old patient showing a highly vascularized intratesticular mass

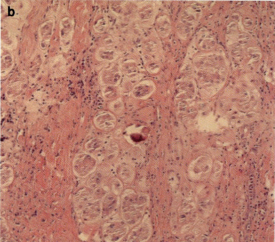

Fig. 9 Large cell calcifying Sertoli cell tumor **a** Ultrasound image showing a markedly hyperechoic intratesticular mass (*astrisks*) with posterior shadowing. **b** Histologic specimen of the enucleated mass

any scrotal problem. It seems it is happening, what is already seen in liver (simple cysts, hemangiomas), gallbladder (asymptomatic stones), kidneys (simple cysts), and thyroid (nodular goiter). Ultrasound is showing the real prevalence of "lesions"; the problem is that we do not know what they are, which is their clinical significance and how to treat them.

Non palpable, indeterminate testicular masses have been reported with prevalences ranging from 0.21 to 1% of cases in four different series (Carmignani et al. 2003; Avci et al. 2008; Powell and Tarter 2006; Toren et al. 2010). Presence of malignancies varied widely, from 0/10 cases (32) to 8/9 of operated subjects (33). Small nodules, with prevalence of benign lesions,

have been reported as a relatively common finding while examining testes of infertile men with ultrasound (Carmignani et al. 2004; Eifler et al. 2008). Orchidectomy as a first approach seems not justified in these patients, and a variety of possible solutions have been suggested. In patients who have small, non-palpable lesions, and in those who have lesions which look benign at imaging (and have not increased tumor markers) a targeted surgical biopsy under ultrasound guidance and simple enucleation if histology shows a benign lesion, can be recommended (Kirkham et al. 2009; Hopps and Goldstein 2002; Browne et al. 2003 Kravets et al. 2006) (Fig. 8). Another choice can be active surveillance, with surgery indicated only to those nodules which show interval growth (Toren et al. 2010; Connolly et al. 2006). However, active surveillance means to follow-up regularly on these patients every three months (Toren et al. 2010), and this can be sometimes difficult. Recently, it has been suggested that surgery may be completely avoided when new US techniques are used. Elastography, a novel technique which evaluates the stiffness of tissues, could potentially identify the "hard" lesions as being more likely malignant, and the "soft" ones as more probably benign. Furthermore, since tumors, either benign or malignant, present internal vascularization, if the nodule is shown to be completely avascular at contrast-enhanced ultrasound, it is very likely to be a benign lesion such as an infarct,

**Fig. 11** Diffuse infiltration of the right testis from recurrence of lymphoma. **a** At ultrasound there is marked hypoechoic unilateral testicular enlargement. **b** At color-Doppler, intraparenchymal vessels run in a linear fashion, and the lesion mimics inflammation. **c** PET study demonstrating the testicular lesion (*astrisks*). No other sites of active disease are identified

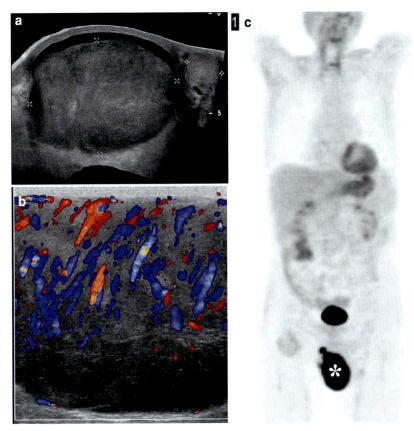

hematoma, or epidermoid cyst (Shah et al. 2010). Again, if tumor markers are not increased, these patients can be put on a watchful waiting program, with surgery indicated only in those lesions which show interval growth.

Percutaneous testicular biopsy is a well-known procedure to evaluate spermatogenic function in infertile men. On the contrary, ultrasound guided transcrotal biospy is not considered a procedure to be performed in patients with testicular masses due to fear of "contamination" of the scrotal wall by tumor seeding along the needle pathway, with consequent possible spread of tumor to inguinal nodes and worsening of the patient prognosis. However, there are no published studies which confirm this hypothesis, and Boileau and Steers reported on a series of patients with "contaminated scrotum" in whom no adverse effects were observed if proper management was instituted after a tumor diagnosis with this manoeuver (Boileau and Steers 1984). However, trascrotal testicular biopsy with fine needles has been described (Garcia-Solano et al. 1998; Verma et al.

1989; Kumar 1998; Assi et al. 2000) and a recent paper has used core-needles to diagnose focal indeterminate intratesticular lesions (Soh et al. 2008). The authors of the latter paper have indicated four clinical scenarios in which the manoeuver seems indicated: lesions with equivocal malignant ultrasound features; discrepancy between radiological and clinical findings; suspected lympho-proliferative disease; atrophic testes, in which it is difficult to differentiate malignancy from heterogeneous testicular texture (Soh et al. 2008).

## 5 Extratesticular Tumors

Extratesticular solid masses are most likely benign, with malignancies encountered in about 3% of cases (Woodward et al. 2003; Akbar et al. 2003; Frates et al. 1997; Lee et al. 2008). Each of the tissues of the scrotum (fascial coverings, epididymis and spermatic cord) can give rise to palpable lumps. The criteria which can help in the differential diagnosis are

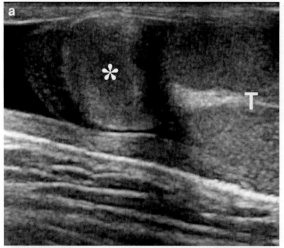

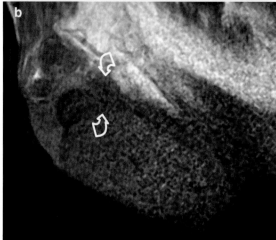

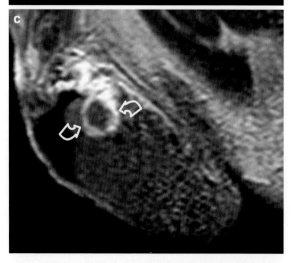

◄ **Fig. 12** Surgically proved adenomatoid tumor of the head of the epididymis. **a** Longitudinal ultrasound view showing a relatively echogenic mass (*astrisks*) at the head of the epididymis. The testis (*T*) is normal. **b, c** Longitidinal T2-weighted and contrast-enhanced MR images showing a relatively hypointense lesion with peripheral enhancement

and laboratory tests. Most of the inflammatory masses, in fact, are associated with acute symptoms and positive laboratory results. Imaging findings are often non-specific and not helpful to differentiate among the different types of lesions and recognize benign from malignant ones. However, there are some cases in which they can be helpful to recognize precisely the nature of the disease process. Paratesticular structures can be involved also by secondary tumors: in a group of 85 patients with non-testicular scrotal neoplasms, 9.4% were found to have lesions of metastatic origin (Lioe and Biggart 1993).

## 5.1 Tumors of the Epididymis

The most common neoplasms of the epididymis are adenomatoid tumors. They are the second in frequency of all extratesticular neoplasms, following only spermatic cord lipomas. Such lesions are benign (Woodward et al. 2003; Akbar et al. 2003; Frates et al. 1997; Lee et al. 2008; Leonhardt and Gooding 1992) and usually seen at US as solid, slightly hyperechoic nodules. At MR imaging too they have non-specific appearance, and seen as epididymal lumps of variable signal intensity (Fig. 12). Cystic-appearing adenomatoid tumors have been described (Akbar et al. 2003).

Leiomyomas are the second most common tumor of the epididymis. They have been described at US as solid, heterogeneous nodules with cystic areas and possible calcifications (Leonhardt and Gooding 1993).

Papillary cystoadenoma of the epididymis is a slow-growing tumor encountered in about 60% of patients with von Hippel-Lindau disease. Sporadic papillary cystoadenoma can be rarely found. They are nodules surrounded by a fibrous capsule and made of multiple cysts lined by papillary fronds. At ultrasound, these can present as predominantly solid lesions, with small internal cystic spaces or may be primarily cystic, with internal vegetations (Akbar et al. 2003; Alexander et al. 1991; Choyke et al. 1997). Up to 40% of such lesions are bilateral, and

localization of the lesion to one of the above mentioned structures and correlation with clinical history

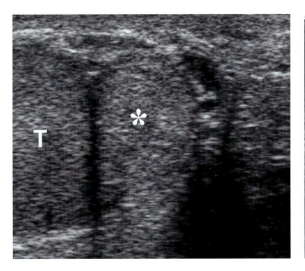

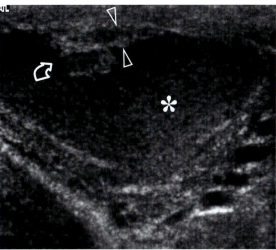

**Fig. 13** Extratesticular Leydig cell tumor at the tail of the epididymis. The lesion (*astrisks*) has a non specific homogeneous echotexture, slightly hyperechoic to the adjacent testis (*T*)

**Fig. 14** Mesotelioma of the tunica vaginalis. Axial scan of the left hemiscrotum showing a thickened portion of the tunica vaginalis (*arrowheads*) with a nodulation (*curved arrow*). There is associated corpuscolated hydrocele (*astrisks*)

this finding is virtually diagnostic of von Hippel-Lindau disease.

Other, more unusual lesions such as extratesticular Leydig cell tumors may be found at the epidydimis. They are usually with non-specific ultrasound pattern (Fig. 13).

Malignant tumors of the epididymis include sarcoma, metastases, and adenocarcinoma, and are rare. It must be remembered that testicular lymphoma can involve the epididymis and the spermatic cord and can be difficult to differentiate from an epididymal inflammatory disease with secondary infiltration of the testis. In lymphomas, however, the testis is more extensively involved than the epididymis, and this can be helpful for the differential diagnosis. Since, most testicular lymphomas occur as a recurrent disease, patient history can also be of help (Woodward et al. 2003).

## 5.2 Tumors of the Tunica Vaginalis

The tunica vaginalis is lined by mesothelial cells, and mesotheliomas have been reported. They are less common than those arising from the pleura and peritoneum; however, lesions of both chest or abdomen and tunica vaginalis can be encountered, and about 50% of patients have a history of asbestos

exposure. They are almost invariably associated with hydrocele, and can be suspected by the presence of irregular thickening of the tunica, with vegetating parietal nodules (Fig. 14). Cystic mesotheliomas have been reported (Woodward et al. 2003; Chien et al. 2000).

Fibrous pseudotumors of the tunica vaginalis are not a real tumor, but a benign fibro inflammatory reaction resulting in nodules (either single or multiple) at the tunica vaginalis or tunica albuginea. At ultrasound, they are seen as solid, hypoechogenic, non specific lesions. MR imaging seems able to recognize such lesions, since they have been reported with intermediate to low signal intensity on both T1- and T2-weighted images, addressing their fibrous nature (Woodward et al. 2003; Saginoya et al. 1996; Krainik et al. 2000).

## 5.3 Tumors of the Spermatic Cord

Most neoplasms of extratesticular structures are benign lipomas originating from the spermatic cord. Most of these lesions have a hyperechogenic structure at ultrasound. However, this is not the case in many patients, and a specific diagnosis may be not possible with this technique. Furthermore, differentiating a hyperchoic lipoma from adjacent fat can be difficult

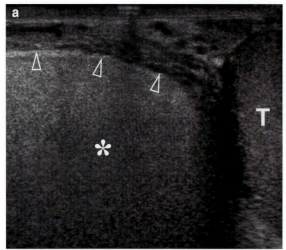

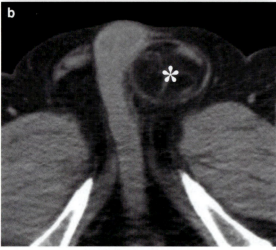

**Fig. 15** Lipoma of the left spermatic cord. **a** Longitudinal ultrasound scan showing a slighly heterogeneous hyperechoic mass in the left inguinal canal (*astrisks*) displacing anteriorly the spermatic vessels (*arrowheads*). Testis (*T*) is normal. **b** The lesion (*astrisks*) presents at unenhanced CT with fat density

with ultrasound alone, and MR imaging is needed to evaluate the full extent of the disease process. Also CT can be used in these cases (Fig. 15). Such tumors have hyperintense signal on both T1-weighted and T2-weighted sequences, and can be differentiated from a hemorrhagic mass with the use of fat suppression sequences. At CT they have hypodense, fatty appearance (Woodward et al. 2003; Akbar et al. 2003). Differentiating a lipoma from a liposarcoma may be difficult at imaging. A liposarcoma can be suspected by a more heterogeneous internal structure; however, excision is needed to establish the diagnosis.

Although rare, other malignant extratesticular masses, such as rhabomyosarcomas, leiomyosarcomas, malignant fibrous histiocytomas and undifferentiated sarcomas can develop.

## References

Akbar SA, Sayyed TA, Jafri SZ et al (2003) Multimodality imaging of paratesticular neoplasms and their rare mimics. Radiographics 23:1461–1476

Alexander JA, Lichtman JB, Varma VA (1991) Ultrasound demonstration of a papillary cystadenoma of the epididymis. J Clin Ultrasound 19:442–445

Assi A, Patetta R, Fava C et al (2000) Fine-needle aspiration of testicular lesions: report of 17 cases. Diagn Cytopathol 23:388–392

Avci A, Erol B, Eken C et al (2008) Nine cases of nonpalpable testicular mass: an incidental finding in a large scale ultrasonography survey. Int J Urol 15:833–836

Baker LL, Hajek PC, Burkhard TK et al (1987a) MR imaging of the scrotum: normal anatomy. Radiology 163:89–92

Baker LL, Hajek PC, Burkhard TK et al (1987b) MR imaging of the scrotum: pathologic conditions. Radiology 163:93–98

Boileau MA, Steers WD (1984) Testis tumors: the clinical significance of the tumor-contaminated scrotum. J Urol 132: 51–54

Browne RF, Jeffers M, McDermott T et al (2003) Technical report. Intra-operative ultrasound-guided needle localization for impalpable testicular lesions. Clin Radiol 58:566–569

Carmignani L, Gadda F, Gazzano G et al (2003) High incidence of benign testicular neoplasms diagnosed by ultrasound. J Urol 170:1783–1786

Carmignani L, Gadda F, Mancini M et al (2004) Detection of testicular ultrasonographic lesions in severe male infertility. J Urol 172:1045–1047

Chien AJ, Strouse PJ, Koo HP (2000) Cystic mesothelioma of the testis in an adolescent patient. J Ultrasound Med 19: 423–425

Choyke PL, Glenn GM, Wagner JP et al (1997) Epididymal cystadenomas in von Hippel-Lindau disease. Urology 49:926–931

Cittadini G, Gauglio C, Pretolesi F et al (2004) Bilateral epididymal cysts of the testis: sonographic and MRI findings. J Clin Ultrasound 32:370–372

Connolly SS, D'Arcy FT, Gough N, et al (2006) Carefully selected intratesticular lesions can be safely managed with serial ultrasonography. BJU Int 98:1005–1007, discussion 1007

Dogra VS, Gottlieb RH, Rubens DJ et al (2001) Testicular epidermoid cysts: sonographic features with histopathologic correlation. J Clin Ultrasound 29:192–196

Dogra VS, Gottlieb RH, Oka M et al (2003) Sonography of the scrotum. Radiology 227:18–36

Drevelengas A, Kalaitzoglou I, Destouni E et al (1999) Bilateral Sertoli cell tumor of the testis: MRI and sonographic appearance. Eur Radiol 9:1934

Eifler JB Jr, King P, Schlegel PN (2008) Incidental testicular lesions found during infertility evaluation are usually benign and may be managed conservatively. J Urol 180:261–264; discussion 265

Eskey CJ, Whitman GJ, Chew FS (1997) Malignant lymphoma of the testis. Am J Roentgenol 169:822

Fabre E, Jira H, Izard V et al (2004) 'Burned-out' primary testicular cancer. BJU Int 94:74–78

Frates MC, Benson CB, DiSalvo DN et al (1997) Solid extratesticular masses evaluated with sonography: pathologic correlation. Radiology 204:43–46

Garcia-Gonzalez R, Pinto J, Val-Bernal JF (2000) Testicular metastases from solid tumors: an autopsy study. Ann Diagn Pathol 4:59–64

Garcia-Solano J, Sanchez-Sanchez C, Montalban-Romero S et al (1998) Fine needle aspiration (FNA) of testicular germ cell tumours; a 10-year experience in a community hospital. Cytopathology 9:248–262

Hamm B (1997) Differential diagnosis of scrotal masses by ultrasound. Eur Radiol 7:668–679

Hopps CV, Goldstein M (2002) Ultrasound guided needle localization and microsurgical exploration for incidental nonpalpable testicular tumors. J Urol 168:1084–1087

Horstman WG, Melson GL, Middleton WD et al (1992) Testicular tumors: findings with color Doppler US. Radiology 185:733–737

Kim W, Rosen MA, Langer JE et al (2007) US MR imaging correlation in pathologic conditions of the scrotum. Radiographics 27:1239–1253

Kirkham AP, Kumar P, Minhas S et al (2009) Targeted testicular excision biopsy: when and how should we try to avoid radical orchidectomy? Clin Radiol 64:1158–1165

Krainik A, Sarrazin JL, Camparo P et al (2000) Fibrous pseudotumor of the epididymis: imaging and pathologic correlation. Eur Radiol 10:1636–1638

Kravets FG, Cohen HL, Sheynkin Y et al (2006) Intraoperative sonographically guided needle localization of nonpalpable testicular tumors. Am J Roentgenol 186:141–143

Kumar PV (1998) Testicular leukemia relapse. Fine needle aspiration findings. Acta Cytol 42:312–316

Langer JE, Ramchandani P, Siegelman ES et al (1999) Epidermoid cysts of the testicle: sonographic and MR imaging features. Am J Roentgenol 173:1295–1299

Lee JC, Bhatt S, Dogra VS (2008) Imaging of the epididymis. Ultrasound Q 24:3–16

Leonhardt WC, Gooding GA (1992) Sonography of intrascrotal adenomatoid tumor. Urology 39:90–92

Leonhardt WC, Gooding GA (1993) Sonography of epididymal leiomyoma. Urology 41:262–264

Lioe TF, Biggart JD (1993) Tumours of the spermatic cord and paratesticular tissue. A clinicopathological study. Br J Urol 71:600–606

Manning MA, Woodward PJ (2010) Testicular epidermoid cysts: sonographic features with clinicopathologic correlation. J Ultrasound Med 29:831–837

Maizlin ZV, Belenky A, Kunichezky M et al (2004) Leydig cell tumors of the testis: gray scale and color Doppler sonographic appearance. J Ultrasound Med 23:959–964

Mazzu D, Jeffrey RB Jr, Ralls PW (1995) Lymphoma and leukemia involving the testicles: findings on gray-scale and color Doppler sonography. Am J Roentgenol 164:645–647

Muglia V, Tucci S Jr, Elias J Jr et al (2002) Magnetic resonance imaging of scrotal diseases: when it makes the difference. Urology 59:419–423

Oyen RH (2002) Scrotal ultrasound. Eur Radiol 12:19–34

Parenti GC, Feletti F, Brandini F et al (2009) Imaging of the scrotum: role of MRI. Radiol Med 114:414–424

Patel MD, Patel BM (2007) Sonographic and magnetic resonance imaging appearance of a burned-out testicular germ cell neoplasm. J Ultrasound Med 26:143–146

Powell TM, Tarter TH (2006) Management of nonpalpable incidental testicular masses. J Urol 176:96–98, discussion 99

Saginoya T, Yamaguchi K, Toda T et al (1996) Fibrous pseudotumor of the scrotum: MR imaging findings. Am J Roentgenol 167:285–286

Serra AD, Hricak H, Coakley FV et al (1998) Inconclusive clinical and ultrasound evaluation of the scrotum: impact of magnetic resonance imaging on patient management and cost. Urology 51:1018–1021

Shah A, Lung PF, Clarke JL et al (2010) Re: new ultrasound techniques for imaging of the indeterminate testicular lesion may avoid surgery completely. Clin Radiol 65:496–497

Shawker TH, Javadpour N, O'Leary T et al (1983) Ultrasonographic detection of "burned-out" primary testicular germ cell tumors in clinically normal testes. J Ultrasound Med 2:477–479

Soh E, Berman LH, Grant JW et al (2008) Ultrasound-guided core-needle biopsy of the testis for focal indeterminate intratesticular lesions. Eur Radiol 18:2990–2996

Tackett RE, Ling D, Catalona WJ et al (1986) High resolution sonography in diagnosing testicular neoplasms: clinical significance of false positive scans. J Urol 135:494–496

Tartar VM, Trambert MA, Balsara ZN et al (1993) Tubular ectasia of the testicle: sonographic and MR imaging appearance. Am J Roentgenol 160:539–542

Tasu JP, Faye N, Eschwege P et al (2003) Imaging of burned-out testis tumor: five new cases and review of the literature. J Ultrasound Med 22:515–521

Toren PJ, Roberts M, Lecker I et al (2010) Small incidentally discovered testicular masses in infertile men–is active surveillance the new standard of care? J Urol 183:1373–1377

Tsili AC, Tsampoulas C, Giannakopoulos X et al (2007) MRI in the histologic characterization of testicular neoplasms. Am J Roentgenol 189:W331–W337

Tsili AC, Argyropoulou MI, Giannakis D et al (2010) MRI in the characterization and local staging of testicular neoplasms. Am J Roentgenol 194:682–689

Verma K, Ram TR, Kapila K (1989) Value of fine needle aspiration cytology in the diagnosis of testicular neoplasms. Acta Cytol 33:631–634

Winter TC (2009) There is a mass in the scrotum-what does it mean? Evaluation of the scrotal mass. Ultrasound Q 25:195–205

Woodward PJ, Sohaey R, O'Donoghue MJ et al (2002) From the archives of the AFIP: tumors and tumorlike lesions of the testis: radiologic-pathologic correlation. Radiographics 22:189–216

Woodward PJ, Schwab CM, Sesterhenn IA (2003) From the archives of the AFIP: extratesticular scrotal masses: radiologic-pathologic correlation. Radiographics 23:215–240

# Imaging Scrotal Lumps in Adults-2: Cysts and Fluid Collections

Massimo Valentino, Libero Barozzi, Pietro Pavlica, and Cristina Rossi

## Contents

M. Valentino (✉)
S.S.D. Radiologia d'Urgenza, Dipartimento di Radiologia e
Diagnostica per Immagini Azienda Ospedaliera,
Universitaria di Parma Ospedale Maggiore,
Via Gramsci 14, 43100 Parma, Italy
e-mail: mvalentino@ao.pr.it

L. Barozzi
Unità Operativa di Radiologia D'Urgenza,
Policlinico S. Orsola-Malpighi, Via Palagi 9,
40138 Bologna, Italy

P. Pavlica
Servizio di Diagnostica per Immagini, Villalba Hospital,
Via di Roncrio 25, 40136 Bologna, Italy

C. Rossi
Dipartimento di Radiologia e Diagnostica
per Immagini Azienda Ospedaliera,
Universitaria di Parma Ospedale Maggiore,
Via Gramsci 14, 43100 Parma, Italy

## Abstract

Scrotal cystic lesions and fluid collections are common incidental findings at ultrasonography performed in symptomatic and asymptomatic men. The majority of cystic lesions are located in the epidydimis, but the testis and the cord are frequently involved. Testicular, albugineal and epidermoid cysts, cystic dysplasia of the rete testis, cysts of the spermatic cord, and cystic appendages are easily detected at ultrasound, which is the method of choice in assessing any fluid containing mass, providing detailed information at high resolution. Magnetic resonance (MR) imaging is a second line procedure and can be used as a problem-solving tool when ultrasound findings are equivocal. Most fluid collections are located in the vaginal sac and can be idiopathic or secondary to trauma, inflammation, or tumor. Ultrasound findings in combination with clinical assessment arc generally sufficient for the final diagnosis, and MR imaging is rarely employed. In this chapter ultrasound and MR appearance of the scrotal cystic lesions and fluid collections are described and differential diagnoses discussed.

## 1 Introduction

There are many fluid scrotal lesions that can simulate a mass in the testis or paratesticular structures. Their incidence in the general population is not well known

**Table 1** Cysts and fluid collections of the scrotum

| Cysts | Epididymal cysts |
|---|---|
| | Testicular cysts |
| |   Tunica albuginea cysts |
| |   Parenchymal testicular cysts |
| | Tubular ectasia of the rete testis |
| | Spermatic cord cysts |
| | Cystic appendages |
| | Testicular abscess |
| Fluid collections | Hydrocele |
| | Hematocele |
| | Arteriovenous malformations |
| | Inguinoscrotal hernia |

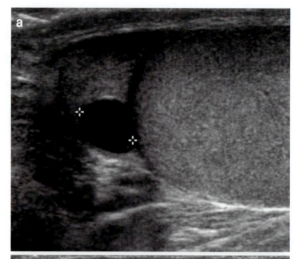

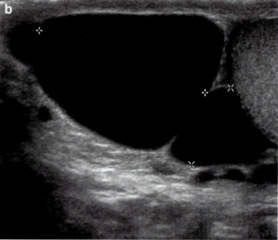

**Fig. 1 a** Simple cyst of the epididymis. Longitudinal ultrasound image of the right scrotum showing typical small fluid collection of the epididymal head, with well-defined margins. **b** Spermatocele. Longitudinal US image of the right scrotum showing a multi-locular cystic mass

because the majority of these disorders are asymptomatic, show a benign behavior and generally do not require surgery.

On the basis of their nature, fluid containing scrotal lumps can be divided into cysts and fluid collections (Table 1).

## 2 Cysts

The majority of scrotal cysts are localized in the epydidimus and, less frequently, in the funicle structures. The testis may occasionally be the site of some cystic lesions that can be confused with a neoplasia (Algaba et al. 2007).

### 2.1 Epididymal Cysts

Epididymal cysts are the most common scrotal masses, being reported in 20–40% of asymptomatic individuals, 29% of whom show more than one cyst (Leung et al. 1984). These masses may be either true cysts, which are lined with epithelium, contain clear serous fluid and are likely to be of lymphatic origin, or they may be spermatoceles, which form from obstruction and dilatation of the efferent ductal system and are filled with thicker, milky fluid containing spermatozoa, lymphocytes and cellular debris (Woodward et al. 2003).

Both true epididymal cysts and spermatoceles appear as anechoic, well-defined masses with increased through-transmission, and are indistinguishable on

ultrasound (Fig. 1). Aspiration of fluid can allow a definitive diagnosis to be made, but this procedure is seldom, if ever, necessary since both lesions are benign and of low clinical value. In a series by Holden and List (1994), epididymal cysts were more common in the general population, accounting for approximately 75% of lesions, but in postvasectomy patients spermatoceles were more frequent (Jarvis and Dubbins 1989). Larger cysts (either true cysts or spermatoceles) may have septations and may be confused with hydroceles. One feature helps differentiate between the two: cysts displace the testis, whereas a hydrocele envelops it (Rifkin et al. 1984).

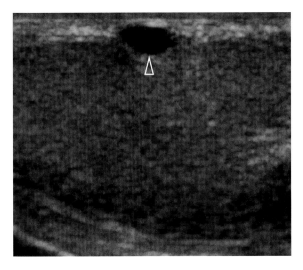

**Fig. 2** Tunica albuginea cyst. Small, anechoic palpable mass along the anterior aspect of the testis within the layers of the tunica (*arrowhead*)

In addition to spermatoceles, another lesion that can be seen in the postvasectomy patient is sperm granuloma, which forms as a foreign body giant cell reaction to extravasated sperm. In an autopsy series, sperm granulomas have been reported in up to 42% of men who have undergone vasectomy and 2.5% of the general population (Bostwick 1997). They can range in size from microscopic to 4 cm, but most of them are less than 1 cm (Ulbright et al. 1999). As for the other cystic formations, sperm granuloma needs to be differentiated from a true neoplasia that must be considered should any content be observed in its interior. Contrast-enhanced MR imaging can be used to document lack of lesion vascularization in these cases.

## 2.2 Cysts of the Tunica Albuginea

These cysts do not usually cause any diagnostic problem, unless they present with complex appearance (Poster et al. 1991). Tunica albuginea cysts typically manifest as small palpable masses, most commonly along the upper anterior or lateral aspect of the testicle, and can be single or multiple. Their origin is uncertain, but they are thought to arise from mesothelial cells (Martinez-Berganza et al. 1998). Ultrasound shows a small, peripherally located, anechoic lesion within the layers of the tunica (Fig. 2). Larger lesions may compress the testicular parenchyma and simulate an intratesticular mass (Dogra et al. 2001).

Less commonly, cysts of the tunica albuginea have internal echoes and raise concern for a neoplasm. At MR imaging, regardless of size, the signal intensity of albugineal cysts follows that of fluid with all pulse sequences. When ultrasound results are equivocal, multiplanar MR imaging can help localize these lesions outside the testis.

## 2.3 Testicular Cysts

Parenchymal testicular cysts are usually nonpalpable and are thus detected incidentally. No treatment is required. Similar to cysts as elsewhere in the body, they are usually well-defined and anechoic with an imperceptible wall (Hamm et al. 1988). At MR imaging testicular cysts shows the signal characteristics of fluid with all pulse sequences (Fig. 3).

When the lesion does not fulfill the typical criteria of a simple cyst and there is the slightest suspicion of an intra-cystic content, a malignant neoplasia should be ruled out (Algaba et al. 2007). Careful inspection is warranted to differentiate benign cysts from cystic testicular neoplasms (Fig. 4) (Kim et al. 2007). Contrast-enhanced MR imaging aids in this diagnosis by demonstrating lack of enhancement within the cyst, while virtually all testicular neoplasms enhance after gadolinium injection.

Testicular epidermoid cysts deserve special consideration. The ultrasound appearance varies according to the maturation, compactness, and quantity of keratin present. The lesion may present as a mass with a target appearance of a central echogenic area surrounded by a hypoechoic periphery, an onion ring appearance of alternating hyperechogenicity and hypoechogenicity, an echogenic mass with dense acoustic shadowing due to calcification, and a well-circumscribed mass with an echogenic rim (Maizlin et al. 2005). Of these, the onion ring pattern is considered characteristic and highly suggestive of an epidermoid cyst, and all reported lesions with this sonographic appearance have been benign. Occasionally, epidermoid cyst may resemble a simple cyst, or a minimally complicated cyst with slightly inhomogeneous content and echogenic rim (Fig. 5). On MR imaging epidermoid cysts may have a similar onion ring appearance, with concentric rings of alternating high and low signal intensity, corresponding to the

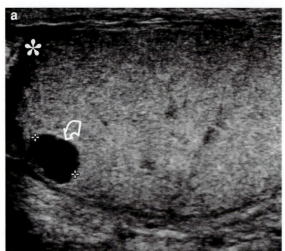

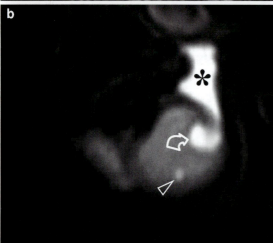

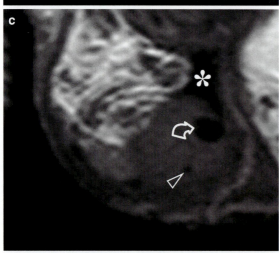

◀**Fig. 3** Testicular cyst. **a** Small non-palpable incidentally detected anechoic lesion with through transmission and no identifiable wall at ultrasound. **b, c** T2-weighted and contrast-enhanced T1-weighted coronal MR images showing high signal intensity and lack of enhancement, consistent with simple cyst. There is an associated hydrocele (*) and another small cyst (*arrowhead*) in the same testis

contrast enhancement is consistent with the avascular nature of these lesions (Langer et al. 1999).

## 3        Tubular Ectasia of the Rete Testis

The rete testis, located in the mediastinum, is composed of a system of numerous seminiferous serpiginous tubules, which drain and connect with the epididymal head. Dilatation of the rete testis is very common, often bilateral, and mostly seen in patients of over 50 years of age. It can be associated with either post-infectious, post-traumatic, or post prostatectomy epididymal obstruction. It has been suggested that possible factors contributing to the development of tubular ectasia of the rete testis include epididymitis, testicular biopsy, and vasectomy (Weingarten et al. 1992; Strauss et al. 2001). Epididymal abnormalities such as spermatoceles or dilated efferent ducts are frequently associated.

The dilated rete testis presents at ultrasound with multiple, low-reflective, oval, or rounded structures that do not demonstrate vascular flow within the mediastinum testis (Fig. 6). Cysts usually measure a few millimetres in diameter but may be as large as 7 cm (Rouviere et al. 1999). At MR imaging the dilated tubules appear hyperintense on T2-weighted images. After administration of gadolinium contrast material, no internal enhancement is seen. Characteristic signal intensity and lack of enhancement can aid in diagnosis (Kim et al. 2007).

Tubular ectasia of the rete testis must be differentiated from cystic dysplasia of the testis, a congenital lesion with complete testicular parenchyma substitution (Fig. 7) described in 1973 by Leissring and Oppenheimer. Cystic dysplasia is usually detected in childhood, and arises during the testicular development with multicystic changes in the seminiferous tubules (Leissring and Oppenheimer 1973). Malunion between the gonadal blastema and mesonephric ducts can explain the origin of this malformation, which is frequently associated with renal malformations.

pathologic finding of multiple layers of keratin debris. In other cases, however, signal intensity characteristics are not specific. The absence of

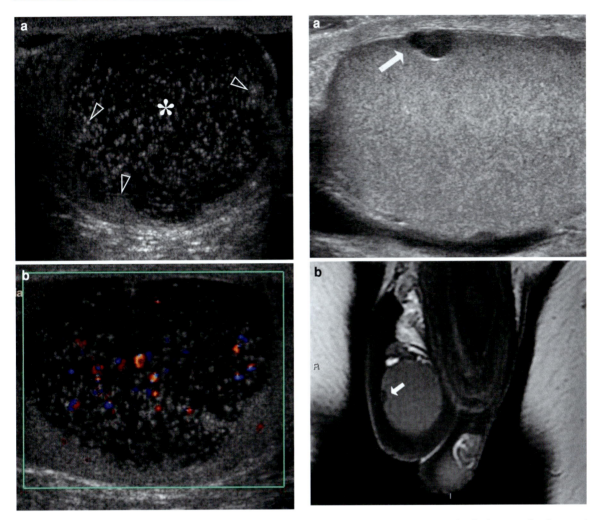

**Fig. 4** Cystic papillary carcinoma of the testis. **a** Sagittal grey-scale ultrasound shows a large cystic mass (*) involving the right testis with multiple areas of high reflectivity demonstrating continuous movement during examination or compression (snowstorm aspect). The wall of the lesion is thickened with multiple sessile excrescences (*arrowheads*). **b** Color Doppler interrogation shows the twinkling phenomenon secondary to the swirling particles

**Fig. 5** Epidermoid cyst. **a** Longitudinal grey-scale ultrasound image showing a small, hypoechoic intratesticular cystic mass with slightly non-homogeneous content and hyperechoic rim (*arrow*). At color Doppler interrogation there was no intralesional flow (not shown). **b** Gadoliniom- enhanced T1-weighted coronal image confirms absence of lesion contrast enhancement (*arrow*)

Associated renal agenesis was described in 41–55% of cases (Mac New et al. 2008).

# 4 Spermatic Cord Cysts

The majority of these cysts do not cause any diagnostic doubts (Fig. 8), except in the case of occasional epidermoid cysts which can simulate a neoplasia (Katergiannakis et al. 2006). Spermatic cord cysts can be unilocular or multilocular depending on their origin, separated from the head of the epididymis and from the didymis. They should not be confused with hydroceles and incarcerated inguinal hernias. Multilocular cysts must be distinguished from the exceptional cystadenomas of probable Müllerian origin (Algaba et al. 2007).

Clinically, epidermoid cysts appear as firm, oval, or lobulated lumps of variable size. They are usually slow growing and asymptomatic (Katergiannakis et al. 2006). At ultrasound, epidermoid cysts appear as ovoid or

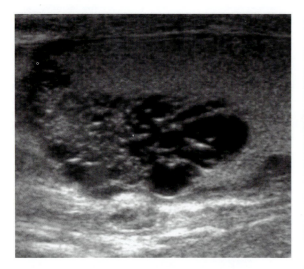

**Fig. 6** Tubular ectasia of the rete testis. Longitudinal ulltrasound view showing multiple cystic or tubular anechoic structures localised in the testicular mediastinum

lobulated masses with well-defined margins. The content is relatively echogenic with hypoechoic foci (Fig. 9). Calcifications are occasionally identified. No vascularity is recognized at color Doppler interrogation, nor CEUS.

At MR imaging, epidermoid cysts present with well-circumscribed masses lacking internal contrast enhancement. A peripheral rim of enhancement may be present (Lee et al. 2010). On T1-weighted images signal intensity is similar or higher compared to muscle, while signal intensity is intermediate to high on T2-weighted images (Tanaka et al. 2000). Irregular low signal intensity areas are recognized on both T1- and T2-weighted images.

## 5 Cystic Appendages

The testicular and epididymal appendages are commonly identified on ultrasound, more easily in the presence of hydrocele or other scrotal fluid collections (Sellars and Sidhu 2003). The appendix testis is a remnant of the Müllerian duct. It is usually sessile and echogenic, but may be pedunculated and with cystic appearance. The appendix epididymis is a remnant of the Wolffian duct. On histopathological examination it is almost invariably cystic, composed of multiple converging ducts. At ultrasound, however, it presents with cystic appearance in only about 36% of cases

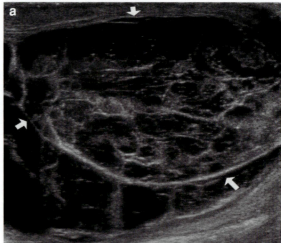

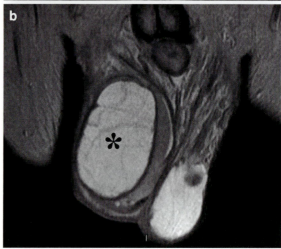

**Fig. 7** Cystic dysplasia of the rete testis. **a** Ultrasound image showing a large heterogeneous, multi-loculated intratesticular mass compressing the parenchyma (*arrows*). **b** Coronal MR image showing the mass containing thin septa with no signs of parenchymal infiltration

(Kantarci et al. 2005). The most common morphology is a pedunculated unilocular cyst (Fig. 10).

## 6 Testicular Abscess

A testicular abscess may develop secondary to severe epididymo-orchitis, or may be secondary to mumps, trauma, or infarction. Ultrasound shows a corpusculated fluid collection (Fig. 11), or a markedly hypoechoic mass with unclear edges, surrounded by a hypoechoic halo. Color Doppler interrogation demonstrates perilesional hyperemia with an absence of blood flow

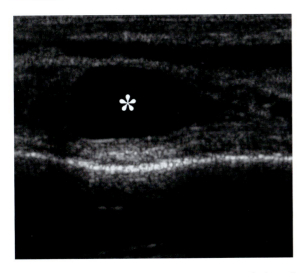

**Fig. 8** Cyst of the spermatic cord. Axial ultrasound view of the inguinal canal showing a cyst with regular rim

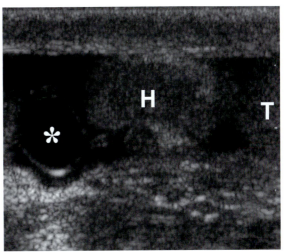

**Fig. 10** Cystic appendix epididymis. Small pedunculated cystic mass arising from the head of the epididymis (*H*). *T* = testis

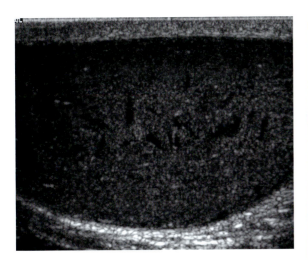

**Fig. 9** Epidermoid cyst of the spermatic cord. Longitudinal ultrasound scan showing a well circumscribed mass with echogenic content containing hypoechoic foci

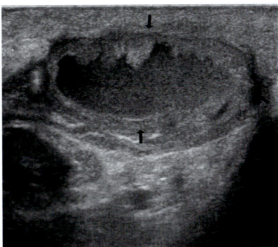

**Fig. 11** Testicular abscess. Ultrasound of the right testis in longitudinal scan. The testis is reduced in size and shows an extensive fluid collection with "dirty shadowing" and thick rim, due to granulomatous reaction, secondary to a long standing abscess

inside the mass. In rare cases gas bubbles are observed in the abscess cavity and they appear as focal hyperechoic spots with posterior shadowing (Pavlica and Barozzi 2001). At MR imaging the abscess is typically hypointense on T1-weighted images and hyperintense on T2-weighted images, compatible with fluid content. T2-weighted images demonstrate a hypointense rim. On contrast-enhanced T1-weighted images the lesion does not enhance, but the surrounding parenchyma shows avid enhancement (Cassidy et al. 2010).

## 7 Fluid Collections

Different kinds of fluid collections are commonly encountered within the scrotum. Among them, hydrocele, inflammatory collections, and hematocele must be differentiated.

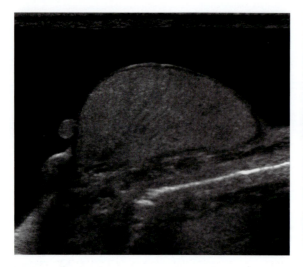

**Fig. 12** Scrotal hydrocele. Very large fluid collections extending from the inguinal area to the scrotum. The testis is normal in size, but compressed and displaced posterior

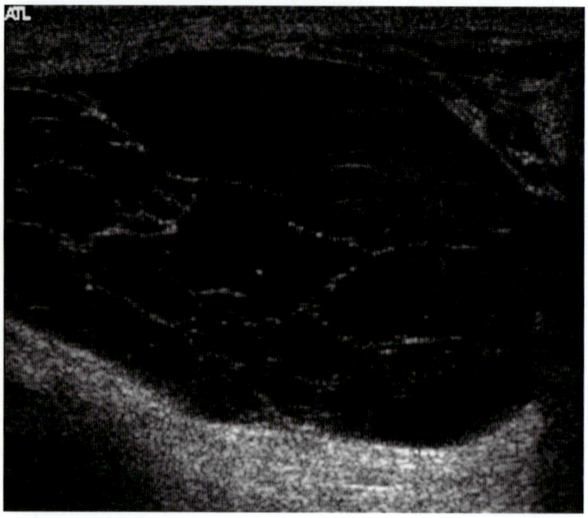

**Fig. 13** Scrotal long standing hydrocele. Scrotal ultrasound in longitudinal scan. Large fluid collection with multiple thin septa and wall thickening

## 7.1  Hydrocele

A minimal amount of fluid is normally present between the parietal and visceral layers of the tunica vaginalis. An abnormal amount of fluid is called a hydrocele. Idiopathic hydrocele, resulting from excessive fluid production or failure of the mesothelial lining to reabsorb the fluid, is frequently observed as the most common cause of scrotal enlargement. In adults, acute hydrocele may occur in conjunction with an inflammatory process (epididymitis or orchitis), as a sequel of trauma or torsion, or in the presence of a testicular tumor. Hydrocele is usually painless, although palpation of the underlying testis is frequently inhibited. The characteristic appearance of an anechoic fluid collection with smooth borders makes the ultrasound diagnosis straightforward (Fig. 12). A chronic hydrocele, which may occur secondary to recurrent inflammation or protracted epididymitis, additionally shows thickening of the wall and is frequently septated (Fig. 13). Scattered reflections may be seen corresponding to fibrin, debris, and inflammatory aggregations (Gooding et al. 1997).

In case of clinically suspected hydrocele, an ultrasound examination may be indicated for (a) confirmation of a fluid collection in patients with unclear clinical findings (b) evaluation of the testis and epididymis if palpation is limited (c) exclusion of a testicular tumor, and (d) reliable differentiation of a hydrocele from a testicular tumor. Sometimes, a massive hydrocele exerts

a pressure effect on the testicular parenchyma mimicking a testicular torsion and may compromise blood flow within the testis. Vascular resistance in intratesticular arteries is increased, and color Doppler interrogation may demonstrate an increase in the caliber of capsular arteries (Mihmanli et al. 2004). In these cases, aspiration of the fluid is mandatory to restore normal blood flow to the testis.

Hydrocele can be the first clinical sign of malignant mesothelioma of the tunica vaginalis, a rare aggressive tumor with a high predilection for metastatic spread, which is usually missed at preoperative imaging. Delayed diagnosis accounts for high recurrence and mortality rates. Aggarwal et al. (2010) described a case of mesothelioma presented with hydrocele, preoperatively diagnosed using scrotal ultrasound underlining the utility of color-Doppler.

## 7.2  Pyocele and Extratesticular Scrotal Abscess

A pyocele may occur as a complication of trauma, surgery, or epididymo-orchitis when the mesothelial lining of the tunica vaginalis is breached and infection ensues. Clinical history and physical examination of a painful scrotum help in making the diagnosis. At ultrasound, a pyocele often appears as a septate or complex heterogeneous fluid collection. A pyocele

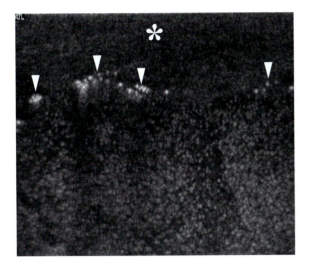

**Fig. 14** Pyocele. Longitudinal ultrasound scan in a patients with acute scrotal pain and swelling showing a corpuscolated fluid collection with reverberation artifacts (*arrowheads*) by presence of air. Thickening of the scrotal wall (*) is associated. Testes were normal (not shown)

organized as an abscess has a well-defined hyperemic wall. Gas bubbles within the fluid collection appear as hyperechoic foci with "dirty shadowing" (Fig. 14). In most cases, conservative treatment with antibiotics is sufficient. However, a scrotal abscess complicated by necrotizing infection of the perineum requires prompt surgery (Garriga et al. 2009).

## 7.3 Hematocele

Hematocele represents an accumulation of blood within the tunica vaginalis sac. It occurs most frequently following trauma or surgery but may also occur spontaneously or, more rarely, in association with clotting disorders, vasculitis or other inflammatory conditions. Haematocele has rarely been described as the presenting feature of malignancy (Mehra et al. 2007). The strength of this association is usually less of an issue than that of differentiating the appearances of haematocele from paratesticular cystic tumors, which may have very similar appearances both clinically and on ultrasound. Particularly with large haematocele, there may also be distortion of the adjacent testis, which can lead to increased suspicion of malignancy. Consequently, haematocele should be included in the differential diagnosis for complex

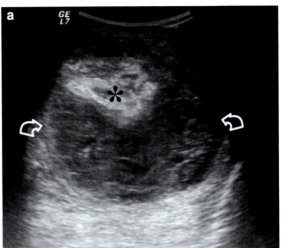

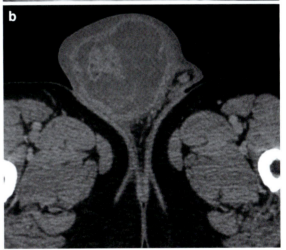

**Fig. 15** Haematocele of the scrotum in a patient with blunt pelvic trauma. **a** Axial ultrasound image of the right hemiscrotum shows a complex slightly echogenic fluid-filled mass, located cranially to the testis (*curved arrows*), enveloping the cord (*). **b** Corresponding CT scan obtained after iodinated contrast administration

cystic masses in the scrotum even in the absence of trauma. In the absence of a clear history of trauma, however, the exclusion of tumor is difficult and surgical exploration may be required.

Haematocele has a variable appearance on ultrasound, with a temporal change in characteristics on repeat ultrasound, as would be expected (Deurdulian et al. 2007). Acutely it is echogenic and becomes more complex and more hypoechoic with age (Fig. 15). Subacute and chronic haematoceles may contain fluid–fluid levels or low-level internal echoes (Dogra et al. 2003).

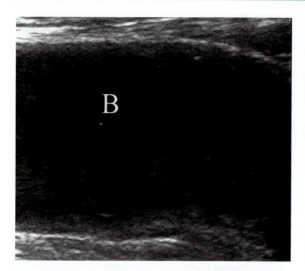

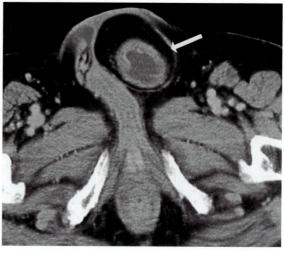

**Fig. 16** Inguinoscrotal hernia. The cord and the upper scrotal sac contain a fluid collection (*B*) due to bowel loop distended by fluid

**Fig. 17** Bladder inguino-scrotal hernia. Contrast-enhanced CT image in axial scan. The cord is distended and contains a fluid filled mass that shows thickened wall, corresponding to the bladder

Whenever ultrasound is not able to furnish a clear diagnosis, MR imaging can be performed since it has higher sensitivity and specificity, allowing a clear demonstration of blood as a collection of high signal intensity on T1-weighted images outside the testis. Especially when spare surgery is required, there may be an increased need to perform MR imaging for a better planning of the intervention.

In post-traumatic injury of the scrotum, CT may be useful in the general evaluation of the patient with pelvic trauma. The scrotal swelling secondary to haematocele or scrotal haematoma is identified as a high-density collection without contrast-enhancement, which is delimited from the residual parenchyma.

## 8    Arteriovenous Malformations

The ultrasound appearance of this uncommon pathological situation is multiple tubular anechoic structures that display vascular flow, readily differentiated from an intratesticular varicocele by lack of retrograde blood flow on the Valsalva manoeuvre. Differentiation from an intra-testicular hemangioma is more difficult; low-resistance flow with elevated peak and diastolic velocities are described in both, but the presence of a draining vein is considered characteristic of an intra-testicular AVM (Deurdulian et al. 2007). Calcification is more suggestive of a hemangioma.

## 9    Inguinoscrotal Hernia

An inguinoscrotal hernia occurs when an intestinal loop or part of the omentum passes into the scrotal cavity through an incompletely obliterated processus vaginalis. Inguinoscrotal hernias are most common in preterm neonates, but they may also develop in adults. The diagnosis can be difficult at physical examination. Ultrasound may be indicated to differentiate an inguinoscrotal hernia from other conditions and to investigate contralateral involvement (Garriga et al. 2009). At ultrasound, intestinal loops within the scrotum appear as a non-homogeneous mass, most commonly hypoechoic due to the fluid content of the bowel (Fig. 16). Peristalsis of bowel loops is possible to detect but the herniated loops are usually filled and without movement. The most useful finding is generally the presence of air bubbles within the cystic-appearing mass, although it can be hard to detect. Color Doppler interrogation may demonstrate vascularity of the intestinal wall. Hernias can also be diagnosed with CT, MR imaging, and even plain radiography if the bowel loops contain gas.

Occasionally, the bladder may herniate into the inguinal and femoral canals, the latter being more frequent in women. A predilection for the right side has been reported. Preoperative recognition is important to avoid complications such as urinary leakage and sepsis.

Retrograde cystography is usually considered the best technique to image scrotal bladder hernia. Diagnosis, however, is possible at ultrasound, CT, and MR imaging in the presence of a fluid-filled lesion in the scrotum (Fig. 17) whose volume and wall thickening changes after micturition. Pointing of the bladder toward the side of the hernia is a useful additional sign (Bacigalupo et al. 2005). Sagittal and coronal can provide better appreciation of the relationships of the herniated bladder, to the adjacent anatomical structures.

# References

Aggarwal P, Sidana A, Mustafa S et al (2010) Preoperative diagnosis of malignant mesothelioma of the tunica vaginalis using Doppler ultrasound. Urology 75:251–252

Algaba F, Mikuz G, Boccon-Gibod L et al (2007) Pseudoneoplastic lesions of the testis and paratesticular structures. Virchows Arch 451:987–997

Bacigalupo LE, Bertolotto M, Barbiera F et al (2005) Imaging of urinary bladder hernias. AJR Am J Roentgenol 184:546–551

Bostwick DG (1997) Spermatic cord and testicular adnexa. In: Bostwick DG, Eble JN (eds) Urologic surgical pathology. Mosby, Philadelphia, pp 647–674

Cassidy FH, Ishioka KM, McMahon CJ et al (2010) MR imaging of scrotal tumors and pseudotumors. Radiographics 30:665–683

Deurdulian C, Mittelstaedt CA, Chong WK et al (2007) US of acute scrotal trauma: optimal technique, imaging findings, and management. Radiographics 27:357–369

Dogra VS, Gottlieb RH, Rubens DJ, et al. (2001) Benign intratesticular cystic lesions: US features. Radiographics, 21:S273–S281

Dogra VS, Gottlieb RH, Oka M et al (2003) Sonography of the scrotum. Radiology 227:18–36

Garriga V, Serrano A, Marin A et al (2009) US of the tunica vaginalis testis: anatomic relationships and pathologic conditions. Radiographics 29:2017–2032

Gooding GA, Leonhardt WC, Marshall G et al (1997) Cholesterol crystals in hydroceles: sonographic detection and possible significance. AJR Am J Roentgenol 169: 527–529

Hamm B, Fobbe F, Loy V (1988) Testicular cysts: differentiation with US and clinical findings. Radiology 168:19–23

Holden A, List A (1994) Extratesticular lesions: a radiological and pathological correlation. Australas Radiol 38:99–105

Jarvis LJ, Dubbins PA (1989) Changes in the epididymis after vasectomy: sonographic findings. AJR Am J Roentgenol 152:531–534

Kantarci F, Ozer H, Adaletli I et al (2005) Cystic appendix epididymis: a sonomorphologic study. Surg Radiol Anat 27:557–561

Katergiannakis V, Lagoudianakis EE, Markogiannakis H et al (2006) Huge epidermoid cyst of the spermatic cord in an adult patient. Int J Urol 13:95–97

Kim W, Rosen MA, Langer JE et al (2007) US MR imaging correlation in pathologic conditions of the scrotum. Radiographics 27:1239–1253

Langer JE, Ramchandani P, Siegelman ES et al (1999) Epidermoid cysts of the testicle: sonographic and MR imaging features. AJR Am J Roentgenol 173:1295–1299

Lee SJ, Lee JH, Jeon SH et al (2010) Multiple epidermoid cysts arising from the extratesticular scrotal, spermatic cord and perineal area. Korean J Urol 51:505–507

Leissring JC, Oppenheimer RO (1973) Cystic dysplasia of the testis: a unique congenital anomaly studied by microdissection. J Urol 110:362–363

Leung ML, Gooding GA, Williams RD (1984) High-resolution sonography of scrotal contents in asymptomatic subjects. AJR Am J Roentgenol 143:161–164

Mac New HG, Terry NE, Fowler CL (2008) Cystic dysplasia of the rete testis. J Pediatr Surg 43:768–770

Maizlin ZV, Belenky A, Baniel J et al (2005) Epidermoid cyst and teratoma of the testis: sonographic and histologic similarities. J Ultrasound Med 24:1403–1409 quiz 1410-1401

Martinez-Berganza MT, Sarria L, Cozcolluela R et al (1998) Cysts of the tunica albuginea: sonographic appearance. AJR Am J Roentgenol 170:183–185

Mehra BR, Thawait AP, Narang RR et al (2007) Adenocarcinoma of the rete testis with uncommon presentation as haematocele. Singapore Med J 48:e311–e313

Mihmanli I, Kantarci F, Kulaksizoglu H et al (2004) Testicular size and vascular resistance before and after hydrocelectomy. AJR Am J Roentgenol 183:1379–1385

Pavlica P, Barozzi L (2001) Imaging of the acute scrotum. Eur Radiol 11:220–228

Poster RB, Spirt BA, Tamsen A et al (1991) Complex tunica albuginea cyst simulating an intratesticular lesion. Urol Radiol 13:129–132

Rifkin MD, Kurtz AB, Goldberg BB (1984) Epididymis examined by ultrasound. Correlation with pathology. Radiology 151:187–190

Rouviere O, Bouvier R, Pangaud C et al (1999) Tubular ectasia of the rete testis: a potential pitfall in scrotal imaging. Eur Radiol 9:1862–1868

Sellars ME, Sidhu PS (2003) Ultrasound appearances of the testicular appendages: pictorial review. Eur Radiol 13:127–135

Strauss S, Belenky A, Cohen M et al (2001) Focal testicular lesion after sperm extraction or aspiration: sonographic appearance simulating testicular tumor. AJR Am J Roentgenol 176:113–115

Tanaka T, Yasumoto R, Kawano M (2000) Epidermoid cyst arising from the spermatic cord area. Int J Urol 7: 277–279

Ulbright TM, Amin MB, Young RH (1999) Miscellaneous primary tumors of the testis, adnexa, and spermatic cord. In: Rosai J, Sobin LH (eds) Atlas of tumor pathology. Armed Forces Institute of Pathology, Washington, pp 235–366

Weingarten BJ, Kellman GM, Middleton WD et al (1992) Tubular ectasia within the mediastinum testis. J Ultrasound Med 11:349–353

Woodward PJ, Schwab CM, Sesterhenn IA (2003) From the archives of the AFIP: extratesticular scrotal masses: radiologic-pathologic correlation. Radiographics 23: 215–240

# Imaging Scrotal Lumps in Children

Brian D. Coley and Venkata R. Jayanthi

## Contents

### Abstract

The discovery of a scrotal mass in a child causes great concern. While the causes of most masses are benign, the history and physical examination may not always be able to discern the etiology. Ultrasound is the most useful imaging tool to define whether or not a mass is present, and most importantly whether it is intratesticular or extra-stesticular. Neoplasms are less common in the pediatric population, and are often of different histologies than in adults. Although ultrasound cannot often diagnose specific tumor types, there are a few benign lesions with sufficiently characteristic ultrasound appearances that can allow consideration for testis sparing surgery, something rarely possible in adults. Understanding the congenital and acquired masses presenting as scrotal lumps in children will improve the imager's ability to assist our clinical colleagues with patient management.

## 1   Introduction

The discovery of a scrotal mass causes concern and alarm in both the patient and parents. While the cause of the mass may be obvious from the history and physical examination, imaging is often required for diagnosis. It is crucial to differentiate between testic-ular and extra-testicular masses. Most pediatric scrotal swelling is due to benign extratesticular causes, but testicular tumors do occur. In evaluating a child with a scrotal mass, ultrasound can confirm that a mass is present, if it is solid or cystic, and whether it is

B. D. Coley (✉)
Department of Radiology,
Nationwide Children's Hospital,
700 Children's Drive, Columbus OH 43205, USA
e-mail: brian.coley@nationwidechildrens.org

V. R. Jayanthi
Department of Pediatric Urology,
Nationwide Children's Hospital,
700 Children's Drive, Columbus OH 43205, USA

M. Bertolotto and C. Trombetta (eds.), *Scrotal Pathology*, Medical Radiology. Diagnostic Imaging,
DOI: 10.1007/174_2011_185, © Springer-Verlag Berlin Heidelberg 2012

intratesticular or paratesticular. Sonography is highly sensitive for the detection of testicular neoplasms, with a negative predictive value approaching 100% (Aso et al. 2005; Dogra et al. 2003; Kennedy et al. 1999). Since there is a greater risk for malignancy with intratesticular masses the determination of site of origin relevant to the clinician for treatment planning; US is 90–100% accurate in differentiating intratesticular from extratesticular processes (Aso et al. 2005; Dogra et al. 2003; Hamm 1997). The histology of some masses can be suspected based upon patient age and sonographic features, but many masses will require tissue sampling or resection for diagnosis.

## 2 Congenital Causes

### 2.1 Polyorchidism

Abnormal division or duplication of the genital ridge (the primordial testis) after the third month of development may result in polyorchidism, a rare anomaly resulting in multiple testes in one hemiscrotum, most commonly triorchidism on the left (Coffin and Dehner 1992; Kogan et al. 1996; Amodio et al. 2004; Coley 2007; Rousso et al. 2006). The ipsilateral testes usually share a common epididymis, vas deferens, and tunica albuginea, although each testis may have its own (Amodio et al. 2004). Polyorchidism usually presents as an incidental asymptomatic scrotal mass. Torsion of one of the duplicated testes occurs in up to 15% of cases, in which case patients present with acute pain (Amodio et al. 2004; Shah et al. 1992). The supernumerary testis may fail to descend normally and may be associated with an inguinal hernia (Amodio et al. 2004). Polyorchid testes may have impaired spermatogenesis, and have an increased risk of malignancy (up to 6%) making clinical or imaging follow-up important (Amodio et al. 2004; Danrad et al. 2004). The contralateral testis may be cryptorchid (15–50%), and there may be an inguinal hernia or hydrocele (Chung and Yao 2002).

Sonographically, the supernumerary testis has normal echogenicity and echotexture, but is often smaller than the normal contralateral testis (Fig. 1). Clinical mimics of polyorchidism include testicular lobulation, splenogonadal fusion, and other paratesticular masses (Amodio et al. 2004; Kao and Gerscovich 2003; Zuppa et al. 2006).

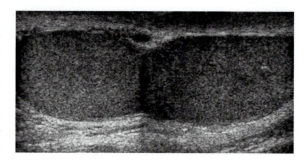

**Fig. 1** Polyorchidism. Longitudinal sonogram of the right scrotum shows two testes with normal echogenicity. There was a normal single left testis

### 2.2 Testicular Ectopia

Testicular ectopia is an anomaly due to an aberration of testicular descent (Marjanovic et al. 2007). Both testes are usually located in the same hemiscrotum, but the crossed testis may be intraabdominal. Patients present with a scrotal mass and contralateral empty scrotum (Marjanovic et al. 2007; Malik et al. 2008). An associated inguinal hernia is present in half of patients, and nearly one-third will have persistent Müllerian duct syndrome (presence of a uterus and sometimes other Müllerian duct derivatives in a male). Twenty percent will have seminal vesicle cysts, renal abnormalities, or hypospadias (Marjanovic et al. 2007). Ectopic testes have sonographic features similar to those of the normal testis, and are easily identified when they are in the scrotum.

### 2.3 Testicular Size Asymmetry

Testicular size asymmetry can be due to congenital causes such as Klinefelter syndrome and endocrine deficiencies (Zeger et al. 2008). Acquired causes include trauma, previous inguinal hernia surgery, torsion, inflammation, varicocele, and radiation therapy. Testicular size asymmetry has also been seen as a transient normal finding in peripubertal patients (Fig. 2). The testicular echogenicity is variable.

### 2.4 Splenogonadal Fusion

Splenogonadal fusion is a rare congenital anomaly with ectopic splenic tissue appearing as a solid mass

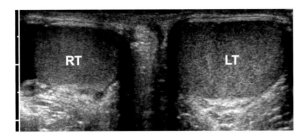

**Fig. 2** Testicular size asymmetry. Transverse sonogram of both testes in a young teenager shows a smaller right testis (*RT*) compared to the left testis (*LT*). There were no parenchymal abnormalities

usually adjacent to the left testis (Cirillo et al. 1999). The ectopic splenic tissue may be an isolated mass (discontinuous form), or may be continuous with a cord of splenic tissue that extends into the left upper quadrant (continuous form) (Varma et al. 2007). Ultrasound shows tissue typically isoechoic to testis and spleen, and is otherwise histologically non-specific unless a connecting cord can be demonstrated (Cirillo et al. 1999; Netto et al. 2004; Stewart et al. 2004).

# 3 Testicular Tumors

## 3.1 Primary Testicular Neoplasms

Primary testicular tumors account for 2% of solid malignant tumors in boys with an incidence of 0.5–2 cases per 100,000 (Agarwal and Palmer 2006; Skoog 1997). Prepubertal tumors are more often benign, and when malignant often have a more favorable clinical course than in older patients (Ciftci et al. 2001; Metcalfe et al. 2003; Ross et al. 2002). Postpubertal tumors are more frequently malignant and have a greater frequency of mixed histology (Agarwal and Palmer 2006).

### 3.1.1 Germ Cell Tumors

Up to 90% of pediatric primary testicular tumors arise from germ cells (Agarwal and Palmer 2006; Skoog 1997; Ciftci et al. 2001; Metcalfe et al. 2003; Ross et al. 2002). Yolk-sac carcinomas and mature teratomas make up the majority of germ cell tumors in the pediatric population, especially in prepubertal patients (Agarwal and Palmer 2006; Skoog 1997; Pohl et al. 2004; Shukla et al. 2004). Less common germ

cell tumors are immature teratomas, embryonal carcinomas, teratocarcinomas, and choriocarcinomas (De Backer et al. 2006). These latter tumors arise universally in pediatric patients. Patients present with painless scrotal enlargement (Agarwal and Palmer 2006; Ciftci et al. 2001; Metcalfe et al. 2003; De Backer et al. 2006), unless complicated by torsion or intratumoral hemorrhage.

Yolk sac tumors usually occur in prepubertal boys (median age, 2 years), and account for 50–75% of germ cell neoplasms (Coley 2007; Agarwal and Palmer 2006; Ciftci et al. 2001; Metcalfe et al. 2003; Pohl et al. 2004; Karmazyn 2010). At presentation, distant metastases are uncommon, with 85% of cases are confined to the scrotum (stage I) (Agarwal and Palmer 2006; De Backer et al. 2006; Grady 2000). Local spread occurs to regional and retroperitoneal lymph nodes. Radical orchiectomy is the treatment of choice. Although as many as 20% of patients may demonstrate a recurrence (detected by imaging or rising alpha fetoprotein levels), with surgical and chemotherapy survival is close to 100% (Wu and Snyder 2004).

The more aggressive embryonal carcinomas, mixed germ cell tumors, teratocarcinomas, and choriocarcinomas usually occur in adolescents or young adults. Elevated serum levels of beta-human chorionic gonadotropin levels are often seen with embryonal cell tumors and teratocarcinomas (Skoog 1997; Ciftci et al. 2001; Ross et al. 2002). Although metastases are less common than in adults, these non-yolk sac germ cell tumors more often have nodal or hematogenous spread (Ciftci et al. 2001; Grady et al. 1995).

Benign mature teratoma accounts for about 25–50% of prepubertal germ cell tumors (Agarwal and Palmer 2006; Ciftci et al. 2001; Metcalfe et al. 2003; Ross et al. 2002; Pohl et al. 2004), usually seen in boys under 4 years of age. Prepubertal teratomas are always benign, and metastatic disease has never been reported (Metcalfe et al. 2003; Ross et al. 2002; Grady 2000). In a prepubertal patient with negative tumor markers and suggestive sonographic findings, testis-sparing surgery can be performed (Metcalfe et al. 2003; Ross et al. 2002). In pubertal patients, however, mixed histologies with malignant elements are often present and the tumors behave more aggressively, necessitating orchiectomy.

Epidermoid cysts are uncommon benign germ cell tumors arising from the ectoderm, accounting for 3%

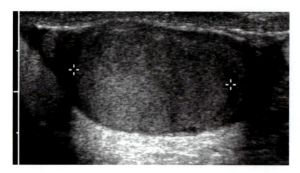

**Fig. 3** Yolk sac tumor. Longitudinal sonogram of the left testis in a 5 month-old with painless left scrotal swelling shows a large solid mass (*cursors*) replacing most of the left testis. Radical orchiectomy was performed

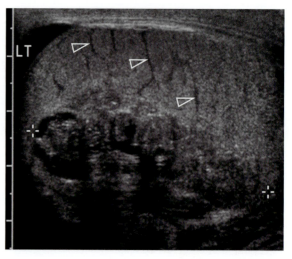

**Fig. 4** Mixed germ cell tumor. Longitudinal sonogram of the left testis in a 16 year-old with painless swelling shows a heterogeneous mass (*cursors*) within the left testis, along with prominence of the interlobular septae (*arrowheads*) indicating edema. Computed tomography demonstrated para-aortic and retroperitoneal metastases

of pediatric testicular tumors (Agarwal and Palmer 2006; Ross et al. 2002; Neumann et al. 1997). Presenting as a painless mass, these tumors often have a sufficiently characteristic appearance, such that testis-sparing surgery is possible (Aso et al. 2005).

Gonadoblastomas are rare germ cell tumors nearly always found in phenotypic females with a karyotype containing an XY cell line (Skoog 1997; Papaioannou et al. 2009). The majority are diagnosed only at surgery to remove dysplastic intra-abdominal gonads. Malignant germ cell elements are found in 10% (Agarwal and Palmer 2006; Papaioannou et al. 2009).

Seminoma is the most common testicular tumor in adults (Ross et al. 2002), but it is rare in children. It is, however, the neoplasm most associated with cryptorchid testes (Berkmen and Alagol 1998). Testis tumors in previously cyptorchid testes usually present in the third decade of life.

### 3.1.1.1  Sonographic Findings

Malignant germ cell tumors are usually well circumscribed with variably heterogeneous echogenicity depending on the presence of calcification, hemorrhage and necrosis (Figs. 3 and 4). However, sometimes they may appear as diffuse testicular enlargement with diffuse parenchymal infiltration (Aso et al. 2005; Dogra et al. 2003; Metcalfe et al. 2003; Ross et al. 2002; Shukla et al. 2004; Woodard et al. 2002). Aggressive tumors may infiltrate the tunica albuginea, producing an irregular testicular contour. Reactive hydroceles are associated finding in 20% of cases (Agarwal and Palmer 2006). Malignant tumors tend to be hyperemic on Doppler imaging, particularly when larger than 1.5 cm (Fig. 5) (Luker and Siegel 1994a). Color

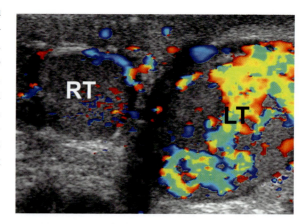

**Fig. 5** Germ cell tumor with hyperemia on color Doppler. Transverse color Doppler images of both testes in a 5-month-old (same patient as in Fig. 3) show tremendous hyperemia within the tumor in the left testis (*LT*). The normal right testis (*RT*) is shown for comparison

Doppler sonography may rarely identify a discrete mass when gray-scale sonography is normal (Luker and Siegel 1994b; Akin et al. 2004). There are no specific gray-scale and Doppler patterns that allow separation of various histological subtypes.

Teratomas appear as complex solid and cystic masses, reflective of their complex composition, and

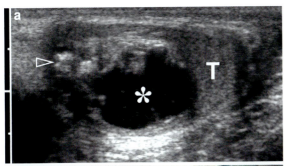

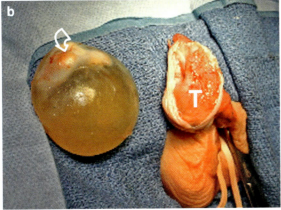

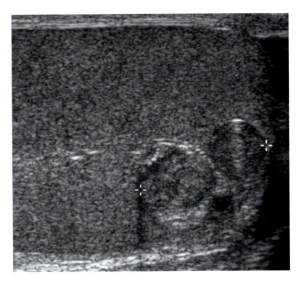

**Fig. 7** Epidermoid. Longitudinal image of the inferior pole of the left testis shows a well-defined bilobed intratesticular mass (*cursors*). The internal contents have a characteristic whorled or lamellated appearance. Testis-spring surgery was performed

**Fig. 6** Benign teratoma. **a** Longitudinal sonogram in a 13-month-old shows a complex mass with solid and cystic (*astrisk*) components as well as echogenic foci representing calcification (*arrowhead*) with normal surrounding testicular parenchyma (*T*). **b** Intraoperative image from another prepubertal patient shows that the testis (*T*) has been bivalved and the translucent cystic teratoma removed intact. There is a solid mural nodule (*curved arrow*) visible within the cystic mass. The testis was normal two years after testis-sparing surgery

often have echogenic foci that can be bone, calcification, or fat (Fig. 6) (Aso et al. 2005; Dogra et al. 2003; Woodard et al. 2002; Frush and Sheldon 1998). These tumors tend to be relatively large compared to the testis, and may produce marked thinning of the remaining testicular parenchyma. Ultrasound tends to underestimate the amount of residual normal testicular tissue, and testis-sparing surgery can result in a normal testis (Patel et al. 2007).

Epidermoid cysts are heterogeneously hypoechoic with well-defined margins. The epithelial lining sheds keratinized debris that often forms a characteristic lamellated or onion-skin appearance, although this is not a universal finding (Fig. 7) (Maizlin et al. 2005; Dogra et al. 2001; Moghe and Brady 1999; Manning and Woodward 2010). They are avascular. In the case of equivocal sonographic findings, magnetic resonance

imaging may be diagnostic and thus allow testis-sparing surgery (Cho et al. 2002; Cittadini et al. 2004).

Gonadoblastomas are usually solid and hypoechoic, although cystic areas occur. Seminomas are usually more homogeneous than other germ cell tumors and appear homogeneously hypoechoic compared with the normal testis. Rarely they are heterogeneous with cystic areas related to necrosis (Dogra et al. 2003).

### 3.1.2 Stromal Tumors

Stromal tumors account for about 10% of pediatric testicular neoplasms (Agarwal and Palmer 2006; Skoog 1997; Ciftci et al. 2001; Ross et al. 2002). Sertoli cell and juvenile granulosa cell tumors each account for about 40%, with Leydig cell tumors accounting for the remaining 20% (Agarwal and Palmer 2006; Ross et al. 2002).

Sertoli cell tumors present as painless masses at a mean age of 6 months (Thomas et al. 2001). Most are hormonally inactive, but they may secrete estrogens causing gynecomastia (Agarwal and Palmer 2006). Bilateral tumors may occur in patients with Peutz–Jeghers syndrome (Aso et al. 2005). Although all tumors reported in boys under the age of 5 years have been benign, malignancy occurs in older boys, so orchiectomy is usually performed.

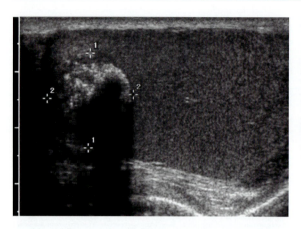

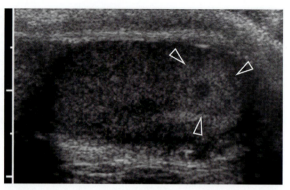

**Fig. 8** Calcifying Sertoli cell tumor. Longitudinal sonogram in a 16 year-old shows a densely calcified mass (*cursors*) in the superior pole of the right testis. Testis-sparing surgery was curative

**Fig. 9** Leydig cell tumor. Longitudinal sonogram of the right testis in a patient with size asymmetry after hernia repair shows a hyperechoic mass (*arrowheads*) with a hypoechoic central area; color Doppler show internal flow. Testis-sparing surgery was curative

Juvenile granulosa cell tumors are hormonally inactive, present in the first months of life, and are associated with chromosomal mosaicism (Yikilmaz and Lee 2007). Radical orchiectomy is the traditional treatment (Agarwal and Palmer 2006), although simple enucleation has been suggested as an acceptable alternative (Shukla et al. 2004).

Leydig cell tumors are typically found in prepubertal boys with a mean age of seven years (Coley 2007). About 30% of tumors produce testosterone with resultant precocious virilization; they have also been associated with Klinefelter's syndrome (Agarwal and Palmer 2006; Skoog 1997; Maizlin et al. 2004; Merlini et al. 2003). Leydig cell tumors are benign in prepubertal patients, and can be treated with testis-sparing tumor resection (Agarwal and Palmer 2006; Merlini et al. 2003).

### 3.1.2.1 Sonographic Findings
Sertoli cell tumors are typically well-circumscribed hypoechoic homogeneous lobular masses. In children, a large-cell calcifying subtype is common and may show large areas of calcification on ultrasound (Fig. 8); they may also be bilateral (Woodard et al. 2002; Maizlin et al. 2004; Ricci et al. 2004; Shin and Outwater 2007). Juvenile granulosa cell tumors typically are multiseptated complex cystic masses with vascular septations, but may rarely be solid (Yikilmaz and Lee 2007; Moore et al. 2003). Leydig cell tumors are typically small solid hypoechoic masses, although some may contain cystic areas or be hyperechoic (Fig. 9) (Woodard et al. 2002; Ricci et al. 2004).

## 3.2 Secondary Testicular Neoplasms

Most pediatric secondary testicular neoplasms are due to leukemia and lymphoma. These are the most common bilateral testicular malignancies, and account for 2–5% of tumors (Agarwal and Palmer 2006). Testicular leukemia may present at initial diagnosis or at any time during treatment, even when patients are in bone marrow remission, with boys with acute lymphoblastic leukemia having testicular involvement in 5–30% of cases at some point during their disease (Dogra et al. 2003; Agarwal and Palmer 2006). The blood–testis barrier limits chemotherapeutic penetration, making the testis second behind the central nervous system as a site of occult and relapsed disease (Dogra et al. 2003; Agarwal and Palmer 2006). Patients present with asymptomatic unilateral or bilateral scrotal enlargement, although occasionally may also have pain.

Testicular lymphoma is almost always due to secondary involvement in non-Hodgkin's lymphoma (Dogra et al. 2003); primary testicular lymphoma is rare in children. Clinically asymptomatic infiltration with Burkitt's lymphoma is seen at autopsy in 5–30% of children (Zwanger-Mendelson et al. 1989). As with leukemia, lymphomatous testicular involvement is usually painless, with pain occurring in only about 5% of children.

At sonography leukemic and lymphomatous infiltration have similar appearances, typically producing enlarged, homogeneous, hypoechoic testes. They usually diffusely replace the testes, but well-circumscribed

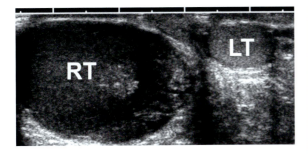

**Fig. 10** Leukemia. Transverse sonogram of both testes in a 10 year-old boy with leukemia shows a diffusely enlarged and hypoechoic right testis (*RT*) indicating diffuse leukemic infiltration. The left testis (*LT*) was normal

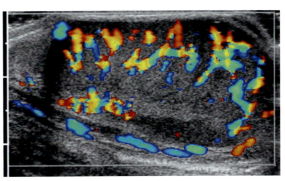

**Fig. 12** Leukemia. Longitudinal sonogram of a patient with testicular involvement with acute lymphocytic leukemia shows marked hyperemia with some irregularity to the course of the vessels through the testicular parenchyma

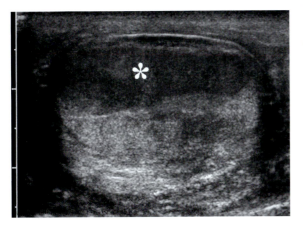

**Fig. 11** Lymphoma. Longitudinal sonogram of a 10 year-old boy shows a large focal hypoechoic mass (*astrisk*) within the left testis

focal hypoechoic masses can occur (Figs. 10 and 11) (Dogra et al. 2003; Agarwal and Palmer 2006; Akin et al. 2004). Involvement is usually bilateral but can be unilateral, and the pattern of involvement may be different in the two testes (Aso et al. 2005; Dogra et al. 2003; Golan et al. 1997; Patriquin 1993). Color Doppler shows hypervascularity (Fig. 12), even with small focal tumors. The hyperemic vessels often appear irregular and disorganized, unlike the more regular vasculature seen in inflammatory conditions (Luker and Siegel 1994a, b; Akin et al. 2004; Mazzu et al. 1995). Rarely, the epididymis is also involved (Ishigami et al. 2004).

Testicular metastases from other primary sites are uncommon, but have been reported with neuroblastoma, Wilms tumor, Langerhans cell histiocytosis, carcinoid, retinoblastoma, and rhabdomyosarcoma (Aso et al. 2005; Luker and Siegel 1994a; Koseoglu

et al. 1999; Stroosma and Delaere 2008; Trobs et al. 2002). Metastases occur from hematogenous or lymphatic dissemination, but direct extension from contiguous tumor may also occur. At sonography, metastases have a variable echogenicity, but are often hypoechoic. They are typically well-defined focal masses, but local invasion of adjacent structures can occur (Aso et al. 2005). Color Doppler usually demonstrates hyperemia (Luker and Siegel 1994a, b; Koseoglu et al. 1999).

## 3.3 Other Testicular Tumors

Non-neoplastic lesions that resemble solid neoplasms include Leydig cell hyperplasia, adrenal rests, hamartomas, hemangiomas, fibromas, and dermoids (Fig. 13) (Ciftci et al. 2001; Carucci et al. 2003; Dogra et al. 2004; Walker et al. 2008; Rubenstein et al. 2004). These benign lesions are usually solid and hypoechoic, but they can be complex or hyperechoic.

Leydig's cell hyperplasia is a rare benign condition. Children usually present between the ages of 5 and 9 years with precocious puberty. Sonography shows multiple hypoechoic or echogenic small testicular nodules (<6 mm), often bilateral (Carucci et al. 2003). Histological examination shows nodules of hyperplastic Leydig cells.

Testicular adrenal rests arise from fetal adrenal cortical cells that migrate with gonadal tissue during fetal development (Dogra et al. 2004). These cells form tumor-like masses in response to increased levels of adrenocortical hormones and are usually found in patients with congenital adrenal hyperplasia, with an

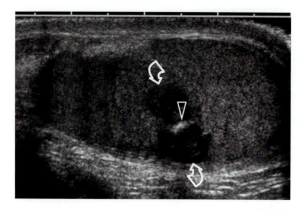

**Fig. 13** Dermoid. Longitudinal sonogram of the right testis in a 2 year-old boy with a palpable mass shows a bilobed hypoechoic mass (*curved arrows*) with a single focus of increased echogenicity (*arrowhead*). Testis-sparing surgery was curative

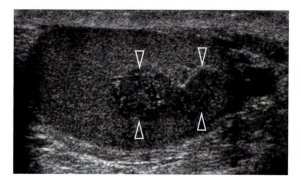

**Fig. 14** Adrenal rests. Longitudinal sonogram of the left testis in a young adult with known congenital adrenal hyperplasia shows lobular hypoechoic masses (*arrowheads*) centrally along the mediastinum testis

incidence of 24–94% (Claahsen-van der Grinten et al. 2007; Stikkelbroeck et al. 2003). At sonography, adrenal rests are round hypoechoic, intratesticular nodules, often bilateral, and most commonly located near the mediastinum testis (Fig. 14) (Dogra et al. 2004; Stikkelbroeck et al. 2003; Avila et al. 1999a, b). Tumor size can vary in response to hormone levels. Adrenal rests appear similar to Leydig cell tumors, but the clinical setting usually clarifies the diagnosis thus avoiding unnecessary surgery (Dogra et al. 2004).

## 4     Paratesticular Tumors

### 4.1     Malignant Lesions

Paratesticular tumors, whether benign or malignant, are uncommon in children and usually arise from the

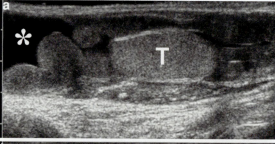

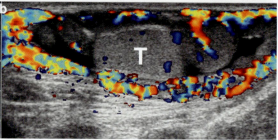

**Fig. 15** Paratesticular rhabdomyosarcoma. **a** Longitudinal sonogram of the right scrotum in a 4 year-old with painless swelling shows a normal testis (*T*) surrounded by lobular soft tissue masses along with a small hydrocele (*astrisks*). **b** Color Doppler image shows tremendous hyperemia in the soft tissue masses with normal flow within the testis (*T*)

epididymis or spermatic cord, and less commonly from the appendix testis or testicular tunics (Sudakoff et al. 2002). While most adult paratesticular tumors are benign, 30% of pediatric paratesticular masses are malignant, the most common being embryonal rhabdomyosarcoma (Aso et al. 2005; Ciftci et al. 2001; Frush and Sheldon 1998; Sung et al. 2006). Patients are generally under 5 years of age and present with a painless rapidly growing mass (Ciftci et al. 2001; Sung et al. 2006). They tend to be large masses, and there is frequently retroperitoneal lymph node spread at diagnosis (Dogra et al. 2003). At sonography paratesticular rhabdomyosarcoma has a variable echogenicity, and may contain areas of necrosis, hemorrhage, or calcification; they are typically hyperemic with color Doppler (Fig. 15). While they tend to be well defined, there may be invasion of the testis and epididymis (Aso et al. 2005).

Other malignant paratesticular tumors include metastatic neuroblastoma, lymphoma, leiomyosarcoma, fibrosarcoma, leukemia, and lymphoma (Dogra et al. 2003; Zwanger-Mendelson et al. 1989; Koseoglu et al. 1999; Karaosmanoglu et al. 2008). The sonographic appearance of these tumors is non-specific, and histology cannot be determined on the basis of sonographic appearance.

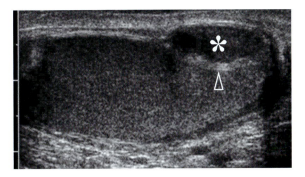

**Fig. 16** Sperm granuloma. Longitudinal sonogram of the right testis in a 16 year-old boy with a tender mass shows a well-circumscribed mass (*astrisk*) inferiorly; color Doppler showed internal flow. The displacement of the tunica albuginea (*arrowhead*) indicates that this mass is paratesticular and not within the testis

## 4.2 Benign Lesions

In children, benign paratesticular masses are usually cystic lesions such as spermatoceles and epididymal or tunica albuginea cysts. Epididymal cystadenomas can be seen in pediatric patients with von Hippel-Lindau disease, appearing as complex cystic masses (Dogra et al. 2003).

Adenomatoid tumors are uncommon in children, but are occasionally found in an older adolescent (Dogra et al. 2003). They are most commonly located in the epididymis, but they may be in the spermatic cord or testicular tunics (Kolgesiz et al. 2003). Sonography shows a variably echogenic solid, well-circumscribed mass (Dogra et al. 2003; Frates et al. 1997).

Other causes of benign paratesticular tumors include fibromas, leiomyomas, hemangiomas, arteriovenous malformation, lipomas, dermoids, neurofibromas, sperm granulomas, and pseudotumor (Sung et al. 2006; Bhatt et al. 2006). The sonographic appearance of these tumors is variable, and solid benign and malignant masses cannot be differentiated by sonographic appearance (Fig. 16); excision or biopsy is required for diagnosis.

## 5 Non-Neoplastic Scrotal Masses

## 5.1 Solid Masses

Meconium periorchitis results from when sterile meconium leaked from in utero bowel perforation

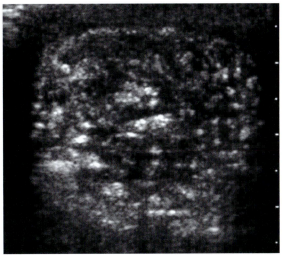

**Fig. 17** Meconium periorchitis. Transverse sonogram of the right scrotum in a newborn with a firm discolored scrotum shows a heterogeneous mass with multiple echogenicities, some of which appear to shadow. Radiographs showed calcifications in the scrotum and abdomen. The right testis was not visible

passes through a patent processus vaginalis where it incites a mass-like inflammatory foreign-body giant-cell reaction (Sung et al. 2006). These masses may be soft at birth, but will eventually become firm and hard with a bluish discoloration of the scrotum. The ipsilateral testis may not be separately palpable (Sung et al. 2006; Varkonyi et al. 2000; Williams et al. 2004). At sonography meconium periorchitis is a complex echogenic mass with areas of shadowing calcification that may obscure the testis (Fig. 17) (Coley 2007). This appearance can be confused with a testicular teratoma, but the diagnosis becomes clear if intra-abdominal calcifications are observed (Varkonyi et al. 2000; Williams et al. 2004; Han et al. 1998). The natural history is for the calcified mass to resolve (Varkonyi et al. 2000).

## 5.2 Cystic Masses

### 5.2.1 Hydrocele

A hydrocele is collection of fluid between the visceral and parietal layers of the tunica vaginalis, and is the most common cause of a painless scrotal swelling in childhood (Bhatt et al. 2006). In neonates and infants, almost all hydroceles are associated with a patent process vaginalis, which allows peritoneal fluid to enter the scrotal sac (Aso et al. 2005; Dogra et al. 2003; Skoog 1997; Chung et al. 1999). The majority of hydroceles are isolated to the scrotum, surround the anterior and lateral aspect of the testis (Aso et al. 2005; Sudakoff et al. 2002), and have a narrow proximal peritoneal communication. Hydroceles can present as a loculated or encysted fluid collection around the spermatic cord if the processus vaginalis closes above the testis and below the internal ring (Chung et al. 1999). Rarely (0.4–3.1% of cases), the hydrocele communicates with the peritoneal cavity and presents as both a scrotal and an intra-abdominal mass (Fenton and McCabe 2002). This occurs when the processus vaginalis is closed at the internal ring and scrotal pressure exceeds abdominal pressure, allowing fluid to flow back into the abdominal cavity (Fenton and McCabe 2002; Cuervo et al. 2009). Clinically, loculated hydroceles and abdominoscrotal hydroceles can resemble inguinal hernias.

In older children and adolescents, hydroceles may be acquired as the result of testicular torsion, trauma, inflammatory processes, and tumors (Aso et al. 2005). Occasionally, patients with ventriculoperitoneal shunts develop hydroceles because cerebrospinal fluid or the shunt itself tracks into the scrotum via a patent process vaginalis (Coley and Kosnik 2006).

At sonography, most hydroceles are thin-walled anechoic fluid collections (Fig. 18) (Chung et al. 1999), but some show low-level echoes due to cholesterol crystals, hemorrhage, or infection (Aso et al. 2005; Dogra et al. 2003; Sudakoff et al. 2002). Chronic hydroceles can be associated with scrotal wall thickening or calcifications. Hydroceles are avascular on Doppler sonography, but transducer movement causing fluid motion or acoustic pressure from the ultrasound beam creating flow patterns (acoustic streaming) can lead to color assignment in the hydrocele (Gerscovich and Kurzrock 2002).

### 5.2.2 Inguinal Hernia

Indirect inguinal hernias are far more common in boys than direct inguinal hernias. An indirect hernia results from the protrusion of intra-abdominal contents through the internal inguinal ring via a patent processus vaginalis.

Since the right processus vaginalis closes later than the left, indirect hernias are more commonly right-sided. The incidence is as high as 4.4% but is

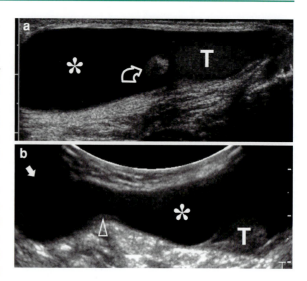

**Fig. 18** Hydroceles. **a** Longitudinal sonogram shows a simple hydrocele (*astrisk*) surrounding the anterior aspect of the testis (*T*), which is normally fixed to the scrotal wall, and the epididymis (*curved arrow*). **b** Extended field of view sonogram shows a large hydrocele (*astrisk*) surrounding the normally fixed testis (*T*), which extends through the inguinal canal (*arrowhead*) into the right lower quadrant (*arrow*)

increased in preterm infants (due to positive pressure ventilation) and in other patients with increased intra-abdominal pressure (Graf et al. 2002). Most hernias are clinically obvious, but sonography can be useful in patients who present with scrotal enlargement of unknown cause (Coley 2007; Graf et al. 2002; Robinson et al. 2006). The hernia may contain small bowel, colon, or omentum (Coley 2007).

Many patients with a clinically apparent unilateral inguinal hernia will have an asymptomatic contralateral patent processus vaginalis (Karmazyn 2010). While repairing the asymptomatic side is controversial, ultrasound can demonstrate these clinically inapparent defects (Graf et al. 2002; Hata et al. 2004). Hernia repair is required to prevent possible bowel incarceration (leading to obstruction) or strangulation (leading to ischemia). There is evidence that inguinal hernias can adversely effect testicular blood flow and function through pressure on the spermatic vessels (Turgut et al. 2007).

The inferior epigastric artery is useful as a landmark for identifying the internal inguinal ring, which lies immediately lateral to the artery at the inguinal ligament (Robinson et al. 2006; Chen et al. 1998; Korenkov et al. 1999). An inguinal canal width of

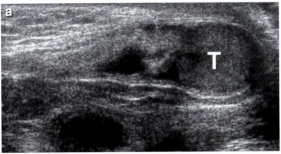

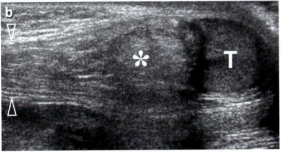

**Fig. 19** Hernia. **a** Longitudinal images of the right inguinal canal at rest show a normal canal and testis (*T*) without an apparent hernia. **b** With Valsalva, there is enlargement of the inguinal canal (*arrowheads*) and hernitaion of intra-abdominal contents (*astrisk*) into the scrotum superior to the testis (*T*)

greater than 4 mm at the internal ring has a sensitivity of 95% in indicating the presence of an indirect hernia (Chen et al. 1998). Raising intra-abdominal pressure by having the patient stand, strain, Valsalva, or cry improves hernia detection and may be the only time that the hernia is visible (Fig. 19). The sonographic appearance of the hernia depends on its content. Fluid-filled bowel will have a characteristic thick-walled tubular appearance, confirmed with the observation of peristalsis (Aso et al. 2005; Sudakoff et al. 2002). Incarcerated but viable bowel will be non-reducible, but will demonstrate normal bowel appearance and have color Doppler flow (Fig. 20). Absent peristalsis or color Doppler flow is concerning for bowel ischemia (Dogra et al. 2003; Coley 2007; Hata et al. 2004). Hernias containing only omentum appear as a complex echogenic paratesticular mass; change in mass shape with Valsalva and identification of omental vessels tracking up the inguinal canal help to clarify the diagnosis. The sonographic findings of hernia can occasionally overlap with those of complex hydroceles and hematoceles, but differentiation is possible when the typical appearance of the bowel wall and peristalsis is.

### 5.2.3 Epididymal Cyst and Spermatocele

Epididymal cysts and spermatoceles are usually incidental findings, but may present as painless palpable masses. Epididymal cysts have no age prediliction, are seen in up to 40% of adults, and occur anywhere along the epididymis (Sudakoff et al. 2002; Chung et al. 1999). While usually an isolated finding, they can be associated with cryptorchidism, cystic fibrosis, and von Hippel–Lindau syndrome (Blau et al. 2002; Homayoon et al. 2004). In children, epididymal cysts may resolve spontaneously (Homayoon et al. 2004). Spermatoceles are seen only after puberty resulting from cystic dilatation of the efferent tubules and are found in the head of the epididymis (Dogra et al. 2003; Chung et al. 1999). Spermatoceles contain spermatozoa and thick, white fluid.

Sonographically, both epididymal cysts and spermatoceles appear as hypoechoic or anechoic thin-walled structures with posterior acoustic enhancement (Fig. 21) (Dogra et al. 2003; Chung et al. 1999). Loculations and septations are occasionally seen. Spermatoceles are more likely to contain internal echoes from spertmatozoa and debris. They are avascular, but color Doppler imaging can show internal motion of this material due to acoustic streaming (Sista and Filly 2008).

### 5.2.4 Hematocele

A hematocele results from blood collecting between the layers of the tunica vaginalis that usually results from scrotal trauma and less commonly from intra-abdominal blood tracking down through a patent processus vaginalis, tumors, surgery, and bleeding disorders (Homayoon et al. 2004). Acute hematoceles are variably heterogeneous and predominantly echogenic, becoming more complex over time with the formation of septations, thickened walls, and even calcifications (Fig. 22) (Sudakoff et al. 2002; Deurdulian et al. 2007). Large hematoceles can displace the testis from its normal position and even result in vascular compromise from compression (Deurdulian et al. 2007).

### 5.2.5 Testicular Cyst

Simple intratesticular cysts are rare in children (Garcia et al. 1999; Garrett et al. 2000). They are composed of a single epithelial layer within a fibrous wall, and usually present as painless masses in children under one year of age (Garcia et al. 1999; Ceylan et al. 2004). Sonographically, testicular cysts are

**Fig. 20** Incarcerated hernia.
**a** Longitudinal composite image of the right inguinal canal and scrotum shows a herniated loop of bowel (*B*) extending into the scrotum superior to the testis (*T*) through an enlarged internal ring (*arrows*). The hernia was not reducible.
**b** Color Doppler image of the herniated bowel loop shows perfusion of the bowel wall, indicating bowel viability.
**c** Intraoperative image in another patient shows a dusky but viable loop of herniated bowel (*B*) delivered through an inguinal incision. The normal testis (*T*) and epididymis (*curved arrow*) have also been brought out and are normal

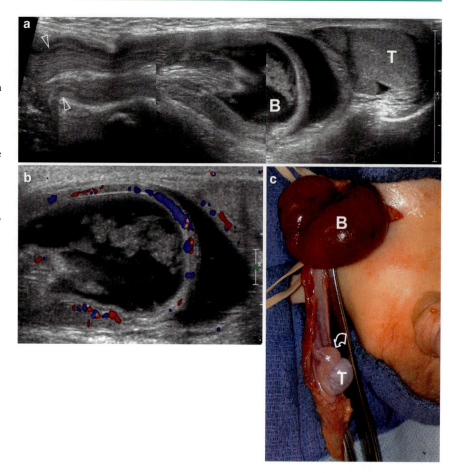

anechoic masses with smooth thin walls and posterior acoustic enhancement, and no solid elements as would be expected with a teratoma (Garcia et al. 1999; Garrett et al. 2000; Ceylan et al. 2004; Honjo et al. 2001). As these cysts grow, they can compress and compromise the surrounding normal parenchyma, so early surgery with simple cyst enucleation is the treatment of choice (Garcia et al. 1999; Ceylan et al. 2004; Upadhyay et al. 1998).

### 5.2.6 Lymphatic Malformation

Lymphatic malformations (lymphangiomas) are congenital malformations characterized by dilated lymphatic channels resulting in multiseptated masses of variably sized cysts. Although uncommon in the scrotum, they are slow-growing painless scrotal masses unless complicated by hemorrhage or infection (Weidman et al. 2002). Sonographically, they usually appear as cystic masses with variably echogenic contents and echogenic septations (Fig. 23) (Chung et al.

1999; Weidman et al. 2002). The cystic components are avascular, while the septations can show flow on color Doppler imaging (Loberant et al. 2002). The multicystic form of this malformation can mimic a complex hydrocele or hematocele. Microcystic lymphatic malformations appear more complex and solid, and can mimic a paratesticular neoplasm (Weidman et al. 2002; Loberant et al. 2002).

### 5.2.7 Pyocele

Pyoceles most commonly arise from the spread of infected intra-abdominal fluid through a patent processus vaginalis, usually from appendicitis or necrotizing enterocolitis (Dogra et al. 2003; Friedman and Sheynkin 1995; Hsieh et al. 1998; Lim et al. 2002; Yasumoto et al. 1998). Less common causes include direct extension from a testicular or epididymal abscess, or secondary infection of a hydrocele. Sonography shows a complex collection with inflammatory changes of scrotal skin thickening and peripheral

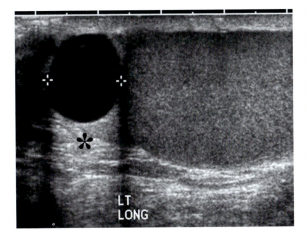

**Fig. 21** Epididymal cyst. Longitudinal sonogram of the left testis and epididymis in a 17 year-old shows a characteristic anechoic cystic mass (*cursors*) with posterior increased through transmission (*astrisk*) within the epididymis

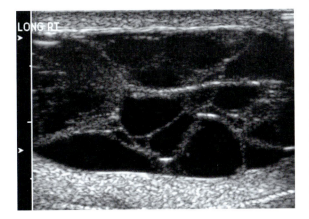

**Fig. 22** Hematocele. Longitudinal sonogram of the right scrotum in a patient with late testicular torsion shows a complex septated cystic collection with areas of anechoic and echogenic fluid

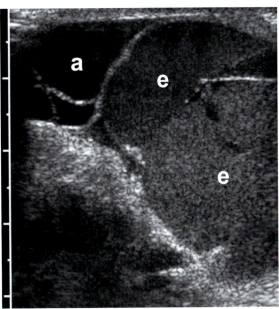

**Fig. 23** Lymphatic malformation. Longitudinal sonogram of the superior left scrotum of a teenager with swelling and discoloration shows a multiseptated cystic mass containing both anechoic fluid *a* and echogenic fluid *e* from hemorrhage

the testis, and if it is cystic or solid. Although the sonographic appearance of most testicular masses is not histologically specific, prepubertal teratomas, epidermoid cysts, and simple cysts often have sufficiently characteristic imaging appearances to allow testis-sparing surgery to be considered. The understanding and recognition of the appearances of pediatric scrotal masses allows the imager to make a significant contribution to patient care.

hyperemia that may involve the testis and epididymis as well (Chung et al. 1999; Srinivasan and Darge 2009).

## 6    Conclusion

When the history and physical examination fail to adequately discern the cause of a child's scrotal swelling, ultrasound is the imaging method of choice. Most scrotal swelling is due to benign extratesticular causes, and pediatric testicular neoplasms are fortunately uncommon. Ultrasound reliably discerns if a mass is present, if it originates within or external to

## References

Agarwal P, Palmer J (2006) Testicular and paratesticular neoplasms in prepubertal males. J Urol 176:875–881

Akin EA, Khati NJ, Hill MC (2004) Ultrasound of the scrotum. Ultrasound Q 20:181–200

Amodio J, Maybody M, Slowotsky C et al (2004) Polyorchidism: report of 3 cases and review of the literature. J Ultrasound Med 23:951–957

Aso C, Enriquez G, Fite M et al (2005) Gray-scale and color Doppler sonography of scrotal disorders in children: an update. RadioGraphics 25:1197–1214

Avila NA, Premkumar A, Merke DP (1999a) Testicular adrenal rest tissue in congenital adrenal hyperplasia: comparison of MR imaging and sonographic findings. AJR 172:1003–1006

Avila NA, Shawker TS, Jones JV et al (1999b) Testicular adrenal rest tissue in congenital adrenal hyperplasia: serial sonographic and clinical findings. AJR 172:1235–1238

Berkmen F, Alagol H (1998) Germinal cell tumors of the testis in cryptorchids. J Exp Clin Cancer Res 17:409–412

Bhatt S, Rubens DJ, Dogra VS (2006) Sonography of benign intrascrotal lesions. Ultrasound Q 22:121–136

Blau H, Freud E, Mussaffi H et al (2002) Urogenital abnormalities in male children with cystic fibrosis. Arch Dis Child 87:135–138

Carucci L, Tirkes A, Pretorius E et al (2003) Testicular Leydig's cell hyperplasia: MR imaging and sonographic findings. AJR 180:501–503

Ceylan H, Karaca I, Sari I et al (2004) Simple testicular cyst: a rare cuase of scrotal swelling in infancy. Int J Urol 11:352–354

Chen KC, Chu CC, Chou TY et al (1998) Ultrasonography for inguinal hernias in boys. J Pediatr Surg 33:1784–1787

Cho J, Chang J, Park B et al (2002) Sonographic and MR imaging findings of testicular epidermoid cysts. AJR 178: 743–748

Chung T, Yao W (2002) Sonographic features of polyorchidism. J Clin Ultrasound 30:106–108

Chung SE, Frush DP, Fordham LA (1999) Sonographic appearances of extratesticular fluid and fluid-containing scrotal masses in infants and children: clues to diagnosis. AJR 173:741–745

Ciftci A, Bingol-Kologlu M, Senocak M et al (2001) Testicular tumors in children. J Pediatr Surg 36:1796–1801

Cirillo RL Jr, Coley BD, Binkovitz LA et al (1999) Sonographic findings in splenogonadal fusion. Pediatr Radiol 29:73–75

Cittadini G, Gauglio C, Pretolesi F et al (2004) Bilateral epidermoid cysts of the testis: sonographic and MRI findings. J Clin Ultrasound 32:370–372

Claahsen-van der Grinten HL, Sweep FCGJ, Blickman JG et al (2007) Prevalence of testicular adrenal rest tumors in male children with congenital adrenal hyperplasia due to 21-hydroxylase deficiency. Eur J Endocrinol 157:339–344

Coffin CM, Dehner LP (1992) The male reproductive system. In: DL Stocker JT (ed) Pediatric pathology. J.B. Lippincott Co., Philadelphia, pp 905–919

Coley BD (2007) Sonography of pediatric scrotal swelling. Sem US, CT, MRI 28:297–306

Coley BD, Kosnik EJ (2006) Abdominal complications of ventriculoperitoneal shunts in children. Sem US, CT, MRI 27:152–160

Cuervo JL, Ibarra H, Molina M (2009) Abdominoscrotal hydrocele: its particular characteristics. J Pediatr Surg 44:1766–1770

Danrad R, Askhker L, Smith w (2004) Polyorchidism: imaging may denote reproductive potential of accessory testicle. Pediatr Radiol 34:492–494

De Backer A, Madern GC, Wolffenbuttel KP et al (2006) Testicular germ cell tumors in children: management and outcome in a series of 20 patients. J Pediatr Urol 2:197–201

Deurdulian C, Mittelstaedt CA, Chong WK et al (2007) US of acute scrotal trauma: optimal technique, imaging findings, and management. RadioGraphics 27:357–369

Dogra V, Gottlieb R, Rubens D et al (2001) Testicular epidermoid cysts: sonographic features with histopathologic correlation. J Clin Ultrasound 29:192–196

Dogra V, Gottlieb R, Oka M et al (2003) Sonography of the scrotum. Radiology 227:18–36

Dogra V, Nathan J, Bhatt S (2004) Sonographic appearance of testicular adrenal rest tissue in congenital adrenal hyperplasia. J Ultrasound Med 23:979–981

Fenton L, McCabe K (2002) Giant unilateral abdominoscrotal hydrocele. Pediatr Radiol 32:882–884

Frates MC, Benson CB, DiSalvo DN et al (1997) Solid extratesticular masses evaluated with sonography: pathologic correlation. Radiology 204:43–46

Friedman SC, Sheynkin YR (1995) Acute scrotal symptoms due to perforated appendix in children: case report and review of literature. Pediatr Emerg Care 11:181–182

Frush DP, Sheldon CA (1998) Diagnostic imaging for pediatric scrotal disorders. RadioGraphics 18:969–985

Garcia CJ, Zuniga S, Rosenberg H et al (1999) Simple intratesticular cysts in children: preoperative sonographic diagnosis and histological correlation. Pediatr Radiol 29:851–855

Garrett JE, Cartwright PC, Snow BW et al (2000) Cystic testicular lesions in the pediatric population. J Urol 163: 928–936

Gerscovich E, Kurzrock E (2002) Acoustic streaming versus venous pseudoaneurysm in a scrotal mass. J Clin Ultrasound 30:569–570

Golan G, Lebensart PD, Lossos IS (1997) Ultrasound diagnosis and follow-up of testicular monocytic leukemia. J Clin Ultrasound 25:453–455

Grady R (2000) Current management of prepubertal yolk sac tumor of the testis. Urol Clin North Am 27:503–508

Grady RW, Ross JH, Kay R (1995) Patterns of metastatic spread in prepubertal yolk sac tumor of the testis. J Urol, 153:1259–

Graf JL, Caty MG, Martin DJ et al (2002) Pediatric hernias. Sem US, CT, MRI 23:197–200

Hamm B (1997) Differential diagnosis of scrotal masses by ultrasound. Eur Radiol 7:668–679

Han K, Mata J, Zaontz MR (1998) Meconium masquerading as a scrotal mass. Br J Urol 82:765–767

Hata S, Takahashi Y, Nakamura T et al (2004) Preoperative sonographic evaluation is a useful method of detecting contralateral patent processus vaginalis in pediatric patients with unilateral inguinal hernia. J Peds Surg 39:1396–1399

Homayoon K, Suhre C, Steinhardt G (2004) Epididymal cysts in children: natural history. J Urol 171:1274–1276

Honjo O, Uemura S, Murakami I (2001) Simple testicular cyst in infants: a case report and review of the literature. Eur J Pediatr Surg 11:425–427

Hsieh DS, Jeng SY, Liu YS (1998) Bilateral idiopathic infantile pyoceles: a case report. Chung Hua I Hsueh Tsa Chih (Taipei) 61:39–43

Ishigami K, Yousef-Zahra D, Abu-Yousef M (2004) Enlargement and hypervascularity of both the epididymis and testis do not exclude involvement with lymphoma or leukemia. J Clin Ultrasound 32:365–369

Kao E, Gerscovich E (2003) Benign testicular lobulation: sonographic findings. J Ultrasound Med 22:299–301

Karaosmanoglu D, Karcaaltincaba M, Balli O et al (2008) Sonographic findings of testicular involvement of neuroblastoma: an unusual clinical association. J Ultrasound Med 26:1785–1787

Karmazyn B (2010) Scrotal Ultrasound. Ultrasound Clinics 5:61–74

Kennedy PT, Elliott JM, Rice PF et al (1999) Ultrasonography of intratesticular lesions: its role in clinical management. Ulster Med J 68:54–58

Kogan S, Hadziselimovic F, Howards SS et al (1996) Pediatric andrology. In: Gillenwater JY, Grayhack JT, Howards SS et al (eds) Adult and pediatric urology, Third edn edn. Mosby, St. Louis, pp 2623–2674

Kolgesiz A, Kantarci F, Kadioglu A et al (2003) Adenomatoid tumor of the tunica vaginalis testis: a special maneuver in diagnosis by ultrasonography. J Ultrasound Med 22:303–305

Korenkov M, Paul A, Troidl H (1999) Color duplex sonography: diagnostic tool in the differentiation of inguinal hernias. J Ultrasound Med 18:565–568

Koseoglu V, Akata D, Kutluk T et al (1999) Neuroblastoma with spermatic cord metastasis in a child: sonographic findings. J Clin Ultrasound 27:287–289

Lim G, Lim S, Jeong Y et al (2002) Infantile scrotal pyocele simulating missed testicular torsion on sonography. J Clin Ultrasound 31:116–118

Loberant N, Chernihovski A, Goldfeld M, et al (2002) Role of Doppler sonography in the diagnosis of cystic lymphangioma of the scrotum. J Clin Ultrasound 384–387

Luker GD, Siegel MJ (1994a) Pediatric testicular tumors: evaluation with gray-scale and color Doppler US. Radiology 191:561–564

Luker GD, Siegel MJ (1994b) Color Doppler sonography of the scrotum in children. AJR 163:649–655

Maizlin ZV, Belenky A, Kunichezky M et al (2004) Leydig cell tumor of the testis: gray scale and color Doppler sonographic appearance. J Ultrasound Med 23:959–964

Maizlin Z, Belenky A, Baniel J et al (2005) Epidermoid cyst and teratoma of the testis: sonographic and histologic similarities. J Ultrasound Med 24:1403–1409

Malik MA, Iqbal Z, Chaudri KM et al (2008) Crossed testicular ectopia. Urology 71:984.e985–e986

Manning MA, Woodward PJ (2010) Testicular epidermoid cysts: sonographic features with clinicopathologic correlation. J Ultrasound Med 29:831–837

Marjanovic ZO, Perovic SV, Slavkovic A et al (2007) Transverse testicular ectopia with and without persistent Mullerian duct syndrome. Int Urol Nephrol 39:1167–1171

Mazzu D, Jeffrey RB, Ralls PW (1995) Lymphoma and leukemia involving the testicles: findings on gray-scale and color Doppler sonography. AJR 164:645–647

Merlini E, Seymandi PL, Betta PG et al (2003) Testis sparing enucleation of a Leydig-cell tumour in a boy. Pediatr Med Chir 25:63–65

Metcalfe P, Farivar-Mohseni H, Farhat W et al (2003) Pediatric testicular tumors: contemporary incidence and efficacy of testicular preserving surgery. J Urol 170:2412–2416

Moghe PK, Brady AP (1999) Ultrasound of testicular epidermoid cysts. Br J Radiol 72:942–945

Moore W, Li S, Rifkin MD (2003) Juvenile granulosal cell tumor of the testicle. Ultrasound Quarterly 19:39–41

Netto J, Perez L, Kelly D et al (2004) Splenogonadal fusion diagnosed by Doppler ultrasonography. Scientific World Journal 4(Suppl 1):253–257

Neumann DP, Abrams GS, Hight DW (1997) Testicular epidermoid cysts in prepubertal children: case report and review of the world literature. J Pediatr Surg 32:1786–1789

Papaioannou G, Sebire NJ, McHugh K (2009) Imaging of the unusual pediatric 'blastomas'. Cancer Imaging 9:1–11

Patel AS, Coley BD, Jayanthi VR (2007) Ultrasonography underestimates the volume of normal parenchyma in benign testicular masses. J Urol 178(4 Pt 2):1730–1732

Patriquin HB (1993) Leukemic infiltration of the testis. In: PA Siegel BA (ed) Pediatric Disease (Fourth series) test and syllabus. American College of Radiology, Reston, VA, pp 667–688

Pohl H, Shukla A, Metcalf P et al (2004) Prepubertal testis tumors: actual prevalence rate of histological types. J Urol 172:2370–2372

Ricci Z, Stein M, Koenigsberg M et al (2004) Unusual sonographic appearance of a Leydig cell tumor of the testis. Pediatr Radiol 34:177–178

Robinson P, Hensor E, Lansdown M et al (2006) Inguinofemoral hernia: accuracy of sonography in patients with indeterminate clinical features. AJR 187:1168–1178

Ross J, Rybicki L, Kay R (2002) Clinical behavior and contemporary management algorithm for prepubertal testis tumors: a summary of the prepubertal testis tumor registry. J Urol 168:1675–1679

Rousso I, Iliopoulos D, Athanasiadou F et al (2006) Congenital bilateral anorchia: hormonal, molecular and imaging study of a case. Genet Mol Res, 5:638–642

Rubenstein R, Dogra V, Seftel A et al (2004) Benign intrascrotal lesions. J Urol 141:1765–1772

Shah S, Miller B, Geisler E (1992) Polyorchidism discovered as testicular torsion. Urology 39:543–544

Shin SL, Outwater EK (2007) Benign large cell calcifying Sertoli cell tumor of the testis in a prepubescent patient. AJR 189:W65–W66

Shukla A, Woodard C, Carr M et al (2004a) Experience with testis sparing surgery for testicular teratoma. J Urol 171:161–163

Shukla A, Huff D, Canning D et al (2004b) Juvenile granulosa cell tumor of the testis: contemporary clinical management and pathological diagnosis. J Urol 171:1900–1902

Sista AK, FILLY RA (2008) Color Doppler sonography in evaluation of spermatoceles: the "falling snow" sign. J Ultrasound Med 27:141–143

Skoog SJ (1997) Benign and malignant pediatric scrotal masses. Pediatr Clin North Am 44:1229–1250

Srinivasan AS, Darge K (2009) Neonatal scrotal abscess: a differential diagnostic challenge for the acute scrotum. Pediatr Radiol 39:91

Stewart V, Sellars M, Somers S et al (2004) Splenogonadal fusion: B-mode and color Doppler sonographic appearances. J Ultrasound Med 23:1087–1090

Stikkelbroeck NM, Suliman HM, Otten BJ et al (2003) Testicular adrenal rests in postpubertal males with congenital adrenal hyperplasia: sonographic and MR features. Eur Radiol 13:1597–1603

Stroosma OB, Delaere KP (2008) Carcinoid tumours of the testis. BJU Int 101:1101–1105

Sudakoff G, Quiroz F, Karcaaltincaba M et al (2002) Scrotal ultrasonography with emphasis on the extratesticular space: anatomy, embryology, and pathology. Ultrasound Quarterly 18:255–273

Sung T, Riedlinger W, Diamond D et al (2006) Solid extratesticular masses in children: radiographic and pathologic correlation. AJR 186:483–490

Thomas J, Ross J, Kay R (2001) Stromal testis tumors in children: a report from the prepubertal testis tumor registry. J Urol 166:2338–2340

Trobs RB, Friedrich T, Lotz I et al (2002) Wilms' tumour metastasis to the testis: long-term survival. Pediatr Surg Int 18:541–542

Turgut AT, Olcucuoglu E, Turan C et al (2007) Preoperative ultrasonographic evaluation of testicular volume and blood flow in patients with inguinal hernias. J Ultrasound Med 26:1657–1666

Upadhyay V, Holmes M, Kolbe A (1998) Gonadal preservation in a simple testicular cyst. Pediatr Surg Int 13:445–446

Varkonyi I, Fliegel C, Rosslein R et al (2000) Meconium periorchitis: case report and literature review. Eur J Pediatr Surg 10:404–407

Varma DR, Sirineni GR, Rao MV et al (2007) Sonographic and CT features of splenogonadal fusion. Pediatr Radiol 37:916–919

Walker RN, Murphy TJ, Wilkerson ML (2008) Testicular hamartomas in a patient with Bannayan-Riley-Ruvalcaba syndrome. J Ultrasound Med 27:1245–1248

Weidman E, Cendron M, Schned A et al (2002) Scrotal lymphangioma: an uncommon cause for a scrotal mass. J Ultrasound Med 21:669–672

Williams H, Abernethy L, Losty P et al (2004) Meconium periorchitis: a rare cause of a paratesticular mass. Pediatr Radiol 34:421–423

Woodard P, Sohaey R, O'Donoghue M et al (2002) Tumors and tumorlike lesions of the testis: radiologic-pathologic correlation. RadioGraphics 22:189–216

Wu H, Snyder H (2004) Pediatric urologic oncology: bladder, prostate, testis. Urol Clin North Am 31:619–627

Yasumoto R, Kawano M, Kawanishi H et al (1998) Left acute scrotum associated with appendicitis. Int J Urol 5:108–110

Yikilmaz A, Lee EY (2007) MRI findings of bilateral juvenile granulosa cell tumors of the testis in a newborn presenting as intraabdominal masses. Pediatr Radiol 37:1031–1034

Zeger MP, Zinn AR, Lahlou N et al (2008) Effect of ascertainment and genetic features on the phenotype of Klinefelter syndrome. J Pediatr 152:716–722

Zuppa AA, Nanni L, Di Gregorio F et al (2006) Complete epididymal separation presenting as polyorchidism. J Clin Ultrasound 34:258–260

Zwanger-Mendelson S, Schneck EH, Doshi V (1989) Burkitt lymphoma involving the epididymis and spermatic cord: sonographic and CT findings. AJR 153:85–86

# The Infertile Male-1: Clinical Features

Giovanni Liguori, Carlo Trombetta, Bernardino de Concilio,
Alessio Zordani, Michele Rizzo, Stefano Bucci,
and Emanuele Belgrano

## Contents

**Abstract**

Male infertility affects 10% of couples and is treatable in many cases. The evaluation of infertility is initiated typically after 1 year of failure to conceive. Clinical evaluation of the infertile man requires a complete medical history, physical examination, and laboratory studies in order to identify and treat correctable causes of subfertility and recognize those who are candidates for assisted reproductive technologies, those who are sterile and should consider adoption or artificial insemination using donor sperm, and those who should undergo genetic screening. Although pregnancies can be achieved without any evaluation other than a semen analysis, this test alone is insufficient to adequately evaluate the male patient. Treatment of correctable male-factor pathology is cost effective, does not increase the risk of multiple births, and can spare the woman invasive procedures and potential complications associated with assisted reproductive technologies.

## 1 Introduction

Infertility, defined as failure to conceive after regular unprotected sexual intercourse over a period of 1 year, continues to be a highly prevalent condition. About 15% of couples are thought to be affected (Templeton 2000; Gnoth et al. 2005). Although arbitrary, the time limit of 12 months is commonly accepted (Rowe 2006). It reflects the fact that the majority (approximately 85%) of couples who have achieved spontaneous pregnancy did so within 12 months. It is not unreasonable, however, to begin a

G. Liguori · C. Trombetta (✉) · B. de Concilio ·
A. Zordani · M. Rizzo · S. Bucci, · E. Belgrano
Department of Urology, University of Trieste,
Ospedale di Cattinara, Strada di Fiume 447,
34124 Trieste, Italy
e-mail: trombcar@units.it

M. Bertolotto and C. Trombetta (eds.), *Scrotal Pathology*, Medical Radiology. Diagnostic Imaging,
DOI: 10.1007/174_2011_186, © Springer-Verlag Berlin Heidelberg 2012

fertility evaluation sooner than 1 year if the woman's age is a factor and delaying the evaluation could further diminish the couple's chance of conceiving. Moreover, in couples with known reproductive disorders, an earlier intervention is also justified.

It is important to recognize that, while in 20–25% of cases the cause of infertility is due to the male partner and in 30–40% the problem is predominantly female, in approximately 30% of cases abnormalities are found in both partners, and in 15% no specific factor could be identified (World Health Organization 1987). In addition, 1–10% of male factor infertility is a result of an underlying, often treatable, but possibly life-threatening medical condition (Honig et al. 1994). Men with infertility are at 17-fold greater risk of having a testis tumor than men in the general population; moreover, pituitary tumors and other forms of acquired hypogonadotropic hypogonadism are not uncommonly detected in men with severe oligospermia or azoospermia. For these reasons, the investigation of the infertile couple must always include the study of both partners: as a matter of fact a male factor is detected in half of the couples with provable abnormalities and, in approximately half of these, there is a female factor as well (Bhasin 2007).

The term "primary male infertility" is used when a man has never impregnated a woman. Impregnation means that conception was attained, independent of the outcome of pregnancy. "Secondary male infertility" is when the man has impregnated a woman, irrespective of whether she is the present partner and irrespective of the outcome of pregnancy. The duration of involuntary infertility is defined as the number of months during which the couple has been having sexual intercourse without the use of any contraceptive method. This gives prognostic information about the couple's future probability of spontaneous conception.

## 2    Physiology

Male fertility needs good erectile function, spermatogenesis, normal endocrine function, and ejaculation. In addition, sexual intercourse timed appropriately to ovulation is an important key to conception. Because of the anxiety and stress that is often associated with couple infertility, male patients often describe difficulty with erections. Any previous history of genitourinary

cancers or pelvic surgeries that may have impaired erectile function should also be addressed. Spermatogenesis has traditionally been described as requiring a 74 day cycle (recent reports suggest it may actually be shorter than this time period). Any insult or intervention will usually require at least one spermatogenic cycle prior to seeing its effect.

FSH and testosterone are essential for normal spermiogenesis. When FSH is elevated, probably the testes are not producing sperm in normal amounts related to various causes including: testicular failure; genetic abnormalities, toxic exposures (including radiation, chemotherapy, and heat). If FSH is elevated by at least twice the upper limit of normal, the probability of finding sperm even on testicular biopsy is very low. This has recently changed with the development of new microsurgical techniques, including microscopic testicular sperm extraction (microTESE). Nonetheless, FSH levels are useful in counseling patients on potential outcomes of the infertility evaluation. If FSH is elevated (greater than twice normal) in a patient with severe oligospermia or azoospermia, the patient must be instructed that advanced reproductive techniques (ART) would most likely be necessary. Testosterone, another crucial hormone, contributes to libido, erectile function, and sperm production.

Obviously, intercourse must be timed to the periovulatory period. Sperms are able to live in the cervical mucus for an average of approximately 48 h. Patients should be instructed to have sexual intercourse near the time of anticipated ovulation.

## 3    Causes of Male Infertility

The etiology of male infertility is commonly multifactorial and the frequency of etiological factors varies among different surveys (Page et al. 1999; de Vries et al. 2001). In general, 15–20% of infertile men are azoospermic (de Vries et al. 2001; Steckel et al. 1993), and 10% have sperm density below 1 million/ml. A specific cause of infertility is not determinable in 40–60% men (Page et al. 1999; Schlegel 1997). Most infertile men have idiopathic oligozoospermia (Kolettis 2003).

Male fertility is a multifaceted process that requires an intact endocrine axis, successful spermatogenesis, adequate sperm delivery to the woman's genital tract, and sperm capable of penetrating the woman's ova. The causes for male infertility are numerous and can affect any one of these processes; as reported in some basic sources of urology, they can be conveniently grouped by effects at one or more of the following levels: pre-testicular, testicular, and post-testicular.

## 3.1 Pre-testicular (Endocrine) Causes

Pre-testicular causes of male infertility are often referred to as endocrine causes. Impairment of fertility in these cases is secondary to hormone deficiency, hormone excess, or receptor abnormality.

Hypogonadotropic hypogonadism results from both pituitary and hypothalamic disorders. Serum testosterone and gonadotropin levels are typically very low, often undetectable. Panhypopituitarism may result from pituitary tumors and the treatment regimens employed.

### 3.1.1 Hypothalamic Disease

Several hypothalamic disorders may be considered. Among them, isolated hypogonadotropic hypogonadism, isolated FSH deficiency, fertile Eunuch Syndrome, and Prader–Willi syndrome.

#### 3.1.1.1 Isolated Hypogonadotropic Hypogonadism

This disease is characterized by low LH, FSH, and testosterone levels. Gonadotropin deficiency may occur in the presence of otherwise normal pituitary function. It may be due to Kallmann syndrome (congenital hypogonadotropic hypogonadism associated with anosmia) or idiopathic hypogonadotropic hypogonadism. Kallmann syndrome is a rare (1:50,000 persons) disorder that occurs in familial and sporadic forms. The X-linked form of the disease is a consequence of a single gene deletion (Xp22.3 region, termed KALIG-1). It may also be autosomally transmitted with sex limitation to males. In either case, it is the consequence of failure of GnRH neurons to migrate from the olfactory area to the hypothalamus during fetal brain development. Clinical findings include anosmia, infertility, and deficient virilization.

#### 3.1.1.2 Isolated FSH Deficiency

In this rare condition, there is insufficient FSH production by the pituitary gland. Patients are normally virilized, as LH is present. Testicular size is normal, and LH and testosterone levels are normal. FSH levels are uniformly low and do not respond to stimulation with GnRH. Sperm counts range from azoospermia to severely low numbers (oligospermia).

#### 3.1.1.3 Fertile Eunuch Syndrome

Isolated LH deficiency occurs rarely in patients with normal FSH levels. These men demonstrate a eunuchoid habitus, large testes, and small-volume ejaculates that may contain a few spermatozoa.

#### 3.1.1.4 Prader–Willi Syndrome

It is a form of hypogonadotropic hypogonadism resulting from hypothalamic dysfunction. In addition to the clinical signs mentioned above for Kallmann's syndrome, obesity, mental retardation, cryptorchidism, and diabetes mellitus may be found. Genetically, deletion of a region on chromosome 15 is often found (Turek 2008).

### 3.1.2 Pituitary Disease

Pituitary function may be affected in cases of pituitary surgery, infarction, tumors, radiation, or infectious diseases.

#### 3.1.2.1 Hyperprolactinemia

Another form of hypogonadotropic hypogonadism is due to elevated levels of circulating prolactin. If hyperprolactinemia occurs, secondary causes such as stress during the blood draw, systemic diseases, and medications should be ruled out. With these causes excluded, the most common and important cause of hyperprolactinemia is a prolactinsecreting pituitary adenoma. Elevated prolactin usually results in decreased FSH, LH, and testosterone levels and causes infertility. Associated symptoms include loss of libido, impotence, galactorrhea, and gynecomastia. Signs and symptoms of other pituitary hormone derangements (adrenocorticotropic hormone, thyroid-stimulating hormone) should also be investigated.

### 3.1.3 Exogenous or Endogenous Hormones

#### 3.1.3.1 Estrogens

An excess of sex steroids, either estrogens or androgens, can cause male infertility due to an imbalance in the testosterone-estrogen ratio. Hepatic cirrhosis increases endogenous estrogens because of augmented aromatase activity within the diseased liver. Likewise, excessive obesity may be associated with testosterone-estrogen imbalance owing to increased peripheral aromatase activity. Less commonly, adrenocortical tumors, Sertoli cell tumors, and interstitial testis tumors may produce estrogens. Excess estrogens mediate infertility by decreasing pituitary gonadotropin secretion and inducing secondary testis failure.

### 3.1.3.2 Anabolic and Androgenic Steroid Abuse

These substances suppress pituitary LH release, leading to decreased intratesticular testosterone production. The end result is severe oligospermia or azoospermia. Although the effects are thought to be reversible, long-term pituitary suppression has been reported. Extremely low, even undetectable FSH and LH levels in a well-virilized patient are the keys to diagnosis.

### 3.1.3.3 Hyper- and Hypothyroidism

Abnormally high or low levels of serum thyroid hormone affect spermatogenesis at the level of both the pituitary and testis. Thyroid balance is important for normal hypothalamic hormone secretion and for normal sex hormone-binding protein levels that govern the testosterone-estrogen ratio. Thyroid abnormalities are a rare cause (0.5%) of male infertility.

## 3.2    Testicular Causes

Testicular causes of subfertility are, at present, largely irreversible. If sperms are observed, however, assisted reproductive technology can provide biological children for affected men.

### 3.2.1    Genetic/Karyotypic Abnormalities

Approximately 7% of men with low sperm counts and 13% with azoospermia have a structural alteration in the long arm of the Y chromosome (Yq). The testis-determining region genes that control testis differentiation are intact, but there may be gross deletions in other regions that may lead to defective spermatogenesis. Abnormalities in chromosomal constitution are well-recognized causes of male infertility. In a study of 1,263 infertile couples, a 6.2% overall incidence of chromosomal abnormalities was detected. In azoospermic men, 21% had significant chromosomal abnormalities. For this reason, Standard karyotype

analysis should be offered to all men with damaged spermatogenesis who are seeking fertility treatment by in vitro fertilization (IVF) or intracytoplasmic sperm injection (ICSI).

The commonest chromosomal abnormality is Klinefelter syndrome (47XXY): the clinical findings may be subtle and easily overlooked. The leg length is disproportionately long to the trunk length and the testicles are small and firm but virilization is often normal. The diagnosis is confirmed by karyotype analysis using a peripheral blood sample. Klinefelter's mosaicism is present in about 15–20% of cases. Low levels of mosaicism may be missed by some laboratories but should be identified if possible because the prospects for sperm recovery are much better than with nonmosaic Klinefelter's syndrome. Paternity with this syndrome is rare but more likely in the mosaic or milder form of the disease. The testes are usually <2 cm in length and always <3.5 cm; biopsies show sclerosis and hyalinization of the seminiferous tubules with normal numbers of Leydig cells. Hormones usually demonstrate decreased testosterone and frankly elevated LH and FSH levels. Serum estradiol levels are commonly elevated. Since testosterone tends to decrease with age, these men will require androgen replacement therapy both for virilization and for normal sexual function.

### 3.2.2    Anatomic Abnormalities

Testicular maldescent is classified according to the position of the testicle. Impalpable testes may be intra-abdominal or atrophic and within the inguinal canal. Intra-abdominal testes are generally positioned within the pelvic cavity, with blood vessels arising from the lower half of the abdominal aorta. Incompletely descended testes may lie within the inguinal canal. Often there is an associated hernia sac. Ectopic testes are defined as those testes that have left the abdominal cavity, but deviated from the normal pathway of descent through the inguinal canal. The most common site for ectopic testis is in the superficial inguinal pouch; in this situation the testis descends through the inguinal canal and lies above the external inguinal ring. The cord including the testicular blood vessels thus run inferiorly from the testicle before entering the superficial inguinal ring to run superiorly into the abdominal cavity. Surgeons need to understand this anatomical relationship to avoid damaging.

### 3.2.3 Gonadotoxins

Chemotherapy, radiation; cigarettes, marijuana, alcohol abuse, heavy metal exposure (lead, mercury), and other toxic/inflammatory insults may temporarily or even permanently suppress spermatogenesis. A proper history will elicit these causes.

### 3.2.4 Varicocele

Varicocele is frequently diagnosed among infertile male population: 35–40% of men with primary and 75–80% of men with secondary infertility (Jarow et al. 1996) according to different authors. Moreover, it is considered the most frequently encountered surgically correctable cause of male infertility, but clear predictive factors of a better outcome after its correction are still lacking. Sperm concentration, motility, and percentage of normal sperm cells are typically altered in infertile men with varicocele (Trombetta et al. 2003). Even the role of varicocele correction in improving these parameters is still debated (Tulloch 1955). As a matter of fact, the association of varicocele with infertility has been recognized for more than 50 years. Varicocele causes a duration-dependent decline in semen analysis parameters due to higher scrotal temperature, reflow of toxic metabolites, local hypoxia, and lack of nutrient factors (Goldstein and Eid 1989).

Several studies have attempted to determine the progression of seminal parameters after surgical correction of varicocele, but the results are yet to be discussed. Although most of them show a significant postoperative improvement in seminal parameters in 55–75% of treated patients (Schiff et al. 2006) recently some authors performed a meta-analysis where every possible beneficial effect of varicocele treatment is denied: this Cochrane Libraries Review failed to offer evidence that treatment of a varicocele in men does improve a couple's chances of spontaneous pregnancy, and the authors suggested that as long as it remains unclear whether a varicocele is "nature's attempt to heal a diseased testis rather than afflict an otherwise healthy one," varicocele correction cannot be recommended (Evers et al. 2009). However, some Italian authors reviewed this study and concluded that its statistical methods were poor and conclusions lacked significance (Ficarra et al. 2006). In contrast with Evers and Collins's meta-analysis, in a recent study we have demonstrated a significant improvement in either sperm concentration

(82% of patients), and motility (73%). Sixty-seven percentage of our patients showed an improvement in both parameters. Each grade of varicocele was associated with a significant improvement in sperm concentration and most of them also in motility and morphology (Liguori et al. 2010).

### 3.2.5 Acquired Testicular Damage

The virus that causes mumps can also infect the testes in 20–30% of males who contract this infection after puberty. There is a high likelihood of testicular damage in such circumstances and this may be irreversible in some cases. Other infections that have been associated with male infertility (Rowe 2006) include tuberculosis, bilharziasis, gonorrhoea, chlamydia, filariasis, typhoid, influenza, brucellosis and syphilis.

Injury to the testes from accidents or even operations can also depress the production of spermatozoa. In torsion of the testis, the testis twists on its cord thereby shutting off its blood supply. If this is diagnosed and untwisted by surgery within a short while the function of the testis may not be adversely affected.

### 3.2.6 Antisperm Antibodies (Testicular Injury, Previous Vasectomy)

The body normally produces antibodies to protect itself from foreign organisms such as bacteria and viruses. Occasionally antibodies against spermatozoa may be produced by the body and they will be found in semen and/or blood. These antisperm antibodies can be produced when there is damage to the testes, infection of the testes and surrounding tissues or obstruction to the transport of spermatozoa along the male genital tract. Antisperm antibodies may bind to spermatozoa and prevent them from moving. The antibodies can also bind several spermatozoa together to form a clump. Even if the motility of spermatozoa is not impaired, these antisperm antibodies may prevent the fertilization of the egg by affected spermatozoa that reach the fallopian tubes. However, the presence of antisperm antibodies does not always signify infertility because many men with these antibodies are able to impregnate their wives. In other words antisperm antibodies reduce fertility but do not prevent conception in every case where they are found; they are a relative rather than an absolute cause of infertility.

### 3.2.7 Idiopathic

A significant proportion of male subfertility currently is unexplained. Idiopathic subfertility occurs in as many as 25% of male partners of infertile couples. In this situation there is no cause found to explain the poor semen parameters.

## 3.3 Post-Testicular Causes

Vasal or epididymal occlusion, ejaculatory duct obstruction, and congenital absence of the vas deferens may be post-testicular causes for infertility.

### 3.3.1 Obstructive Azoospermia

Obstruction to the flow of spermatozoa from the testis to the exterior results in azoospermia. Vasal or epididymal occlusion may be congenital or acquired. The seminal fluid volume will be of normal quantity because very little of it is contributed by the vasal and epididymal component. Congenital epididymal obstruction is typically located at the vasal-epididymal junction. Acquired causes are numerous, the most common being vasectomy. Inflammation of the vas and epididymis may lead to scarring and point occlusions, most commonly in the epididymis. Tuberculous vasitis and epididymitis may completely obliterate large luminal sections, making reconstruction impossible. Young's syndrome is characterized by bronchiectasis and gradual epididymal obstruction by inspissated epididymal secretions. It is unclear whether Young's syndrome is also a mild form of cystic fibrosis. The testis size and consistency are normal, as spermatogenesis is unaffected. Serum FSH, LH, and testosterone are all within an adequate range, reflecting an uncompromised spermatogenic and androgenic axis. The epididymis may be firm and full, which can be appreciated only with careful and thoughtful physical examination.

When no sperm is found in the ejaculate of the patient with a semen volume of less than 1 mL, either ejaculatory duct obstruction or one of the syndromes of vasal aplasia will usually be the cause.

#### 3.3.1.1 Ejaculatory Duct Obstruction

This condition may result from both acquired and congenital causes. Congenital midline prostatic cysts may be of müllerian origin and can outwardly compress the terminal portions of the ejaculatory ducts as they course through the prostate. These are easily seen with TRUS. Prior prostatic inflammation may result in scarring and occlusion of the ejaculatory ducts. In this circumstance, no intraprostatic dilation of the ducts will be seen, although there will be vasal ampullary and seminal vesicle dilation. Complete ejaculatory duct occlusion is manifested by low-volume azoospermia, but partial ejaculatory duct obstruction may present as severe oligoasthenospermia out of proportion to what might be expected from the testis size and consistency coupled with the hormonal data.

#### 3.3.1.2 Congenital Absence of the Vas Deferens

Congenital bilateral absence of the vas deferens (CBAVD) and congenital unilateral absence of the vas deferens (CUAVD) are clinically mild forms of a phenotypic spectrum that includes cystic fibrosis. The presence of abnormalities (e.g., mutations, deletions of base pairs) in both the maternal and paternal copies of the cystic fibrosis transmembrane conductance regulator (CFTR) gene leads to defective protein action. Pulmonary and pancreatic ductal secretions are thick and tenacious as a consequence, and disease becomes manifest. In addition, nearly all male patients with cystic fibrosis have bilateral vasal aplasia and are infertile. CBAVD and CUAVD are limited, "mild" clinical expressions of CFTR dysfunction in which no pulmonary or pancreatic pathology is evident but vasal absence is still present. Cystic fibrosis mutation analysis is critical before commencement of infertility treatment for both partners to define and refine their risk, as a couple, of transmitting maternal and paternal CFTR gene anomalies. TRUS images seminal vesicle anatomic abnormalities, including aplasia, hypoplasia, or cystic dysplasia. The vasal ampullae are typically absent.

### 3.3.2 Male Accessory Gland Infection

The accessory glands (seminal vesicles, prostate and Cowper's glands) may become infected with organisms that cause the sexually transmitted diseases such as gonorrhoea, syphilis, chlamydia and non-specific urethritis. Urinary tract infections can secondarily affect the accessory glands. These infections may affect the contribution of these glands to seminal fluid. They can also extend to the vas deferens and epididymis, and cause their blockage. Testicular infection will affect the production of spermatozoa as well as lead to the production of antisperm antibodies.

## 3.4 Retrograde Ejaculation

If semen is propelled backwards into the bladder, rather than forward and out of the penis, there is no intravaginal deposition of semen. The bladder sphincters are closed at the time of ejaculation thereby preventing semen from passing backwards into the bladder. Diseases such as diabetes mellitus and multiple sclerosis may impair the closure of these sphincters leading to retrograde ejaculation. Operations around the bladder neck such as simple prostatectomy (removal of part of or the whole prostate gland) or transurethral resection of the prostate can also cause this problem. Moreover many drugs have been implicated on occasions.

## 3.5 Infrequent Sexual Intercourse

Some couples may present with infertility because they do not have intercourse frequently enough to ensure that spermatozoa are present in the female genital tract around the time of ovulation. The optimal frequency of sexual intercourse is unknown. However, if it happens at least three times a week there is a reasonable chance that this will be adequate for conception. Patterns of sexual activity amongst couples show a wide variation. Some may not maintain a high frequency of sexual intercourse for a long period of time for many reasons. It is important for these particular couples to ensure that they increase their sexual activity around the time of ovulation.

## 3.6 Wrong Timing of Sexual Intercourse

Some couples may concentrate their sexual activity at the wrong time of the menstrual/ovarian cycle. It has been known for a couple to have sexual intercourse only at the time of menstruation or soon afterwards because they believed that, that was when the woman was most fertile.

## 3.7 Sexual Dysfunction

Sexual dysfunction stemming from low libido or impotence is a frequent cause of infertility.

In ejaculatory failure, the man may have an erection but is unable to ejaculate during sexual intercourse.

## 3.8 Premature Ejaculation

Premature ejaculation can only be regarded as a cause of infertility if ejaculation occurs outside the vagina. If intravaginal ejaculation always take place, other causes for the infertility have to be looked for. At the same time the couple in question can seek psychosexual assistance to enable the man to achieve better control over the timing of his ejaculation so as to allow his wife adequate time to enjoy the sexual act and hopefully reach an orgasm.

## 4 Diagnosis

## 4.1 History

For all men with infertility, a complete history and physical examination is recommended to identify potentially correctable causes of male factor infertility. The evaluation of male infertility should proceed in concert with the female. The goals of male evaluation are to discover correctable causes of infertility, categorize the chance of successful sperm retrieval (for men who do not have sperm in the ejaculate), and identify significant medical problems associated with infertility.

The duration of the infertility, previous evaluation and treatment, previous pregnancies (for either partner), and any difficulty establishing these pregnancies should be documented. Inadequate frequency or timing of intercourse, sexual dysfunction, and lubricant use can impede pregnancy. The optimal frequency of intercourse is every day or every other day around the expected time of ovulation (Wilcox et al. 1995). Because nearly all commercially available lubricants are spermatotoxic, their use is discouraged.

A thorough history includes information about not only medical and surgical problems, but also about developmental issues, occupational and social habits, and exposures. Remember that sperm production is very sensitive to overall body health and problems that make the body ill will often affect spermatogenesis. The surgical history should include questions regarding a history of cryptorchidism and patient's age at the time of repair. Cryptorchidism can cause oligospermia or even azoospermia, if bilateral. Correction of hypospadias, chordee, or hernia should also be ascertained as well as any surgery on the bladder neck, urethra, rectum, or pelvis. A history of urethral strictures and/or sexually transmitted diseases may result in urethral and ductal obstruction causing reduced sperm counts. Men who have been treated for testicular cancer or Hodgkin's lymphoma may have reduced sperm counts related to their disease as well as treatments such as chemotherapy and radiation. Surgery for testicular cancer may include retroperitoneal lymph node dissections and this can injure the sympathetic nerves involved in ejaculation.

Most patients do not have a significant medical history, but some specific risk factors may be recognized. Diabetes mellitus can cause erectile and ejaculatory dysfunction. Previous disorders of the testes, such as cryptorchidism or spermatic cord torsion, or a history of inguinal, scrotal, or retroperitoneal surgery, are associated with subfertility (Sigman et al. 1997).

## 4.2 Physical Examination

Emphasis is placed on a thorough genitourinary examination. The male patient should be examined in a warm room. Normal virilization should be noted. The presence of gynecomastia should prompt questions regarding marijuana use or an evaluation for a prolactin producing pituitary tumor. The phallus may reveal hypospadias, chordee, plaques, or venereal lesions. Normal testicular size is 20 cm$^3$ and the testicle should be firm but not hard, not unlike the feel of a hard boiled egg. An orchidometer can be used to assess size. A normal testicle is at least 2.5 × 3 × 4 cm. Since 80% of testis volume is determined by spermatogenesis, testis atrophy is likely associated with decreased sperm production. Palpation of the epididymides and vas deferens might reveal induration, fullness or nodules indicative of infections, or obstruction. Careful delineation of each vas deferens may reveal agenesis, atresia, or injury (remember that 80% of men with CBAVD have at least one cystic fibrosis mutation). The spermatic cords should be examined for asymmetry suggestive of a lipoma or varicocele. Clinically significant varicoceles are diagnosed exclusively by physical examination. Lastly, a rectal examination is

important in identifying large cysts, infections, or dilated seminal vesicles (Shefi and Turek 2006).

## 4.3 Semen Analysis

Semen analysis is the cornerstone of male fertility assessment and is often the trigger to refer patients for a specialist opinion. If the semen analysis is normal, it is unlikely that other laboratory testing will be needed or useful. An abnormal semen analysis suggests that the probability of achieving fertility is lower than normal. Two semen analyses, performed with 2–3 days of sexual abstinence, are sought due to the large variability in semen parameters in healthy men. There is recent debate concerning precisely which values are considered "normal". The World Health Organization 1999 currently recommends 20 million sperm/mL and 50% motility as normal. The formal evaluation of sperm shape is termed morphologic assessment. In general, the percentage of sperm with normal morphology has the greatest discriminatory power in distinguishing fertile from infertile semen, although no particular value is diagnostic of fertility or infertility. Sperm morphology complements the routine semen analysis in the male evaluation and better estimates the chances of fertility. Semen analysis will be better and largely discussed in the chapter entitled: "The Infertile Male-2. Sperm Analysis".

## 4.4 Hormonal Evaluation

Male subfertility caused by correctable endocrinopathies is rare. As such, hormone testing for all subfertile men is not necessary. Current recommendations for endocrine evaluation of the infertile male are: a) sperm concentration <10 million sperm/mL; b) erectile dysfunction; c) other clinical signs or symptoms suggestive of low testosterone or unrelated endocrinopathy. The initial evaluation should include serum testosterone and follicle stimulating hormone (FSH) levels. This evaluation is usually adequate to assess the pituitary–testicular axis in the majority of cases.

If hypogonadism is suspected based on the semen analysis (severe oligospermia or azoospermia), evaluation of morning follicle-stimulating hormone (FSH) and total serum testosterone levels can help distinguish between primary and secondary causes.

**Table 1** Current indications for genetic testing of infertile male

| |
|---|
| Severe oligoasthenospermia in a couple considering in vitro fertilization (IVF) and intracytoplasmic sperm injection (ICSI) (Y microdeletion assay and karyotype analysis) |
| Azoospermia with testis atrophy in a couple considering testis sperm extraction with IVF and ICSI (Y microdeletion assay and karyotype analysis) |
| Azoospermia or very low sperm concentration with at least one absent vas deferens on physical examination (cystic fibrosis gene mutations) |
| Azoospermia with evidence of normal spermatogenesis (cystic fibrosis gene mutations) |

Elevated levels of FSH in the presence of low testosterone levels correlate with primary hypogonadism. Low levels of both hormones suggest secondary hypogonadism. If the testosterone level is low, a repeat testosterone (total and possibly free testosterone) with luteinizing hormone (LH) and prolactin serum levels in a morning blood draw is advised. Although an endocrinopathy is found in 10% of tested men, clinically significant endocrinopathies are detected in <2% of men (Bhasin 2007). In the setting of subfertility, a low level may indicate an underlying FSH deficiency, such as which occurs with hypogonadotropic hypogonadism (Rowe et al. 1993).

Normal testosterone, normal LH, and elevated FSH levels in an azoospermic or severely oligozoospermic man are suggestive of primary spermatogenic failure. These men should undergo measurement of testicular volume, karyotyping, and screening for Yq microdeletions.

## 4.5 Genetic Evaluation

The number of genes that may have a bearing on human fertility is progressively increasing. Thus, genetic testing should be performed in men with severe oligospermia, with detection of genetic anomalies increasing as sperm concentration decreases. Deletion of regions on the Y chromosome (microdeletions) occurs in 6% of men with severely low sperm counts and 15% of men with no sperm counts (Foresta et al. 2001). Deletion of the DAZ (deleted in azoospermia) gene in the AZFc region is the most commonly observed microdeletion in infertile men. In addition, 2% of men with low counts and 15–20% of men with no sperm counts will harbor chromosomal abnormalities detected by cytogenetic analysis (karyotype). Patients at highest risk for abnormal cytogenetic findings include men with small, atrophic testes, elevated FSH levels, and azoospermia. These include

conditions such as Klinefelter syndrome and translocations of non-sex chromosomes. Current indications for genetic testing of infertile males (Turek 2005) are outlined in Table 1. Similarly, genetic testing is indicated for infertile men who present with cystic fibrosis or congenital absence of the vas deferens. Approximately 80% of men without palpable vasa will harbor a cystic fibrosis gene mutation.

## 4.6 Other Testing

### 4.6.1 Anti-Sperm Antibodies

The testis is an immunologically privileged site, probably because of the blood-testis barrier. Autoimmune infertility may result when the blood-testis barrier is broken and the body is exposed to sperm antigens.

Testing for antisperm antibodies is indicated if: a) the semen analysis reveals aggregates of sperm; b) there is isolated asthenospermia; c) there is a risk of autoimmune infertility (i.e. prior torsion or testis injury); or d) there is unexplained infertility with a normal routine semen analysis. Usually performed with antibody coated, polyacrylamide spheres, an anti-sperm antibodies test with at least 50% of sperm bound with antibodies is considered clinically significant. Occurring in 5–10% of infertile men, it is thought that antibodies bound to the sperm head might interfere with sperm-egg interaction, penetration and fertilization, whereas tail bound antibodies may be more likely to affect sperm transport through the female reproductive tract (Francavilla et al. 2007).

## References

Bhasin S (2007) Approach to the infertile man. J Clin Endocrinol Metab 92:1995–2004

de Vries JW, Repping S, Oates R et al (2001) Absence of deleted in azoospermia (DAZ) genes in spermatozoa of infertile men with somatic DAZ deletions. Fertil Steril 75:476–479

Evers JH, Collins J, Clarke J (2009) Surgery or embolisation for varicoceles in subfertile men. Cochrane Database Syst Rev:CD000479

Ficarra V, Cerruto MA, Liguori G et al (2006) Treatment of varicocele in subfertile men: the cochrane review–a contrary opinion. Eur Urol 49:258–263

Foresta C, Moro E, Ferlin A (2001) Y chromosome microdeletions and alterations of spermatogenesis. Endocr Rev 22:226–239

Francavilla F, Santucci R, Barbonetti A et al (2007) Naturally-occurring antisperm antibodies in men: interference with fertility and clinical implications. An update. Front Biosci 12:2890–2911

Gnoth C, Godehardt E, Frank-Herrmann P et al (2005) Definition and prevalence of subfertility and infertility. Hum Reprod 20:1144–1147

Goldstein M, Eid JF (1989) Elevation of intratesticular and scrotal skin surface temperature in men with varicocele. J Urol 142:743–745

Honig SC, Lipshultz LI, Jarow J (1994) Significant medical pathology uncovered by a comprehensive male infertility evaluation. Fertil Steril 62:1028–1034

Jarow JP, Coburn M, Sigman M (1996) Incidence of varicoceles in men with primary and secondary infertility. Urology 47:73–76

Kolettis PN (2003) Evaluation of the subfertile man. Am Fam Physician 67:2165–2172

Liguori G, Ollandini G, Pomara G et al (2010) Role of renospermatic basal reflow and age on semen quality improvement after sclerotization of varicocele. Urology 75:1074–1078

Page DC, Silber S, Brown LG (1999) Men with infertility caused by AZFc deletion can produce sons by intracytoplasmic sperm injection, but are likely to transmit the deletion and infertility. Hum Reprod 14:1722–1726

Rowe T (2006) Fertility and a woman's age. J Reprod Med 51:157–163

Rowe PJ, Comhaire FH, Hargreave TB et al (1993) WHO manual for the standardized investigation diagnosis and management of the infertile male. Cambridge University Press, New York

Schiff JD, Li PS, Goldstein M (2006) Correlation of ultrasound-measured venous size and reversal of flow with Valsalva with improvement in semen-analysis parameters after varicocelectomy. Fertil Steril 86:250–252

Schlegel PN (1997) Is assisted reproduction the optimal treatment for varicocele-associated male infertility? A cost-effectiveness analysis. Urology 49:83–90

Shefi S, Turek PJ (2006) Definition and current evaluation of subfertile men. Int Braz J Urol 32:385–397

Sigman M, Lipshultz LI, Howards SS (1997) Evaluation of the subfertile male. In: Lipshultz SSHLI (ed) Infertility in the male, 3rd edn. Mosby, St. Louis, pp 173–193

Steckel J, Dicker AP, Goldstein M (1993) Relationship between varicocele size and response to varicocelectomy. J Urol 149:769–771

Templeton A (2000) Infertility and the establishment of pregnancy–overview. Br Med Bull 56:577–587

Trombetta C, Liguori G, Bucci S et al (2003) Percutaneous treatment of varicocele. Urol Int 70:113–118

Tulloch WS (1955) Varicocele in subfertility; results of treatment. Br Med J 2:356–358

Turek PJ (2005) Practical approaches to the diagnosis and management of male infertility. Nat Clin Pract Urol 2:226–238

Turek PJ (2008) Male infertility. In: Tanagho EA, McAninch JW (eds) Smith's general urology, 17th edn. McGraw-Hill, New York, pp 684–716

Wilcox AJ, Weinberg CR, Baird DD (1995) Timing of sexual intercourse in relation to ovulation. Effects on the probability of conception, survival of the pregnancy, and sex of the baby. N Engl J Med 333:1517–1521

World Health Organization (1987) Towards more objectivity in diagnosis and management of male infertility. Int J Androl 7(Suppl 1):1–53

World Health Organization (1999) WHO laboratory manual for the examination of human semen and sperm-cervical mucus interaction. Cambridge University Press, Cambridge

# The Infertile Male-2: Sperm Analysis

Loredana Gandini, Andrea Lenzi, and Francesco Lombardo

## Contents

L. Gandini (✉) · A. Lenzi · F. Lombardo
Department of Experimental Medicine,
V Medical Clinic, University of Rome "La Sapienza",
Viale del Policlinico 155, 00161 Rome, Italy
e-mail: loredana.gandini@uniroma1.it

**Abstract**

Semen analysis remains the most important diagnostic tool for the study of male infertility. For this reason, as well as the ease with which it can be performed, this analysis should be among the first steps in cases of suspected infertility, carried out before subjecting the female partner to long and complex diagnostic tests. The test's efficacy depends on the experience and ability of the seminologist, who must first carry out a subjective analysis of fundamental parameters such as motility and morphology. Laboratories specializing in these analyses have applied different criteria for the evaluation of sperm parameters, making it extremely difficult to compare their results. Despite the considerable progress made in the standardization of semen analysis, there are still marked intra- and inter laboratory differences. The demand for regular internal and external laboratory quality control systems has become so great that the latest edition of the WHO manual includes, for the first time, a lengthy paragraph on quality control techniques.

## 1   Introduction

Semen analysis is the most important laboratory test for establishing the reproductive potential of the male partner in a couple. It is also an essential part of the evaluation of reproductive and urogenital health. As part of an appropriate diagnostic procedure, it enables suitable medical or surgical treatment to be planned and guides the couple in the choice towards assisted reproduction. It is also necessary in

M. Bertolotto and C. Trombetta (eds.), *Scrotal Pathology,* Medical Radiology. Diagnostic Imaging,
DOI: 10.1007/174_2011_187, © Springer-Verlag Berlin Heidelberg 2012

establishing the need for sperm banking in the event of any diseases requiring treatment that might result in sterility (Lamb 2010). Despite this, semen analysis is often still carried out by non-specialist staff, as if it did not require any specific skills.

Reference standards have been available both from the WHO (1999, 2010) and national and international scientific societies for many years, with a common protocol for the standardization of test procedures. As with all laboratory tests, semen analysis should be broken down into the pre-analysis, analysis, and post-analysis phases. All phases require the equal attention of both the laboratory seminologist and the clinician interpreting them.

## 2 Pre-analysis: Standards for the Collection of the Semen Sample

As is already the case with other biological samples, procedures for the collection of semen samples need to be standardised and should be clearly communicated to patients. These standards concern days of sexual abstinence, collection methods, the container, and procedures for consignment.

Two possibilities are suggested for the minimum and maximum number of days of abstinence from ejaculation before the collection: a broader range of 2–7 days and a more restrictive range of 3–5 days, enabling an evaluation less subject to random variations. This is essential to reduce the variability of sperm quantity and quality and enables comparison against both previous and subsequent analyses as well as against the reference values.

The semen sample must be collected by masturbation. Where this is impossible or the patient objects, collection in suitable non-cytotoxic condoms may be permitted. Samples should be collected in the laboratory, especially if there are medical or legal reasons for their collection (e.g. sperm banking, paternity testing). However, collection elsewhere (e.g. at home) for psychological or organisational reasons is acceptable.

The best container is a sterile plastic jar. The sample must be consigned within 30–60 min of ejaculation, if collected other than at the laboratory, and must be protected from extremes of temperature and carried without upturning the container, to avoid leaking and minimise cell trauma.

These recommendations may be disregarded only if the analysis is urgently required prior to surgery or the start of chemotherapy or radiotherapy, or in the event of the patient's near or complete inability to ejaculate.

The container is now placed in an incubator (35–37°C) to enable liquefaction and transfer from the collection jar to a graduated conical test tube. These standards are essential to avoid artefacts and errors in the subsequent analytical phase.

## 3 Analysis

The analytical phase consists of macroscopic and microscopic examination.

### 3.1 Macroscopic Examination

This phase evaluates volume, pH, appearance, liquefaction and viscosity. These variables should be examined at 1 or 2 h after ejaculation, and in any case after liquefaction is complete.

Volume is measured in mL and is an essential parameter for the subsequent evaluation of total sperm count. In addition, reduced semen volumes could indicate partial or complete obstruction of the seminal tract, while high volumes might suggest genital tract inflammation.

pH is evaluated using short range pH paper (between pH 6 and 10). A pH <7 in association with low volume might point to a diagnosis of impaired seminal vesicle secretion, while values >8 are sometimes associated with hypersecretory inflammatory conditions.

Normal semen has a white opalescent appearance. It might be more transparent if there is a low sperm concentration, pink, red or red–brown when red blood cells are present, milk-white if consisting only of prostate secretions, and yellowish white in the case of pyospermia, or in patients taking substances containing pigments.

Semen liquefaction takes between 10 and 60 min, and is defined on this basis as normal, delayed or incomplete, in the case of persistent grains or streaks.

Viscosity is assessed by letting the semen drip from a pipette. It is defined as normal if it leaves the sample as small discrete drops, raised in the case of a continuous thread, which may indicate an acute or chronic inflammatory disease, and reduced if there are rapidly forming drops, caused by a reduced sperm concentration.

## 3.2 Microscopic Examination

The microscopic examination evaluates the sperm and other cells as well as non-cellular elements.

### 3.2.1 Evaluation of Sperm

Sperm evaluation requires the assessment of three parameters: number, motility and morphology. The number must be evaluated both as concentration per mL and as total sperm number, in order to establish the testicular spermatogenetic activity, which is closely related to the hormone situation. After evaluation of raw semen, a cell counting chamber is used. If there are no suspended sperm, the ejaculate must be centrifuged and the sperm looked for in the pellet. The patient may be defined as azoospermic only if no sperm are found in the entire pellet. The diagnosis of azoospermia must be confirmed by two or three repetitions of the analysis (Oates and Amos 2008). WHO (1999) gives reference values for sperm number of $20 \times 10^6$/mL and $40 \times 10^6$ per ejaculate. In contrast, WHO (2010) indicates the lower reference limit for sperm concentration as $15 \times 10^6$/mL and for total sperm number as $39 \times 10^6$ per ejaculate.

Sperm motility is quantified as a percentage using a $20\times$ or $25\times$ objective at a set time after ejaculation (1 or 2 h), but in any case once liquefaction is complete. In samples with a low sperm concentration, the assessment must be repeated on a number of new slides. Motility may also be evaluated using Computer Aided Sperm Analysis (CASA system). However, this cannot replace the microscopic examination and is used mainly for research purposes (Lenzi 1997). Motility is defined both qualitatively and quantitatively. WHO (1999) gives the lower reference limit for total motility as $\geq 50\%$; WHO (2010) distinguishes between progressive motility, non-progressive motility and immotility and considers the lower reference limit for total motility as 40%. Impaired motility is found in almost all urogenital diseases and is therefore not a pathognomonic sign. Only in the case of immotility may a genetic disease related to microtubular

impairment (primary ciliary dyskinesia) be suspected, sometimes correlated with Kartagener syndrome.

Sperm morphology may be evaluated on raw semen using a $40\times$ objective and on a fixed, stained preparation (May-Grünwald-Giemsa, Diff Quick, Papan icolau) with a $100\times$ objective (Fig. 1). Abnormal sperm are described on the basis of the section in which the abnormality is located: head, neck or tail (WHO 1999, 2010). According to WHO (1999), the subject is considered still potentially fertile with an abnormal sperm count of up to 70%, while WHO (2010) increases this to 96%. This percentage seems unreasonably high and has led to debate over the clinical significance of this parameter among andrologists worldwide (Menkveld 2010).

Like motility, impaired sperm morphology is not associated with any specific urogenital diseases. Where the sample contains <100,000/mL of sperm or contains sperm in the pellet alone, the motility and morphology cannot be quantified as a percentage, and must be described under the observations.

### 3.2.2 Evaluation of Non-Sperm Elements

The presence and characteristics of the following components are evaluated: leucocytes, red blood cells, spermatogenetic cells, exfoliated epithelial cells, and sperm agglutination.

The leucocytes consist mainly of neutrophils, and are evaluated in millions/mL. Concentrations above $1 \times 10^6$/mL are considered an important indicator of genital tract inflammation (Moretti et al. 2009).

There should be no red blood cells in the ejaculate; if present, they are a sign of micro-bleeding or inflammatory disease, or very rarely of prostate diseases such as hypertrophy or cancer. Spermatogenetic cells are always present and mainly consist of spermatocytes and spermatids, and more rarely, spermatogonia. Exfoliated epithelial cells originate from the genitourinary tract and may be isolated or present in small clusters. They are defined as rare, present or numerous, and in the latter case may only be a sign of an inflammatory disease.

Semen may contain clusters of mixed cells (sperm and leucocytes or other cells) (non-specific aggregation) or agglutinations of sperm alone. In the latter case, if microscopic examination reveals agglutination of motile sperm, this may indicate the presence of antisperm antibodies. Agglutination is evaluated on raw semen and defined as rare, present or severe.

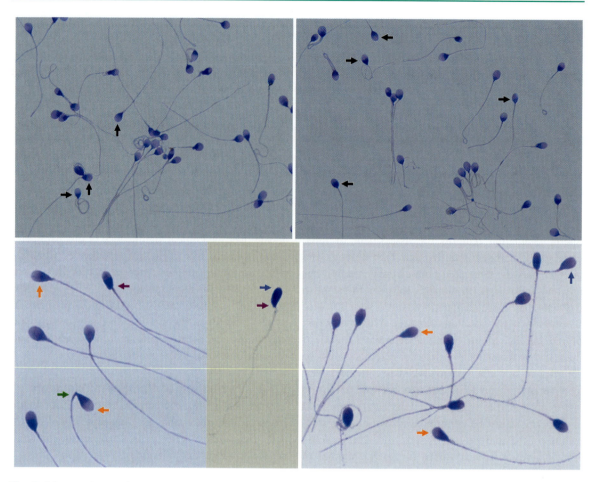

**Fig. 1** Microscopic examination of sperm stained with May-Grünwald-Giemsa showing normal (*black arrows*) and abnormal morphology (*coloured arrows*)

**Table 1** Nomenclature related to semen

| Term | Explanation |
| --- | --- |
| Normozoospermia | Normal sperm concentration, motility and morphology |
| Oligozoospermia | Reduced sperm concentration |
| Cryptozoospermia | Very low numbers of sperm in the ejaculate, sometimes evident only after sample centrifugation |
| Azoospermia | Absence of sperm in the ejaculate |
| Asthenozoospermia | Quantitative and qualitative impairment of motility |
| Teratozoospermia | High percentage of sperm with abnormal morphology |
| Oligoasthenoteratozoospermia | Low sperm number and low percentage of motile, morphologically normal sperm in the ejaculate. High percentage of sperm with abnormal morphology |
| Necrozoospermia | Low percentage of motile sperm in the ejaculate |
| Haemospermia | Presence of erythrocytes in the ejaculate |
| Leukospermia | Presence of leukocytes in the ejaculate |
| Aspermia | Absence of ejaculate: may or may not be associated with anorgasmia or retrograde ejaculation |

For the clinical interpretation of semen analysis data, knowledge of the currently used terminology is useful (Table 1).

## 4 Post-Analysis

Semen analysis reports must be as complete as possible, taking into account their medical or legal significance, and describe all parameters. So-called "fertility indices" must never be included in the report, as they have long been considered not only devoid of any clinical significance but often even misleading.

Given the complexity of the semen analysis, the seminology laboratory should have a good internal quality control system involving both intra-and inter-seminologist control (Gandini et al. 2000; Pacey 2010). Where possible, it should participate in an external quality control program involving the blind evaluation of concentration and sperm morphology of the semen samples provided and the evaluation of sperm motility in videotapes or DVDs (Cooper et al. 2007).

In conclusion, it should be stressed that sperm analysis carried out according to the above standards is not a simple, routine laboratory test but requires a training period that should be certified by a suitable number of analyses carried out under the guidance of an expert seminologist (Gandini et al. 2004).

## References

Cooper TG, Hellenkemper B, Nieschlag E (2007) External quality control for semen analysis in Germany–Qualitäts-kontrolle der Deutschen Gesellschaft für Andrologie (QuaD-EGA). The first 5 years. J Reprod med Endokrinol 4:331–335

Gandini L, Menditto A, Chiodo F et al (2000) From the European Academy of Andrology. Italian pilot study for an external quality control scheme in semen analysis and antisperm antibiotics detection. Int J Androl 23:1–3

Gandini L, Lombardo F, Dondero F et al (2004) Atlante di Seminologia. Carocci Editore, Roma

Lamb DJ (2010) Semen analysis in 21st century medicine: the need for sperm function testing. Asian J Androl 12:64–70

Lenzi A (1997) Computer-aided semen analysis (CASA) 10 years later: a test-bed for the European scientific andrological community. Int J Androl 20:1–2

Menkveld R (2010) Clinical significance of the low normal sperm morphology value as proposed in the fifth edition of the WHO laboratory manual for the examination and processing of human semen. Asian J Androl 12:47–58

Moretti E, Cosci I, Spreafico A et al (2009) Semen characteristics and inflammatory mediators in infertile men with different clinical diagnoses. Int J Androl 32:637–646

Oates RD, Amos JA (2008) Evaluation of the azoospermic male. Fertil Steril 90(Suppl 5):S74–S77

Pacey AA (2010) Quality assurance and quality control in the laboratory andrology. Asian J Androl 12:21–25

WHO (1999) Laboratory manual for the examination of human semen and semen-cervical mucus interaction. Cambridge University Press, Cambridge

WHO (2010) Laboratory manual for the examination and processing of human semen. World Health Organization, Geneva

# The Infertile Male-3: Endocrinological Evaluation

Francesco Lotti, Giovanni Corona, Csilla Gabriella Krausz,
Gianni Forti, and Mario Maggi

## Contents

F. Lotti (✉) · G. Corona · C. G. Krausz · G. Forti ·
M. Maggi
Sexual Medicine and Andrology Unit,
Department of Clinical Physiopathology,
University of Florence,
Viale Pieraccini 6, 50139 Florence, Italy
e-mail: flottimd@yahoo.it; francesco.lotti@dfc.unifi.it

**Abstract**

About 14% of European couples suffer from reproductive health disorders, which can result in infertility. In 50% of involuntarily childless couples a male infertility associated factor is found together with abnormal semen parameters. The etiology of male infertility can be related to several congenital or acquired factors acting at pre-testicular (10%), testicular (75%), or post-testicular (15%) level. In 30–40% of cases, no male infertility associated factor is found (idiopathic male infertility). Idiopathic male infertility may be explained by several factors, including endocrine disruption as a result of environmental pollution, reactive oxygen species or genetic abnormalities. The diagnostic work up of the infertile male should include careful medical and reproductive history collection, physical examination, sperm analysis, and hormone evaluation followed by second and, when useful, third level examinations. The general endocrinologist can easily perform a first-line diagnostic evaluation of the infertile couple as the hormonal assessment has an important role in the initial workup of both partners, and semen analysis can be easily interpreted. It is also rather obvious that if the infertility has an endocrine cause the endocrinologist has an important role in the treatment. On the other hand, further diagnostic work up of the couple requires appropriate knowledge of the physiology and pathology of the male and female reproductive tract as well as of second- and third-level diagnostic procedures.

M. Bertolotto and C. Trombetta (eds.), *Scrotal Pathology*, Medical Radiology. Diagnostic Imaging,
DOI: 10.1007/174_2011_188, © Springer-Verlag Berlin Heidelberg 2012

# 1 Introduction

The prevalence of infertile couples differs according to the definition of couple infertility. Since about 84% of fertile couples successfully conceive within 1 year (te Velde et al. 2000), the most commonly used definition for couple infertility is "lack of pregnancy after 1 year of unprotected regular intercourses" (Krausz and Forti 2000). According to this definition, the prevalence of infertile couples is estimated about 10–15% in Western countries (Krausz and Forti 2000; ESHRE Capri Workshop Group 1996). Furthermore, the diagnostic work up of infertile couple is generally suggested to be initiated after 1 year of regular unprotected intercourses. An earlier evaluation may be performed if known male or female risk factors exist (ESHRE Capri Workshop Group 1996). However, about half of the couples who do not conceive at the first year will do so during the second year of regular unprotected intercourses (te Velde et al. 2000). In line with these data, the European Society of Human Reproduction and Embriology (ESHRE) defines couple infertility as "lack of pregnancy within 2 years of regular coital exposure". According to ESHRE definition, the prevalence of infertile couples within Europe and North America is approximately 5–6% (Forti and Krausz 1998). A multicenter study carried out by the World Health Organization (1987) found that the cause of couple infertility was predominantly male (pure male factor) in 20% of cases, female (pure female factor) in 38%, both partners presented abnormalities in 27% and in the remaining 15% no clear cause was identified (unexplained infertility). However, some Authors report a higher percentage of male factor (30% of cases), while female factor, infertility due to abnormalities detected in both partners and an unexplained infertility represent approximately 35, 20, and 15% of cases of couple infertility, respectively (Forti and Krausz 1998). About 14% of European couples suffer from reproductive health disorders which can result in infertility. In 50% of involuntarily childless couples a male infertility associated factor is found together with abnormal semen parameters (World Health Organization 2000; Dohle et al. 2010). A fertile partner may compensate for the fertility problem of the men and thus infertility usually becomes manifest if both partners have reduced fertility (World Health Organization 2000;

Dohle et al. 2010). As a male factor for infertility, pure or combined with a female factor, is considered affecting about half of infertile couples, it must be assumed that approximately 7% of all men have fertility problems (Forti and Krausz 1998).

# 2 Etiology of Male Infertility and Endocrine Involvement

The etiology of male infertility can be related to several congenital or acquired factors acting at pre-testicular (10%), testicular (75%), or post-testicular (15%) level (Table 1) (Nieschlag et al. 2010). These factors affect sperm and semen production, quality and/or transport/emission with several mechanisms. Genetic factors can be identified in 15–20% of cases of male infertility and are involved in each etiologic category (Nieschlag et al. 2010; Nuti and Krausz 2008). Patients with azoospermia and severe oligozoospermia are mandatory candidates for genetic screening (Nieschlag et al. 2010). The most relevant genetic factors affecting male fertility are karyotype abnormalities, Y chromosome microdeletions, CFTR (cystic fibrosis transmembrane conductance regulator protein) gene mutation in congenital bilateral absence of vas deferens (CBAVD), and those involved in congenital hypogonadotropic hypogonadism or primitive testicular failure. Some of them are currently part of the diagnostic work up of selected groups of patients (Table 2) (Nieschlag et al. 2010; Nuti and Krausz 2008; Root 2010; Lenzi et al. 2009). According to the updated guidelines on male infertility of the European Academy of Urology (Dohle et al. 2010), male fertility can be reduced as a result of: congenital or acquired urogenital abnormalities, urogenital tract infections, endocrine disturbances, genetic abnormalities, immunological factors, and increased scrotal temperature (e.g., as a consequence of varicocele) (World Health Organization 1987; Dohle et al. 2010). In 30–40% of cases, no male infertility associated factor is found (idiopathic male infertility). These men present with no previous history of fertility problems and have normal findings on physical examination and endocrine laboratory testing. Semen analysis, however, reveals oligo- and/or astheno- and/or teratozoospermia (Dohle et al. 2010). Idiopathic male infertility may be explained by several factors, including endocrine disruption as a result

**Table 1** Classification of male infertility

| Aetiology | Treatment |
|---|---|
| **Pre-testicular (10%)** | |
| *Endocrine (gonadotropins deficiency)* | |
| Congenital (e.g., Kallmann's syndrome, congenital hypogonadotropic hypogonadism) | Medical |
| Acquired (pituitary or brain tumor, post-trauma, empty sella, iatrogenic, hyperprolactinemia) | Medical/surgical |
| *Coital disorders* | |
| Erectile dysfunction | Medical/ARTs |
| Ejaculatory disorders | |
| Idiopathic | |
| **Testicular (75%)** | |
| *Congenital* | |
| Anorchia | No therapy |
| Cryptorchidism | Medical and/or surgical before 2 years; ARTs |
| *Genetic* | |
| Klinefelter syndrome and its variants | (micro)TESE + ICSI |
| Y chromosome deletions | (micro)TESE + ICSI |
| monogenic anomalies | |
| *Varicocele* | Surgery in selected cases; (ARTs) |
| Antispermatogenetic agents (environmental, drugs) | Identification and elimination of the noxa; (ARTs) |
| Chemotherapy | Cryoconservation of sperm + ARTs |
| Irradiation | Cryoconservation of sperm + ARTs |
| Vascular torsion | Depending on the grade of spermatogenetic failure; (ARTs) |
| Trauma | Depending on the grade of spermatogenetic failure; (ARTs) |
| Orchitis | Depending on the grade of spermatogenetic failure; (ARTs) |
| Idiopathic | |
| **Post-testicular (15%)** | |
| *Obstructive* | |
| Epididymal (congenital or post-infective, bilateral) | TESE + ICSI |
| Vasal (genetic o post-vasectomy) | TESE + ICSI |
| Male accessory gland infections (MAGI) | Antibiotic treatment |
| *Immunological (Idiopathic or secondary)* | (Medical) or ARTs |
| *Idiopathic* | |
| **Idiopathic (about 40% of all)** | ARTs |

Classification of male infertility based on localization of cause and treatment options. *ARTs* = assisted reproductive techniques; *TESE* = testicular sperm extraction; *ICSI* = intra cytoplasmatic sperm injection

of environmental pollution, reactive oxygen species, or genetic abnormalities (Dohle et al. 2010). A study performed on 12,945 patients (Nieschlag et al. 2010) reports idiopathic male infertility in 30% and hypogonadism as the main endocrine cause of male infertility in 10.1% of the subjects studied. 1,146 of those patients (11.2%) were azoospermic, and the percentage of hypogonadism as the leading diagnosis in these patients was 16.4% (Nieschlag et al. 2010). Table 3 provides an overview of the frequency of individual disorders as they may occur in a large center of andrology/reproductive medicine.

**Table 2** Diagnostic genetic testing in male infertility and therapeutic options

| Gene or region | Indication for testing | Therapeutic options |
| --- | --- | --- |
| | **Hypogonadotropic hypogonadism** | |
| KAL-1 | Kallmann syndrome | Hormone therapy or ARTs |
| KAL-2 (FGFR1) | Kallmann syndrome or normoosmic IHH | |
| PROK2/PROK2R | Kallmann syndrome or normoosmic IHH | |
| FGF8 | Kallmann syndrome or normoosmic IHH | |
| GnRH/GnRHR | IHH (normoosmic) | |
| KiSS1/GPR54 | IHH (normoosmic) | |
| TAC3/TAC3R | IHH (normoosmic) | |
| FSH | Isolated FSH deficiency | |
| LH | Isolated LH deficiency | |
| | **Primitive testicular dysfunction** | |
| Chromosomal abnormalities | Azoo or $<10 \times 10^6$ sp/ml | ARTs (IUI, IVF or ICSI) |
| Y chromosome microdeletions (AZFa, AZFb, AZFc) | Azoo or $<5 \times 10^6$ sp/ml | |
| gr-gr deletion (partial AZFc) | Oligozoospermia ($<20 \times 10^6$ sp/ml) | |
| AR mutations | Hypoandrogenized infertile man, hypospadia | |
| | **Congenital post-testicular forms** | |
| CFTR | Congenital absence of vas deferens (uni- or bilateral) | ARTs (IVF or ICSI) |
| | Idiopathic epididymal obstruction | |

Diagnostic genetic testing in male infertility and therapeutic options. *IHH* idiopathic hypogonadotrophic hypogonadism; *ART* assisted reproductive techniques; *IUI* intrauterine insemination; *IVF* in vitro fertilization; *ICSI* intracytoplasmic sperm injection; *sp* spermatozoa

## 3      Diagnostic work up of the Infertile Male

The diagnostic work up of the infertile male should include careful medical and reproductive history collection, physical examination, sperm analysis and hormone evaluation followed by second and, when useful, third level examinations.

## 3.1    Medical and Reproductive History

History is focused on the identification of risk factors or behavior patterns which could affect fertility. Onset of puberty, voice mutation, and the beginning and the trend of beard growth have to be recorded (Krausz and Forti 2000; Nieschlag et al. 2010; Grumbach and Styne 2003). Male puberty usually occurs between 9

and 14 years, and the first sign of the onset of puberty is represented by testicular volume increasing >4 ml, as detected by Prader orchidometer (Grumbach and Styne 2003; Partsch et al. 2002). Delayed puberty can be related to constitutional delay of puberty, hypogonadotropic hypogonadism (e.g., Kallmann syndrome) as well to hypergonadotropic hypogonadism (e.g., Klinefelter syndrome), while early puberty could suggest the presence of a cerebral tumor which sometimes is associated to hypogonadotropic hypogonadism (Lenzi et al. 2009; Grumbach and Styne 2003; Partsch et al. 2002; Traggiai and Stanhope 2002; Lanfranco et al. 2004). Hypo- or anosmia suggests the presence of Kalmann syndrome (Krausz and Forti 2000; Nieschlag et al. 2010; Lenzi et al. 2009; Grumbach and Styne 2003). Any testicular maldescendent, the age at which medical therapy or surgery for cryptorchidism were carried out, herniotomy (for possible subsequent testicular damage) has

**Table 3** Percentage distribution of diagnoses of 12,945 patients attending the Institute of Reproductive Medicine of the University of Münster

| Diagnosis | Unselected patients ($N = 12945$) | Azoospermic patients ($N = 1146$) |
|---|---|---|
| *All* | 100% | 11.2% |
| *Infertility of known (possible) cause* | 42.6 | 42.6 |
| Maldescended testes (current/former) | 8.4 | 17.2 |
| Varicocele | 14.8 | 10.9 |
| Infection | 9.3 | 10.5 |
| Autoantibodies against sperm | 3.9 | – |
| Testicular tumor | 1.2 | 2.8 |
| Others | 5.0 | 1.2 |
| *Idiopathic infertility* | 30.0 | 13.3 |
| *Hypogonadism* | 10.1 | 16.4 |
| Klinefelter syndrome (47, XXY) | 2.6 | 13.7 |
| XX-male | 0.1 | 0.6 |
| Primary hypogonadism of unknown cause | 2.3 | 0.8 |
| Secondary (hypogonadotropic) hypogonadism | 1.6 | 1.9 |
| Kallmann syndrome | 0.3 | 0.5 |
| Idiopathic hypogonadotropic hypogonadism | 0.4 | 0.4 |
| Residual after pituitary surgery | <1.0 | 0.3 |
| Others | 0.8 | 0.8 |
| Late-onset hypogonadism | 2.2 | – |
| Constitutional delay of puberty | 1.4 | – |
| *General/systemic disease* | 2.2 | 0.5 |
| *Cryopreservation due to malignant disease* | 7.8 | 12.5 |
| Testicular tumor | 5.0 | 4.3 |
| Lymphoma | 1.5 | 4.6 |
| Leukemia | 0.7 | 2.2 |
| Sarcoma | 0.6 | 0.9 |
| *Disturbance of erection/ejaculation* | 2.4 | – |
| *Obstruction* | 2.2 | 10.3 |
| Vasectomy | 0.9 | 5.3 |
| Cystic fibrosis, CBAVD | 0.5 | 3.1 |
| Others | 0.8 | 1.9 |
| *Gynecomastia* | 1.5 | 0.2 |
| *Y-chromosomal deletion* | 0.3 | 1.6 |
| *Other chromosomal aberrations* | 0.2 | 1.3 |
| Translocations | 0.1 | 0.3 |
| Others | <0.1 | 0.3 |
| *Others* | 0.7 | 1.3 |

Percentage distribution of diagnoses of 12,945 patients attending the Institute of Reproductive Medicine of the University of Münster based on the clinical databank Androbase® . 1446 (=11.2%) of these patients were azoospermic. In the event of several diseases, only the leading diagnosis was included. Adapted with permission from: Tüttelmann F and Nieschlag E (2010), Chap. 4, Table 4.2, p 90. *CBAVD* = congenital bilateral absence of vas deferens to be recorded (Krausz and Forti 2000; Forti and Krausz 1998; Nieschlag et al. 2010; Grumbach and Styne 2003). Gonadal exposure to exogenous toxins, occupational exposure to heat and chemicals which may impair spermatogenesis and testicular testosterone production should be carefully recorded (Krausz and Forti 2000; Forti and Krausz 1998; Nieschlag et al. 2010; Grumbach and Styne 2003). Intake of anabolic steroids, especially in athletic males, and use of toxic drugs (e.g., sulfasalazine, cytostatic agents, antibiotics) should be investigated (Krausz and Forti 2000; Forti and Krausz 1998; Nieschlag et al. 2010; Grumbach and Styne 2003). Systemic diseases, previous chemo/radiotherapy, alcohol and/or nicotine abuse should be ruled out (Krausz and Forti 2000; Forti and Krausz 1998; Nieschlag et al. 2010; Grumbach and Styne 2003). The family medical history could provide important information for a possible genetic cause of hypogonadism and infertility (Krausz and Forti 2000; Forti and Krausz 1998; Nieschlag et al. 2010; Grumbach and Styne 2003). The patient should be asked about familiarity for infertility, recurrent abortion, and malformations. Furthermore, reproductive history and risk factors for infertility or hypogonadism should be ruled out (Krausz and Forti 2000; Forti and Krausz 1998; Nieschlag et al. 2010; Grumbach and Styne 2003). The patient should be asked for duration of infertility and prior fertility (eventually with previous partner) (Krausz and Forti 2000; Forti and Krausz 1998; Nieschlag et al. 2010; Grumbach and Styne 2003). Impaired libido, erectile dysfunction, reduction of spontaneous erections, and reduction of the volume of ejaculate should be investigated: because sexual desire, the beginning and the end of erection process, and male accessory glands (prostate, seminal vesicles) are modulated by testosterone, their alteration suggests the presence of hypogonadism (Krausz and Forti 2000; Nieschlag et al. 2010; Grumbach and Styne 2003; Morelli et al. 2007; Morelli et al. 2005; Vignozzi et al. 2005; Corona and Maggi 2010; Corona et al. 2004a). Ejaculatory time, coital frequency, and timing should be investigated (Krausz and Forti 2000; Nieschlag et al. 2010; Grumbach and Styne 2003). Both thyroidal hormones and testosterone levels have been observed to be associated with ejaculatory dysfunction (Corona et al. 2004b, 2006a, 2008, 2010; Carani et al. 2005; Cihan et al. 2009). In particular, hyperthyroidism has been associated to premature ejaculation while hypothyroidism has been related to delayed ejaculation (Corona et al. 2004b, 2006a, 2010; Carani et al. 2005; Cihan et al. 2009). In addition, specific treatment of those thyroidal dysfunctions are associated to the reduction of the prevalence of the relative ejaculatory dysfunction (Corona et al. 2010; Carani et al. 2005; Cihan et al. 2009). Furthermore, high testosterone levels seem to play a facilitatory role in the control of ejaculatory reflex while hypogonadism is associated with an overall lower propensity to ejaculate (Corona et al. 2006a, 2008, 2010). Finally, it has been reported that subjects with low prolactin levels (e.g., in the lower quartile of the normal range) show a higher risk of premature ejaculation (Corona et al. 2009a) while subjects with high prolactin levels in the normal range (i.e., excluding subjects with pathological hyperprolactinaemia) more often report ejaculatory latency (Corona et al. 2010). It has been speculated that basal PRL could mirror an impaired central serotoninergic pathway, and it is well known that central serotonin is the main central drive controlling ejaculation. Therefore, prolactin measurement is suggested in subjects with ejaculatory dysfunction, because it might reflect the central serotoninergic tone (Corona et al. 2009a, 2010). Prostatitis has been reported as a cause of acquired premature ejaculation (Jannini and Lenzi 2005; Screponi et al. 2001; El-Nashaar and Shamloul 2007; Lotti et al. 2009). In addition, we recently suggested varicocele as a possible cause of acquired premature ejaculation, mediated by prostatitis induction (Lotti et al. 2009).

Orchitis, testicular trauma, inguinal surgery, cryptorchidism, and varicocele should be investigated. In fact, they have been variously related to testicular damage, leading to a reduction in sperm parameters, quantity and quality and in testicular testosterone production (Krausz and Forti 2000; Forti and Krausz 1998; Nieschlag et al. 2010; Grumbach and Styne 2003; Forti et al. 2003). In addition, cryptorchidism is associated to a higher risk of testicular cancer, also in the opposite descended testis (Nieschlag et al. 2010; Grumbach and Styne 2003).

Finally, sexually transmitted diseases, male accessory gland infections (MAGI, e.g., prostatitis, prostato–vesiculitis, prostato–vesicular–epididymitis), and recurrent urogenital infections should be ruled out, because they have been variously associated to affect sperm parameters (Krausz and Forti 2000;

Forti and Krausz 1998; Nieschlag et al. 2010; Pellati et al. 2008; Rowe et al. 1993; Krause 2008).

## 3.2 Physical Examination

Physical examination should include evaluation of secondary sex characteristics such as hair distribution, body proportions, voice, breast development, and investigating for the presence of gynecomastia (Krausz and Forti 2000; Nieschlag et al. 2010; Grumbach and Styne 2003). Rapidly developing gynecomastia may indicate an endocrinologically active testicular tumor (Krausz and Forti 2000; Nieschlag et al. 2010; Grumbach and Styne 2003). Conversely, during puberty, uni- or bilateral gynecomastia is a frequent finding, usually benign, often characterized by spontaneous resolution (Grumbach and Styne 2003). Furthermore, careful palpation of the testes is obligatory, and it should be completed by scrotal ultrasound if a testicular mass is suspected (Nieschlag et al. 2010; Grumbach and Styne 2003). Particular focus should be given to the genitalia. Examination of the penis including the location of urethral meatus and the presence of surgical or traumatic penile scars and induration plaques should be performed (Krausz and Forti 2000; Nieschlag et al. 2010; Grumbach and Styne 2003). The finding of hypospadia may be due to mutations in the androgen receptor gene (Nieschlag et al. 2010; Grumbach and Styne 2003). A severe curvature of the penis due to La Peyronie disease could impair sexual intercourse (Nieschlag et al. 2010; Grumbach and Styne 2003). Measurement of testicular volume by Prader orchidometer is extremely useful for the andrologist (Krausz and Forti 2000; Forti and Krausz 1998; Nieschlag et al. 2010; Grumbach and Styne 2003): in fact, testis volume is significantly related to reproductive and hormonal function. A Prader volume <14 ml has been associated with abnormalities of sperm count, motility, and morphology, while <12 ml is related to a mild abnormality in Leydig cells function (Takihara et al. 1987); moreover testis volume is significantly related to spermatozoa TESE (TEsticular Sperm Extraction) retrieval in the testis of azoospermic patients, with a reduction of 50% of the retrieval chances if testis Prader volume is <15 ml (Seo and Ko 2001). The seminiferous tubules represent approximately 80–85% of the testicular mass.

Moreover, a testicular volume <15 ml suggests a significant impairment of the seminiferous tubules (Forti and Krausz 1998). Small firm testis, with typical eunocoid features are indicative for Klinefelter syndrome (Krausz and Forti 2000; Forti and Krausz 1998; Nieschlag et al. 2010; Grumbach and Styne 2003; Lanfranco et al. 2004). On the other hand, an eunocoid habitus with infantile genitalia, sparse or nearly absent body hair, gynecomastia, and low testicular volume is typical of congenital gonadotrophin deficiency (Krausz and Forti 2000; Forti and Krausz 1998; Nieschlag et al. 2010; Grumbach and Styne 2003). Palpation of the testes should be performed in order to exclude the presence of testicular mass, because infertile patients are usually young and testicular tumors are the most frequent tumors in the young male, in particular between 15 and 34 years (Woodward et al. 2002). Palpation of the epididymides (for cysts, consistency, and size) and vas deferens should be performed, expecially looking for total or segmental absence (Krausz and Forti 2000; Forti and Krausz 1998; Nieschlag et al. 2010; Grumbach and Styne 2003). Furthermore, palpation of the spermatic cord and varicocele evaluation should be performed (Krausz and Forti 2000; Forti and Krausz 1998; Nieschlag et al. 2010; Grumbach and Styne 2003). Finally, digito-rectal examination gives some important informations: the presence of an enlarged or tender prostate, possibly associated to pain and/or fever, could be related to prostate inflammation; conversely, a reduced prostate volume could be related to hypogonadism, because prostate is a plastic androgen dependent gland (Krausz and Forti 2000; Forti and Krausz 1998; Nieschlag et al. 2010; Grumbach and Styne 2003). In addition, it must be underlined that finding firm nodules related to tumors in the prostate of young subjects (<50 years), as usually are males complaining for couple infertility, is extremely rare (Brooks et al. 2010). Conversely, firm palpatory prostate findings could be related to calcifications, which can be better investigated by transrectal ultrasound.

## 3.3 Semen Analysis

This test is very important to diagnose and define the severity of male factor for infertility (Krausz and Forti 2000; Forti and Krausz 1998; Nieschlag et al. 2010).

Semen analysis should be performed according to the WHO (2010) recommended procedure. This analysis will provide sperm concentration, motility, morphology and semen parameters such as semen volume, pH, and viscosity. Reference ranges for sperm parameters have been recently updated (World Health Organization 2010). Sperm parameters should be considered abnormal after the evaluation of at least two semen analyses. Normal values help to identify patients supposed to induce a pregnancy with high probability; however, excepted severe oligozoospermia or azoospermia, the predictive value of subnormal semen parameters is limited. In fact, it should be considered that severe disturbances of semen parameters may still be compatible with couple fertility since a highly fertile female partner may compensate for male subfertility. In other words, couple fertility depends on the fertility potential of the two members of the couple (Krausz and Forti 2000; Forti and Krausz 1998; Dohle et al. 2010; Nieschlag et al. 2010). Some pre-analytical factors could interfere with the reliability of the analysis, such as inappropriate collection or transport of semen (the specimen should be kept at body temperature during transport; the abstinence period should be between 2 and 5 days, no loss of ejaculate during collection should occur), and antibiotic therapy or presence of fever months before semen collection (Krausz and Forti 2000; Forti and Krausz 1998; Dohle et al. 2010; Nieschlag et al. 2010). It should be underscored that spermatogenesis takes almost 3 months in human to be completed, so the effect of an exogenous noxae may persist over 2–3 months (Krausz and Forti 2000; Forti and Krausz 1998; Nieschlag et al. 2010). Analytical factors may also alter the reliability of the examination; for this reason laboratories should adequate to a quality control program. In azoospermia, after centrifugation of the semen sample, a careful analysis of the pellet is also necessary in order to distinguish between azoospermia (complete absence of spermatozoa both in the ejaculate and in the pellet) and cryptozoospermia (absence of spermatozoa in the ejaculate but detection of spermatozoa in the pellet) (Krausz and Forti 2000; Forti and Krausz 1998; Nieschlag et al. 2010). When azoospermia is present, obstruction should be distinguished from seminiferous tubular damage. A reduced bilateral testicular volume (<15 ml), with normal volume ejaculate (>2 mL) and high FSH is indicative of damaged spermatogenesis (Krausz and

Forti 2000; Forti and Krausz 1998; Nieschlag et al. 2010). Obstructive azoospermia is usually characterized by a normal testicular volume and normal FSH levels (Krausz and Forti 2000; Forti and Krausz 1998; Nieschlag et al. 2010). In these patients, very simple semen parameters such as low volume of the ejaculate, and acidic pH can suggest congenital bilateral absence of vas deferens (CBAVD) and/or seminal vesicles, a condition that is associated with a high incidence of mutations in the cystic fibrosis gene (CFTR), acquired bilateral ejaculatory duct obstruction or the presence of a dysembriogenetic or acquired prostatic cysts compressing ab extrinseco both ejaculatory ducts. The last two cases are rare and could be characterized by several degrees of moderate-severe oligospermia (Krausz and Forti 2000; Forti and Krausz 1998; Nieschlag et al. 2010). In oligo- and/or astheno- and/or teratozoospermic patients, immunological infertility and/or male accessory glands infection (MAGI) should be suspected. If the percentage of motile spermatozoa coated by antisperm antibodies is more than 50%, a pure immunological factor is likely and titration of sperm antibodies in serum will help to confirm the diagnosis. If semen is characterized by high viscosity, high pH (around 8), and leukocytospermia (more than $10^6$ leukocytes/ml), MAGI should be considered (Krausz and Forti 2000; Forti and Krausz 1998; Nieschlag et al. 2010).

## 3.4 Hormonal Parameters

The most important hormonal measurement in the infertile male, both from the diagnostic and prognostic point of view, is serum FSH. High FSH levels and normal LH and testosterone levels are present in the majority of normally virilized infertile men with sperm concentration lower than $5 \times 10^6$/mL and are usually related to the entity of spermatogenetic damage (Forti and Krausz 1998; Bergmann et al. 1994). Some Authors (Andersson et al. 2004) report that FSH >7 U/L has a specificity of 95% and a sensitivity of 57%, with an overall accuracy of 85% in discriminating between idiopathic infertile men and a reference group of proven fertile normozoospermic men. However, definitions of cut-off levels are always the result of a compromise between a high sensitivity and a high specificity that includes considerations on how many false-positive and false-negative cases one

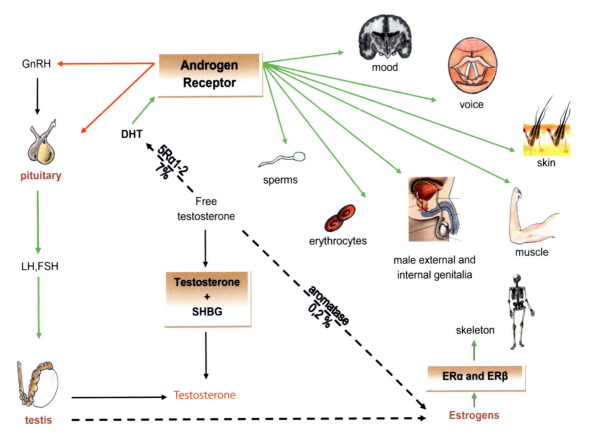

**Fig. 1** Testosterone formation and activity in the male. *Green arrows* represent stimulatory pathways, *red arrows* represent inhibitory ones. *SHBG* sex hormone binding globulin, *ER* = estrogen receptor, *DHT* = dihydrotestosterone, 5αR1 and 2 = 5α reductase type 1 and 5α reductase type 2

will accept. However, a cut-off of 7–8 U/L could be considered a good compromise (still with some overlap of the FSH values) in discriminating infertile men with disturbed spermatogenesis versus normozoospermic men (Andersson et al. 2004). Serum inhibin B levels have been recently reported to be inversely related to FSH in infertile men, suggesting that inhibin B levels reflect Sertoli cell function (Forti and Krausz 1998; Anawalt et al. 1996). However, the diagnostic value of inhibin B measurement in the routine assessment of male infertility has still to be evaluated (Forti and Krausz 1998; Andersson et al. 2004).

Low testosterone levels suggest the presence of hypogonadism, which etiology has to be well elucidated, and which is usually related to hypothalamic/pituitary or to testicular affections frequently associated to an impaired sperm production or function (Forti and Krausz 1998; Nieschlag et al. 2010; Grumbach and Styne 2003). Testosterone exerts biological actions in part by itself, and in part through its reduction or aromatization to dihydrotestosterone (DHT) and estrogens, respectively (Nieschlag et al. 2010; Grumbach and Styne 2003; Morelli et al. 2007; Corona and Maggi 2010). Testosterone biological actions are represented in Fig. 1. Circulating testosterone binds with high affinity to a carrier protein, sex hormone binding globulin (SHBG) (45%), and with lower affinity to albumin (50%). The fraction of Testosterone unbound to SHBG and albumin (about 5% of total testosterone) is termed free testosterone, and is thought to represent the bioactive fraction of total testosterone (Nieschlag et al. 2010; Grumbach and Styne 2003). Measurement of free testosterone represents the cornerstone of evaluating the androgen state. However, it is not an easy task, because the commercially available direct methods, based on a labeled testosterone analogue, are often unreliable and separation of unbound testosterone fraction at equilibrium dialysis is technically very difficult. Therefore, at the present time the gold standard method for free testosterone determination is the calculation of the free fraction (Rosner et al. 2007), as derived from measurement of its total fraction and its carrier protein SHBG, and considering albumin levels, according to a standard formula (Vermeulen et al. 1999) (Vermeulen's formula, available at http://www.issam.ch/freetesto.htm). Testosterone acts modulating sexual desire, positively controls both the initiation and the end of the erectile process, and timely adjusts the erectile process as a function of sexual desire (Nieschlag et al. 2010; Grumbach and Styne 2003; Morelli et al. 2007; Morelli et al. 2005; Vignozzi et al. 2005; Corona and Maggi 2010; Corona et al. 2004a). Furthermore, testosterone acts on muscle mass and strength, on the distribution of lean and fat mass, on glicometabolic parameters, on mood, on bone density, on erythropoiesis, on voice tone, on hair and beard growth, on sebaceous glands. Finally, it acts on androgen dependent male accessory glands (prostate, seminal vesicles) and improves spermatogenesis (Nieschlag et al. 2010; Grumbach and Styne 2003). Testosterone deficiency and sperm failure is termed male hypogonadism (Nieschlag et al. 2010; Grumbach and Styne 2003; Morelli et al. 2007). Hypogonadism in patients with sexual dysfunction can be assessed using a simple, brief (12 items) structured interview named AN-DROTEST© (Corona et al. 2006b), which provides scores useful for the screening of hypogonadism, defined as low total testosterone (<10.4 nmol/L, 300 ng/dL), with an overall accuracy of 74%. On the other hand, erectile dysfunction can be investigated using a brief (13 items) structured interview, SIEDY (Structured Interview on Erectile DYsfunction) (Petrone et al. 2003), a multidimentional instrument for the identification and quantification of the organic, relational, and intrapsychic components of erectile dysfunction. The diagnosis of treatable hypogonadism requires the presence of symptoms and signs suggestive of testosterone deficiency (hypoactive sexual desire, erectile dysfunction, decreased muscle mass and strength, increased body fat, decreased bone mineral density and ostheoporosis, decreased vitality, and depressed

mood) corroborated with low serum testosterone levels, such as circulating total testosterone below 8 nmol/L (231 ng/dL) or free testosterone (measured by equilibrium dialysis method or calculated according to Vermeulen's formula (Vermeulen et al. 1999)) below 180 pmol/L (52 pg/mL) (Wang et al. 2009). A testosterone treatment trial should be considered when total testosterone is >8 and <12 nmol/L (346 ng/dL) or free testosterone below 225 pmol/L (65 pg/mL) in the presence of typical hypogonadal symptoms (Wang et al. 2009). Moreover, SHBG should be measured especially when total testosterone is between 8 and 12 nmol/L or if high levels are suspected, as in presence of hepatic disease (e.g., hepatitis) or hepatic stimulation (e.g., some antiepileptic drugs such as carbamazepine, hyperthyroidism, increased oestrogens/androgens ratio) (Nieschlag et al. 2010; Grumbach and Styne 2003; Wang et al. 2009).

Low testosterone levels associated to low LH and FSH levels suggest the presence of hypogonadotropic hypogonadism, congenital or more often acquired, e.g., testis failure due to a hypothalamic or pituitary gonodotropin release deficiency, which might be associated to a pituitary tumor (more often a prolactinoma or a non-functioning pituitary tumor) as well to a brain tumor or an empty sella (Nieschlag et al. 2010; Grumbach and Styne 2003). If patient's history and phenotype are suggestive for a congenital hypogonadotropic hypogonadism, genetic causes should be ruled out (Root 2010; Lenzi et al. 2009). Magnetic resonance imaging of the whole brain and the pituitary gland should be performed in order to exclude malignant tumors and pituitary tumors (Nieschlag et al. 2010; Grumbach and Styne 2003). On the other side, low testosterone levels associated with high levels of FSH and LH (hypergonadotropic or primary hypogonadism) suggest primary testicular failure that might be due to congenital (e.g., Klinefelter syndrome, which is quite frequent, with an overall prevalence of 1/500 newborns) or acquired causes (Nieschlag et al. 2010; Grumbach and Styne 2003).

Male hypogonadism is classically considered as a partial or total disruption of the cross talk among hypothalamus, pituitary gland, and testis (Nieschlag et al. 2010; Grumbach and Styne 2003). Accordingly, the classic taxonomy of hypogonadism includes defects of various nature and degree occurring at each one of these levels. This classification does not take

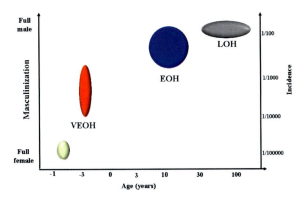

**Fig. 2** Characteristics of male hypogonadism, reported according to the age of onset of the disease and the patient's phenotype. Schematic prevalence in male population is also shown. Size of ellipsis reflects on *abscissa* (*log scale*): age of onset and on *ordinates* (*log scale*): incidence (*right axis*) or female to male phenotype (*left axis*, arbitrary unit). *VEOH* very early onset hypogonadism, i.e., starting during foetal life for absence of testosterone formation or activity (examples are: Leydig cell hypoplasia type 2, complete androgen insensitivity or absence of 17 beta-hydroxysteroid dehydrogenase, *yellow ellipsis*) or impaired secretion or activity of GnRH (for causes see Table 1, *red ellipsis*). *EOH* early onset hypogonadism (i.e., peri-pubertal onset, as in Klinefelter's syndrome, *blue ellipsis*). *LOH* late onset hypogonadism, i.e., in adulthood or aging (*grey ellipsis*)

into consideration signs and symptoms (Morelli et al. 2007). Signs and symptoms of hypogonadism are indeed quite similar irrespective to the different sites of origin of the disease. However, they are deeply different depending on the age of hypogonadism onset. In other words, the phenotype of the hypogonadal patient is more often affected by the age of onset than by the site of origin (Morelli et al. 2007). Figure 2 illustrates this point and proposes a new classification of hypogonadism, based on symptoms and prevalence in the general population. In the case of a very early onset hypogonadism (VEOH), e.g., during early foetal life, symptoms would be even dramatic, spanning from an almost complete female phenotype (complete androgen insensitivity or enzymatic defects blocking androgen synthesis) to various defects in virilization (micropenis, hypospadia, cryptorchidism), as in the case of impaired secretion or activity of GnRH. Differences in the severity of the expression of VEOH phenotype reside in the presence or absence of a temporary GnRH-independent/hCG-dependent testosterone secretion from the foetal testis (Morelli et al. 2007). In the case of a peri-pubertally appearance of the hypogonadism (early onset hypogonadism, EOH),

because of milder central or peripheral defects (as in Klinefelter's syndrome), there might be a delay in the onset of puberty with an overall eunochoidal phenotype, including scant body hair, high-pitched voice, small testis, penis, and prostate (Morelli et al. 2007). In the case of late onset hypogonadism (LOH), symptoms will be relatively mild, insidious, and difficult to be recognized and, therefore, treated. In addition, in the case of LOH, the site of origin is often unclear, resulting from a mixed contribution of testicular and hypothalamic/pituitary failure (Morelli et al. 2007). While EOH and, in particular, VEOH are rather uncommon problems (although not so rare, spanning from 1:500 for Klinefelter's syndrome to 1:100,000 for complete androgen insensitivity syndrome, CAIS) and more appropriately treated by dedicated specialists, LOH is a very common disorder. Therefore, physicians should become more and more confident with its nature and symptoms (Morelli et al. 2007).

Using this approach (medical history and physical examination with testicular volume assessment, semen analysis, and hormone measurement), a definite diagnosis of the cause of male infertility can be obtained in approximately 70% of cases (Behre et al. 1994).

## 4 Second Level Examinations

Second level examinations should be performed to further elucidate the etiology of male factor when first level examinations are not conclusive for a diagnosis or when anatomical or functional abnormalities of the genital tract or genetic abnormalities are suspected, and they are selected on the basis of clinical suspect and semen phenotype.

### 4.1 Genetic Assessment

Chromosome abnormalities are much more frequent in infertile males (5.3%) than in the general population (0.6%) (Forti and Krausz 1998; Egozcue 1989); therefore, karyotype must be performed in men with azoospermia and severe oligozoospermia if FSH levels are increased and testicular volume is markedly reduced (Egozcue 1989). The most frequent abnormalities are sex chromosome aneuploidies such as the 47, XXY and the 47, XYY karyotype (1:500 and 1:750 newborns, respectively), autosomal Robertsonian translocations, and other types of translocations (Krausz and Forti 2000; Forti and Krausz 1998; Nieschlag et al. 2010). In azoospermic and severe oligozoospermic patients ($<5 \times 10^6$ spermatozoa/ml), microdeletions of the Y chromosome should be investigated because their frequency in this population ranges between 3 and 18% (Forti and Krausz 1998). Microdeletions of the Y chromosome are clinically relevant deletions occurring on the long arm of the Y chromosome and remove partially or, more often, completely, one or more AZF regions (classically divided into three AZospermia Factor regions, AZFa, AZFb, and AZFc). Y microdeletion is the most frequently known molecular genetic cause of severe impairment of spermatogenesis. Its frequency is about 10% in non-obstructive azoospermic and 3–5% in idiopathic severe oligozoospermic men (Krausz and Degl'Innocenti 2006). The identification of Y microdeletions is not only relevant for the diagnosis but it may also have prognostic value prior testicular biopsy (TESE) (Brandell et al. 1998; Krausz et al. 2000). In fact, complete AZFa and AZFb deletions of the Y chromosome are associated to a chance of finding spermatozoa at TESE that is virtually zero; moreover, TESE should not be proposed.

In patients with CBAVD, which is now considered a mild form of cystic fibrosis, screening for cystic fibrosis gene mutations should be performed since mutations of this gene have been reported in approximately 70–80% of such patients, the most frequent being the $\Delta F$ 508 mutation (Chillon et al. 1995). Due to the high carrier frequency in Europe and North America (1:25) genetic screening should also be done in the female partner especially if an assisted reproductive technique (ART) attempt is planned (Forti and Krausz 1998; Nieschlag et al. 2010).

If congenital hypogonadothropic hypogonadism is suspected, specific genetic investigation should be performed (Root 2010; Lenzi et al. 2009).

## 4.2 Microbiological Examination of Sperm and Urine and Urethral Swab

These examinations should be performed if an infection is suspected, especially if MAGI is suspected (Nieschlag et al. 2010; Pellati et al. 2008; Rowe et al. 1993; Krause 2008). It should be considered that only in 10–15% of cases germs are found for a specific antibiotic therapy. In addition, it should be underscored that antibiotic therapy could have a negative impact on sperm parameters for a few months, according to the knowledge that spermatogenesis takes almost 3 months in human to be completed (Krausz and Forti 2000; Forti and Krausz 1998; Nieschlag et al. 2010). So, even if antibiotic therapy has long term positive effect on sperm parameters by contrasting infections, they may exert an acute negative impact on sperm parameters.

## 4.3 Scrotal and Transrectal Color-Doppler Ultrasound

Ultrasound has become a more and more useful technique which helps investigating the cause of semen abnormalities and evaluating the presence of scrotal or prostato–vesicular abnormalities (Behre et al. 1995). Scrotal color-Doppler ultrasound should be performed in order to evaluate testis localization, volume, echogenicity, homogeneity, and tumors (Behre et al. 1995; Isidori and Lenzi 2008). The volume of the testis measured by ultrasound positively correlates with sperm count (Behre et al. 2000). It means that the finding of low testis volume is usually predictive for low sperm count. Prader measure of testicular volume is considered about 4 ml higher than the value measured by ultrasound (Carlsen et al. 2000). For this reason, since a testicular volume of 14–15 ml is considered a value discriminating between well and less functioning testicle, it can be assumed that a testicular volume assessed by ultrasound lower than 10–11 ml should be associated to reduced sperm parameters, and maybe to reduced testosterone levels. Furthermore, inhomogeneity of the testis should be interpreted as a pathological finding, related to a reduced testicular function (Lenz et al. 1993). Changes in echogenicity and consistency of the testis are correlated to reduced semen production. In contrast, steroid hormone production may still be normal even in a severely abnormal testis (Isidori and Lenzi 2008). Cryptorchid testis is often inhomogeneous and hypoechoic and is associated to the presence of abnormal sperm parameters, reduced testosterone levels, and high FSH levels (Nieschlag et al. 2010; Isidori and Lenzi 2008). Microlithiasis (>5 calcifications with size 1–3 mm, 56) is supposed to correlate with a higher incidence of testicular tumors (Cast et al. 2000; Bach et al. 2001) and to worse sperm parameters (Thomas et al. 2000), but the argument is still debated (Otite et al. 2001; Peterson et al. 2001; Kessaris and Mellinger 1994). In addition, small calcifications can be observed in Klinefelter syndrome (Aizenstein et al. 1997). Epididymis inhomogeneity, hypo- or hyper-echogenicity, and coarse epididymal calcifications, especially of the tail, suggest the presence of chronic inflammations (Isidori and Lenzi 2008; Woodward et al. 2003; Lee et al. 2008). Epididymal subobstruction can be found at ultrasonography evaluation (Woodward et al. 2003). Varicocele should usually be investigated, and the severity grade should be indicated by the physician (Liguori et al. 2004). The presence of the varicocele has been associated with an impairment in the spermatogenesis and of the hormonal function (Jarow 2001). Furthermore, the possibility to revert infertility through varicocele treatment is still under debate (Evers et al. 2009; Ficarra et al. 2006). In a recent study (Lotti et al. 2009) we found that subjects with severe varicocele showed higher LH, FSH, and prolactin levels with a total testosterone not significantly different from the rest of the sample, suggesting a compensated hypergonadotropic hypogonadism with a androgens/estrogens imbalance determining higher prolactin levels.

Transrectal ultrasound gives informations about prostate, seminal vesicles and the final part of the vas deferens (Nieschlag et al. 2010; Behre et al. 1995). Prostate and seminal vesicles are Testosterone targets; therefore, in the presence of a low volume of the glands, testosterone deficiency should be suspected (Nieschlag et al. 2010; Grumbach and Styne 2003). An enlarged, asymmetric, and hypoechoic prostate, the presence of calcifications, and high periprostatic plexus are considered ultrasound signs of inflammation (Vicari 1999). Furthermore, hyperaemia of the gland is another sign of inflammation (Cho et al. 2000). Seminal vesicle hypoplasia can be found associated to CBAVD in subjects with CFTR mutations as well as in testosterone deficiency (Nieschlag et al. 2010), while seminal vesicles enlargement, thickening, and calcifications of the gland epithelium and areas of endocapsulation with thick septa are considered signs of inflammation of the glands (Vicari 1999). Evaluation of the seminal vesicles should be performed before and after ejaculation, in order to assess the presence of intraprostatic uni- or

bilateral subobstruction, to avoid the bias of the sexual abstinence on seminal vesicle size and to be sure that a finding observed before ejaculation (for example areas of endocapsulation) are still present after ejaculation. Dysembriogenetic or acquired cysts can be found and should be distinguished in otricolar or mullerian cysts, the latter eventually communicating with ejaculatory duct (McDermott et al. 1995). Obstruction, dilatation, or calcifications of the ejaculatory ducts could be observed, the latter eventually associated to ejaculatory pain and hemospermia (Nieschlag et al. 2010). Vas deferens ampullae should be investigated, even if scrotal ultrasound demonstrates the presence of the proximal part of the vas deferens, because not only complete but also partial absence of vas deferens has been described. Finally, cysts of the ejaculatory ducts and/or seminal vesicles could associate with the presence of CFTR mutation, that should be ruled out (Behre et al. 1995; Futterer et al. 2008; Kim and Lipshultz 1996; Older and Watson 1996; Kim et al. 2009; Vohra and Morgentaler 1997).

# 5 Third Level Examinations

Third level examinations should be performed to finally understand the etiology of male factor when first and second level examinations are not conclusive for a diagnosis or when systemic anatomical or functional abnormalities related to the clinical and hormonal abnormalities are suspected.

## 5.1 Testicular Biopsy

Nowadays, testicular biopsy (TESE) can be considered more a therapeutic than a diagnostic procedure (Forti and Krausz 1998). Testicular sperms can be obtained from testicular biopsies of men with azoospermia caused by obstruction, incomplete maturation arrest, or Sertoli Cell Only Syndrome type II and can be successfully used for ICSI treatment (Silber et al. 1996). There is no general agreement concerning the most successful way for testicular sperm retrieval. Some authors found open testicular biopsy to be the best way, related to better results compared to fine-needle testicular aspiration (Friedler et al. 1997). MicroTESE is nowadays considered the best technique for testicular sperm retrieval (Schlegel 1999). Cryopreservation of a fraction of retrieved testicular spermatozoa is suggested for further ICSI (Intra Cytoplasmic Sperm Injection) cycles (Forti and Krausz 1998).

## 5.2 Pituitary Function Evaluation

If hypogonadotropic hypogonadism is diagnosed, pituitary function evaluation should be performed (Grumbach and Styne 2003). First of all, ACTH and plasmatic morning cortisol should be assessed in order to avoid central adrenal insufficiency. If low ACTH and low plasmatic morning cortisol are found, sometimes in presence of central adrenal insufficiency stigmate (e.g., low glycemia levels, low arterial pressure and weakness, mild to moderate hyponatremia and hyperkalemia), central adrenal insufficiency is plausible, and substitutive therapy must be started. When plasmatic morning cortisol values are not surely diagnostic for central adrenal insufficiency presence, ACTH test should be performed in order to evaluate pituitary ACTH reserve and response to stress (Grumbach and Styne 2003). Prolactin (PRL) should be evaluated when hypogonadotropic hypogonadism is present. Hyperprolactinemia, determined by several causes (Grumbach and Styne 2003), can induce hypogonadism by reducing GnRH, LH, and FSH pulses, or, when determined by a macroprolactinoma, through a damage of LH and FSH secreting cells compressed against the inextensible sella turcica, so reducing the drive on spermatogenetic tubules and Leydig cells (Grumbach and Styne 2003). In presence of hyperprolactinemia the physician should evaluate the presence of a pituitary adenoma (hypersecreting prolactin or just compressing the pituitary stalk), the use of drugs interfering with dopamine receptors, and all the other causes of abnormally high PRL levels (Grumbach and Styne 2003). Furthermore, TSH, FT3, and FT4 should be investigated in order to find out the presence of a central hypothyroidism (Grumbach and Styne 2003). Finally, GH and IGF1 should be investigated in order to find out the presence of GH deficit (Grumbach and Styne 2003).

## 5.3 GnRH Test

This test has been suggested to determine the gonadotropin reserve capacity of the pituitary and is particularly indicated for low-normal LH and FSH values, which cannot always be differentiated from pathologically low basal values (Nieschlag et al. 2010). Nowadays GnRH test is considered useful only in the diagnostic management of early puberty in order to discriminate between GnRH-dependent and GnRH-independent early puberty (Partsch et al. 2002), while it is considered useless for other diagnostic purposes (e.g., investigating delayed puberty—in particular constitutional delay of growth versus hypogonadotropic hypogonadism, hypotalamic or pituitary origin of hypogonadotropic hypogonadism, pituitary gonadotropins reserve evaluation). (Grumbach and Styne 2003; Partsch et al. 2002; De Martino et al. 2003). Some Authors propose GnRH test for the evaluation of the efficacy of medical therapy with GnRH analogues used for treating central early puberty (Partsch et al. 2002).

## 5.4 hCG Test

The endocrine reserve capacity of the testis can be tested by stimulation with human chorionic gonadotropin (hCG). hCG has predominantly LH activity and stimulates testosterone production of the Leydig cells. Today, the test is predominantly used for differentiation between bilateral cryptorchidism or ectopy of the testis (rise in testosterone levels present, but diminished) and anorchia (absent testosterone rise) (Nieschlag et al. 2010).

## 5.5 Glicometabolic Evaluation

Glycemia, insulinemia, total cholesterol, HDL, LDL, and tryglicerides should be evaluated to discover metabolic syndrome, dyslipidemia, or diabetes that are related to hypogonadism (usually associated to normal gonadotropin levels) (Corona et al. 2006c, 2007, 2009b) and abnormalities in spermatogenesis (Kasturi et al. 2008).

## 5.6 Magnetic Resonance Imaging of the Brain and of Pituitary Region

When hypogonadotropic hypogonadism is certain or highly suspected, MR imaging of the whole brain and of the pituitary gland should be performed in order to exclude the presence of malignant tumors and pituitary tumors causing hormonal abnormalities (Nieschlag et al. 2010; Grumbach and Styne 2003).

## 5.7 Abdomen Imaging

Hepatic ultrasound evaluation should be performed when high SHBG levels are found and hepatic disease is suspected (Nieschlag et al. 2010; Grumbach and Styne 2003). Hepatotropic viruses should be investigated at the same time. Renal and urinary tract evaluation should be performed when seminal vesicles (one or both) absence or seminal vesicles giant cysts and/or vas deferens absence (CBAVD) has been observed, or when cryptorchidism has been referred or is present: renal absence, dysgenesis or renal/urinary tract abnormalities can be revealed (Kim et al. 2009; Lissens and Liebaers 1997; Pappis et al. 1988). When cryptorchidism is present, the hidden testicle must be found out. Sometimes it is very difficult to find a cryptorchid testicle, especially when it is in the inguinal channel or in abdomen. Moreover, when testes are unpalpable, pelvic MR imaging is the imaging method of choice (Nieschlag et al. 2010).

## 5.8 Dual energy X-ray Absorptiometry

Dual energy X-ray Absorptiometry (DXA) applied to the lumbar spine and proximal femur has become the method of choice for determining bone density (Nieschlag et al. 2010). It should be performed when hypogonadism has been ruled out because testosterone has a positive effect on bone density and its deficiency is associated with osteopenia or osteoporosis (Nieschlag et al. 2010; Grumbach and Styne 2003).

## 6 Brief Evaluation of the Treatment of Infertile Men

In contrast to infertile females, only a small percentage of infertile or subfertile males can undergo a rationale, effective treatment. Before considering specific treatments, however, we must remember that expectant management can be an option if the duration of infertility is less than 3 years and the woman's age is less than 30 years because the fecundity of the woman can often compensate for the presence of low sperm concentration (even $<5 \times 10^6$/ml) and motility (20%) (Forti and Krausz 1998; Collins et al. 1993; Collins et al. 1995).

Rationale treatment (medical or surgical) should be performed when possible. If a specific cause of male infertility or hypogonadism is found and can be removed, it should be removed. For example, hypogonadism due to hyperprolactinemia can often be restored by medical therapy; sometimes the damage of LH and FSH cells cannot be reversed, or surgery is necessary for massive macroprolactinomas, with high risk of secondary persistent hypogonadism (Grumbach and Styne 2003). If hypogonadotropic hypogonadism is found, gonadotropin therapy can be performed, which may be associated to an increment in testicular volume and in sperm and testosterone production (Grumbach and Styne 2003). If hypergonadotropic hypogonadism is found, testicular biopsy (TESE or microTESE) for possible spermatozoa retrieval could be performed. Even if often no spermatozoa are found, nowadays some Authors report sperm retrieval even in Klinefelter patients, which will be used for ICSI technique. Then, testosterone substitutive treatment should be performed (Nieschlag et al. 2010; Grumbach and Styne 2003). If severe varicocele is found, surgical solution could be performed, with amelioration of sperm parameters, even if there is still debate on the opportunity of surgical correction of varicocele to improve couple's chance of conception in couples with otherwise unexplained subfertility (Forti et al. 2003; Evers et al. 2009; Ficarra et al. 2006). If infection of the sex accessory glands is present, appropriate treatment with antibiotics must be performed in both partners (Forti and Krausz 1998; Nieschlag et al. 2010). If distal obstructive azoospermia is documented, testicular biopsy and IVF (In Vitro Fertilization)/ICSI should be performed (Forti and Krausz 1998; Nieschlag et al. 2010). In patients with idiopathic semen abnormalities, different kinds of empirical pharmacological treatments, e.g., tamoxifene, especially if FSH is in the normal range, can be tried (Forti and Krausz 1998; Nieschlag et al. 2010). More than 30% of couples with unexplained infertility will become pregnant within 3 years of expectant management (Collins et al. 1995). However, in case of long-standing, unexplained infertility, with a female partner more than 30 years old, it is difficult to apply this approach. The most effective treatment seems to be superovulation combined with assisted reproductive techniques, sometimes using fresh or cryopreserved semen obtained by TESE or microTESE technique (Forti and Krausz 1998; Nieschlag et al. 2010).

# 7    Conclusions

The general endocrinologist can easily perform a first-line diagnostic evaluation of the infertile couple as the hormonal assessment has an important role in the initial workup of both partners, and semen analysis can be easily interpreted. It is also rather obvious that if the infertility has an endocrine cause (e.g., hypogonadotropic hypogonadism, polycystic ovarian syndrome, or hyperprolactinaemia) the endocrinologist has an important role in the treatment. On the other hand, further diagnostic work up of the couple requires appropriate knowledge of the physiology and pathology of the male and female reproductive tract as well as of second- and third-level diagnostic procedures.

# References

Aizenstein RI, Hibbeln JF, Sagireddy B et al (1997) Klinefelter's syndrome associated with testicular microlithiasis and mediastinal germ-cell neoplasm. J Clin Ultrasound 25: 508–510

Anawalt BD, Bebb RA, Matsumoto AM et al (1996) Serum inhibin B levels reflect sertoli cell function in normal men and men with testicular dysfunction. J Clin Endocrinol Metab 81:3341–3345

Andersson AM, Petersen JH, Jorgensen N et al (2004) Serum inhibin B and follicle-stimulating hormone levels as tools in the evaluation of infertile men: significance of adequate reference values from proven fertile men. J Clin Endocrinol Metab 89:2873–2879

Bach AM, Hann LE, Hadar O et al (2001) Testicular microlithiasis: what is its association with testicular cancer? Radiology 220:70–75

Behre HM, Kliesch S, Meschede D et al (1994) Hypogonadismus und infertilitat des mannes. In: Gerok W, Hartmann F, Prfcundschuh M et al (eds) Klinik der gegenwart. Urban und Scwarzenberg, Munchen, pp 1–73

Behre HM, Kliesch S, Schadel F et al (1995) Clinical relevance of scrotal and transrectal ultrasonography in andrological patients. Int J Androl 18(Suppl 2):27–31

Behre HM, Yeung CH, Holstein AF et al (2000) Diagnosis of male infertility and hypogonadism. In: Nieschlag E, Behre HM (eds) Andrology: male reproductive health and dysfunction, 2nd edn. Springer, Heidelberg, pp 90–124

Bergmann M, Behre HM, Nieschlag E (1994) Serum FSH and testicular morphology in male infertility. Clin Endocrinol (Oxf) 40:133–136

Brandell RA, Mielnik A, Liotta D et al (1998) AZFb deletions predict the absence of spermatozoa with testicular sperm extraction: preliminary report of a prognostic genetic test. Hum Reprod 13:2812–2815

Brooks DD, Wolf A, Smith RA et al (2010) Prostate cancer screening 2010: updated recommendations from the American cancer society. J Natl Med Assoc 102:423–429

Carani C, Isidori AM, Granata A et al (2005) Multicenter study on the prevalence of sexual symptoms in male hypo- and hyperthyroid patients. J Clin Endocrinol Metab 90:6472–6479

Carlsen E, Andersen AG, Buchreitz L et al (2000) Inter-observer variation in the results of the clinical andrological examination including estimation of testicular size. Int J Androl 23:248–253

Cast JE, Nelson WM, Early AS et al (2000) Testicular microlithiasis: prevalence and tumor risk in a population referred for scrotal sonography. AJR Am J Roentgenol 175:1703–1706

Chillon M, Casals T, Mercier B et al (1995) Mutations in the cystic fibrosis gene in patients with congenital absence of the vas deferens. N Engl J Med 332:1475–1480

Cho IR, Keener TS, Nghiem HV et al (2000) Prostate blood flow characteristics in the chronic prostatitis/pelvic pain syndrome. J Urol 163:1130–1133

Cihan A, Demir O, Demir T et al (2009) The relationship between premature ejaculation and hyperthyroidism. J Urol 181:1273–1280

Collins JA, Burrows EA, Willan AR (1993) Occupation and the follow-up of infertile couples. Fertil Steril 60:477–485

Collins JA, Burrows EA, Wilan AR (1995) The prognosis for live birth among untreated infertile couples. Fertil Steril 64:22–28

Corona G, Maggi M (2010) The role of testosterone in erectile dysfunction. Nat Rev Urol 7:46–56

Corona G, Mannucci E, Petrone L et al (2004a) Psychobiological correlates of hypoactive sexual desire in patients with erectile dysfunction. Int J Impot Res 16:275–281

Corona G, Petrone L, Mannucci E et al (2004b) Psychobiological correlates of rapid ejaculation in patients attending an andrologic unit for sexual dysfunctions. Eur Urol 46:615–622

Corona G, Mannucci E, Petrone L et al (2006a) Psychobiological correlates of delayed ejaculation in male patients with sexual dysfunctions. J Androl 27:453–458

Corona G, Mannucci E, Petrone L et al (2006b) ANDROTEST: a structured interview for the screening of hypogonadism in patients with sexual dysfunction. J Sex Med 3:706–715

Corona G, Mannucci E, Petrone L et al (2006c) Association of hypogonadism and type II diabetes in men attending an outpatient erectile dysfunction clinic. Int J Impot Res 18:190–197

Corona G, Mannucci E, Petrone L et al (2007) NCEP-ATPIII-defined metabolic syndrome, type 2 diabetes mellitus, and prevalence of hypogonadism in male patients with sexual dysfunction. J Sex Med 4:1038–1045

Corona G, Jannini EA, Mannucci E et al (2008) Different testosterone levels are associated with ejaculatory dysfunction. J Sex Med 5:1991–1998

Corona G, Mannucci E, Jannini EA et al (2009a) Hypoprolactinemia: a new clinical syndrome in patients with sexual dysfunction. J Sex Med 6:1457–1466

Corona G, Mannucci E, Forti G et al (2009b) Hypogonadism, ED, metabolic syndrome and obesity: a pathological link supporting cardiovascular diseases. Int J Androl 32:587–598

Corona G, Jannini EA, Lotti F et al (2010) Premature and delayed ejaculation: two ends of a single continuum influenced by hormonal milieu. Int J Androl doi:10.1111/j.1365-2605 2010.01059.x

De Martino MU, Pastore R, Caprio M et al (2003) Dynamic testing in the evaluation of male gonadal function. J Endocrinol Invest 26:107–113

Dohle GR, Diemer T, Giwercman A et al (2010) Guidelines on male infertility. AUA Guidelines

Egozcue J (1989) Chromosomal aspects of male infertility. In: Serio M (ed) Perspectives in andrology. Raven Press, New York, pp 341–346

El-Nashaar A, Shamloul R (2007) Antibiotic treatment can delay ejaculation in patients with premature ejaculation and chronic bacterial prostatitis. J Sex Med 4:491–496

ESHRE Capri Workshop Group (1996) Guidelines to the prevalence, diagnosis, tratment and management of infertility. Hum Reprod 11:1775–1807

Evers JH, Collins J, Clarke J (2009) Surgery or embolisation for varicoceles in subfertile men. Cochrane Database Syst Rev:CD000479

Ficarra V, Cerruto MA, Liguori G et al (2006) Treatment of varicocele in subfertile men: the cochrane review–a contrary opinion. Eur Urol 49:258–263

Forti G, Krausz C (1998) Clinical review 100: evaluation and treatment of the infertile couple. J Clin Endocrinol Metab 83:4177–4188

Forti G, Krausz C, Cilotti A et al (2003) Varicocele and infertility. J Endocrinol Invest 26:564–569

Friedler S, Raziel A, Strassburger D et al (1997) Testicular sperm retrieval by percutaneous fine needle sperm aspiration compared with testicular sperm extraction by open biopsy in men with non-obstructive azoospermia. Hum Reprod 12:1488–1493

Futterer JJ, Heijmink SW, Spermon JR (2008) Imaging the male reproductive tract: current trends and future directions. Radiol Clin North Am 46:133–147 vii

Grumbach MM, Styne DM (2003) Puberty: ontogeny, neuroendocrinology, physiology, and disorders. In: Larsen PR, Kronenberg HM, Melmed S et al (eds) Williams textbook of endocrinology, 10th edn. Saunders, Philadelphia, pp 1115–1286

Isidori AM, Lenzi A (2008) Scrotal ultrasound: morphological and functional atlas. Forum Service Editore srl, Genova

Jannini EA, Lenzi A (2005) Ejaculatory disorders: epidemiology and current approaches to definition, classification and subtyping. World J Urol 23:68–75

Jarow JP (2001) Effects of varicocele on male fertility. Hum Reprod Update 7:59–64

Kasturi SS, Tannir J, Brannigan RE (2008) The metabolic syndrome and male infertility. J Androl 29:251–259

Kessaris DN, Mellinger BC (1994) Incidence and implication of testicular microlithiasis detected by scrotal duplex sonography in a select group of infertile men. J Urol 152:1560–1561

Kim ED, Lipshultz LI (1996) Role of ultrasound in the assessment of male infertility. J Clin Ultrasound 24:437–453

Kim B, Kawashima A, Ryu JA et al (2009) Imaging of the seminal vesicle and vas deferens. Radiographics 29:1105–1121

Krause W (2008) Male accessory gland infection. Andrologia 40:113–116

Krausz C, Degl'Innocenti S (2006) Y chromosome and male infertility: update, 2006. Front Biosci 11:3049–3061

Krausz C, Forti G (2000) Clinical aspects of male infertility. Results Probl Cell Differ 28:1–21

Krausz C, Quintana-Murci L, McElreavey K (2000) Prognostic value of Y deletion analysis: what is the clinical prognostic value of Y chromosome microdeletion analysis? Hum Reprod 15:1431–1434

Lanfranco F, Kamischke A, Zitzmann M et al (2004) Klinefelter's syndrome. Lancet 364:273–283

Lee JC, Bhatt S, Dogra VS (2008) Imaging of the epididymis. Ultrasound Q 24:3–16

Lenz S, Giwercman A, Elsborg A et al (1993) Ultrasonic testicular texture and size in 444 men from the general population: correlation to semen quality. Eur Urol 24:231–238

Lenzi A, Balercia G, Bellastella A et al (2009) Epidemiology, diagnosis, and treatment of male hypogonadotropic hypogonadism. J Endocrinol Invest 32:934–938

Liguori G, Trombetta C, Garaffa G et al (2004) Color doppler ultrasound investigation of varicocele. World J Urol 22:378–381

Lissens W, Liebaers I (1997) The genetics of male infertility in relation to cystic fibrosis. Baillieres Clin Obstet Gynaecol 11:797–817

Lotti F, Corona G, Mancini M et al (2009) The association between varicocele, premature ejaculation and prostatitis symptoms: possible mechanisms. J Sex Med 6:2878–2887

McDermott VG, Meakem TJ 3rd, Stolpen AH et al (1995) Prostatic and periprostatic cysts: findings on MR imaging. AJR Am J Roentgenol 164:123–127

Morelli A, Filippi S, Zhang XH et al (2005) Peripheral regulatory mechanisms in erection. Int J Androl 28(Suppl 2):23–27

Morelli A, Corona G, Filippi S et al (2007) Which patients with sexual dysfunction are suitable for testosterone replacement therapy? J Endocrinol Invest 30:880–888

Nieschlag E, Behre HM, Nieschlag S (2010) Andrology: male reproductive health and dysfunction. Springer, Berlin

Nuti F, Krausz C (2008) Gene polymorphisms/mutations relevant to abnormal spermatogenesis. Reprod Biomed Online 16:504–513

Older RA, Watson LR (1996) Ultrasound anatomy of the normal male reproductive tract. J Clin Ultrasound 24:389–404

Otite U, Webb JA, Oliver RT et al (2001) Testicular microlithiasis: is it a benign condition with malignant potential? Eur Urol 40:538–542

Pappis CH, Argianas SA, Bousgas D et al (1988) Unsuspected urological anomalies in asymptomatic cryptorchid boys. Pediatr Radiol 18:51–53

Partsch CJ, Heger S, Sippell WG (2002) Management and outcome of central precocious puberty. Clin Endocrinol (Oxf) 56:129–148

Pellati D, Mylonakis I, Bertoloni G et al (2008) Genital tract infections and infertility. Eur J Obstet Gynecol Reprod Biol 140:3–11

Peterson AC, Bauman JM, Light DE et al (2001) The prevalence of testicular microlithiasis in an asymptomatic population of men 18 to 35 years old. J Urol 166:2061–2064

Petrone L, Mannucci E, Corona G et al (2003) Structured interview on erectile dysfunction (SIEDY): a new, multi-dimensional instrument for quantification of pathogenetic issues on erectile dysfunction. Int J Impot Res 15:210–220

Root AW (2010) Reversible isolated hypogonadotropic hypo-gonadism due to mutations in the neurokinin B regulation of gonadotropin-releasing hormone release. J Clin Endocrinol Metab 95:2625–2629

Rosner W, Auchus RJ, Azziz R et al (2007) Position statement: utility, limitations, and pitfalls in measuring testosterone: an endocrine society position statement. J Clin Endocrinol Metab 92:405–413

Rowe PJ, Comhaire FH, Hargreave TB et al (1993) WHO manual for the standardized investigation and diagnosis of the infertile couple. Cambridge University Press, Cambridge

Schlegel PN (1999) Testicular sperm extraction: microdissec-tion improves sperm yield with minimal tissue excision. Hum Reprod 14:131–135

Screponi E, Carosa E, Di Stasi SM et al (2001) Prevalence of chronic prostatitis in men with premature ejaculation. Urology 58:198–202

Seo JT, Ko WJ (2001) Predictive factors of successful testicular sperm recovery in non-obstructive azoospermia patients. Int J Androl 24:306–310

Silber SJ, van Steirteghem A, Nagy Z et al (1996) Normal pregnancies resulting from testicular sperm extraction and intracytoplasmic sperm injection for azoospermia due to maturation arrest. Fertil Steril 66:110–117

Takihara H, Cosentino MJ, Sakatoku J et al (1987) Significance of testicular size measurement in andrology: II. Correlation of testicular size with testicular function. J Urol 137:416–419

te Velde ER, Eijkemans R, Habbema HD (2000) Variation in couple fecundity and time to pregnancy, an essential concept in human reproduction. Lancet 355:1928–1929

Thomas K, Wood SJ, Thompson AJ et al (2000) The incidence and significance of testicular microlithiasis in a subfertile population. Br J Radiol 73:494–497

Traggiai C, Stanhope R (2002) Delayed puberty. Best Pract Res Clin Endocrinol Metab 16:139–151

Tüttelmann F and Nieschlag E (2010) Classification of andro-logical disorders. In: Nieschlag E, Behre HM, Nieschlag S (eds) Andrology, male reproductive health and dysfunction, 3rd edn. Springer, Berlin

World Health Organization (2000) WHO manual for the standardised investigation and diagnosis of the infertile couple. Cambridge University Press, Cambridge

Vermeulen A, Verdonck L, Kaufman JM (1999) A critical evaluation of simple methods for the estimation of free testosterone in serum. J Clin Endocrinol Metab 84:3666–3672

Vicari E (1999) Seminal leukocyte concentration and related specific reactive oxygen species production in patients with male accessory gland infections. Hum Reprod 14:2025–2030

Vignozzi L, Corona G, Petrone L et al (2005) Testosterone and sexual activity. J Endocrinol Invest 28:39–44

Vohra S, Morgentaler A (1997) Congenital anomalies of the vas deferens, epididymis, and seminal vesicles. Urology 49:313–321

Wang C, Nieschlag E, Swerdloff R et al (2009) ISA, ISSAM, EAU, EAA and ASA recommendations: investigation, treatment and monitoring of late-onset hypogonadism in males. Int J Impot Res 21:1–8

Woodward PJ, Sohaey R, O'Donoghue MJ et al (2002) From the archives of the AFIP: tumors and tumorlike lesions of the testis: radiologic-pathologic correlation. Radiographics 22:189–216

Woodward PJ, Schwab CM, Sesterhenn IA (2003) From the archives of the AFIP: extratesticular scrotal masses: radio-logic-pathologic correlation. Radiographics 23:215–240

World Health Organization (1987) Towards more objectivity in diagnosis and management of male infertility. Int J Androl 7:1–53

World Health Organization (2010) WHO laboratory manual for the examination and processing of human semen. World Health Organization, Geneva

# The Infertile Male-4: Management of Obstructive Azoospermia

Giovanni Liguori, Carlo Trombetta, Alessio Zordani, Renata Napoli, Giangiacomo Ollandini, Giorgio Mazzon, Bernardino de Concilio, and Emanuele Belgrano

## Contents

### Abstract

Azoospermia is the total absence of spermatozoa in the ejaculate. It is found in 10–15% of male infertility cases and is caused by a testicular insufficiency in the majority of patients. Obstructive azoospermia is less frequent and arises in 15–20% of men with azoospermia. Most causes of male infertility are treatable, and many treatments restore the ability to father a children naturally. In case of vasal or epididymal obstruction, microsurgical reconstruction of the seminal pathways, if possible, remains the safest and most cost-effective treatment option for these patients, allowing natural conception in many cases. Not all men with obstructive azoospermia are treatable by microsurgical reconstruction. In such situations, various sperm-retrieval techniques can be employed to take sperm for use with in vitro fertilization (IVF) via intracytoplasmic sperm injection (ICSI).

## 1 Introduction

Azoospermia is defined as the total absence of spermatozoa in the ejaculate. It is found in 10–15% of male infertility cases and is caused by a testicular insufficiency in the majority of patients. Obstructive azoospermia is less frequent and arises in 15–20% of patients. The most common cause is previous vasectomy. Other causes are epididymal, vessel, or ejaculatory duct pathology relating to genitourinary infection, iatrogenic injury during scrotal or inguinal surgery, and congenital anomalies (Sheynkin et al. 1998).

G. Liguori · C. Trombetta (✉) · A. Zordani · R. Napoli ·
G. Ollandini · G. Mazzon · B. de Concilio · E. Belgrano
Department of Urology, University of Trieste,
Ospedale di Cattinara, Strada di Fiume 447,
34124 Trieste, Italy
e-mail: trombcar@units.it

M. Bertolotto and C. Trombetta (eds.), *Scrotal Pathology*, Medical Radiology. Diagnostic Imaging,
DOI: 10.1007/174_2011_189, © Springer-Verlag Berlin Heidelberg 2012

Most causes of male infertility are treatable, and many treatments restore the ability to father a children naturally.

## 2 Clinical Presentation

Men with obstructive azoospermia present with normal size testes and normal FSH. On examination, enlargement of the epididymis can be found and sometimes the vas deferens appears to be absent, due to congenital factors or previous inguinal or scrotal surgery. Although obstructions in primary infertile men are commonly present at the epididymal level, other sites of obstruction are the ejaculatory ducts and the vas deferens.

In 25% of men with a suspected obstruction, no spermatozoa are found in the epididymis during scrotal exploration, indicating that there is an intra-testicular obstruction (Practice Committee of the American Society for Reproductive Medicine 2008a).

Moreover, clinical management of obstructive azoospermia must also take into account any concomitant infertility factors in the female partner. As a result, both partners should be examined before making a specific treatment proposal.

## 3 Treatment Options for Obstructive Azoospermia

Men with obstructive azoospermia may father children in one of two ways:
- Surgical correction of the obstruction.
- Retrieval of sperm directly from the epididymis or the testis followed by in vitro fertilization (IVF) or intracytoplasmatic sperm injection.

In case of vasal or epididymal obstruction, microsurgical reconstruction of the seminal pathways, if possible, remains the safest and most cost-effective treatment option for these patients, allowing natural conception in many cases (Donovan et al. 1998; Pavlovich and Schlegel 1997; Kolettis and Thomas 1997). The surgical management of obstructive azoospermia depends on the site of obstruction: if obstruction is present at the level of the vas deferens or epididymis microsurgery is indicated; on the contrary, ejaculatory duct obstruction is treated by transurethral resection of the ejaculatory ducts

(TURED) (Practice Committee of the American Society for Reproductive Medicine 2008a).

## 3.1 Transurethral Resection of the Ejaculatory Ducts

Ejaculatory duct obstruction is suspected when the ejaculate volume is <2.0 mL and no sperm or fructose is present. Clinical suspicion can be confirmed by TRUS demonstration of dilated seminal vesicles or dilated ejaculatory ducts.

Transurethral resection of the ejaculatory ducts is performed cystoscopically. A small resectoscope and electrocautery loop are inserted, and the verumontanum is resected in the midline. Since the area of resection is at the prostatic apex, near the external urethral sphincter and the rectum, careful positioning of the resectoscope is essential. There is convincing evidence from several large studies of patients treated for infertility that 65–70% of men show significant improvement in semen quality after TURED and that a 20–30% pregnancy rate can be expected. The complication rate from TURED is approximately 20%. Most complications are self-limited and include hematospermia, hematuria, urinary tract infection, epididymitis, and a watery ejaculate. Rarely reported complications include retrograde ejaculation, rectal perforation, and urinary incontinence.

## 3.2 Microsurgical Reconstruction of the Vas Deferens and Epididymis

Microsurgical reconstruction to correct male infertility, although usually performed for vasectomy reversal, is also performed to correct other types of iatrogenic, congenital, and post inflammatory obstruction.

Microsurgical reconstruction of the seminal pathways may be accomplished via anastomosis of the vasal ends (vasovasostomy) or anastomosis of the abdominal end of the vas deferens to the epididymis (vasoepididymostomy).

Before surgery, it is necessary for the surgeon to alert the cryobank laboratory personnel: as a matter of fact intraoperative retrieval of sperms from the vas, epididymis or testis is performed in order to cryo-preserve sperm for possible later use for IVF/ICSI in case of microsurgery failure.

### 3.2.1 Vasovasostomy or Vasoepididymostomy

Vasovasostomy almost always is performed for the reversal of an elective vasectomy (6% of men who undergo vasectomy ultimately request reversal), but, vasovasostomy is not always a feasible option to restore vasal patency; as a matter of fact if epididymal obstruction is present, whether primary or secondary to chronic vasal obstruction, a vasoepididymostomy is required proximal to the obstruction to restore continuity for sperm transport (Goldstein et al. 1998).

Every procedure begins with the careful dissection of the vas deferens with an intact sheath and meticulous preservation of the blood supply. Once the site of the previous vasectomy has been identified, the vas is transected perpendicularly on the abdominal and testicular limbs as close as possible to the obstructed segment to preserve vasal length and the fluid is examined under a separate bench light microscope to determine whether vasovasostomy or vasoepididymostomy is indicated. If copious, clear, watery fluid is identified or if intact sperm or sperm parts are identified, then vasovasostomy is indicated.

### 3.2.2 Vasovasostomy

Vasovasostomy represents the simplest form of microsurgical reconstruction of the reproductive tract. The microsurgical anastomosis may be performed with either a modified one-layer or a two-layer technique. The modified one-layer anastomosis (Schmidt 1978) is performed using six to eight interrupted full thickness sutures of 9–0 nylon placed equidistantly around the circumference of each end of the vas, followed by the placement of more superficial outer muscular layer sutures of 9–0 nylon between adjacent full thickness sutures.

The two-layer end-to-side microsurgical anastomosis (Belker 1980) is performed by placing six to eight interrupted sutures of 10–0 nylon through the mucosa of each end of the vas, followed by the placement of approximately eight interrupted sutures of 9–0 nylon through the outer muscular layer of the vas (Fig. 1). A folding vas approximating clamp is useful to perform this anastomosis (Belker et al. 1991).

The one-layer technique is performed in patients in whom there is little difference in the diameters of vas deferens between the distal and the proximal sides. Nevertheless, to simplify the surgical procedure and to shorten the duration of the operation, the one-layer

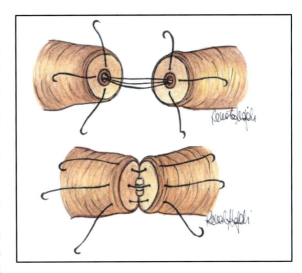

**Fig. 1** Vasovasostomy. Inner mucosal edges are approximated with interrupted 10–0 nylon sutures and outer muscular edges are approximated with interrupted 9–0 nylon sutures

technique might be sufficient for vasectomy reversal. In vasovasostomy after herniorrhaphy, when there used to be a large difference in the diameters of the vas deferens between the distal and the proximal sides because of the long duration of obstruction, the two-layer technique is required to ensure the precise attachment of the mucosa of the vas deferens. When compared with the fertility rate (42–50%) for patients who underwent vasectomy reversal with duration <10 years, the results for the patients who underwent vasectomy reversal with duration >10 years after vasectomy showed markedly poor results (37%) (Nagler and Jung 2009). Known inhibiting factors of pregnancy after vasovasostomy include stricture and obstruction of the seminal tract at the anastomotic site; ruptured ductus epididymis caused by occlusion or back pressure and secondary obstruction of ruptured ductus epididymidis. Antisperm antibodies have also been reported to play a role (Royle et al. 1981).

### 3.2.3 Vasoepididymostomy

This procedure is performed by creating vertical scrotal incisions that are adequately long to extrude the scrotal contents. Otherwise the testicles are exposed by means of an infrapubic incision according to Kelami.

The presence of active spermatogenesis is an obvious prerequisite to this surgical procedure and, if a testis biopsy has not already been carried out before this surgery, it can be done in a standard fashion and the tissue examined under the microscope (400×) for the presence of sperm, some of which may be motile.

It is necessary to prove that the vasa are patent. For this reason a 27-gauge needle is inserted into the lumen of the vas, pointing away from the testicle and a vasography is carried out: a vasogram involves the injection of contrast media into the vas toward the bladder from the scrotum.

Vasography can delineate the proximal vas deferens, seminal vesicle and ejaculatory duct anatomy and determine whether obstruction is present (Fig. 2). The procedure begins by first freeing up the abdominal limb of the vas deferens that will be used for the anastomosis. Mobilization of the vas with meticulous preservation of blood supply is necessary to create a tension-free anastomosis. For this purpose the vas must be prepared to the level of the ring and drawn through an opening in the tunica vaginalis: Then the vas is brought to the epididymis in a straight-line fashion and the posterior edge of the epididymal tunic is sewed to the posterior edge of the vasal muscularis with interrupted 9–0 nylon sutures in order to position the lumen of the vas adjacent to the selected epididymal tubule (Kolettis 2008).

The results of vasoepididymostomy are increasingly successful, the lower the anastomosis is performed in the epididymis (Jarow et al. 1997). While it is important to perform the anastomosis at the lowest possible epididymal level, the level must be at a point in the epididymis at which spermatozoa are present in the epididymal tubular fluid, which assures that the anastomosis will be performed above the obstruction in the epididymis. Although vasovasostomy may have a successful result despite the intraoperative absence of spermatozoa from the vas fluid, vasoepididymostomy will never be successful when performed at an epididymal level at which spermatozoa are absent from the epididymal tubular fluid (Niederberger and Ross 1993).

Multiple anastomotic techniques have been described, although three variations are currently used: direct end-to-end, direct end-to-side, and end-to-side intussusceptions (HAJ and Khera 2007; Belgrano et al. 1984).

Of all the modifications reported in literature, intussusception vasoepididymostomy anastomotic techniques have had the greatest impact on clinical practice and are now used widely by urologic microsurgeons.

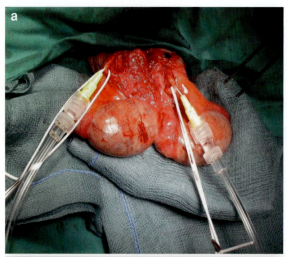

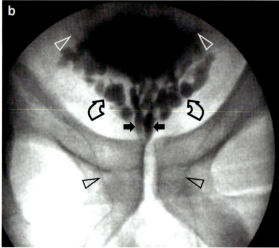

**Fig. 2** Vasography. **a** A 27-gauge needle is inserted into the lumen of the vas, pointing away from the testicle and the iodinated contrast media is injected into the vas toward the bladder from the scrotum. **b** X-ray showing the vas deferens (*arrowheads*), seminal vesicle (*curved arrows*) and ejaculatory duct anatomy (*black arrows*). In this case distal obstruction is not present

Berger (1998) first described the use of an invagination vasoepididymostomy in clinical practice. He described a triangulation intussusception technique using three double-armed 10–0 nylon sutures, which would be equivalent to six luminal sutures. In a series of 12 men who underwent bilateral vasoepididymostomy with this technique, the patency rate was 92%.

Marmar (2000) then described a two-suture intussusceptions vasoepididymostomy technique that many regarded as another significant advance: the sutures were placed transversely in the epididymal tubule with a single, simultaneous needle placement.

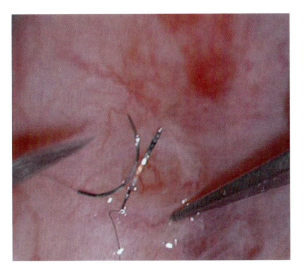

**Fig. 3** Transversal two-suture intussusceptions vasoepididymostomy. The sutures were placed transversely in the epididymal tubule with a single, simultaneous needle placement

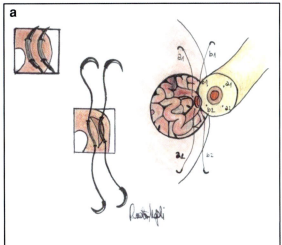

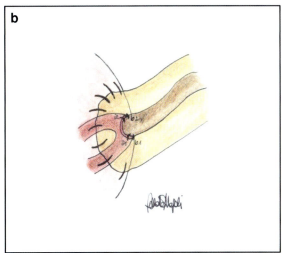

**Fig. 4** Longitudinal two-suture longitudinal end-to-side vasoepididymostomy technique. **a** Two sutures are placed longitudinally on epididymal tubule to achieve four-point anastomosis; opening is created on epididymal tubule after confirmation of sperm appearance in epididymal tubule. **b** Epididymal tubule is intussuscepted into lumen of vas by four sutures that are placed to the mucosa of the vas; then 9–0 nylon sutures are placed on tunic of epididymis to secure watertight anastomosis

The Cornell group has also reported on a two-suture method. In their study, the sutures were placed longitudinally rather than transversely (Chan et al. 2003). This maneuver was then followed by a tubulotomy cut between the sutures. After the epididymal fluid is tested for sperm and aspirated into micropipettes for cryopreservation, the two needles within the epididymal tubule are pulled through, and all four needles are placed through the vas lumen at the marked locations. Tying down the sutures allows the epididymal tubule to be intussuscepted into the vasal lumen, completing the anastomosis (Figs. 3, 4). The patency rate with the longitudinal intussusception vasoepididymostomy approach was over 90% in a recent clinical series, and intussusception is the preferred method for all vasoepididymostomies (Chan et al. 2005).

## 3.3 Sperm Retrieval Techniques

Not all men with obstructive azoospermia are tractable by microsurgical reconstruction. In such situations, various sperm-retrieval techniques can be employed to take sperm for use with in vitro fertilization (IVF) via intracytoplasmic sperm injection (ICSI). For obstructive azoospermia, fertilization and pregnancy rates are comparable with those achieved with ejaculated sperm. The results with frozen testicular sperm are comparable to those obtained with fresh testicular sperm.

Sperm retrieval with IVF/ICSI offers the possibility of early achievement of a relatively high live delivery rate, but any couple considering IVF/ICSI should be apprised of the risks involved in this type of treatment. These include the possibility of ovarian hyperstimulation, the potential complications of oocyte retrieval and the risks and consequences of multiple gestations (Schlegel and Girardi 1997).

In men with obstructive azoospermia, sperm may be retrieved from either the epididymis or the testis via a variety of percutaneous, open, or microsurgical techniques.

The microsurgical techniques may also be used concomitantly with reconstructive procedures as a means to obtain sperm for cryopreservation in the event the attempt at reconstruction is not successful.

The obvious advantages of percutaneous acquisition are the minimally invasive nature of this method and the ability to sample multiple sites within the testes with minimal potential for harm to the testis. The obvious disadvantage is that the area of tissue sampled is decreased, markedly compared with the open biopsy.

### 3.3.1 Sperm Retrieval Techniques

According to the Practice Committee of American Society for Reproductive Medicine Guidelines, since only 20–40% of couples conceive after attempted vasoepididymostomy despite patency rates of 60–80%, it is reasonable to consider sperm retrieval at the time of surgical reconstruction (Practice Committee of the American Society for Reproductive Medicine 2008b). If motile sperm are found at the site of reconstruction, they may be aspirated and cryopreserved. Alternatively, sperm may be retrieved via testicular biopsy.

The first successful attempt at ICSI using epididymal sperm (MESA or microsurgical epididymal sperm aspiration) was reported by Silber et al. (1994) and Tournaye et al. (1994). Many reports have shown that the cause of obstruction is not important when considering the success rate with MESA. The MESA procedure is performed under general anaesthesia. After exposure, a dilated tubule of the epididymis is microsurgically opened and its fluid examined for the presence of motile spermatozoa. The best quality sperm are typically found in the proximal epididymis close to the testis. Puncture sites may be closed or cauterized. Performing aspiration under direct vision with the aid of the operating microscope allows for procurement of a large number of good quality, motile sperm from the epididymal tubules (Nudell et al. 1998).

An alternative method for epididymal aspiration of sperm is PESA (percutaneous epididymal sperm aspiration), being less invasive and less costly than MESA.

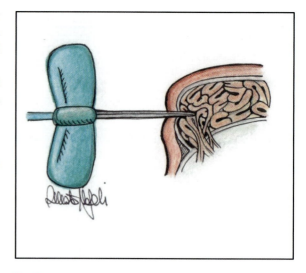

**Fig. 5** PESA: a needle is introduced through the skin into the epididymis and is then aspirated

Epididymal aspiration also can be performed without surgical scrotal exploration, repeatedly, easily, and at low cost, without an operating microscope or expertise in microsurgery. PESA can be performed under local anesthesia. This technique is indicated in patients with obstructive azoospermia who were unable to undergo or who decided against surgical reconstruction. A needle is introduced through the skin into the epididymis and is then aspirated (Fig. 5). Multiple punctures may be required to obtain sufficient fluid. However, the number of sperm retrieved is often not sufficient to allow for cryopreservation, so repeat procedures may be warranted for multiple IVF cycles. In addition, there is a risk for development of scrotal hematoma or injury to the epididymal or testicular vessels given the blind nature of this procedure.

Despite the good results with MESA and PESA, many studies have shown that ICSI with testicular spermatozoa retrieved by TESE (testicular sperm extraction) can also be successfully applied in almost all cases of azoospermia (Trombetta et al. 2000). The most popular methods of sperm retrieval are conventional "open biopsy" retrieval (TESE), FNA (fine needle aspiration) or TESA (testicular sperm aspiration). In patients with normal spermatogenesis it seems that FNA and TESE give comparable results (Tournaye 1997).

The choice of sperm retrieval method in men with obstructive azoospermia depends primarily on the experience and preference of both the physician who will perform the retrieval and the IVF laboratory embryologist. There are not enough data to conclude that either the technique of sperm retrieval (open or percutaneous) or the source of sperm (testicular, epididymal, vasal, or seminal vesicular) significantly affects pregnancy rates.

Moreover, epididymal and testicular sperm could be frozen, stored and subsequently used in future ICSI cycles. For obstructive azoospermia, fertilization and pregnancy rates are comparable with those using ejaculated spermatozoa, and results with frozen sperm are comparable to those obtained with fresh testicular sperm.

Cryopreservation of sperm is an essential technique in the treatment of infertile couples wherein the man has obstructive azoospermia. Whenever available, excess retrieved spermatozoa should be cryopreserved to avoid unnecessary subsequent sperm retrieval procedures (Practice Committee of the American Society for Reproductive Medicine 2008b).

The results achieved with retrieved sperm and ICSI are excellent. Contemporary pregnancy rates of 24–64% have been achieved using sperm retrieved from azoospermic men (Craft et al. 1995; Palermo et al. 1999). Maternal factors (maternal age, oocyte number, and oocyte quality) alone are now considered the principal determinants of outcomes achieved with ART and ICSI for couples with infertility related to obstructive azoospermia (Silber et al. 1997).

## 4    Conclusion

Microsurgical reconstruction should be offered to men having a repairable reproductive tract obstruction and is preferable to sperm retrieval with IVF/ICSI in men with prior vasectomy if the obstructive interval is less than 15 years and no female fertility risk factors are present. If an epididymal obstruction is present, the decision to use either microsurgical reconstruction or sperm retrieval with IVF/ICSI should be individualized.

Vasoepididymostomy should be performed by an expert in reproductive microsurgery.

Sperm retrieval with ART is an alternative to microsurgical repair for men with correctable reproductive tract obstruction and represents the only treatment that can offer men with irreparable obstruction, the opportunity to have their own genetic children. Almost all men with obstructive azoospermia have abundant sperm in the testes that can be retrieved successfully using a variety of different techniques.

Sperm retrieval/ICSI is preferred to surgical treatment when (1) advanced female age is present, (2) female factors requiring IVF are present (3) the chance for success with sperm retrieval/ICSI exceeds the chance for success with surgical treatment or (4) sperm retrieval/ICSI is preferred by the couple for financial reasons.

## References

Belgrano E, Puppo P, Trombetta C et al (1984) Monolateral tubulovasostomy. Report of four cases. J Androl 5:330–333

Belker AM (1980) Microsurgical two-layer vasovasostomy. Simplified technique using hinged, folding-approximating clamp. Urology 16:376–381

Belker AM, Thomas AJ Jr, Fuchs EF et al (1991) Results of 1, 469 microsurgical vasectomy reversals by the vasovasostomy Study Group. J Urol 145:505–511

Berger RE (1998) Triangulation end-to-side vasoepididymostomy. J Urol 159:1951–1953

Chan PT, Li PS, Goldstein M (2003) Microsurgical vasoepididymostomy: a prospective randomized study of 3 intussusception techniques in rats. J Urol 169:1924–1929

Chan PT, Brandell RA, Goldstein M (2005) Prospective analysis of outcomes after microsurgical intussusception vasoepididymostomy. BJU Int 96:598–601

Craft IL, Khalifa Y, Boulos A et al (1995) Factors influencing the outcome of in vitro fertilization with percutaneous aspirated epididymal spermatozoa and intracytoplasmic sperm injection in azoospermic men. Hum Reprod 10:1791–1794

Donovan JF Jr, DiBaise M, Sparks AE et al (1998) Comparison of microscopic epididymal sperm aspiration and intracytoplasmic sperm injection/in vitro fertilization with repeat microscopic reconstruction following vasectomy: is second attempt vas reversal worth the effort? Hum Reprod 13:387–393

Goldstein M, Li PS, Matthews GJ (1998) Microsurgical vasovasostomy: the microdot technique of precision suture placement. J Urol 159:188–190

Lipshultz LHAJ, Khera M (2007) Surgical management of male infertility. In: Wein AJ, Kavoussi LR, Novick AC et al (eds) Campbell-Walsh Urology, 9th edn. Saunders Elsevier, Philadelphia

Jarow JP, Oates RD, Buch JP et al (1997) Effect of level of anastomosis and quality of intraepididymal sperm on the outcome of end-to-side epididymovasostomy. Urology 49:590–595

Kolettis PN (2008) Restructuring reconstructive techniques—advances in reconstructive techniques. Urol Clin North Am 35:229–234, viii-ix

Kolettis PN, Thomas AJ Jr (1997) Vasoepididymostomy for vasectomy reversal: a critical assessment in the era of intracytoplasmic sperm injection. J Urol 158:467–470

Marmar JL (2000) Modified vasoepididymostomy with simultaneous double needle placement, tubulotomy and tubular invagination. J Urol 163:483–486

Nagler HM, Jung H (2009) Factors predicting successful microsurgical vasectomy reversal. Urol Clin North Am 36:383–390

Niederberger C, Ross LS (1993) Microsurgical epididymovasostomy: predictors of success. J Urol 149:1364–1367

Nudell DM, Conaghan J, Pedersen RA et al (1998) The mini-micro-epididymal sperm aspiration for sperm retrieval: a study of urological outcomes. Hum Reprod 13:1260–1265

Palermo GD, Schlegel PN, Hariprashad JJ et al (1999) Fertilization and pregnancy outcome with intracytoplasmic sperm injection for azoospermic men. Hum Reprod 14:741–748

Pavlovich CP, Schlegel PN (1997) Fertility options after vasectomy: a cost-effectiveness analysis. Fertil Steril 67:133–141

Practice Committee of the American Society for Reproductive Medicine (2008a) The management of infertility due to obstructive azoospermia. Fertil Steril 90:S121–S124

Practice Committee of the American Society for Reproductive Medicine (2008b) Sperm retrieval for obstructive azoospermia. Fertil Steril 90:S213–S218

Royle MG, Parslow JM, Kingscott MM et al (1981) Reversal of vasectomy: the effects of sperm antibodies on subsequent fertility. Br J Urol 53:654–659

Schlegel PN, Girardi SK (1997) Clinical review 87: In vitro fertilization for male factor infertility. J Clin Endocrinol Metab 82:709–716

Schmidt SS (1978) Vasovasostomy. Urol Clin North Am 5:585–592

Sheynkin YR, Hendin BN, Schlegel PN et al (1998) Microsurgical repair of iatrogenic injury to the vas deferens. J Urol 159:139–141

Silber SJ, Nagy ZP, Liu J et al (1994) Conventional in vitro fertilization versus intracytoplasmic sperm injection for patients requiring microsurgical sperm aspiration. Hum Reprod 9:1705–1709

Silber SJ, Nagy Z, Devroey P et al (1997) The effect of female age and ovarian reserve on pregnancy rate in male infertility: treatment of azoospermia with sperm retrieval and intracytoplasmic sperm injection. Hum Reprod 12:2693–2700

Tournaye H (1997) Use of testicular sperm for the treatment of male infertility. Baillieres Clin Obstet Gynaecol 11:753–762

Tournaye H, Devroey P, Liu J et al (1994) Microsurgical epididymal sperm aspiration and intracytoplasmic sperm injection: a new effective approach to infertility as a result of congenital bilateral absence of the vas deferens. Fertil Steril 61:1045–1051

Trombetta C, Liguori G, Gianaroli L et al (2000) Testicular sperm extraction combined with cryopreservation of testicular tissue in the treatment of azoospermia. Urol Int 65:15–20

# The Infertile Male-5: Management of Non-Obstructive Azoospermia

Mirco Castiglioni, Elisabetta M. Colpi, Fabrizio I. Scroppo, and Giovanni M. Colpi

## Contents

M. Castiglioni · G. M. Colpi (✉)
Andro-Urology Unit and IVF Center,
University of Milan, Ospedale San Paolo,
Via A Di Rudiní 8, 20142 Milan, Italy
e-mail: gmcolpi@yahoo.com

E. M. Colpi
Biogenesi IVF Center, Istituti Clinici Zucchi,
Via Zucchi 24, 20052 Monza, Italy

F. I. Scroppo
Urology Unit, Ospedale di Circolo e Fondazione Macchi,
Via Borri 57, Varese 21100, Italy

### Abstract

Surgical testicular sperm retrieval for intra-cytoplasmic sperm injection purposes is the only possibility of biological fathering in case of non-obstructive azoospermia (NOA). Successful retrieval only correlates with histology, not with FSH values or testicular volume. Testicular sperm extraction (TESE) (mean of successful retrievals in the literature: 52.7%) is the technique of choice: we had successful retrievals in 100% of cases of hypospermatogenesis with >5 spermatids/tubule (spd/tub), 81.8% of cases of hypospermatogenesis with <4 spd/tub, 50% of cases of maturation arrest, and 25% of cases of histologically pure Sertoli cell only syndrome. Microsurgical TESE (MicroTESE) has been reported to increase successful retrievals: from 16.7 to 45% for standard TESE to 42.9–63.6% for MicroTESE, depending on the distribution of testicular histology in the various case studies. TeFNA does not appear to be indicated in NOA, both because of its low success rates—which, in practice, are only positive in hypospermatogenesis, and because it is unable to detect any carcinomas in situ. Previous surgery of left varicocele in NOA could increase the chances of subsequent recovery.

## 1 Introduction

The absence of spermatozoa within the ejaculate is called azoospermia. According to etiology it is classified as pre-testicular, due to hypogonadotropic hypogonadism (with low FSH and low LH, normal or low serum testosterone); testicular: non-obstructive

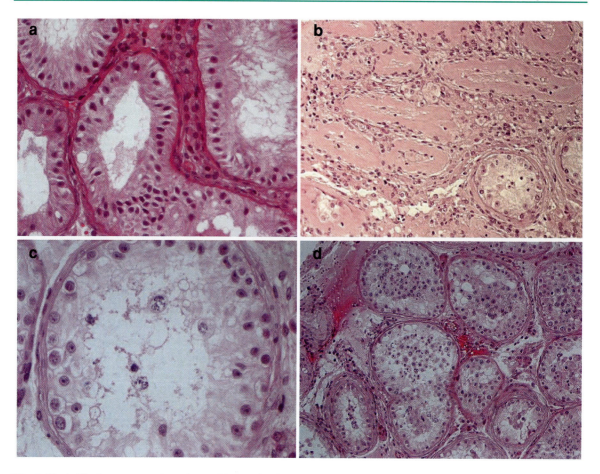

**Fig. 1** Testis histology patterns in patients with non-obstrictive azoospermia. **a** Complete Sertoli cell only syndrome (SCOS); **b** Incomplete SCOS with tubular hyalinization; **c** Maturation arrest; **d** Hypospermatogenesis

azoospermia (NOA); and post-testicular: obstructive azoospermia.

Testicular failure is responsible for non-obstructive azoospermia, it affects 10% of infertile men and is diagnosed in 49–93% of azoospermic patients (Jarow et al. 1989; Matsumiya et al. 1994; Jarvi et al. 2010). Pre-testicular azoospermia is very rare, accounting for about 2% of azoospermia cases and the diagnosis is quite simple.

The clinical diagnosis of NOA is a diagnosis of exclusion that is an obstruction must be ruled out as the cause of the absence of spermatozoa within the ejaculate. Apart from the unquestionable cases of deferential agenesis, clinical diagnosis is often based only on data from clinical history, clinical examination, and laboratory tests (e.g., history of cryptorchidism; chromosomal abnormalities such as Klinefelter syndrome, translocations and microdeletions; previous gonadotoxic therapies, small testicular size, high FSH, and presence of germ cells within the semen after centrifugation). Diagnosis remains mainly presumptive in some cases (Jarow et al. 1989; Palermo et al. 1999; Ezeh 2000; Raman and Schlegel 2003). Most often, the cause of NOA is not identifiable (Chan and Schlegel 2000).

Differential diagnosis is based only upon a testis histological examination, showing normal spermatogenesis in case of obstructive azoospermia and abnormal patterns in case of non-obstructive azoospermia; unfortunately this datum is available only following a testicular biopsy, therefore it is retrospective.

Retrieving sperm in a patient with NOA depends only on the presence of foci of preserved spermatogenesis within the testis. Testis histology may present one of the following four predominant patterns (Fig. 1):

- Complete Sertoli-cell only syndrome, when the tubules are only populated by Sertoli cells;

- Incomplete Sertoli cell only syndrome, when only few tubules contain germ cells, and the majority of them have only Sertoli cells;
- Maturation arrest, characterized by a halt of the maturation sequence of the spermatogenesis;
- Hypospermatogenesis, characterized by tubules with a severely reduced population of germ cells and a poor order of spermatogenesis.

After the introduction of intracytoplasmic sperm injection (ICSI) the chance to become genetic fathers has also been offered to patients with NOA owing to the possibility of retrieving sperm from their own dysfunctional testes (Palermo et al. 1999). Since a correspondence between etiological factors and histological pattern has not yet been demonstrated, a successful sperm retrieval with consequent pregnancy cannot be excluded in almost all patients (in fact, there are no chances of sperm recovery only in subjects with NOA having AZFa and AZFb microdeletions) (Hopps et al. 2003). These observations suggest that nearly all cases of male factor infertility can potentially be treated (Schlegel and Kaufman 2007).

A hypogonadotropic hypogonadism should be ruled out before proposing a surgical sperm retrieval; in fact, a substitution treatment with gonadotropins may restore spermatogenesis and thus sperm within the ejaculate (Meseguer et al. 2004).

Another clinical situation worth considering when dealing with NOA is a concomitant varicocele. Varicocele is estimated to be associated with azoospermia in 5–10% of cases and many studies seem to suggest varicocele surgery in these patients (Matthews et al. 1998; Kim et al. 1999). In such cases, testicular biopsies have shown isolated areas of preserved spermatogenesis (Jow et al. 1993).

After the first ones (Mehan 1976; Czaplicki et al. 1979), several authors have reported the appearance of spermatozoa in the ejaculate following the correction of varicocele. Recently, a meta-analysis demonstrated that after varicocele repair 39.1% patients had motile sperm in the ejaculate (Weedin et al. 2010). In this instance, in order to prevent a possible worsening, semen should be immediately cryopreserved (Pasqualotto et al. 2006). Moreover, ICSI performed using motile ejaculated sperm is more successful than ICSI with sperm obtained by surgical testicular sperm extraction (TESE) (Aboulghar et al. 1997). Also in patients with NOA and varicocele

where no motile sperm was achieved from the ejaculate, a significant difference was demonstrated as regards to positive sperm retrieval rate by microsurgical TESE (see Sect. 2.3 MicroTESE), as well as to pregnancy rate and to live birth rate, in varicocele-treated patients with NOA compared to those untreated (Haydardedeoglu et al. 2010).

## 2    Sperm Retrieval in NOA

Least invasive, least damaging, best recovery: this is the ideal technique. A technique that allows, with the least damage to the testicle, to recover the greater number of viable spermatozoa able to fertilize all the available oocytes and to freeze the remainder for new attempts in the future, in case of failure. None of the currently available techniques fulfill these criteria. Sperm retrieval from a patient with NOA for fresh use in intracytoplasmic sperm injection is obviously "the ideal one". When retrieved, sperm of patients with NOA used for fresh insemination has the same potential to achieve fertilization and pregnancy via intracytoplasmic sperm injection as sperm retrieved in patients with obstructive azoospermia (Kanto et al. 2008); however, we never know previously if there will be a positive retrieval, so that we are always compelled in practice to cryopreserve the gametes (the so called CryoTESE) (Verheyen et al. 2004; Ishikawa et al. 2009).

Three techniques are currently used for testicular sperm retrieval in subjects with NOA: testicular fine needle aspiration (TeFNA), TESE, and microsurgical dissection of testicular tissue or MicroTESE.

### 2.1    TeFNA

In cases of obstructive azoospermia, mostly when no recanalization surgery is planned, TeFNA is frequently the preferred option to finely retrieve sperm for intracytoplasmic sperm injection, even if often unsuitable for cryopreservation (Sereni et al. 2008). On the contrary, TeFNA results in NOA cases are far from being so good. Positive retrieval rates are very low, such as 21.1% (median) in a review (Colpi et al. 2005) and even lower (10%) in a more recent study (El-Haggar et al. 2008), and are mainly related to testicular histological patterns of hypospermatogenesis (Aridogan et al. 2003; Ezeh et al. 1998).

Furthermore, providing only samples suitable for cytology (Bergmann 2006), TeFNA is not recommended by the European Association of Urology (EAU) guidelines in NOA (Dohle et al. 2010): in fact, it does not allow to detect carcinomas in situ and testicular malignancies, whose prevalence in NOA population is significantly higher (Jacobsen et al. 2000; Mancini et al. 2007).

TeFNA is a simple technique, which can be performed under local anesthesia on an outpatient basis. Using a 20 ml plastic syringe for aspiration, a 21-G Butterfly™ needle is inserted directly into the testicular tissue (Fig. 2). After aspiration, the needle is removed and flushed with culture medium into a test-tube. Upon removal of the needle, to facilitate haemostatis, a moderate pressure should be maintained on the testis at the insertion point. The procedure may be repeated several times (Bourne et al. 1995). Although TeFNA is a blind technique, its complications are very rare, including intratesticular hematoma, hematocele, and puncture of the epididymis (which might compromise any attempt of subsequent microsurgical vasoepididymostomy).

In a rat experimental model Shufaro et al. (2002) reported severe, progressive, and irreversible damage on the architecture of the tubules in the needle's path following TeFNA, eventually leading to widespread tubular atrophy. In contrast, TESE causes localized scarring and fibrosis, leaving most of the remaining testicles intact.

## 2.2 TESE

TESE is the most commonly used surgical sperm retrieval method. Originally devised by Silber in 1995 for patients with obstructive azoospermia where microsurgical epididymal sperm aspiration (MESA) had resulted unsuccessful, it is now currently employed in patients with NOA as well. Usually, a single TESE is performed from each testis, but, in order to increase the success rate, some urologists perform multiple TESE procedures on the same side (Ezeh et al. 1998). Under local anesthesia, TESE is performed either with a complete testicular exposure or with a small scrotal opening, the so called "window" technique (Fig. 3). The scrotal wall is incised, the tunica vaginalis opened, a 5–10 mm incision is made in an avascular area of the tunica albuginea, and some

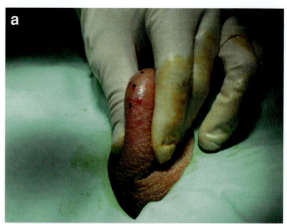
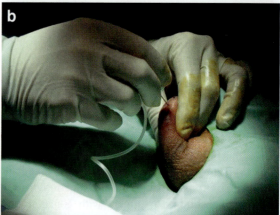
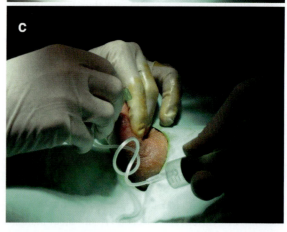

**Fig. 2** Testicular fine needle aspiration (TeFNA). **a** The points of needle insertion are marked. **b** A 21G butterfly needle is inserted into the testicular tissue. **c** Aspiration

of the emerging testicular parenchyma is removed and given for sperm search to the biologist.

A smaller chip (about 5 × 3 × 2 mm) is taken and sent to the pathologist for histological examination after fixation in Bouin's solution. Antisepsis with

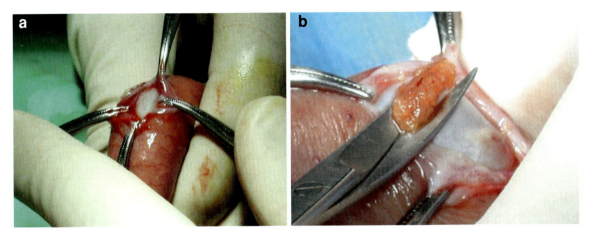

**Fig. 3** Testicular sperm extraction (TESE). **a** Window technique. A small scrotal wall incision is performed to expose the testis. **b** After having opened the tunica vaginalis, and incised the tunica albuginea a fragment of emerging testicular tissue is excised

Ringer solution containing gentamycin, careful haemostasis of the bleeding subalbugineal vessels (if any), and closure of the albuginea, the tunica vaginalis, the dartos, and the skin in close succession, bring the procedure to an end.

In our experience, eschewing any minimal gauze scraping to the tunica albuginea and injecting 1.5 mg of betamethasone solution inside the vaginal cavity will prevent adhesions, markedly reduce postoperative pain and ease any subsequent TESE repetition or microsurgical vasoepididymostomy.

Positive sperm retrieval rate in patients with NOA by TESE (49.5–52.7% according to a review by Colpi et al. (2005) is significantly more successful than by TeFNA (Hauser et al. 2006). For this reason, TESE is the recommended sperm retrieval technique for patients with NOA according to the EAU guidelines (Dohle et al. 2010). High recovery rates can also be assured with a second iterative TESE (Vernaeve et al. 2006). Multiple TESE has been reported to increase the overall success rate compared to single TESE (49 versus 37.5%), but the sperm retrieval rate was significantly different in all histopathological groups, except for Sertoli cell only syndrome, tubular sclerosis, and Klinefelter's pattern (Amer et al. 1999).

Rare surgical complications of TESE are local infection, scrotal hematoma, and subsequent testosterone deficiency in NOA patients with very small testes (Pantke et al. 2008). There is some concern indeed about the decline in testosterone after surgery. A large-scale comparative study showed that serum testosterone levels dropped to 80% of pre-operative levels in both the TESE and MicroTESE groups at 3–6 months after the procedure and that the levels rose back to 85% after 12 months and to 95% after 18 months (Ramasamy et al. 2005). A "de novo" androgen deficiency was seen in 16% of patients (Everaert et al. 2006). However, more recent studies have shown that testosterone level decline is significant only in Klinefelter patients (30–35% less than the baseline). (Takada et al. 2008; Ishikawa et al. 2009).

## 2.3  MicroTESE

"Sperm extraction by open biopsy (TESE) is much more efficient than fine needle aspiration (TEFNA), however it carries potential risks of injury to the testis and often removes unnecessarily large volumes of testicular parenchyma". Based on these simple considerations, in 1999 Peter Schlegel introduced a new concept in the field of male infertility treatment, the microsurgical dissection TESE or MicroTESE (Schlegel 1999).

The major advantages of MicroTESE are: (a) the identification, by the operative microscope, of individual clumps of tubules with better spermatogenesis (the seminiferous tubules can be carefully looked over at ×24 magnification in order to identify the larger, whitish, and opaque tubules—if any—in which spermatogenesis is active); (b) the excision of single tubules, so providing the biologist with less testicular tissue to dissect in order to find spermatozoa; (c) the best visualization of the subalbugineal terminal

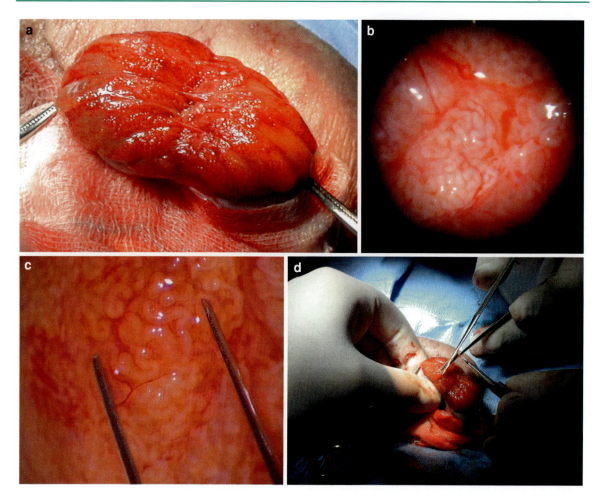

**Fig. 4** Microsurgical dissection of testicular tissue (MicroTESE). **a** Bivalve opening of the testis. **b** Tissue inspection under the microscope to search for areas with larger tubules. **c, d** Microretrievals of groups (**c**) or individual (**d**) seminiferous tubules

vessels, which allows their optimal preservation and minimal damage to the testis blood supply. Thus, it combines the advantages of an invasive limited approach with those of an open biopsy.

Usually performed under general or spinal anesthesia, MicroTESE requires a long equatorial incision of the tunica albuginea, approximately for three quarters of testicular circumference, preserving as much as possible the predominantly transversal subalbugineal vessels. Hemostasis of the few bleeding ones is done with a microsurgical bipolar thermal device. The testis is opened like a book by gently separating the lobular tissue of both sides with a spatula. A very small subalbugineal chip is removed, fixed in Bouin's solution and sent to the pathologist for histology. Then, the tissue is carefully inspected

under the microscope at ×10–24 magnification to search for areas with dilated tubules, from which numerous "microretrievals" of groups of or individual seminiferous tubules are performed (Fig. 4). Otherwise, in the case of homogeneous tubular size, a sort of testicular mapping must be performed, exciding at different depth levels from the albuginea to the hilum inside the parenchyma those tubules which are closest to the blood vessels (Colpi et al. 2005). About 30 testicular draws are usually obtained from each testis. Only afterward, in order to avoid damage to the recovered gametes, the testicular tissue surfaces are irrigated for antisepsis with Ringer solution plus 80 mg gentamycin/100 ml. Haemostasis on the parenchyma is then performed by gently pressing it for 2–3 min, by using a gauze wet with the same antibiotic solution and, if necessary, using the bipolar thermal device. Albugineal incision is repaired with continuous suture (Vicryl^TM 5-0), followed by closure of tunica vaginalis (into cavity of which infusion of betamethasone solution will prevent pain and adhesions), dartos, and skin.

Several not randomized studies have been published on the comparison between MicroTESE and TESE. Almost all of them show better positive sperm retrieval rates by MicroTESE than by TESE (even by multiple TESE), reporting rarer complications (Ramasamy et al. 2005; Schlegel 1999; Dardashti et al. 2000; Amer et al. 2000; Okada et al. 2002; Okubo et al. 2002; Tsujimura 2007; Donoso et al. 2007), even in cases of repeated procedures on the same testicle (Talas et al. 2007). A previous failure with TESE does not exclude a successful MicroTESE, but could even be an indication to do the latter (Ramasamy and Schlegel 2007).

The last Cochrane update about "Techniques for surgical retrieval of sperm prior to intracytoplasmic sperm injection for azoospermia" confirmed the conclusions of the previous one (Van Peperstraten et al. 2006), that "There is insufficient evidence to recommend any specific sperm retrieval technique for azoospermic men undergoing intracytoplasmic sperm injection" (Van Peperstraten et al. 2008). However, a meta-analysis of 25 articles identified from Cochrane Library and Medline from 1990 to 2008 assessed that "MicroTESE is the best sperm retrieval technique" (sperm retrieval rate: 54 versus 35.7% with TESE) (Yang et al. 2008). In 2009 the first RCT confirmed that MicroTESE is significantly more effective than TESE in retrieving sperm in patients with NOA (Colpi et al. 2009). In this study, MicroTESE achieved a higher sperm retrieval rate than TESE for every class of testicular volume, and when FSH was higher than normal (>N), but resulted significantly better when FSH $\geq$ 3N. Therefore, at least in these patients, MicroTESE should be the preferred choice. At this moment, another study of ours shows by a multivariate analysis that MicroTESE has a significantly higher retrieval rate than TESE in all cases where FSH > N and testicular volume is <7.1 ml (35.6 versus 22.3%) (Colpi and Castiglioni 2009).

Obviously, MicroTESE is more expensive than TESE, due to longer operative time, special sutures, and instruments. Morever it requires a learning curve, which correlates with the results (Ishikawa et al. 2010).

With MicroTESE the damage to testis blood supply is minimal (Dardashti et al. 2000), and in our experience ultrasonographic follow-up does not reveal any significant damage to testicular parenchyma or vascularization (Colpi et al. 2005).

## 2.4 Sperm Search in TESE or MicroTESE Samples

The microfragments of the testicular tissue are collected into a sterile Petri dish together with 0.5 ml of sperm washing medium^TM. The tissue must be reduced to fine particles using microscissors and then repeatedly passed through a 24G angiocatheter for 3–5′ to obtain a cloudy suspension. Some aliquots of this latter are carefully examined under the microscope to check for sperm and other germ cells. This search may take up to 4 h. In the case the count in the fluid is at least 100 sperm/mm$^3$, an eosin-nigrosin live/dead stain test may be carried out, too.

## 2.5 Predictors of Sperm Retrieval

It is crucial for the clinician to provide any azoospermic patient before surgery with comprehensive and realistic information about the probability of successful recovery.

Many parameters have been investigated as a predictor for sperm retrieval such as testicular volume and FSH (Hibi et al. 2005; Ziaee et al. 2006; Ravizzini et al. 2008; Turunc et al. 2010), vascularization according to Doppler-ultrasonography findings (Souza et al. 2005; Herwig et al. 2007), molecular markers in seminal plasma (Haraguchi et al. 2009), and in the testis (Bonaparte et al. 2010), seminal plasma inhibin B, and anti-Müllerian hormone (Duvilla et al. 2008; Toulis et al. 2010). Serum FSH and inhibin B are widely used, in the daily clinical practice, as predictors of normal spermatogenesis, but while both FSH and inhibin B are not rarely able to differentiate non-obstructive from obstructive azoospermia (Mitchell et al. 2010), none of them can be unquestionably accepted as a predictor for positive sperm recovery before TESE or MicroTESE procedures (Adamopoulos and Koukkou 2010). The higher is FSH, the lower is the probability of a positive sperm retrieval: however, we found sperm by TESE or MicroTESE even in few cases where FSH was higher than six times the maximum value of the normal range. The only reliable predictor is testis histopathology (Tournaye et al. 1996; Tournaye et al. 1997; Su et al. 1999; Silber 2000; Anniballo et al. 2000; Zheng et al. 2000; Seo and Ko 2001), unfortunately the only one unavailable before surgery.

Also TeFNA was proposed as a diagnostic tool prior to TESE in suspected NOA cases with testicular volume greater than 12 ml, obtaining a sperm recovery suitable to intracytoplasmic sperm injection in 45.9% of patients: however, hystology was not reported (Houwen et al. 2008). In a series of 50 NOA cases submitted by us to TESE where orchidometry was larger than 12 ml, sperm recovery was positive in 30 cases (60%); histology showed hypospermatogenesis in 18 (60%) of the 30 positive and in none of the 20 negative cases (Colpi and Castiglioni 2009). Therefore, it can be assumed that in patients with NOA presenting a histologic pattern of hypospermatogenesis, the probability of finding sperm by TESE is similar to that of patients with NOA.

Anyway, good clinical practice warns against performing a pre-TESE testicular biopsy only devoted to histology (Tsujimura 2007).

In conclusion, at the moment no reliable predictor of a successful sperm retrieval in NOA cases is available to the andrologist.

## 3    ICSI Results in Patients with NOA

The fathering prognosis is significantly worse for NOA compared to patients with obstructive azoospermia (Vernaeve et al. 2003). In fact, first of all, sperm can be recovered only in about 50% of non-obstructive versus virtually in 100% of subjects with obstructive azoospermia. In addition, when used for intracytoplasmic sperm injection, the fertilization rate of NOA sperm is 57 versus 80.5% of obstructive azoospermia sperm (Palermo et al. 1999) and the birth rate 19 versus 28% (Sousa et al. 2002), respectively. This means that since the beginning a couple with a NOA male has grossly about one-third of the fathering probability of a couple with obstructive azoospermia. Also miscarriage rate is higher for couples with NOA compared to those with obstructive azoospermia (11.5 versus 2.5%) (Borges et al. 2002). These results were confirmed by a meta-analysis (Nicopoullos et al. 2004). In addition,

referring to other relevant clinical data, like preterm deliveries and prenatal abnormal karyotypes, a negative rate trend related to NOA when compared to obstructive azoospermia was reported by Varnaeve et al. (2003). A systematic review by Woldringh et al. (2010) confirmed these data, suggesting the need for a comprehensive data collection from all the assisted reproductive technologies (ART) Centers regarding also the most precise information about the health status of ICSI-conceived children during their growth, their puberty, and their own reproductive age. Even in patients with NOA, intracytoplasmic sperm injection results significantly depend on the severity of spermatogenetic damage: the lower is the mean number of mature spermatids per tubular section at histological examination, the lower are the oocyte fertilization rate and the cleavage rate (Colpi et al. unpublished data on ICSI with TESE frozen/thawed sperm).

Controversial data are reported in the literature about intracytoplasmic sperm injection results from fresh compared to frozen/thawed sperm in patients with NOA (Sousa et al. 2002; Wald et al. 2006). Anyway, in the latest years a sort of consensus has grown about the better ICSI results achievable using fresh TESE sperm (Verheyen et al. 2004): Verheyen et al. (2004) and Konc et al. (2008) found different embryo-transfer rate; Hauser et al. (2005) found more favorable implantation rates.

On the other hand, when coping with a NOA male and the option of using donor's semen is refused by the couple or forbidden by the Country law, the ethical need to avoid an ovarian hormonal stimulation, which could result useless at all in the case of a contemporary unsuccessful testicular sperm retrieval, suggests to perform a preliminary TESE with a precautionary cryopreservation of the recovered spermatozoa: in this case, of necessity the following intracytoplasmic sperm injection will be carried out using frozen/thawed sperm.

How to meet so conflicting clinical needs remain today a problem to be solved.

## References

Aboulghar MA, Mansour RT, Serour GI et al (1997) Fertilization and pregnancy rates after intracytoplasmic sperm injection using ejaculate semen and surgically retrieved sperm. Fertil Steril 68:108–111

Adamopoulos DA, Koukkou EG (2010) 'Value of FSH and inhibin-B measurements in the diagnosis of azoospermia'—a clinician's overview. Int J Androl 33:e109–e113

Amer M, Haggar SE, Moustafa T et al (1999) Testicular sperm extraction: impact of testicular histology on outcome, number of biopsies to be performed and optimal time for repetition. Hum Reprod 14:3030–3034

Amer M, Ateyah A, Hany R et al (2000) Prospective comparative study between microsurgical and conventional testicular sperm extraction in non-obstructive azoospermia: follow-up by serial ultrasound examinations. Hum Reprod 15:653–656

Anniballo R, Ubaldi F, Cobellis L et al (2000) Criteria predicting the absence of spermatozoa in the Sertoli cell-only syndrome can be used to improve success rates of sperm retrieval. Hum Reprod 15:2269–2277

Aridogan IA, Bayazit Y, Yaman M et al (2003) Comparison of fine-needle aspiration and open biopsy of testis in sperm retrieval and histopathologic diagnosis. Andrologia 35:121–125

Bergmann M (2006) Evaluation of testicular biopsy samples from the clinical perspective. In: Schill WB, Comhaire FH, Hargreave TB (eds). Springer, Berlin, pp 454–461

Bonaparte E, Moretti M, Colpi GM et al (2010) ESX1 gene expression as a robust marker of residual spermatogenesis in azoospermic men. Hum Reprod 25:1398–1403

Borges E Jr, Rossi-Ferragut LM, Pasqualotto FF et al (2002) Testicular sperm results in elevated miscarriage rates compared to epididymal sperm in azoospermic patients. Sao Paulo Med J 120:122–126

Bourne H, Watkins W, Speirs A et al (1995) Pregnancies after intracytoplasmic injection of sperm collected by fine needle biopsy of the testis. Fertil Steril 64:433–436

Chan PT, Schlegel PN (2000) Nonobstructive azoospermia. Curr Opin Urol 10:617–624

Colpi GM, Castiglioni M (2009) Testicular microsurgery in NOA patients. NAFA Annual Meeting, Aarhus

Colpi GM, Piediferro G, Nerva F et al (2005) Sperm retrieval for intra-cytoplasmic sperm injection in non-obstructive azoospermia. Minerva Urol Nefrol 57:99–107

Colpi GM, Colpi EM, Piediferro G et al (2009) Microsurgical TESE versus conventional TESE for ICSI in non-obstructive azoospermia: a randomized controlled study. Reprod Biomed Online 18:315–319

Czaplicki M, Bablok L, Janczewski Z (1979) Varicocelectomy in patients with azoospermia. Arch Androl 3:51–55

Dardashti K, Williams RH, Goldstein M (2000) Microsurgical testis biopsy: a novel technique for retrieval of testicular tissue. J Urol 163:1206–1207

Dohle GR, Diemer T, Giwercman A et al (2010) Guidelines on male infertility. European Association of Urology Guidelines

Donoso P, Tournaye H, Devroey P (2007) Which is the best sperm retrieval technique for non-obstructive azoospermia? A systematic review. Hum Reprod Update 13:539–549

Duvilla E, Lejeune H, Trombert-Paviot B et al (2008) Significance of inhibin B and anti-Mullerian hormone in seminal plasma: a preliminary study. Fertil Steril 89:444–448

El-Haggar S, Mostafa T, Abdel Nasser T et al (2008) Fine needle aspiration vs. mTESE in non-obstructive azoospermia. Int J Androl 31:595–601

Everaert K, De Croo I, Kerckhaert W et al (2006) Long term effects of micro-surgical testicular sperm extraction on androgen status in patients with non obstructive azoospermia. BMC Urol 6:9

Ezeh UI (2000) Beyond the clinical classification of azoospermia: opinion. Hum Reprod 15:2356–2359

Ezeh UI, Moore HD, Cooke ID (1998) A prospective study of multiple needle biopsies versus a single open biopsy for testicular sperm extraction in men with non-obstructive azoospermia. Hum Reprod 13:3075–3080

Haraguchi T, Ishikawa T, Yamaguchi K et al (2009) Cyclin and protamine as prognostic molecular marker for testicular sperm extraction in patients with azoospermia. Fertil Steril 91:1424–1426

Hauser R, Yogev L, Amit A et al (2005) Severe hypospermatogenesis in cases of nonobstructive azoospermia: should we use fresh or frozen testicular spermatozoa? J Androl 26:772–778

Hauser R, Yogev L, Paz G et al (2006) Comparison of efficacy of two techniques for testicular sperm retrieval in nonobstructive azoospermia: multifocal testicular sperm extraction versus multifocal testicular sperm aspiration. J Androl 27:28–33

Haydardedeoglu B, Turunc T, Kilicdag EB et al (2010) The effect of prior varicocelectomy in patients with nonobstructive azoospermia on intracytoplasmic sperm injection outcomes: a retrospective pilot study. Urology 75:83–86

Herwig R, Tosun K, Schuster A et al (2007) Tissue perfusion-controlled guided biopsies are essential for the outcome of testicular sperm extraction. Fertil Steril 87:1071–1076

Hibi H, Ohori T, Yamada Y et al (2005) Probability of sperm recovery in non-obstructive azoospermic patients presenting with testes volume less than 10 ml/FSH level exceeding 20 mIU/ml. Arch Androl 51:225–231

Hopps CV, Mielnik A, Goldstein M et al (2003) Detection of sperm in men with Y chromosome microdeletions of the AZFa, AZFb and AZFc regions. Hum Reprod 18:1660–1665

Houwen J, Lundin K, Soderlund B et al (2008) Efficacy of percutaneous needle aspiration and open biopsy for sperm retrieval in men with non-obstructive azoospermia. Acta Obstet Gynecol Scand 87:1033–1038

Ishikawa T, Shiotani M, Izumi Y et al (2009a) Fertilization and pregnancy using cryopreserved testicular sperm for intracytoplasmic sperm injection with azoospermia. Fertil Steril 92:174–179

Ishikawa T, Yamaguchi K, Chiba K et al (2009b) Serum hormones in patients with nonobstructive azoospermia after microdissection testicular sperm extraction. J Urol 182:1495–1499

Ishikawa T, Nose R, Yamaguchi K et al (2010) Learning curves of microdissection testicular sperm extraction for nonobstructive azoospermia. Fertil Steril 94:1008–1011

Jacobsen R, Bostofte E, Engholm G et al (2000) Risk of testicular cancer in men with abnormal semen characteristics: cohort study. BMJ 321:789–792

Jarow JP, Espeland MA, Lipshultz LI (1989) Evaluation of the azoospermic patient. J Urol 142:62–65

Jarvi K, Lo K, Fischer A et al (2010) CUA guideline: the workup of azoospermic males. Can Urol Assoc J 4:163–167

Jow WW, Steckel J, Schlegel PN et al (1993) Motile sperm in human testis biopsy specimens. J Androl 14:194–198

Kanto S, Sugawara J, Masuda H, et al (2008) Fresh motile testicular sperm retrieved from nonobstructive azoospermic patients has the same potential to achieve fertilization and pregnancy via ICSI as sperm retrieved from obstructive azoospermic patients. Fertil Steril 90(2010):e2015–2017

Kim ED, Leibman BB, Grinblat DM et al (1999) Varicocele repair improves semen parameters in azoospermic men with spermatogenic failure. J Urol 162:737–740

Konc J, Kanyo K, Cseh S (2008) The effect of condition/state of testicular spermatozoa injected to the outcome of TESE-ICSI-ET cycles. Eur J Obstet Gynecol Reprod Biol 141:39–43

Mancini M, Carmignani L, Gazzano G et al (2007) High prevalence of testicular cancer in azoospermic men without spermatogenesis. Hum Reprod 22:1042–1046

Matsumiya K, Namiki M, Takahara S et al (1994) Clinical study of azoospermia. Int J Androl 17:140–142

Matthews GJ, Matthews ED, Goldstein M (1998) Induction of spermatogenesis and achievement of pregnancy after microsurgical varicocelectomy in men with azoospermia and severe oligoasthenospermia. Fertil Steril 70:71–75

Mehan DJ (1976) Results of ligation of internal spermatic vein in the treatment of infertility in azoospermic patients. Fertil Steril 27:110–114

Meseguer M, Garrido N, Remohi J et al (2004) Testicular sperm extraction (TESE) and intracytoplasmic sperm injection (ICSI) in hypogonadotropic hypogonadism with persistent azoospermia after hormonal therapy. J Assist Reprod Genet 21:91–94

Mitchell V, Robin G, Boitrelle F et al (2010) Correlation between testicular sperm extraction outcomes and clinical, endocrine and testicular histology parameters in 120 azoospermic men with normal serum FSH levels. Int J Androl

Nicopoullos JD, Gilling-Smith C, Almeida PA et al (2004) Use of surgical sperm retrieval in azoospermic men: a meta-analysis. Fertil Steril 82:691–701

Okada H, Dobashi M, Yamazaki T et al (2002) Conventional versus microdissection testicular sperm extraction for nonobstructive azoospermia. J Urol 168:1063–1067

Okubo K, Ogura K, Ichioka K et al (2002) Testicular sperm extraction for non-obstructive azoospermia: results with conventional and microsurgical techniques. Hinyokika Kiyo 48:275–280

Palermo GD, Schlegel PN, Hariprashad JJ et al (1999) Fertilization and pregnancy outcome with intracytoplasmic sperm injection for azoospermic men. Hum Reprod 14:741–748

Pantke P, Diemer T, Marconi M et al (2008) Testicular sperm retrieval in azoospermic men. Eur Urol S7:703–714

Pasqualotto FF, Sobreiro BP, Hallak J et al (2006) Induction of spermatogenesis in azoospermic men after varicocelectomy repair: an update. Fertil Steril 85:635–639

Raman JD, Schlegel PN (2003) Testicular sperm extraction with intracytoplasmic sperm injection is successful for the treatment of nonobstructive azoospermia associated with cryptorchidism. J Urol 170:1287–1290

Ramasamy R, Schlegel PN (2007) Microdissection testicular sperm extraction: effect of prior biopsy on success of sperm retrieval. J Urol 177:1447–1449

Ramasamy R, Yagan N, Schlegel PN (2005) Structural and functional changes to the testis after conventional versus microdissection testicular sperm extraction. Urology 65:1190–1194

Ravizzini P, Carizza C, Abdelmassih V et al (2008) Microdissection testicular sperm extraction and IVF-ICSI outcome in nonobstructive azoospermia. Andrologia 40:219–226

Schlegel PN (1999) Testicular sperm extraction: microdissection improves sperm yield with minimal tissue excision. Hum Reprod 14:131–135

Schlegel PN, Kaufman J (2007) Surgical treatment of male infertility. In: Kandeel FR (ed) Male reproductive dysfunction: pathophysiology and treatment. Marcel-Dekker, New York, pp 365–384

Seo JT, Ko WJ (2001) Predictive factors of successful testicular sperm recovery in non-obstructive azoospermia patients. Int J Androl 24:306–310

Sereni E, Bonu MA, Fava L et al (2008) Freezing spermatozoa obtained by testicular fine needle aspiration: a new technique. Reprod Biomed Online 16:89–95

Shufaro Y, Prus D, Laufer N et al (2002) Impact of repeated testicular fine needle aspirations (TEFNA) and testicular sperm extraction (TESE) on the microscopic morphology of the testis: an animal model. Hum Reprod 17:1795–1799

Silber SJ (2000) Microsurgical TESE and the distribution of spermatogenesis in non-obstructive azoospermia. Hum Reprod 15:2278–2284

Sousa M, Cremades N, Silva J et al (2002) Predictive value of testicular histology in secretory azoospermic subgroups and clinical outcome after microinjection of fresh and frozen-thawed sperm and spermatids. Hum Reprod 17:1800–1810

Souza CA, Cunha-Filho JS, Fagundes P et al (2005) Sperm recovery prediction in azoospermic patients using Doppler ultrasonography. Int Urol Nephrol 37:535–540

Su LM, Palermo GD, Goldstein M et al (1999) Testicular sperm extraction with intracytoplasmic sperm injection for non-obstructive azoospermia: testicular histology can predict success of sperm retrieval. J Urol 161:112–116

Takada S, Tsujimura A, Ueda T et al (2008) Androgen decline in patients with nonobstructive azoospemia after microdissection testicular sperm extraction. Urology 72:114–118

Talas H, Yaman O, Aydos K (2007) Outcome of repeated micro-surgical testicular sperm extraction in patients with non-obstructive azoospermia. Asian J Androl 9:668–673

Toulis KA, Iliadou PK, Venetis CA et al (2010) Inhibin B and anti-Mullerian hormone as markers of persistent spermatogenesis in men with non-obstructive azoospermia: a meta-analysis of diagnostic accuracy studies. Hum Reprod Update 16:713–724

Tournaye H, Liu J, Nagy PZ et al (1996) Correlation between testicular histology and outcome after intracytoplasmic sperm injection using testicular spermatozoa. Hum Reprod 11:127–132

Tournaye H, Verheyen G, Nagy P et al (1997) Are there any predictive factors for successful testicular sperm recovery in azoospermic patients? Hum Reprod 12:80–86

Tsujimura A (2007) Microdissection testicular sperm extraction: prediction, outcome, and complications. Int J Urol 14:883–889

Turunc T, Gul U, Haydardedeoglu B et al (2010) Conventional testicular sperm extraction combined with the microdissection technique in nonobstructive azoospermic patients: a prospective comparative study. Fertil Steril 94:2157–2160

Van Peperstraten A, Proctor ML, Johnson NP et al (2006) Techniques for surgical retrieval of sperm prior to ICSI for azoospermia. Cochrane Database Syst Rev 3:CD002807

Van Peperstraten A, Proctor ML, Johnson NP et al (2008) Techniques for surgical retrieval of sperm prior to intracytoplasmic sperm injection (ICSI) for azoospermia. Cochrane Database Syst Rev: CD002807

Verheyen G, Vernaeve V, Van Landuyt L et al (2004) Should diagnostic testicular sperm retrieval followed by cryopreservation for later ICSI be the procedure of choice for all patients with non-obstructive azoospermia? Hum Reprod 19:2822–2830

Vernaeve V, Tournaye H, Osmanagaoglu K et al (2003a) Intracytoplasmic sperm injection with testicular spermatozoa is less successful in men with nonobstructive azoospermia than in men with obstructive azoospermia. Fertil Steril 79:529–533

Vernaeve V, Bonduelle M, Tournaye H et al (2003b) Pregnancy outcome and neonatal data of children born after ICSI using testicular sperm in obstructive and non-obstructive azoospermia. Hum Reprod 18:2093–2097

Vernaeve V, Verheyen G, Goossens A et al (2006) How successful is repeat testicular sperm extraction in patients with azoospermia? Hum Reprod 21:1551–1554

Wald M, Ross LS, Prins GS et al (2006) Analysis of outcomes of cryopreserved surgically retrieved sperm for IVF/ICSI. J Androl 27:60–65

Weedin JW, Khera M, Lipshultz LI (2010) Varicocele repair in patients with nonobstructive azoospermia: a meta-analysis. J Urol 183:2309–2315

Woldringh GH, Besselink DE, Tillema AH et al (2010) Karyotyping, congenital anomalies and follow-up of children after intracytoplasmic sperm injection with non-ejaculated sperm: a systematic review. Hum Reprod Update 16:12–19

Yang J, Liu JH, Zou XF et al (2008) Sperm retrieval and the predictive parameter of non-obstructive azoospermia: a meta-analysis of literatures 1990 to 2008. Zhonghua Yi Xue Za Zhi 88:2131–2135

Zheng J, Huang X, Li C (2000) Predictive factors for successful sperm recovery in azoospermia patients. Zhonghua Wai Ke Za Zhi 38:366–368

Ziaee SA, Ezzatnegad M, Nowroozi M et al (2006) Prediction of successful sperm retrieval in patients with nonobstructive azoospermia. Urol J 3:92–96

# Imaging the Infertile Male-1: Varicocele

Giovanni Liguori, Stefano Bucci, Carlo Trombetta,
Boris Brkljačić, and Michele Bertolotto

## Contents

G. Liguori · S. Bucci · C. Trombetta
Department Urology, University of Trieste,
Ospedale di Cattinara, Strada di Fiume 447,
34124 Trieste, Italy

B. Brkljačić
Department of Diagnostic and Interventional Radiology,
Dubrava University Hospital, Avenija Gojka Šuška 6,
HR-10000 Zagreb, Croatia

M. Bertolotto (✉)
Department of Radiology, University of Trieste,
Ospedale di Cattinara, Strada di Fiume 447,
34124 Trieste, Italy
e-mail: bertolot@units.it

**Abstract**

Color Doppler ultrasound is the imaging modality of choice to evaluate patients with varicocele. In order to assess correctly the extension of the disease and the characteristics of flow, the patient should be examined supine and while standing, at rest and during Valsalva's maneuver. Several classifications can be used to grade varicocele based on position of the dilated vessels and characteristics of flow. Besides color Doppler ultrasound, spectral analysis is important to assess reflux duration. Experimental studies showed that varicocele causes flow changes in the testicular flows, but investigation in men requires validation. While extratesticular varicocele is relatively common, intratesticular varicocele is rare. Abdominal masses may not cause compressible secondary varicocele. CT and MR imaging are usually not indicated for evaluation of varicocele, but this condition may be recognized in case of examinations performed for other purposes. Scintigraphy and thermography have no current clinical role, while venography is usually performed as a part of percutaneous sclerotherapy.

## 1 Introduction

Varicocele is defined as an abnormal venous dilatation of the pampiniformis plexus. It is actually considered the most common correctable cause of male infertility, even though the mechanisms responsible for infertility are still unclear. It affects approximately 15% of the general population (Meacham et al. 1994)

M. Bertolotto and C. Trombetta (eds.), *Scrotal Pathology,* Medical Radiology. Diagnostic Imaging,
DOI: 10.1007/174_2011_191, © Springer-Verlag Berlin Heidelberg 2012

and up to 40% of men with infertility (Carlsen et al. 2000; Naughton et al. 2001; Shafik et al. 1990). About 80% of affected patients, however, have normal semen parameters.

Varicocele is assessed and graded clinically using the criteria introduced by Dubin and Amelar (1970), but this evaluation is highly subjective and strongly depends on the expertise of the physician (Beddy et al. 2005), since dartos hyperactivity and contraction of the cremaster muscle induced by palpation or Valsalva's maneuver may mimic or mask testicular venous distension (Liguori et al. 2004). The subjectivity of the clinical grading for varicocele is confirmed by Hargreave and Liakatas (1991), who found disagreement in 26% of patients examined by two experienced clinicians, and by a multicenter study on 141 sub-fertile men sponsored by the World Health Organization (1985), which showed that compared with venography clinical assessment of varicocele was approximately 50% sensitive, with a false positive rate of 23%. Using color Doppler ultrasound, Niedzielski et al. (1997) found reflux in only 39% of patients in whom varicocele was suspected on clinical evaluation.

Since clinical diagnosis and grading of varicocele are limited, several imaging methods have been introduced to evaluate this disease, including gray-scale and color Doppler ultrasound, thermography, venography, scintigraphy, CT, and MR imaging. Color Doppler ultrasound is currently the imaging modality of choice. Other methods are necessary in selected cases only.

## 2  Gray-Scale Ultrasound

The ultrasound appearance of varicocele consists of multiple, hypoechoic, serpiginous, tubular structures of varying size larger than 2–3 mm in diameter that are usually best visualized superior and/or lateral to the testis. When large, a varicocele can extend posteriorly and inferiorly to the testis (Beddy et al. 2005; Dogra et al. 2003). The size of dilated veins usually increases in the upright position and with a Valsalva's maneuver. Low-level internal echoes are often detected in the dilated veins (Fig. 1), consistent with slow flow (Dogra et al. 2003; Pearl and Hill 2007). Echoes are mobile during respiratory movements, during manual compression, and with a Valsalva's maneuver.

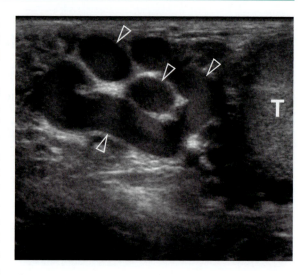

**Fig. 1** Gray-scale appearance of varicocele. Multiple, hypoechoic serpiginous dilated veins (*arrowheads*) larger than 2–3 mm are visible superior to the testis (*T*). Veins contain low-level internal echoes

Different threshold values of venous size are used for the diagnosis of varicocele. Most authors consider a cut-off value of 3 mm, but Gonda et al. (1987) reported a 95% sensitivity with a cut-off of 2 mm. Therefore, a diagnosis based only on the diameter of the vessels is characterized by a high number of false positives and negatives. Moreover, variability makes it difficult to compare the results of diagnostic modalities and treatments.

Besides evaluation of varices, gray-scale ultrasound allows assessment of the testis as well. Accurate and objective measurement of testicular volume can be obtained more accurately than with physical examination or using an orchidometer.

A strong association between clinical varicoceles and testicular damage was found, as reflected by testicular size (Jarow 2001; Sakamoto et al. 2008; Marks et al. 1986). According to Sigman and Jarow (1997), testicular hypotrophy is associated with a significantly decreased total motile sperm count and higher-grade varicoceles. Zini et al. (1997) showed that left sub-clinical varicocele may also be associated with decreased left testicular volume. Finally, Marks et al. (1986) showed that in patients with varicocele a lack of testicular hypotrophy results in a higher postoperative pregnancy rate.

Other studies, however, did not find a close relationship between testicular volume and subclinical varicocele (Sakamoto et al. 2008), nor a correlation

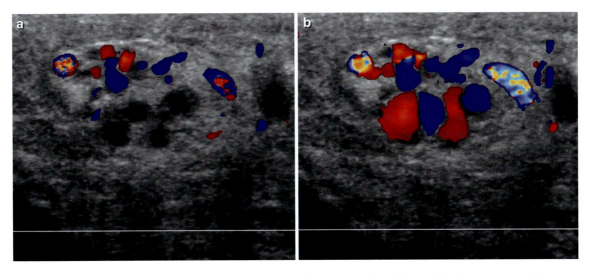

**Fig. 2** Sarteschi's Grade I varicocele. Color doppler images obtained at rest (**a**) and during Valsalva's maneuver (**b**) showing dilated veins of the spermatic cord with reflux during Valsalva at the inguinal channel

between testicular hypotrophy and clinical grading (Alukal et al. 2005).

## 3 Color Doppler Ultrasound

At present, color Doppler ultrasound is the imaging modality of choice for detection and grading varicocele (Callea et al. 1997; Aydos et al. 1993; Chiou et al. 1997; Eskew et al. 1993; Lund and Nielsen 1994; Sarteschi et al. 1993; Tasci et al. 2001; Winkelbauer et al. 1994); it is more sensitive than clinical examination, and can detect up to 93% of the reflux subsequently confirmed by spermatic venography (Petros et al. 1991).

In order to obtain a suitable evaluation of flow changes in the spermatic veins, ultrasound should be performed in the supine and then the upright positions, with and without a Valsalva's maneuver.

Diagnosis is reached in case of prolonged venous flow augmentation or reflux. This must be differentiated from the mild and transient flow augmentation that can be seen with a Valsalva's maneuver in normal men, lasting less than 1 s. According to Sarteschi and to the majority of investigators, we believe that in order to make a correct diagnosis of varicocele it is necessary to detect a prolonged reflux that must be longer than 2 s. Other authors, however, use a threshold value of 1 s to distinguish between physiological reflux and varicocele (Sakamoto et al. 2008).

Several classifications have been used for grading varicocele. We use the score system introduced by Sarteschi et al. (1993) which divides varicocele into five grades according to the characteristics of the reflux, to its length, and to changes during Valsalva's maneuver.

According to Sarteschi, Grade 1 varicocele is characterized by the detection of a prolonged reflux in vessels in the inguinal channel only during Valsalva's maneuver, while scrotal varicosity is not evident in the previous gray-scale study (Fig. 2). Grade 2 is characterized by a small varicosity that reaches the superior pole of the testis and whose diameter increases during Valsalva's maneuver. Color Doppler interrogation clearly demonstrates the presence of a venous reflux in the supratesticular region only during Valsalva (Fig. 3). Grade 3 is characterized by vessels that appear enlarged to the inferior pole of the testis when the patient is evaluated in a standing position. Color Doppler ultrasound demonstrates a clear reflux only during Valsalva's maneuver (Fig. 4). Grade 4 is diagnosed if vessels appear enlarged, even if the patient is studied in a supine position; dilatation increases in an upright position and during Valsalva's maneuver (Fig. 5). Enhancement of the venous reflux during Valsalva's maneuver is the criterion that allows the distinction between this grade from the previous and the next one. Hypotrophy of the testis is common at this stage. Grade 5 is characterized by an evident venous ectasia even in the supine position. Color Doppler

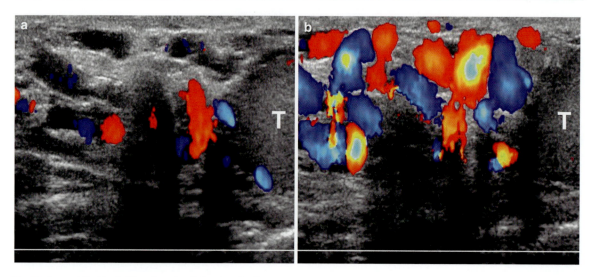

**Fig. 3** Sarteschi's Grade II varicocele. Color doppler images obtained at rest (**a**) and during Valsalva's maneuver (**b**) showing dilated veins in the supratesticular region with reflux during Valsalva ($T$ = testis)

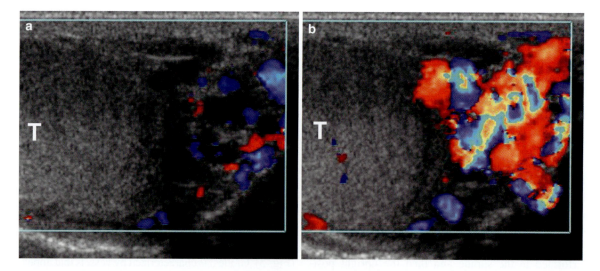

**Fig. 4** Sarteschi's Grade III varicocele. Color doppler images obtained at rest (**a**) and during Valsalva's maneuver (**b**) showing dilated veins to the inferior pole of the testis ($T$) with reflux during Valsalva

interrogation demonstrates basal venous reflux that does not change substantially while standing and during Valsalva's maneuver.

Sarteschi's classification for varicocele is the most commonly used system in Europe. Other authors, however, suggested different score systems. Hoekstra and Witt (1995) and Hirsh et al. (1980), for instance, suggested two similar classifications, which score varicocele in 4 and 3 degrees, respectively (Tables 1, 2). Oyen (2002) scores 3 degrees for varicocele mainly

based on the length of reflux at pulsed Doppler interrogation (Table 3).

## 4 Spectral Doppler Analysis

Precise duration of the reflux can be only measured at pulsed Doppler interrogation (Liguori et al. 2004; Cornud et al. 1999). Brief reflux lasting less than a second is physiological. Permanent reflux is not

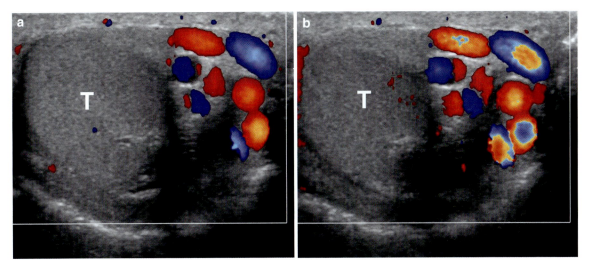

**Fig. 5** Sarteschi's Grade IV varicocele. Color Doppler images obtained in supine position at rest (**a**) and while standing during Valsalva's maneuver (**b**). Dilated veins with reflux are visible also at rest. Reflux increases while standing during Valsalva (*T* = testis)

**Table 1** Hoekstra's classification for varicocele at color doppler ultrasound

| | |
|---|---|
| Grade 0 | No dilated vein |
| Grade 1 | Dilated veins <2.5 mm in diameter without flow reversal after Valsalva maneuver |
| Grade 2 | Dilated and tortuous veins 2.5–3.5 mm in diameter and flow reversal after Valsalva maneuver |
| Grade 3 | Dilated and tortuous veins >3.5 mm in diameter and flow reversal after Valsalva maneuver |

**Table 2** Hirsh's classification for varicocele at color doppler ultrasound

| | |
|---|---|
| Grade 1 | No spontaneous venous reflux, but inducible reflux with Valsalva maneuver |
| Grade 2 | Intermittent spontaneous venous reflux |
| Grade 3 | Continuous spontaneous venous reflux |

**Table 3** Oyen's classification for varicocele at color doppler and PW-doppler ultrasound

| | |
|---|---|
| Grade 1 | Slight reflux (<2 s) during Valsalva |
| Grade 2 | Reflux (>2 s) during Valsalva, but no continuous reflux during the Valsalva maneuver |
| Grade 3 | Reflux in rest during normal respiration or continuously during the entire Valsalva maneuver |

palpable in only 20% of cases, lasts more than 2 s, and has a plateau aspect throughout the abdominal strain (Fig. 6). It does not correlate with the diameter of the spermatic vein (Cornud et al. 1999). Intermediate reflux is never palpable and lasts 1–2 s in most cases. It keeps decreasing during the Valsalva maneuver, and stops before the end of the maneuver. It has been suggested that, in the absence of palpable varicocele, only permanent reflux should be termed subclinical varicoceles, because the Doppler features and changes after treatment are identical to those of palpable varicocele (Cornud et al. 1999).

## 5    Patient Reporting

A correct ultrasound evaluation of patients with varicocele must integrate findings at gray-scale, color Doppler and pulsed Doppler analysis. Since classification may change in the different medical centers, a

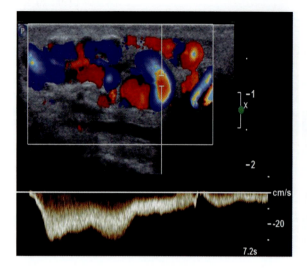

**Fig. 6** Spectral Doppler analysis in varicocele showing a reflux during Valsalva lasting approximately 5 s

detailed description of ultrasound and Doppler features is necessary to warrant the correct evaluation of patients in every case. Regardless of the classification used, a series of gray-scale, color Doppler and spectral Doppler parameters should be enclosed in the medical report:

1. Size and position of the varices at gray-scale ultrasound while supine; size changes while standing and during Valsalva's maneuver;
2. Presence of flow at color Dppler interrogation while supine and during spontaneous breathing at the level of the inguinal channel, in the suprastesticular region, and around the testis; flow changes in the same positions while standing and during Valsalva's maneuver;
3. Length and waveform characteristics of reflux at duplex Doppler interrogation while the patient is supine, while standing, and during Valsalva's maneuver;
4. Size and echotexture of both testes;
5. Incidental findings.

## 6    Bilateral Varicocele

Based on several methods of examination, including venography, Gat et al. (2004) showed that prevalence of bilateral varicocele is probably much higher than originally thought. In fact, many communicating vessels exist between the left and right testicular

venous systems, either in the abdomen, in the pelvis, or in the scrotum. After the detection of left varicocele, it is therefore, necessary to study the contralateral side in order to detect any coexistence of contralateral venous ectasia and blood reflux.

In case of bilateral scrotal venous ectasia, it is mandatory to distinguish, by the use of color Doppler interrogation of the right inguinal channel, between the so-called "false" and "real" bilateral varicocele, because these two situations require two different types of treatment (Liguori et al. 2004; Sarteschi et al. 2003). False bilateral varicocele is characterized by absence of reflux in the right inguinal channel. Scrotal venous ectasia is fed by the contralateral varicosity through communicant transsectal vessels. In case of false bilateral varicocele correction on the left side usually leads to the regression of the right ectasia as well. Bilateral treatment is not recommended. Conversely, in real bilateral varicocele venous ectasia is due to right gonadic vein reflux which is identified using color Doppler ultrasound. In these cases bilateral treatment must be performed. The limitation of this approach is that multiple communications between the right and the left testicular veins exist also in the abdomen and pelvis, which may be responsible for a "false" bilateral varicocele which cannot be diagnosed using color Doppler ultrasound.

## 7    Outcome After Varicocele Correction

There is increasing evidence that preoperative color Doppler ultrasound may be a useful tool for predicting the outcome of varicocele correction (Shiraishi et al. 2003; Hussein 2006; Liguori et al. 2010). Liguori et al. (2010) evaluated 113 patients with left unilateral varicocele before and after correction using retrograde or anterograde sclerotization. During a postoperative control performed at least 3 months after the procedure seminal quality improved among the entire population, regardless of patient age, and a better improvement in sperm density was found in patients with varicocele of Grades 3–5, following the Sarteschi's classification, compared to patients with varicocele of Grades 1–2. They concluded that evidence of venous basal renospermatic reflow at preoperative color Doppler ultrasound is the main predictive factor of a better seminal response to varicocele correction.

## 8      Intratesticular Varicocele

Varicocele may rarely be intratesticular as well, within the mediastinum testis or in a subcapsular location. Less than 100 cases have been reported till now (Atasoy and Fitoz 2001; Weiss et al. 1992; Ozcan et al. 1997; Das et al. 1999; Abduljaleel et al. 2006; Mehta and Dogra 1998; DemIrbas et al. 2001; Tetreau et al. 2007; Morvay and Nagy 1998; Diamond et al. 2004; Bucci et al. 2008; Conti et al. 2005). Some authors report a prevalent dilatation of the mediastinal veins (Das et al. 1999; Tetreau et al. 2007), while others do not (Atasoy and Fitoz 2001). Intratesticular varicocele is bilateral in approximately 25% of published cases (Tetreau et al. 2007). It is usually idiopathic, but can be also secondary to conditions producing renal vein obstruction, such as tumors, or renal vein thrombosis (Abduljaleel et al. 2006). Association with cryptorchidism and previous orcheopexy has been reported (Tetreau et al. 2007; O'Donnell and Dewbury 1998; Erdogan et al. 2003).

With the exception of Das et al. (1999) the different series report a high prevalence of left sided intratesticular and associated extratesticular varicocele, usually of high degree, and of testicular hypotrophy.

Incidence of intratesticular varicocele varies in the different studies between 0.4 and 2% of patients with proved clinically suspected extratesticular varicocele (Das et al. 1999; Tetreau et al. 2007; Morvay and Nagy 1998; Diamond et al. 2004; Bucci et al. 2008; Conti et al. 2005). Preoperative recognition is important because spermatic cord compression during sclerotheraphy is recommended in order to prevent gonadal damage (DemIrbas et al. 2001; Bucci et al. 2008).

The appearance of intratesticular varicocele at grayscale and color Doppler interrogation is similar to that already described for the extratesticular form (Fig. 7). Many authors report that intratesticular veins of 2 mm or greater in diameter show increased flow velocities during Valsalva maneuver. Others, however, consider any intratesticular venous structure showing reflux during the Valsalva maneuver, regardless of the diameter. In fact, obviously dilated intratesticular veins that show conspicuous reflux may be identified whose if the diameter is smaller than 2 mm.

Differential diagnosis between intratesticular varicocele and other hypo/anechoic lesions in the testes, such as cysts, tubular ectasia of rete testis, hematoma,

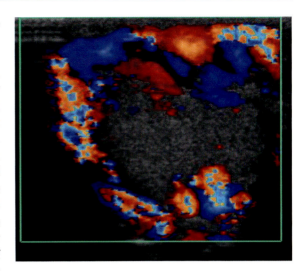

**Fig. 7** Intratesticular varicocele. Dilated veins are appreciable within the testis showing flows at rest in the supine position (*not show*n) that increase during Valsalva

focal infection, and cystic intratesticular neoplasm is straightforward, since these lesions do not show flow at color Doppler interrogation. Differentiation with other intratesticular vascular pathologies is possible. Arterial pseudoaneurysms are usually post-traumatic and display a characteristic yin-and-yang flow pattern, distinct from the venous flow of a varicocele (Dee et al. 2000) while intratesticular arteriovenous malformation or hemangiomas characteristically show high-velocity arterial waveforms (Yilmaz and Arslan 2009; Bhatt et al. 2006).

## 9      Secondary Varicocele

Increased pressure on the spermatic vein caused by various disease processes such as hydronephrosis, cirrhosis, or an abdominal mass may cause secondary varicocele. Flow characteristics are different from most idiopathic forms, because secondary varicocele is constantly evident while supine, and presents basal reflux that does not change substantially during Valsalva's maneuver (Sarteschi's Grade 5). Neoplasm is the most likely cause of Grade 5 varicocele in men over 40 years of age (Dogra et al. 2003; Graif et al. 2000). Detection of a newly developing Grade 5 varicocele on either the right or left side in older men should, therefore, prompt the investigation for a mass (Fig. 8).

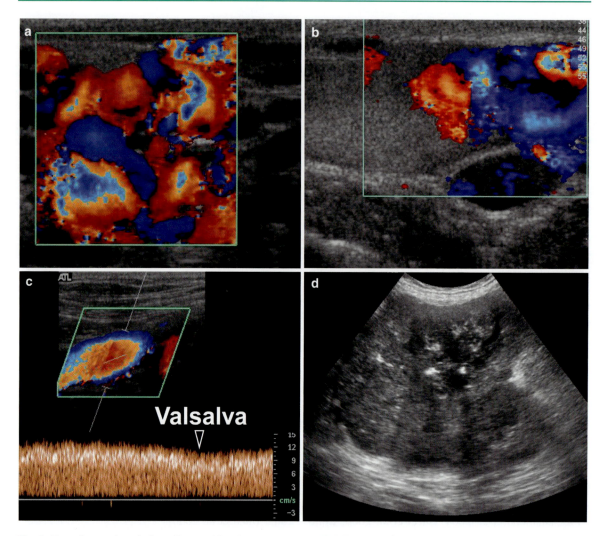

**Fig. 8** Secondary varicocele in a 63 year-old patient presenting with a left scrotal lump. **a** Color Doppler ultrasound of the left spermatic cord shows markedly dilated pampiniform plexus with basal reflux. **b** Color Doppler interrogation of the left hemiscrotum shows associated extratesticular and intratesticular varicocele. **c** Doppler interrogation of the left spermatic vein obtained in an upright position shows basal reflux that does not change during Valsalva maneuver. **d** Ultrasound interrogation of the left kidney shows a large renal tumor

## 10 Evaluation of Testicular Flows

Experimental studies in rats with induced varicocele show that this condition causes chronic precapillary vasoconstriction and decreased nutrient blood flow to the testes resulting in reduced ATP concentration, defective energy metabolism at the mitochondrial level, and eventually impaired spermatogenesis (Harrison et al. 1983, 1986; Sweeney et al. 1991; Hsu et al. 1994). Evaluation of testicular blood flow may, therefore, have a role also in assessment of infertile men with varicocele.

Several investigations used color Doppler ultrasound and spectral analysis to evaluate vascular changes in testes of patients with varicocele. Ross et al. (1994) failed to find significant alteration in testicular blood flow. Biagiotti et al. (2002) evaluated azoospermic/oligo-asthenospermic patients. They found that patients with varicocele, either fertile or not, had the highest peak systolic velocity and RI values. Tarhan et al. (2003) found that the mean flow velocity and arterial blood flow in the testicular artery, calculated multiplying the mean arterial velocity by the cross-sectional area of the artery, were significantly lower in the patients with varicocele, compared with a control group of 44 fertile normal volunteers. They found no statistically significant differences between PSV, EDV, RI and PI of the varicocele and of the control group. In the patient group, however, also the median testicular volume was significantly lower than in the control group. Further investigation is, therefore, necessary to understand whether these changes are due to varicocele, or rather due to testicular hypotrophy. Ünsal et al. (2007) evaluated 15 patients with clinical left-sided varicocele and 34 control patients without varicocele or with subclinical varicocele. In the left testicle of patients with clinical varicocele they found statistically significant increase in RI and PI, suggesting that these parameters may be an indicator of altered testicular microcirculation.

Testicular blood flow measurements have been obtained before and after treatment of varicocele, to evaluate whether different procedures might have effect on testicular vasculature. Tanriverdi et al. (2006) evaluated 56 patients clinically diagnosed with varicocele. The patients were randomized in two groups of 28 patients who underwent high-ligation surgery and microsurgery, respectively. No differences were found between preoperative and postoperative RI, PSV, and EDV of the two groups, suggesting that no significant impairment in testicular circulation results using these different surgical techniques.

As a result from these studies, there is an increasing evidence that varicocele may cause changes in testicular flows in men. However, arterial spectral Doppler analysis is performed at various locations in the different studies, including the spermatic cord, trunk, testicular hilum, capsular and intratesticular arteries (Ross et al. 1994; Biagiotti et al. 2002; Tarhan et al. 2003; Ünsal et al. 2007; Grasso Leanza et al. 1997). Standardization of the sampling site is, therefore, needed to obtain comparable results and extrapolate cut-off values for the different Doppler parameters that may have a practical use in the clinical management of patients.

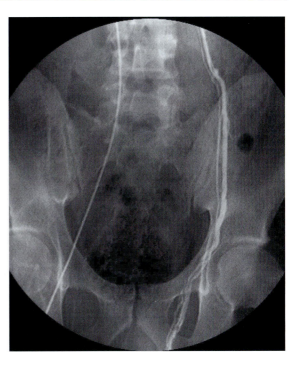

**Fig. 9** Super selective venography of the left internal spermatic vein demonstrates a clear reflux and filling of a duplicated vein in the upper and lower retroperitoneal segments; moreover, small collateral channels that are parallel to the internal spermatic vein are well evident

## 11    Other Imaging Techniques

Besides color Doppler ultrasound, several imaging techniques can be used in imaging varicocele. Scintigraphy and thermography have been widely used in the past, but currently have no established clinical indications. Venography is currently indicated in selective cases only. MR imaging and CT are of limited clinical use for various reasons, including cost, availability, lack of randomized controlled studies, and lack of outcome data demonstrating that they are equally or more effective compared to venography and color Doppler ultrasound.

### 11.1    Scintigraphy

Scintigraphy allows the noninvasive evaluation of reflux through the internal spermatic vein, which may be useful in planning therapy. Moreover, comparison

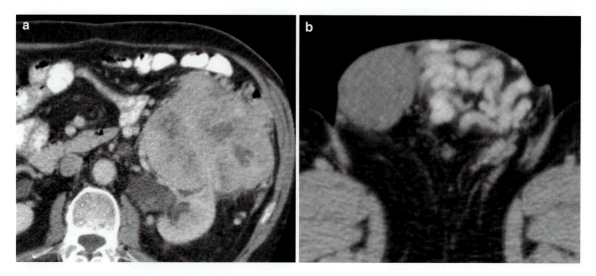

**Fig. 10** Appearance of varicocele at contrast-enhanced CT. Same patient of Fig. 8. CT scan performed to evaluate the left renal tumor shows the mass (**a**) and associated secondary varicocele (**b**)

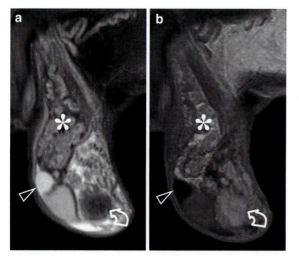

**Fig. 11** Appearance of varicocele at MR imaging. T2-weighted sagittal scan **a** and gadolinium-enhanced T1-weighted sagittal scan **b** of the left hemiscrotum performed for characterization of an extratesticular scrotal lesion show the mass (*curved arrow*), a cyst of the head of the epididymis (*arrowhead*), and associated varicocele (*asterisk*)

of features obtained before and after therapeutic interventions allows to verify adequacy of treatment or severity of recurrence (Geatti et al. 1991). Scintigraphy, however, is time consuming, and requires use of ionizing radiation. It has largely been superseded by color Doppler ultrasound.

## 11.2 Thermography

Thermographic assessment of varicocele was first reported in 1979, and widely used for several years. Subsequent studies have found contact termography to be unreliable and to have little clinical utility (sensitivity 97%, specificity 9%) (Basile-Fasolo et al. 1986; Trum et al. 1996). As a consequence, this technique has largely been superseded by ultrasound. Some authors, however, claim use of thermography, combined with ultrasonography, to improve diagnosis of right-sided and bilateral varicocele (Gat et al. 2003, 2005).

## 11.3 Venography

Venography shows, in real time, the direction of blood flow in the spermatic veins (Gat et al. 2005), and is generally considered to be the best diagnostic test for varicocele. However, it is time consuming, it requires use of ionizing radiation, and it is an invasive procedure with risks.

In patients with varicocele venography shows enlarged internal spermatic vein with reflux into the abdominal, inguinal, scrotal, or pelvic portions (Fig. 9). Collaterals and anastomotic channels can be identified. Similar to color Doppler ultrasound, the degree of reflux can be classified in five degrees

(Marsman 1985). In our institution venography is currently performed only as part of percutaneous sclerotheraphy of the internal spermatic vein.

## 11.4 CT and MRI

Varicocele can be identified incidentally in MRI and CT investigations performed for other purposes (Figs. 10, 11). Published case reports describe the use of gadolinium-enhanced, three-dimensional, phase-contrast magnetic resonance angiography to evaluate recurrent varicoceles (von Heijne 1997; Varma et al. 1998). This technique has been suggested as an alternative to spermatic venography; however, it is unlikely to achieve routine use. The appearance of intratesticular varicocele at MRI has been described in a case report in which this technique did not add significantly to color Doppler ultrasound.

## References

Abduljaleel PM, Al-Mulhim F, Nouman A et al (2006) Intratesticular varicocele and extratesticular varicocele in a patient with nephrotic syndrome complicated by left renal vein thrombosis. Ann Saudi Med 26:228–230

Alukal JP, Zurakowski D, Atala A et al (2005) Testicular hypotrophy does not correlate with grade of adolescent varicocele. J Urol 174:2367–2370 discussion 2370

Atasoy C, Fitoz S (2001) Gray-scale and color Doppler sonographic findings in intratesticular varicocele. J Clin Ultrasound 29:369–373

Aydos K, Baltaci S, Salih M et al (1993) Use of color Doppler sonography in the evaluation of varicoceles. Eur Urol 24:221–225

Basile-Fasolo C, Izzo PL, Canale D et al (1986) Doppler sonography, contact scrotal thermography and venography: a comparative study in evaluation of subclinical varicocele. Int J Fertil 30:62–64

Beddy P, Geoghegan T, Browne RF et al (2005) Testicular varicoceles. Clin Radiol 60:1248–1255

Bhatt S, Rubens DJ, Dogra VS (2006) Sonography of benign intrascrotal lesions. Ultrasound Q 22:121–136

Biagiotti G, Cavallini G, Modenini F et al (2002) Spermatogenesis and spectral echo-colour Doppler traces from the main testicular artery. BJU Int 90:903–908

Bucci S, Liguori G, Amodeo A et al (2008) Intratesticular varicocele: evaluation using gray scale and color Doppler ultrasound. World J Urol 26:87–89

Callea A, Berardi B, Dilorenzo V et al (1997) Echo-color Doppler in the topographic study of varicocele. Arch Ital Urol Androl 69:189–192

Carlsen E, Andersen AG, Buchreitz L et al (2000) Inter-observer variation in the results of the clinical andrological examination including estimation of testicular size. Int J Androl 23:248–253

Chiou RK, Anderson JC, Wobig RK et al (1997) Color Doppler ultrasound criteria to diagnose varicoceles: correlation of a new scoring system with physical examination. Urology 50:953–956

Conti E, Fasolo PP, Sebastiani G et al (2005) Color Doppler sonography in the intratesticular varicocele. Arch Ital Urol Androl 77:63–65

Cornud F, Belin X, Amar E et al (1999) Varicocele: strategies in diagnosis and treatment. Eur Radiol 9:536–545

Das KM, Prasad K, Szmigielski W et al (1999) Intratesticular varicocele: evaluation using conventional and Doppler sonography. Am J Roentgenol 173:1079–1083

Dee KE, Deck AJ, Waitches GM (2000) Intratesticular pseudo-aneurysm after blunt trauma. Am J Roentgenol 174:1136

DemIrbas M, Ellergezen A, BI CY et al (2001) Intratesticular varicocele treated with percutaneous embolization. Urology 58:1058

Diamond DA, Roth JA, Cilento BG et al (2004) Intratesticular varicocele in adolescents: a reversible anechoic lesion of the testis. J Urol 171:381–383

Dogra VS, Gottlieb RH, Oka M et al (2003) Sonography of the scrotum. Radiology 227:18–36

Dubin L, Amelar RD (1970) Varicocele size and results of varicocelectomy in selected subfertile men with varicocele. Fertil Steril 21:606–609

Erdogan N, Ekmekcioglu O, Baykara M (2003) Bilateral intratesticular varicocele in a patient with a history of bilateral cryptorchidism. Turk J Med Sci 33:117–119

Eskew LA, Watson NE, Wolfman N et al (1993) Ultrasonographic diagnosis of varicoceles. Fertil Steril 60:693–697

Gat Y, Zukerman ZV, Bachar GN et al (2003) Adolescent varicocele: is it a unilateral disease? Urology 62:742–746 discussion 746–747

Gat Y, Bachar GN, Zukerman Z et al (2004) Varicocele: a bilateral disease. Fertil Steril 81:424–429

Gat Y, Zukerman Z, Chakraborty J et al (2005) Varicocele, hypoxia and male infertility. Fluid Mechanics analysis of the impaired testicular venous drainage system. Hum Reprod 20:2614–2619

Geatti O, Gasparini D, Shapiro B (1991) A comparison of scintigraphy, thermography, ultrasound and phlebography in grading of clinical varicocele. J Nucl Med 32:2092–2097

Gonda RL Jr, Karo JJ, Forte RA et al (1987) Diagnosis of subclinical varicocele in infertility. Am J Roentgenol 148:71–75

Graif M, Hauser R, Hirshebein A et al (2000) Varicocele and the testicular-renal venous route: hemodynamic Doppler sonographic investigation. J Ultrasound Med 19:627–631

Grasso Leanza F, Pepe P, Panella P et al (1997) Volocimetric evaluation of spermatic vessels with echo color Doppler in patients with idiopathic varicocele. Minerva Urol Nefrol 49:179–182

Hargreave TB, Liakatas J (1991) Physical examination for varicocele. Br J Urol 67:328

Harrison RM, Lewis RW, Roberts JA (1983) Testicular blood flow and fluid dynamics in monkeys with surgically induced varicoceles. J Androl 4:256–260

Harrison RM, Lewis RW, Roberts JA (1986) Pathophysiology of varicocele in nonhuman primates: long-term seminal and testicular changes. Fertil Steril 46:500–510

Hirsh AV, Cameron KM, Tyler JP et al (1980) The Doppler assessment of varicoceles and internal spermatic vein reflux in infertile men. Br J Urol 52:50–56

Hoekstra T, Witt MA (1995) The correlation of internal spermatic vein palpability with ultrasonographic diameter and reversal of venous flow. J Urol 153:82–84

Hsu HS, Chang LS, Chen MT et al (1994) Decreased blood flow and defective energy metabolism in the varicocele-bearing testicles of rats. Eur Urol 25:71–75

Hussein AF (2006) The role of color Doppler ultrasound in prediction of the outcome of microsurgical subinguinal varicocelectomy. J Urol 176:2141–2145

Jarow JP (2001) Effects of varicocele on male fertility. Hum Reprod Update 7:59–64

Liguori G, Trombetta C, Garaffa G et al (2004) Color Doppler ultrasound investigation of varicocele. World J Urol 22:378–381

Liguori G, Ollandini G, Pomara G et al (2010) Role of renospermatic basal reflow and age on semen quality improvement after sclerotization of varicocele. Urology 75:1074–1078

Lund L, Nielsen AH (1994) Color Doppler sonography in the assessment of varicocele testis. Scand J Urol Nephrol 28:281–285

Marks JL, McMahon R, Lipshultz LI (1986) Predictive parameters of successful varicocele repair. J Urol 136:609–612

Marsman JW (1985) Clinical versus subclinical varicocele: venographic findings and improvement of fertility after embolization. Radiology 155:635–638

Meacham RB, Townsend RR, Rademacher D et al (1994) The incidence of varicoceles in the general population when evaluated by physical examination, gray scale sonography and color Doppler sonography. J Urol 151:1535–1538

Mehta AL, Dogra VS (1998) Intratesticular varicocele. J Clin Ultrasound 26:49–51

Morvay Z, Nagy E (1998) The diagnosis and treatment of intratesticular varicocele. Cardiovasc Intervent Radiol 21:76–78

Naughton CK, Nangia AK, Agarwal A (2001) Pathophysiology of varicoceles in male infertility. Hum Reprod Update 7:473–481

Niedzielski J, Paduch D, Raczynski P (1997) Assessment of adolescent varicocele. Pediatr Surg Int 12:410–413

O'Donnell PG, Dewbury KC (1998) The ultrasound appearances of intratesticular varicocoele. Br J Radiol 71:324–325

Oyen RH (2002) Scrotal ultrasound. Eur Radiol 12:19–34

Ozcan H, Aytac S, Yagci C et al (1997) Color Doppler ultrasonographic findings in intratesticular varicocele. J Clin Ultrasound 25:325–329

Pearl MS, Hill MC (2007) Ultrasound of the scrotum. Semin Ultrasound CT MR 28:225–248

Petros JA, Andriole GL, Middleton WD et al (1991) Correlation of testicular color Doppler ultrasonography, physical examination and venography in the detection of left varicoceles in men with infertility. J Urol 145:785–788

Ross JA, Watson NE Jr, Jarow JP (1994) The effect of varicoceles on testicular blood flow in man. Urology 44:535–539

Sakamoto H, Ogawa Y, Yoshida H (2008) Relationship between testicular volume and varicocele in patients with infertility. Urology 71:104–109

Sarteschi LM, Paoli R, Bianchini M et al (1993) Lo studio del varicocele con eco-color Doppler. G Ital Ultrasonologia 4:43–49

Sarteschi LM, Liguori G, Trombetta C (2003) Varicocele. In: Sarteschi LM, Menchini-Fabris GF (eds) Ecografia andrologica, 1st edn edn. Athena Srl, Modena, pp 139–155

Shafik A, Moftah A, Olfat S et al (1990) Testicular veins: anatomy and role in varicocelogenesis and other pathologic conditions. Urology 35:175–182

Shiraishi K, Naito K, Takihara H (2003) Indication of varicocelectomy in the era of assisted reproductive technology: prediction of treatment outcome by noninvasive diagnostic methods. Arch Androl 49:475–478

Sigman M, Jarow JP (1997) Ipsilateral testicular hypotrophy is associated with decreased sperm counts in infertile men with varicoceles. J Urol 158:605–607

Sweeney TE, Rozum JS, Desjardins C et al (1991) Microvascular pressure distribution in the hamster testis. Am J Physiol 260:H1581–H1589

Tanriverdi O, Miroglu C, Horasanli K et al (2006) Testicular blood flow measurements and mean resistive index values after microsurgical and high ligation varicocelectomy. Urology 67:1262–1265

Tarhan S, Gumus B, Gunduz I et al (2003) Effect of varicocele on testicular artery blood flow in men–color Doppler investigation. Scand J Urol Nephrol 37:38–42

Tasci AI, Resim S, Caskurlu T et al (2001) Color Doppler ultrasonography and spectral analysis of venous flow in diagnosis of varicocele. Eur Urol 39:316–321

Tetreau R, Julian P, Lyonnet D et al (2007) Intratesticular varicocele: an easy diagnosis but unclear physiopathologic characteristics. J Ultrasound Med 26:1767–1773

Trum JW, Gubler FM, Laan R et al (1996) The value of palpation, varicoscreen contact thermography and colour Doppler ultrasound in the diagnosis of varicocele. Hum Reprod 11:1232–1235

Ünsal A, Turgut AT, Taşkin F et al (2007) Resistance and pulsatility index increase in capsular branches of testicular artery: Indicator of impaired testicular microcirculation in varicocele? J Clin Ultrasound 35:191–195

Varma MK, Ho VB, Haggerty M et al (1998) MR venography as a diagnostic tool in the assessment of recurrent varicocele in an adolescent. Pediatr Radiol 28:636–637

von Heijne A (1997) Recurrent varicocele. Demonstration by 3D phase-contrast MR angiography. Acta Radiol 38:1020–1022

Weiss AJ, Kellman GM, Middleton WD et al (1992) Intratesticular varicocele: sonographic findings in two patients. Am J Roentgenol 158:1061–1063

Winkelbauer FW, Ammann ME, Karnel F et al (1994) Doppler sonography of varicocele: long-term follow-up after venography and transcatheter sclerotherapy. J Ultrasound Med 13:953–958

World Health Organization (1985) Comparison among different methods for the diagnosis of varicocele. Fertil Steril 43:575–582

Yilmaz C, Arslan M (2009) Intrascrotal arteriovenous malformation simulating varicocele. Am J Roentgenol 192: W351

Zini A, Buckspan M, Berardinucci D et al (1997) The influence of clinical and subclinical varicocele on testicular volume. Fertil Steril 68:671–674

# Imaging the Infertile Male-2: Obstructive Syndromes and Other Disorders

Min Hoan Moon and Seung Hyup Kim

## Contents

**Abstract**

The evaluation of infertile men *begins with a detailed* clinical history and physical examination and then proceeds to laboratory test including semen analysis, hormonal assays, sperm function test, and genetic test. Imaging studies can be used selectively as part of the comprehensive evaluation of male infertility. In this chapter, we review the spectrum of diseases responsible for male infertility, discuss appropriate imaging modalities to be proven for specific clinical settings, and illustrate characteristic imaging findings that permit specific diagnosis. We also discuss how imaging studies may be used to distinguish defects of sperm production from obstruction of sperm passage. The discussion is divided into three main categories: obstruction in sperm passage, impairment in sperm function, and defect in sperm genesis.

M. H. Moon (✉)
Department of Radiology,
Seoul Metropolitan Boramae Medical Center,
Seoul National University, College of Medicine,
39 Boramae-Gil, Dongjak-Gu,
Seoul 156-707, Korea
e-mail: mmhoan@gmail.com

S. H. Kim
Department of Radiology,
Seoul National University Hospital,
#28 Yongon-dong, Chongno-gu,
Seoul 110-744, Korea

## 1 Introduction

Infertility is defined as the case in which there is a failure in pregnancy in spite of unprotected intercourse of 12 months. Infertility is caused by either male factors or female factors. Male factors are found in up to 50% of infertile couples and the sole causes of infertility in 30% (Macleod 1951; Brugh and Lipshultz 2004). The evaluation of infertile men *begins with a detailed* clinical history and physical examination and then proceeds to laboratory test including semen analysis, hormonal assays, sperm function test, and genetic test. Imaging studies can be

M. Bertolotto and C. Trombetta (eds.), *Scrotal Pathology*, Medical Radiology. Diagnostic Imaging,
DOI: 10.1007/174_2011_192, © Springer-Verlag Berlin Heidelberg 2012

**Table 1** The causes of disturbance in sperm passage according to obstruction level

| Obstruction level | Condition | | |
|---|---|---|---|
| Epididymis | | Chronic epididymitis | |
| Vas deferens | Scrotal portion | Operation, trauma, iatrogenic | |
| | Inguinal portion | Operation, trauma, iatrogenic | |
| | Pelvic portion | CAVD[*] | |
| Ejaculatory duct | | Ejaculatory duct obstruction | Inflammation associated |
| | | | Midline cysts |

*Congenital absence of the vas deferens

used selectively as part of the comprehensive evaluation of male infertility. In this chapter, we review the spectrum of diseases responsible for male infertility, discuss appropriate imaging modalities to be proven for specific clinical settings, and illustrate characteristic imaging findings that permit specific diagnosis. We also discuss how imaging studies may be used to distinguish defects of sperm production from obstruction of sperm passage. The discussion is divided into three main categories: obstruction in sperm passage, impairment in sperm function, and defect in sperm genesis.

## 2 Obstruction in Sperm Passage

Infertile men with obstruction in sperm passage typically have normal-sized testes and a normal serum FSH. Imaging studies are used to identify the location of the obstruction. Although obstructions occur anywhere along the genital duct (Table 1), evaluation of the proximal and distal genital duct can reveal most of the conditions causing obstruction in sperm passage because the middle genital duct is a rare site of obstruction. Scrotal ultrasound and transrectal ultrasound are the imaging techniques of choice to demonstrate the pathologies causing proximal genital duct obstructions (e.g., chronic epididymitis) and those causing distal genital duct obstruction (e.g., congenital absence of the vas deferens (CAVD) or ejaculatory duct obstruction), respectively.

### 2.1 Chronic Epididymitis

Epididymitis is a common cause of acute scrotal pain and, if chronic, it may affect male fertility through post-inflammatory obstruction of the epididymal ducts (Breeland et al. 1981). Scrotal ultrasound is the imaging technique most frequently used to assess intrascrotal abnormalities. On scrotal ultrasound, chronic epididymitis appears as focal or diffuse enlargement of the epididymis with variable echogenecity and calcifications (Fig. 1). A range of organisms are implicated in the development of chronic epididymitis. Among these, tuberculous epididymitis tends to involve the tail portion of the epididymis in comparison with nontuberculous epididymitis (Kim et al. 1993). Because the determination of obstruction site may have important implications for planning of appropriate treatments (Brugh and Lipshultz 2004), it is advisable to assess the possible obstruction site as well as the presence or absence of chronic epididymitis.

### 2.2 Congenital Absence of the Vas Deferens

Men with CAVD can be divided into two groups according to their association with cystic fibrosis; the cases with mutation in cystic fibrosis transmembrane regulator gene (CFTR gene) (Quinzii and Castellani 2000; Daudin et al. 2000) versus the cases without mutation in CFTR gene. The former is usually bilateral and is not associated with other genitourinary

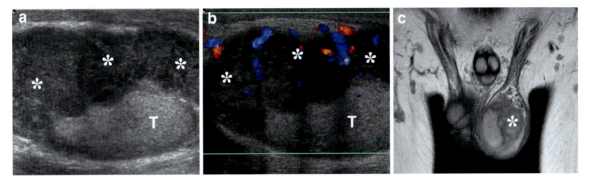

**Fig. 1** Chronic epididymitis in a 31 year-old man. Longitudinal gray-year old manscale (**a**) and color Doppler (**b**) ultrasound images of the left scrotum show diffusely enlarged, hypoechoic epididymis (*) with increased vascularity in the paratesticular area. Note that the enlarged epididymis encroaches on the left testis (*T*). **c** T2-weighted MR image in coronal plane shows diffusely enlarged left epididymis with low signal intensity (*) in the paratesticular area

abnormalities except for seminal vesicle agenesis or hypoplasia. The presumed mechanism for CAVD with the mutation in CFTR gene is that the mutation in CFTR gene causes abnormal glycoprotein secretion from the epididymis and leads to subsequent obstruction in a distal genital duct, with progressive distal genital duct atrophy (Tizzano et al. 1994). Transrectal ultrasound is the procedure of choice for demonstrating absence of the vas deferens (Fig. 2). CAVD irrelevant to CFTR gene is a developmental anomaly of the Wolffian duct. It is usually unilateral and often has association with ipsilateral genitourinary anomaly such as renal agenesis or seminal vesicle cyst (Fig. 3).

## 2.3 Ejaculatory Duct Obstruction: Inflammation Associated

Ejaculatory duct obstructions, one of the important causes of male infertility, usually occur as a complication of seminal vesiculitis or prostatitis. In the past, the standard method of imaging for ejaculatory duct obstruction was vasography, but its invasiveness and the risk of vasal scarring have narrowed its clinical use in the evaluation of ejaculatory duct obstruction. Instead, transrectal ultrasound has become the most popular alternative to vasography because of its noninvasiveness and relatively low cost. Transrectal ultrasound supports of the diagnosis of ejaculatory duct obstruction by demonstrating ejaculatory duct cysts, echogenic lines along the course of the ejaculatory duct, luminal distension of the ejaculatory duct or seminal vesicle, or stones causing ejaculatory duct obstruction (Fig. 4). However, such transrectal ultrasound imaging findings should be interpreted with caution because anatomical abnormalities, depicted by transrectal ultrasound, do not have consistent causal relationship with ejaculatory duct obstruction (Colpi et al. 1997; Purohit et al. 2004).

## 2.4 Ejaculatory Duct Obstruction: Midline Cysts

In infertile men with suspicion of ejaculatory duct obstruction, cystic lesions located at prostatic midline are commonly identified by transrectal ultrasound scan. Based on their embryologic origin, the cystic lesions can be classified into utricular cysts, Müllerian duct cysts, and ejaculatory duct cysts. Utricular cysts derive from a dilatation of the prostatic utricle and are often associated with other malformations, such as hypospadia or virilization defect (Nghiem et al. 1990). Müllerian duct cysts arise from the embryologic remnants of the Müllerian duct. Unlike utricular cysts, Müllerian duct cysts do not communicate with the prostatic urethra and are usually larger than utricular cysts. Ejaculatory duct cysts are of Wolffian duct origin and contain spermatozoa in their content.

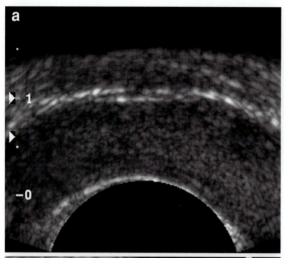

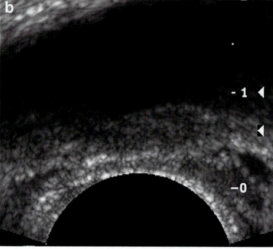

**Fig. 2** Congenital absence of the bilateral vas deferens in a 28 year-old infertile man: **a** transverse ultrasound image of the prostate base, **b** transverse ultrasound image above the level of the prostate base showing absence of both vas deferens and seminal vesicles

Ejaculatory duct cysts are the consequence of diverticulum formation from the obstruction of the ejaculatory duct, whereas both utricular cysts and Müllerian duct cysts may cause compression and displacement of the ejaculatory ducts, resulting in obstruction. Transrectal ultrasound findings of those cystic lesions are similar irrespective of their embryologic origin and appear as teardrop- or oval-shaped cysts behind the verumontanum along the midline of the prostate gland (Fig. 5).

## 3 Impairments in Sperm Function

Infertile men with impairments in sperm function are generally presented with decreased sperm motility (asthenozoospermia) or abnormal sperm morphology (teratozoospermia). A variety of causes have been found to cause impairments in sperm function and radiologically identifiable causes include varicocele and Kartagener syndrome.

### 3.1 Varicocele

Varicocele is defined as abnormal dilatation of the pampiniform plexus and is the most frequent cause of male infertility. Varicocele accounts for 40% of primary infertility and 45–80% of secondary infertility (Brugh and Lipshultz 2004; Brugh et al. 2003). Left-sided varicocele is more common than right-sided varicocele by a ratio of 10:1. It is unclear how varicocele will affect male fertility, but the most commonly accepted theory is that varicoceles increase scrotal temperature and subsequent hyperthermia interferes with normal spermatogenesis, leading to oligospermia, decreased sperm motility, or abnormal sperm morphology (Takihara et al. 1991). Scrotal ultrasound is the standard method in the diagnosis of varicoceles. On gray-scale ultrasound, varicoceles appear as multiple anechoic serpiginous tubular structures of various sizes, along the course of the spermatic cord or in the paratesticular area. Use of color or pulsed Doppler ultrasound facilitates the diagnosis of varicocele by demonstrating excessive color flow and retrograde filling during the Valsalva maneuver (Fig. 6). It has to be noted, however, that transient reflux during Valsalva maneuver should not be mistaken for presence of varicoceles. Scanning with the patients standing often may improve detection of varicoceles that is not apparent in recumbent position.

### 3.2 Primary Ciliary Dyskinesia

Primary ciliary dyskinesia, also known as immotile ciliary syndrome, is a rare autosomal-recessive disorder of ciliary dysfunction that leads to impaired mucociliary clearance and clinical disease of upper and lower

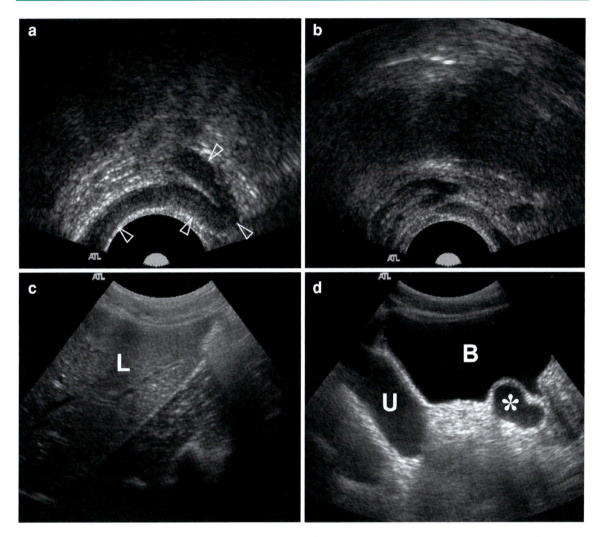

**Fig. 3** Congenital absence of the unilateral vas deferens in a 23 year-old man: **a** oblique ultrasound image along the long axis of the left vas deferens shows the left vas deferens of a tubular, hypoechoic structure (*arrowheads*). **b** oblique ultrasound image along the presumed long axis of the right vas deferens shows absence of the right vas deferens, **c** the right kidney is not demonstrated on transabdominal ultrasound scan, suggestive of right renal agenesis. *L*, liver, **d** longitudinal ultrasound image of the pelvis shows that the right remnant distal ureter (*U*) is dilated with concurrent ureterocele formation (*)

airway infection (Noone et al. 2004). In approximately half of cases, primary ciliary dyskinesia is associated with situs inversus (reversal of the internal organs). Kartagener syndrome is a subgroup of primary ciliary dyskinesia characterized by the clinical triad of sinusitis, bronchiectasis, and situs inversus (Kartagener and Stucki 1962). Because the tail of the sperm has a core structure identical to that of the cilia, primary ciliary dyskinesia results in poor sperm motility that leads to male infertility (Afzelius 1979). Sinus and chest radiographs can detect characteristic airway changes of primary ciliary dyskinesia such as sinusitis, bronchiectasis, and situs inversus (Fig. 7). High-resolution CT scan of the chest can be performed to detect early and subtle abnormalities of airways which can be missed by routine chest radiographs (Kennedy et al. 2007). The diagnosis of immotile cilia syndrome is made by electron microscopic ultrastructural analysis of samples of nasal or airway mucosa acquired with minimally invasive techniques (Afzelius 1976).

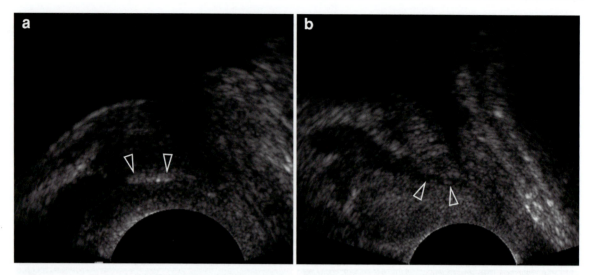

**Fig. 4** US imaging of ejaculatory duct obstruction. **a** Longitudinal ultrasound images through the prostate shows echogenic lines (*arrowheads*) along the course of the left ejaculatory duct. Diffuse calcification or fibrosis may be underlying pathologic changes responsible for the echogenic lines. **b** Luminal distension (*arrowheads*) of the ejaculatory duct is another ultrasound imaging finding suggestive of ejaculatory duct obstruction. The lumen of the ejaculatory duct normally is not apparent with transrectal ultrasound scan

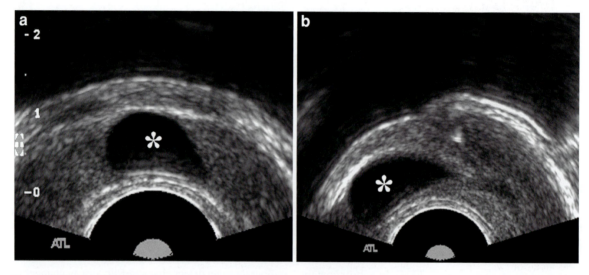

**Fig. 5** Midline cyst in a 53 year-old man. The cyst (*) is seen as a round- or oval-shaped anechoic lesion on the transverse scan (**a**) and as teardrop- or oval-shaped cysts on the longitudinal scan (**b**) behind the verumontanum along the midline of the prostate gland

## 4    Defects in Sperm Production

Defects in sperm production are caused by either primary or secondary testicular failure (Table 2). The results of initial endocrine evaluation are helpful in distinguishing primary testicular failure from secondary testicular failure. Primary testicular failure results from end-organ failure and shows an elevated serum FSH level and a normal or low serum testosterone. Secondary testicular failure results from hormonal imbalance of the hypothalamic-pituitary–gonadal axis and presents with low serum testosterone and low serum level of LH and FSH. For secondary testicular failure, cross-sectional imaging including CT or MR can *provide specific* imaging features that,

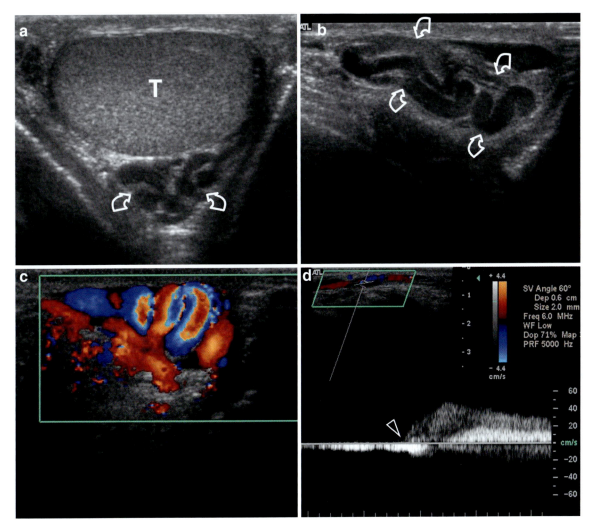

**Fig. 6** Varicocele in a 16 year-old man. **a–b** Transverse (**a**) and longitudinal (**b**) ultrasound images of the left hemiscrotum show multiple anechoic structures (*curved arrows*) in the paratesticular area. *T*, testis. **c** Color Doppler ultrasound image shows intense blood flow signals within the anechoic structure during the Valsalva maneuver. **d** Pulsed-wave Doppler image shows a venous waveform with marked reflux during the Valsalva maneuver (*arrowhead*)

in association with clinical findings, allow a specific diagnosis to be made. In contrast, imaging studies in primary testicular failure are of limited value because men with primary testicular failure manifest by non-specific radiographic changes of small testes, irrespective of underlying etiology.

## 4.1 Primary Testicular Failure

The men with primary testicular failure can have a variety of underlying pathologies ranging from chromosomal abnormalities (numerical or structural) to congenital or infection (Table 2). As mentioned above, imaging studies are usually not helpful in making a specific diagnosis of primary testicular failure, except for undescended testis (Fig. 8). Instead, the role of imaging in the evaluation of primary testicular failure is to differentiate primary testicular failure from obstruction in sperm passage. For this purpose, scrotal ultrasound, a first-line diagnostic modality for male infertility, is especially useful in two ways; one with measurements of testis volume and the other with the evaluation of the epididymis (Moon et al. 2006). Testis volumes can be calculated by using the empiric formula of Lambert (1951): length * height * width * 0.71.

**Fig. 7** Kartagener syndrome in a 31 year-old man. **a** Chest PA shows right-sided cardiac shadow (*arrowhead*), suggestive of dextrocardia. Note that the stomach gas (*curved arrow*) is also seen in the right upper abdomen. **b** Waters Caldwell view obtained in a same patient reveals chronic inflammation (*) of the maxillary sinus. These imaging findings are compatible with Kartagener syndrome

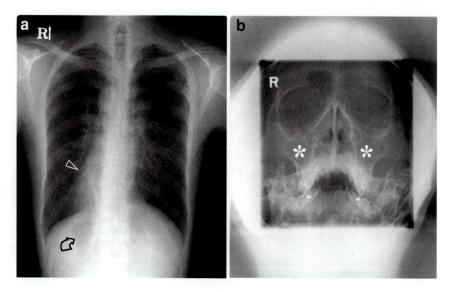

**Table 2** The classification and causes of defects in sperm production

| Classification | Specific diagnosis |
|---|---|
| Primary testicular failure | Y microdeletion |
| | Klinefelter syndrome |
| | Orchitis (viral or bacterial) |
| | Undescended testis |
| Secondary testicular failure | Hemochromatosis |
| | Kallmann syndrome |
| | Hyperprolactinemia |
| | Congenital adrenal hyperplasia |
| | Androgen insensitivity syndrome |
| | Exposure to gonadotoxin |

According to our experience, testes with a volume of <10 ml are likely to have primary testicular failure, whereas those with a volume of more than 15 ml are likely to have obstruction in sperm passage. Intermediate-sized testis with a volume of 10–15 ml has the possibility of both primary testicular failure and obstruction in sperm passage. The evaluation of the epididymis is also helpful in distinguishing primary testicular failure from obstruction in sperm passage in that it can directly demonstrate pathologies of the proximal genital duct and may also detect secondary changes of the proximal genital duct caused by the distal genital duct obstruction. Epididymal abnormalities suggestive of obstruction in sperm passage include tubular ectasia, tapering, absence, or inflammatory mass formation (Fig. 9).

## 4.2 Hemochromatosis

Hemochromatosis is a disorder of abnormal iron metabolism characterized by excess iron deposition in parenchymal cells that leads to cellular damage and organ dysfunction. Hemochromatosis can be classified as primary (or genetic) hemochromatosis and secondary (or acquired) hemochromatosis. Primary hemochromatosis is an autosomal recessive disorder in that the increase of intestinal iron absorption leads to iron deposition whereas, in secondary hemochromatosis, iron deposition ensues from dietary iron overload, commonly in the form of repeated blood transfusion. Excess iron deposition in the anterior lobe of the pituitary gland leads to male infertility in the form of hypogonadotropic hypogonadism (Siminoski et al. 1990; Bhansali et al. 1992). Magnetic resonance imaging is the most reliable imaging method in the diagnosis

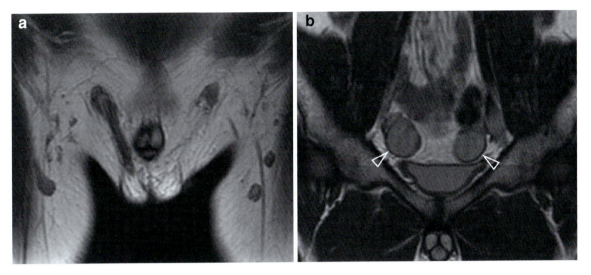

**Fig. 8** Bilateral undescended testes in a 21-year-old man. **a** Coronal T2-weighted image shows absence of both testes within the scrotal sac and inguinal canal. **b** Coronal T2-weighted image obtained posterior to (**a**) shows bilateral intraabdominal undescended testes (*arrowheads*) in the supravesical area

**Fig. 9** Epididymal abnormalities suggestive of obstruction in sperm passage. **a–b** In a 40-year old man proved to be inflammatory-associated azoospermia, caudal portion of the left hemiscrotum shows enlarged epididymal tail (*) with heterogeneous echogenecity (**a**). Color Doppler ultrasound image (**b**) demonstrates increased blood flow signal within the enlarged epididymal tail. **c** In a 30 year-old man proved to be a patient with congenital absence of the vas deferens (CAVD) longitudinal ultrasound image of the right hemiscrotum shows multiple cysts in the epididymal head. **d** In a 28 year-old man proved to be CAVD patient, longitudinal ultrasound image through the left epididymal body shows abrupt narrowing (*arrowhead*) in the proximal to mid portion of the epididymal body

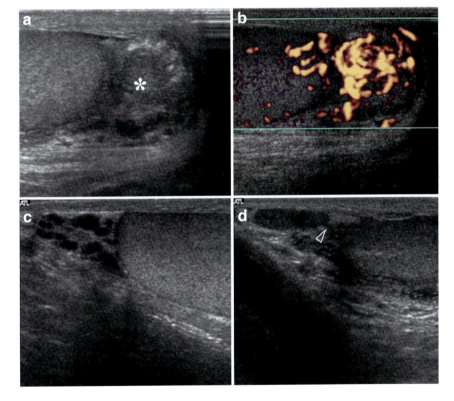

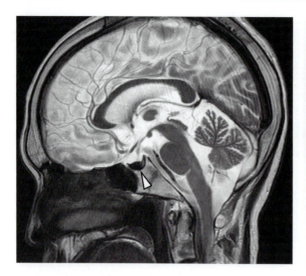

**Fig. 10** Hemochromatosis in a 23 year-old man. Sagittal T2-weighted image shows dark signal intensity (*arrowhead*) of the pituitary gland. Paramagnetic effect caused by iron deposition leads to this signal loss of the pituitary gland on T2-weighted image

of hemochromatosis. Paramagnetic effect caused by iron deposition leads to signal loss of the pituitary gland on T2-weighted image (Fig. 10) (Sparacia et al. 1998).

## 4.3   Kallmann Syndrome

Idiopathic hypogonadotropic hypogonadism is defined as the cases in which abnormal synthesis and release of gonadotropin-releasing hormone without an anatomic cause lead to hypogonadism. Kallmann syndrome, a subtype of idiopathic hypogonadotropic hypogonadism associated with anosmia, is the most common X-linked disorder in male infertility, with an incidence of 1 in 10,000–60,000 (Bick et al. 1992). The diagnosis of Kallmann syndrome is suspected when infertile men with azoospermia or oligospermia are associated with anosmia or hyposmia. The central to the imaging of infertile men suspected of Kallmann syndrome is to demonstrate the absence or hypoplasia of olfactory bulbs and tracts that can best be evaluated with magnetic resonance imaging (Fig. 11) (Yousem et al. 1996).

## 4.4   Hyperprolactinemia

Hyperprolactinemia suppresses gonadotropin releasing hormone from the hypothalamus, causing a

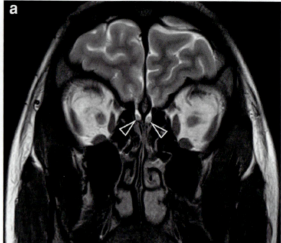

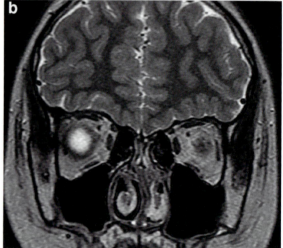

**Fig. 11** MR imaging of Kallmann syndrome. **a** Coronal T2-weighted image of a normal volunteer demonstrates normal olfactory tracts (*arrowheads*). **b** Coronal T2-weighted image in a 28 year-old infertile man with anosmia shows absence of the olfactory tracts, suggesting the diagnosis of Kallmann syndrome

decrease in luteinizing hormone and follicle-stimulating hormone, ultimately leading to oligospermia or azoospermia. Hyperprolactinemia can be suspected in infertile men when they manifest by decreased libido, impotence, galactorrhea, or gynecomastia. The major cause of hyperprolactinemia is prolactinoma that is the most common functional pituitary adenoma. Pituitary macroadenomas (above 10 mm in diameter) can be easily demonstrated with conventional magnetic resonance imaging after contrast administration (Fig. 12). However, for assessment of pituitary microadenomas (below 10 mm in diameter), dynamic study with intravenous bolus injection of contrast medium is

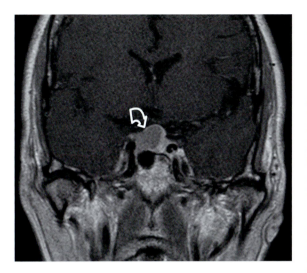

**Fig. 12** Pituitary macroadenoma in a 33 year-old man. Coronal T1-weighted contrast-enhanced image shows macroadenoma (*curved arrow*) on the right side of the pituitary gland

needed to delineate the tumor from the normal pituitary gland (Fig. 13). The normal pituitary gland and stalk have strong enhancement in the early phase of dynamic imaging, whereas microadenomas have relatively weak enhancement (Bartynski and Lin 1997).

## 4.5 Congenital Adrenal Hyperplasia

*Congenital adrenal hyperplasia* is a group of autosomal recessive disorders with a deficiency of one of adrenocortical enzyme necessary for cortisol synthesis. More than 90% of cases are caused by a deficiency of 21-hydroxylase. The deficiency leads to a lack of cortisol production and a subsequent overproduction of adrenocorticotropic hormone (ACTH) through loss of negative feedback to the pituitary gland. The elevated ACTH level promotes the secretion of adrenal androgens that inhibit the release of luteinizing hormone and follicle-stimulating hormone, leading to hypogonadotropic hypogonadism. Computed tomography is widely used in the evaluation of the adrenal gland. Congenital adrenal hyperplasia appears as diffuse enlargement of both adrenal glands with preservation of normal configuration (Fig. 14) (Johnson et al. 2009). However, the presence of normal-sized adrenal glands does not exclude the diagnosis of congenital adrenal hyperplasia (Sivit et al. 1991; CA et al. 1988). Testicular adrenal rest is

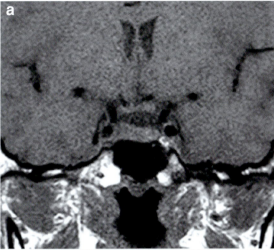

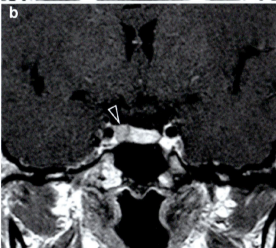

**Fig. 13** Pituitary microadenoma in a 25 year-old man. **a** Prior to contrast material administration, a pituitary microadenoma is not clearly visualized on coronal T1-weighted image. **b** In the early phase of dynamic imaging, coronal T1-weighted image shows strong enhancement of the normal pituitary gland whereas pituitary microadenoma (*arrowhead*) shows relatively weak enhancement

aberrant adrenal tissue that become trapped within the developing gonad during prenatal life and, if testicular adrenal rest is exposed to elevated levels of ACTH, the testicular adrenal rest can enlarge to form masses and mimic multifocal testicular malignancy.

## 4.6 Androgen Insensitivity Syndrome

Androgen insensitivity (testicular feminization) syndrome is a rare syndrome that lacks functional

**Fig. 14** Congenital adrenal hyperplasia with testicular adrenal rest in an 18 year-old man. **a–b** axial (**a**) and coronal (**b**) postcontrast CT images show bilateral enlarged adrenal glands (*arrowheads*). **c** Longitudinal ultrasound image of the left scrotum shows a large low echoic intratesticular mass (*). Note that small residual testis (*T*) is seen in the inferior portion of the left scrotum. **d** Axial T2-weighted image of the scrotum shows bilateral intratesticular masses of low signal intensity (*). Note residual testis of high signal intensity (*curved arrows*)

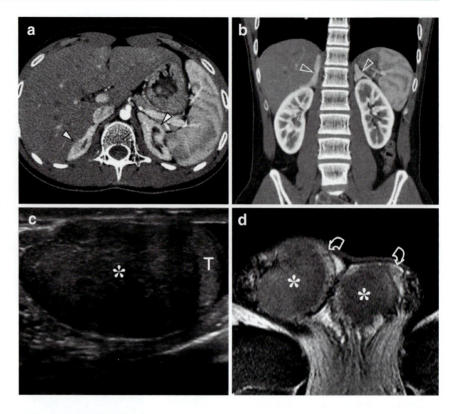

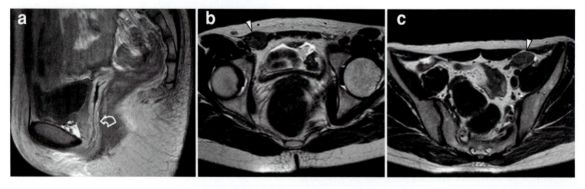

**Fig. 15** MR imaging of androgen insensitivity syndrome. **a** On sagittal T1-weighted contrast-enhanced image, the uterus is absent and the vagina (*curved arrow*) ends as a blind pouch. Note that the external genitalia looks female. **b–c** Axial T2-weighted images show right undescended testis (*arrowhead* in **b**) in the inguinal canal and left intraabdominal undescended testis (*arrowhead* in **c**)

androgen receptor and leads to an absence of wolffian duct derivatives and development of a female phenotype (Coulam et al. 1984; Rutgers and Scully 1991). Because the patients with androgen insensitivity syndrome usually present with a female phenotype without genital ambiguity, the diagnosis is usually made at puberty during workup for amenorrhea. The role of imaging is to assess the internal genitalia and to provide clinician androgen insensitivity syndrome as a possible cause of infertility. Ultrasound, computed tomography, and magnetic resonance imaging not only can demonstrate the absence of müllerian duct derivatives but also can show undescended testes in the inguinal canal or abdomen (Fig. 15) (Gambino et al. 1992; Gale 1983).

# References

Afzelius BA (1976) A human syndrome caused by immotile cilia. Science 193:317–319

Afzelius BA (1979) The immotile-cilia syndrome and other ciliary diseases. Int Rev Exp Pathol 19:1–43

Bartynski WS, Lin L (1997) Dynamic and conventional spin-echo MR of pituitary microlesions. AJNR Am J Neuroradiol 18:965–972

Bhansali A, Banerjee PK, Dash S et al (1992) Pituitary and testicular involvement in primary haemochromatosis. A case report. J Assoc Physicians India 40:757–759

Bick D, Franco B, Sherins RJ et al (1992) Brief report: intragenic deletion of the KALIG-1 gene in Kallmann's syndrome. N Engl J Med 326:1752–1755

Breeland E, Cohen MS, Warner RS et al (1981) Epididymal obstruction in azoospermic males. Infertility 4:49–66

Brugh VM 3rd, Lipshultz LI (2004) Male factor infertility: evaluation and management. Med Clin North Am 88:367–385

Brugh VM 3rd, Matschke HM, Lipshultz LI (2003) Male factor infertility. Endocrinol Metab Clin North Am 32:689–707

CA BryanPJ, Morrison SC et al (1988) US findings in adrenogenital syndrome. J US Med 7:675–679

Colpi GM, Negri L, Nappi RE et al (1997) Is transrectal ultrasonography a reliable diagnostic approach in ejaculatory duct sub-obstruction? Hum Reprod 12:2186–2191

Coulam CB, Graham ML 2nd, Spelsberg TC (1984) Androgen insensitivity syndrome: gonadal androgen receptor activity. Am J Obstet Gynecol 150:531–533

Daudin M, Bieth E, Bujan L et al (2000) Congenital bilateral absence of the vas deferens: clinical characteristics, biological parameters, cystic fibrosis transmembrane conductance regulator gene mutations, and implications for genetic counseling. Fertil Steril 74:1164–1174

Gale ME (1983) Hermaphroditism demonstrated by computed tomography. AJR Am J Roentgenol 141:99–100

Gambino J, Caldwell B, Dietrich R et al (1992) Congenital disorders of sexual differentiation: MR findings. AJR Am J Roentgenol 158:363–367

Johnson PT, Horton KM, Fishman EK (2009) Adrenal imaging with MDCT: nonneoplastic disease. AJR Am J Roentgenol 193:1128–1135

Kartagener M, Stucki P (1962) Bronchiectasis with situs inversus. Arch Pediatr 79:193–207

Kennedy MP, Noone PG, Leigh MW et al (2007) High-resolution CT of patients with primary ciliary dyskinesia. AJR Am J Roentgenol 188:1232–1238

Kim SH, Pollack HM, Cho KS et al (1993) Tuberculous epididymitis and epididymo-orchitis: sonographic findings. J Urol 150:81–84

Lambert B (1951) The frequency of mumps and of mumps orchitis and the consequences for sexuality and fertility. Acta Genet Stat Med 2:1–166

Macleod J (1951) Semen quality in 1000 men of known fertility and in 800 cases of infertile marriage. Fertil Steril 2:115–139

Moon MH, Kim SH, Cho JY et al (2006) Scrotal US for evaluation of infertile men with azoospermia. Radiology 239:168–173

Nghiem HT, Kellman GM, Sandberg SA et al (1990) Cystic lesions of the prostate. Radiographics 10:635–650

Noone PG, Leigh MW, Sannuti A et al (2004) Primary ciliary dyskinesia: diagnostic and phenotypic features. Am J Respir Crit Care Med 169:459–467

Purohit RS, Wu DS, Shinohara K et al (2004) A prospective comparison of 3 diagnostic methods to evaluate ejaculatory duct obstruction. J Urol 171:232–235 discussion 235–236

Quinzii C, Castellani C (2000) The cystic fibrosis transmembrane regulator gene and male infertility. J Endocrinol Invest 23:684–689

Rutgers JL, Scully RE (1991) The androgen insensitivity syndrome (testicular feminization): a clinicopathologic study of 43 cases. Int J Gynecol Pathol 10:126–144

Siminoski K, D'Costa M, Walfish PG (1990) Hypogonadotropic hypogonadism in idiopathic hemochromatosis: evidence for combined hypothalamic and pituitary involvement. J Endocrinol Invest 13:849–853

Sivit CJ, Hung W, Taylor GA et al (1991) Sonography in neonatal congenital adrenal hyperplasia. AJR Am J Roentgenol 156:141–143

Sparacia G, Banco A, Midiri M et al (1998) MR imaging technique for the diagnosis of pituitary iron overload in patients with transfusion-dependent beta-thalassemia major. AJNR Am J Neuroradiol 19:1905–1907

Takihara H, Sakatoku J, Cockett AT (1991) The pathophysiology of varicocele in male infertility. Fertil Steril 55:861–868

Tizzano EF, Silver MM, Chitayat D et al (1994) Differential cellular expression of cystic fibrosis transmembrane regulator in human reproductive tissues. Clues for the infertility in patients with cystic fibrosis. Am J Pathol 144:906–914

Yousem DM, Geckle RJ, Bilker W et al (1996) MR evaluation of patients with congenital hyposmia or anosmia. AJR Am J Roentgenol 166:439–443

# Undescended Testis: Prevalence and Clinical Features

Francesco M. Minuto, Mara Boschetti, and Umberto Goglia

## Contents

**Abstract**

Undescended testis is the most common congenital abnormality of the male urogenital tract being present in about 3% of full term and in up to 30% of preterm newborn infants. In general this condition is transient, as in the majority of cases the testes descend into the scrotum within the first months of life. The diagnosis is primarily based on clinical examination and subsequent morphological approach and endocrine tests. The latter are particularly useful for differentiation of cryptorchidism from anorchia and the vanishing testis syndrome. The undescended testis can cause an impairment of normal spermatogenesis. The risk of developing a testicular tumor is four times higher than normal in undescended testis, particularly in intra-abdominal testes. Early diagnosis and management are needed to preserve fertility and improve early detection of testicular malignancy.

## 1 Introduction

Undescended testis, the most common genital malformation in male population, is due to the failure of migration of at least one testicle from abdomen to the scrotum.

Two major forms of undescended testis are recognized: **true cryptorchidism** (when the testis is found in the physiological migration path), and **ectopia testis** (when the testis is found outside the normal pathway of descent). When no testes are evident by any diagnostic approach the term "anorchia" is used.

F. M. Minuto (✉) · M. Boschetti · U. Goglia
Department of Endocrinology and Medical Sciences,
University of Genova, Viale Benedetto XV 6,
16132 Genoa, Italy
e-mail: minuto@unige.it

M. Bertolotto and C. Trombetta (eds.), *Scrotal Pathology*, Medical Radiology. Diagnostic Imaging,
DOI: 10.1007/174_2011_193, © Springer-Verlag Berlin Heidelberg 2012

Undescended testis is a multifactorial disease involving genetic, endocrine, and environmental factors, not clearly elucidated yet, which could be involved in any of the different phases of maturation and migration of testes.

The diagnosis is primarily based on clinical examination and subsequent morphological approach and endocrine tests (basal gonadotropins, basal and stimulated testosterone levels). The latter are particularly useful for differentiation of cryptorchidism from anorchia and the vanishing testis syndrome.

Undescended testis can cause an impairment of normal spermatogenesis, oligo- and astenozoospermia. The risk of developing a testicular tumor is four times higher than normal in undescended testis, particularly in intra-abdominal testes.

## 2    Definition and Prevalence

Undescended (maldescended) testis is consequence of the failure of at least one testicle to move from the abdominal cavity, through the inguinal canal into the scrotum. It is the most common genital malformation in male population, being present in about 3% of full term and in about 30% of premature newborn infants (Ferlin et al. 2008). In general this condition is transient, as in the vast majority of cases the testes descend into the scrotum within the first 3 months of life (Toppari and Kaleva 1999; Mathers et al. 2009) so that the incidence after the first year of life is <1%.

A practical approach to this syndrome is an accurate use of nomenclature. When the testis is found intra-abdominally or in the inguinal canal the term **undescended testis** testis is the most appropriate as the testis is present but it is not in the scrotum. In the case of a not palpable testis (either located intra-abdominally or absent) the term **cryptorchidism** (from the ancient Greek "κρυπθος"—hidden—and "ορχις"—testicle) can be used, while the term *anorchia* is used when no testes are evidenced by any diagnostic approach. Other anomalies of testicular descent involve migration of the testes in a position out of the physiological migration path (*ectopia testis*).

## 3    Factors Involved in Testicular Descent

The specific mechanism causing the undescended testis is partly obscure, but there is evidence about a multifactorial origin of this condition. Indeed genetic, endocrine, and environmental factors are involved (Virtanen et al. 2007; Feng et al. 2009; Ferlin et al. 2009).

Male gonadal maturation leads to testis migration into the scrotum from the urogenital ridge: this process is called testicular descent. The testis must descend from the abdomen to an extracorporeal position in order to reach a lower temperature for spermatogenesis. The decrease of intratesticular temperature, as compared with abdominal temperature is in the order of 2–4°C.

Two mesentery ligaments attached to the developing gonad, the **cranial suspensory**, and the **gubernacular ligaments** seem to play major roles in this process.

During the *transabdominal phase* (between the 10 and the 23 week of gestation) the testes gradually move from their original position in the urogenital ridge to the inguinal region.

The process of transabdominal descent occurs in parallel with the shortening of the gubernacular ligament, differentiation and eversion of the cremasteric muscle. The *second phase* occurs at weeks 24–34 and consists in the caudal extension of the gubernaculum, its involution and protrusion into the scrotal sac, in the development of the processus vaginalis, and dilation of the inguinal canal by the gubernacular bulb. By consequence, the intra-abdominal pressure pushes the testis through the canal.

These two phases are regulated by different factors. During the first phase the insulin-like peptide 3 (**INSL3**) stimulates the differentiation of the gubernacular ligament and migration to the low abdominal position. In the second phase **androgens** cause regression of the cranial suspensory ligament and, in concert with other factors, produce the testicular descent into the scrotal sac.

# 4    Classification and Clinical Features

The classification and the different implications of cryptorchidism are mainly dependent on the site where the testis is found at the end of the maturation process. According to physical examination it is possible to describe **true cryptorchidism** and **ectopic testis** (Fig. 1).

## 4.1    True Cryptorchidism

This condition includes the vast majority of cases. The testis is found in the migration path and, according to its position it is identified in the abdomen, in the inguinal canal, or in the upper portion of the scrotum.

### 4.1.1    Intra-Abdominal Cryptorchidism
It represents the 10% of cases of cryptorchidism. In the bilateral intra-abdominal testis it is often impossible to find testicular tissue and the differential diagnosis between cryptorchidism and female pseudohermafroditism is possible only by the chromosomal karyotype assessment. Sometimes the testes are located just above the internal inguinal ring.

### 4.1.2    Canalicular Cryptorchidism
In this case (20%) the testicular tissue is in the inguinal canal and may move between the canal and the upper scrotum. Testes may be small and sometimes they are able to get outside the external inguinal ring; sometimes it is possible to palpate and to manipulate them in order to produce the temporary descent into the scrotum.

### 4.1.3    High scrotal Cryptorchidism
'High scrotal testis' or 'gliding testis' is the most frequent type of cryptorchidism (40%). It is usually considered a mild form of undescended testis. It is defined as a testis which can be manipulated through the scrotal entrance into a high, but unstable, scrotal position, while further traction on cord structures is painful. After release, the testis retracts immediately

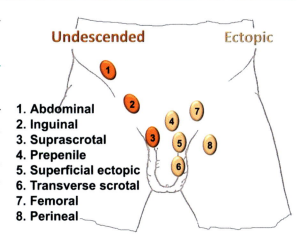

**Fig. 1** Cryptorchidism. Possible anatomical location of the undescended testis along the physiological path (1–3) and in ectopic location (4–8)

to the groin region. The retraction can make diagnosis and classification difficult.

### 4.1.4    Retractile Testis
It is a physiological condition (hypermobile testis), due to *cremasteric reflex*; recognizing the high scrotal testis from the retractile testis is particularly important because the latter does not require treatment.

### 4.1.5    Obstructed Testis
It represents the 30% of cases and consists in a testis whose descent has been prevented by fascial bands between the inguinal pouch and the scrotum.

## 4.2    Ectopic Testis

It is a rare disease, caused by an abnormality of the gubernaculum, which is attached outside the normal pathway of descent, producing the ectopic location. The testis can be found in the perineum, the femoral canal, the inguinal pouch, and the suprapubic area (Larsen 2003).

# 5    Diagnosis

The *differential diagnosis* of undescended testis is with anorchia and vanishing testis syndrome.

In prepubertal children with nonpalpable gonads, **testosterone**, **LH**, and **FSH** in serum should be measured to evaluate the hormonal asset, and the karyotype should be assessed to exclude a genetic disease; a *stimulation test with hCG* is required in case of suspected bilateral anorchia because if the response of testosterone is absent the surgical exploration is useless. Also the measurement of serum Anti Mullerian Hormone/Mullerian Inhibiting Substance (**AMH/MIS**) can be useful to determine testicular status in differentiating anorchia from undescended testis and serving as a measure of testicular integrity in children with intersexual anomalies.

## 6    Sequelae

### 6.1    Effects on Fertility

As the normal position of testis in the scrotum is essential to assure a normal spermatogenesis, cryptorchidism is associated with defective spermatogenesis. Indeed, an history of cryptorchidism is present in about 10% of infertile males and in about 20% of azoospermic men. Impaired spermatogenesis is more frequent in bilateral and in abdominal cryptorchidism but can also be found in subjects with one cryptorchid and one normally descended testis. **Oligospermia** and **azoospermia** are present in 70–80% of subjects with bilateral and in 40–50% of subjects with unilateral cryptorchidism.

The age of orchidopexy influences the spermatogenesis but a well-timed surgery does not resolve the risk of infertility, as only about 60% of males with a history of surgical correction of bilateral cryptorchidism during early childhood are fertile (Larsen 2003; Foresta et al. 2008).

### 6.2    Risk of Testicular Tumors

Cryptorchidism represents one of the most important risk factor for the development of **testicular tumors** (four times the general population). About 10% of testicular tumors arise in undescended testes being the greatest risk associated with intra-abdominal testes. Surgical correction of cryptorchidism does not remove the risk and in a fifth of tumors associated with unilateral cryptorchidism the malignancy arises

from the contralateral normally descended scrotal testis. Indeed a fetal *testicular disgenesis syndrome* (**TDS**), characterized by congenital cryptorchidism, infertility, and development of testicular malignancy during adult age has been described (Main et al. 2009).

In a study in 300 men with previous orchidopexy, subsequent testicular biopsy revealed a testicular intraepithelial neoplasia in 1.7%, thus routine testicular biopsy at the time of orchidopexy in childhood is not recommended (Giwercman et al. 1989). Therefore, in operated cryptorchid patients a lifelong follow-up (considering that the maximum incidence of these tumors is between 15 and 40 years of age) with periodic examination of the testes is recommended.

## 7    Medical Therapy

Intra-abdominal testis requires surgical correction. The testes that cannot be brought into the scrotum should be removed. The surgical therapy is indicated also in obstructed and ectopic testes.

In canalicular or high scrotal testes the role of medical therapy is discussed. Large randomized trials have shown that treatment of boys with hCG, GNRH, or both produce the descent of testes in about 20% of cases but increase apoptosis of germ cells with possible negative effects on fertility in the adult age (Larsen 2003).

## References

Feng S, Ferlin A, Truong A et al (2009) INSL3/RXFP2 signaling in testicular descent. Ann N Y Acad Sci 1160:197–204

Ferlin A, Zuccarello D, Zuccarello B et al (2008) Genetic alterations associated with cryptorchidism. JAMA 300:2271–2276

Ferlin A, Zuccarello D, Garolla A et al (2009) Mutations in INSL3 and RXFP2 genes in cryptorchid boys. Ann N Y Acad Sci 1160:213–214

Foresta C, Zuccarello D, Garolla A et al (2008) Role of hormones, genes, and environment in human cryptorchidism. Endocr Rev 29:560–580

Giwercman A, Bruun E, Frimodt-Moller C et al (1989) Prevalence of carcinoma in situ and other histopathological abnormalities in testes of men with a history of cryptorchidism. J Urol 142:998–1001 (discussion 1001–1002)

Larsen PR (2003) Williams textbook of endocrinology. Saunders Elsevier, Philadelphia

Main KM, Skakkebaek NE, Toppari J (2009) Cryptorchidism as part of the testicular dysgenesis syndrome: the environmental connection. Endocr Dev 14:167–173

Mathers MJ, Sperling H, Rubben H et al (2009) The undescended testis: diagnosis, treatment and long-term consequences. Dtsch Arztebl Int 106:527–532

Toppari J, Kaleva M (1999) Maldescendus testis. Horm Res 51:261–269

Virtanen HE, Cortes D, Rajpert-De Meyts E et al (2007) Development and descent of the testis in relation to cryptorchidism. Acta Paediatr 96:622–627

# The Undescended Testis Management: Microsurgery and Laparoscopy

Andrea Lissiani, Giuseppe Ocello, and Carlo Trombetta

## Contents

**Abstract**

The mainstay of therapy for undescended testes is surgical treatment within the first years of life in order to avoid ongoing testicular degenerative changes. The surgical therapy for the palpable undescended testis is orchidopexy and when the testis is non-palpable the laparoscopic approach is considered both as a diagnostic tool as well as an important therapeutic solution. In this article the different aspects of the laparoscopic approach to undescended testis will be described and discussed.

## 1 Introduction

Cryptorchidism, sometimes also referred as "undescended testis", is commonly defined as the absence of the testicle in the scrotum and regards 1/150 of full-term newborns. In 80% of the cryptorchid cases the testicle can be found in the groin while only in the remaining 20% the testicle is non-palpable (Levitt et al. 1978).

The diagnostic modalities available to locate the non-palpable testis can be divided into "non-invasive" and "minimally-invasive". Non-invasive techniques are represented by ultrasound, CT and MR imaging; on the contrary arteriography, venography and laparoscopy are considered as minimally-invasive techniques. However, all the radiological evaluations have been found to be insufficiently sensitive to locate the testicle. Since 1976 Cortesi has proven that laparoscopy is the most affordable option among all the other diagnostic solutions (Cortesi et al. 1976). Moreover further data suggest that laparoscopic

A. Lissiani · G. Ocello · C. Trombetta (✉)
Department of Urology, University of Trieste,
Ospedale di Cattinara, Strada di Fiume 447,
34124 Trieste, Italy
e-mail: trombcar@units.it

M. Bertolotto and C. Trombetta (eds.), *Scrotal Pathology*, Medical Radiology. Diagnostic Imaging,
DOI: 10.1007/174_2011_194, © Springer-Verlag Berlin Heidelberg 2012

outcomes in identification and management of non-palpable testis are superior to those of open surgical approaches (Docimo 1995).

A non-palpable testis can be described at the time of diagnosis as absent (vanishing), intra-abdominal or inside the inguinal canal (intra-canalicular) (Cisek et al. 1998). In the presence of an intra-abdominal testis, laparoscopy is recommended not only for examination of the testicle but also for its removal in case of an adult patient with a normal contralateral gonad in order to prevent malignant transformation, or to perform an orchidopexy whenever possible (Jordan and Winslow 1994).

Huff clearly showed the development of abnormal histologic changes after 12 months thus resulting in recommendation for orchidopexy (Huff et al. 1987). Recent studies suggest that the optimal timing for orchidopexy is at 6 months as it emphasizes the anatomical advantages of the children's small size coupled with the real chances for spontaneous descent (Elder 2004). On the contrary the role of orchidopexy in older child is less well defined regarding the fertility potential; nevertheless its usefulness must be considered for the androgen production. Adult healthy males with unilateral undescended testis are recommended to undergo orchiectomy (Oh et al. 2002).

Actually, it is worldwide approved that only laparoscopy can definitely diagnose the presence or absence of intra-abdominal testis (Baker et al. 2001).

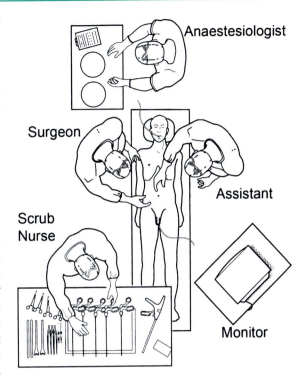

**Fig. 1** Operating room setup and surgical team positions for a left-sided laparoscopic orchidopexy

## 2 Preoperative Preparation

The patient is informed of the standard laparoscopic risks of bleeding, infection, injury of intra-abdominal viscera or vessels as well as the specific risks of testicular atrophy in case of injury of the gonadal vessels or vas deferens. The need for orchiectomy or the potential for conversion to an open procedure are also explained.

Under general anesthesia, the patient is placed in supine position with the monitor at the foot of the bed. The primary surgeon stands on the opposite side of the affected testis while the assistant surgeon lies contralateral. The scrub nurse stands on the same side of the primary surgeon (Fig. 1).

The standard instrumentation includes a 0° laparoscope, an atraumatic grasper, a monopolar scissor, a clip applier and a needle-holder. If available the harmonic scalpel may come in help, even if it is not mandatory and also quite expensive. Both in pediatric and adult patients, the procedure can easily be carried out with three 5 mm trocars even if sometimes a 10 mm trocar can be useful, especially in the adult. In pediatric departments 3 or 2 mm instruments are widely available. In case of orchidopexy a fourth port is sometimes used for the delivery of the testis.

The first trocar is placed in the periumbilical region according to the preferred open Hasson approach or, less commonly, with the Veress needle. After the pneumoperitoneum is created, the laparoscope is inserted and the peritoneal cavity inspected. Usually two other 5 mm ports are sufficient to complete the procedure: they can be placed both along the pararectal line just underneath the umbilicus in a symmetrical fashion or asymmetrically towards the affected groin depending on the size of the patient (Fig. 2). The preparation is completed setting the peritoneal pressure from 10 to 12 mmHg and placing the bed in Trendelenburg position.

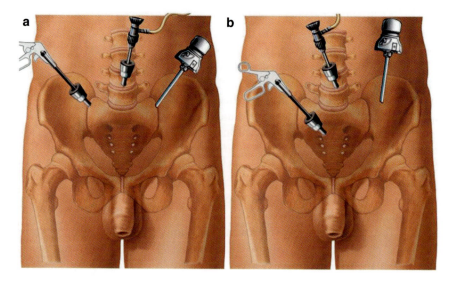

**Fig. 2** Trocars placement for laparoscopic orchydopexy: **a** pediatric patient, **b** adult or small patient

## 3    Diagnostic Procedure

Begin the exploration of the peritoneal cavity with a brief inspection at the inner inguinal ring: the normal aspect is marked by the confluence of the spermatic vessels laterally with the vas deferens medially. The umbilical artery and the external iliac vessels along with the epigastric vessels are also usually seen at this point (Fig. 3). The spermatic vessels are useful to guide the surgeon to the testis which can be anywhere along the path of the normal testicular descent from the renal hilum to the inguinal ring.

  Depending on the findings, different scenarios are possible:

- Normal spermatic vessels and normal vas deferens exit the internal inguinal ring which can be
  - *Closed* is advisable to explore the groin for a possible atrophic remnant which needs to be removed as in 10% of the cases it contains germ cells that may be responsible of undergoing malignant change.
  - *Open* a viable intra-canalicular or peeping testis can be present and can be revealed by gentle pressure over the groin. Otherwise the groin must be inspected for atrophic testis.
- *Blind-ending vas deferens is identified without blind-ending spermatic vessels* a dysjunction between the testis and the Wolfian structures occurred so further laparoscopic exploration is required to identify the gonadal vessels.

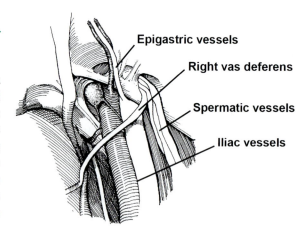

**Fig. 3** Laparoscopic view. Normal anatomical relationships during inspection of the abdominal wall. The normal right vas deferens joins the normal spermatic vessels at the inner inguinal ring

- *Blind-ending vas deferens and blind-ending spermatic vessels are identified* these findings are pathognomonic for the vanishing testis and no further exploration is required.
- *Intra-abdominal testis is located*
  - *Near the inguinal ring or below the iliac vessels* one-stage laparoscopic orchidopexy is appropriate.
  - *Far from the inguinal ring with short vascular pedicle* two-stage laparoscopic orchidopexy should be considered.

  Data show that 50% of all cases are represented by intra-abdominal or peeping testis, 30% are atrophic remnants and the remaining 20% vanishing testis.

## 4   Therapeutic Procedure

The spermatic vessels and the vas deferens compound the two sides of a triangle where the testis is the apex: the opening of this triangle allows the access to the pedicle mobilization (Fig. 4).

A peritoneotomy is made to surround the internal inguinal ring. Grasping the apex of the peritoneum just distally to the testis and retracting it cranially, exposes the gubernaculum and its vascularization in order to thin it and cut it across. Attention must be paid to identify and avoid injury to a long looping vas deferens. The testis is then further bluntly mobilized freeing as much as possible its vas deferens and spermatic vessels. The preservation of the triangle of peritoneum between the vas and vessels usually ensures further blood supply to these structures. At this time, if the testicle can be pulled towards the opposite internal inguinal ring, then the mobilization is sufficient to place the testicle inside the ipsilateral hemiscrotum in a tension-free fashion following a path, which is medial to the umbilical artery and lateral to the bladder.

After adequate mobilization is achieved, a subdartoic pouch must be created through a hemiscrotal incision. A simple and safe solution adopted to deliver the testicle into the hemiscrotum is carried out by placing a 10 mm trocar from the scrotal incision. An atraumatic grasper is inserted through the port and the testis is grasped at the gubernaculum and smoothly extracted while removing the trocar under direct visual control from the inside to avoid torsion. Alternatively, a grasper can be directly inserted inside the abdominal cavity from the scrotal incision passing over the symphysis pubis. Fixation of the testicle into the Dartos pouch and control for active bleeding are done at the end of the procedure.

In case of high testis, the Prentiss maneuver can be considered. After high retroperitoneal mobilization of the spermatic vessels, a new inguinal canal is created by passing a grasper medially to the epigastric vessels and laterally to the umbilical artery all through the anterior abdominal wall fascia just above the pubic tubercle.

If mobilization is inadequate even after wide proximal dissection, then consider switching to a two-stage Fowler–Stephens orchidopexy (Fowler and Stephens 1959; Caldamone and Amaral 1994). As a

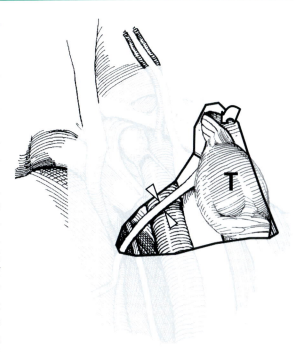

**Fig. 4** Laparoscopic view of an intra-abdominal testis located at the inner inguinal ring. The vas deferens (*arrowheads*) and spermatic vessels (*curved arrow*) are the two sides of a triangle where the testis is placed at its apex (T). The opening of this triangle is necessary to begin the pedicle mobilization

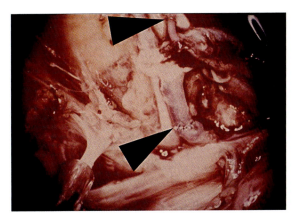

**Fig. 5** Microsurgical anastomosis (*arrowheads*) of the spermatic vessels with the inferior epigastric vessels

general guideline, a testicle more than 2 cm away from the internal inguinal ring is at risk for a tension-free orchidopexy whereas a distance superior to 4 cm between the testis and inguinal ring necessarily requires a vessels transaction. In stage one, the spermatic vessels are proximally clipped with a 5 mm

**Table 1** Comparison of open versus laparoscopic orchidopexy success rates from two large series

|  | Primary orchidopexy | | Two-stage Fowler Stephens orchidopexy | |
| --- | --- | --- | --- | --- |
|  | Patients | Success rate (%) | Patients | Success rate (%) |
| Open procedure (Docimo 1995) | 80 | 81.3 | 56 | 76.8 |
| Lap procedure (Baker et al. 2001) | 178 | 97.2 | 58 | 87.9 |

clip applier. After 6 months stage two is carried out: at this time a collateral blood supply develops by means of the deferential and cremasteric arteries. Nevertheless do not forget to inform the patient that atrophy may occur during this period and orchiectomy could be necessary. With the same placement of the ports as before, the previously clipped vessels are transected and the testis is mobilized on the vas deferens. Great care must be taken to preserve all perivasal tissue and the peritoneal triangle. Placement of the testicle in the scrotal pouch is the same as described for primary orchidopexy.

In selected cases microvascular autotransplantation might be considered, mostly in the presence of variability of collateral vascular supply that could compromise the Fowler–Stephens procedure. This technique has first been described by Silber and Kelly (1976) and then modified by Wacksman et al. (1996). After accurate laparoscopic preparation and transposition of the inferior epigastric vessels, the spermatic vessels are anastomosed with the inferior epigastric artery and vein under loupe magnification by means of the operative microscope (Fig. 5). Even if a direct end-to-end anastomosis is described, in our experience an end-to-side anastomosis in an interrupted fashion using 9–10/0 prolene stitches is advisable (Giuliani et al. 1984).

## 5 Complications

Incidence of acute testicular atrophy may vary from 3 to 13% in case of primary orchidopexy or two-stage Fowler–Stephens orchidopexy, respectively and depends on excessive skeletonization of the spermatic vessels, extreme use of electrocautery, inadvertent torsion of the spermatic vessels during the descent of the testicle inside scrotal pouch or a result of the transaction of the vessels during the Fowler–Stephens procedure (Docimo 1995; Lindgren et al. 1999). Other operative complications are quite uncommon and include the following: injury to the abdominal

viscera (in case of blind insertion of the first trocar when performed after Veress needle insufflations), injury to the bladder (especially during the Prentiss maneuver if the catheter drainage has not been verified), bleeding due to damage of great vessels (which could even require emergent conversion to open laparotomy), mechanical injury to the vas deferens during mobilization, and indirect inguinal hernia (Esposito et al. 2003; Metwalli and Cheng 2002).

## 6 Postoperative Management

Diet is advanced early and the patient can be discharged within 24–48 h. Oral narcotics may be necessary for the first few days. Straddle activities are prohibited for the next 4 weeks. Postoperative follow-ups are carried out at 1 week, 1 month and 6 months after surgery.

## 7 Surgical Results

As for all new techniques, also validation of laparoscopic management of undescended testicle needs to be compared to the gold standard of open surgical approach. Large published series confirmed the overall superiority of the laparoscopic orchidopexy over the open counterpart both in the preservation and division of the spermatic vessels where success rate is defined as absence of testicular atrophy and adequate scrotal position (Baker et al. 2001; Chang et al. 2001). The most compromising results are obviously obtained in primary orchidopexy whether open or laparoscopic (Table 1).

## 8 Conclusions

Laparoscopy is gaining more support in every urological field every day. Also in the management of non-palpable testicle the advantages of laparoscopic approach, represented mainly by improvement in visualization and mobilization of critical structures, outweigh the disadvantages. On the other hand, many series have been reported the identification of intra-abdominal testis after negative open exploration. For these many reasons, laparoscopy is becoming world-wide the standard procedure in both evaluation and therapeutic solution for undescended testicle, clearly overcoming the traditional open counterpart.

# References

Baker LA, Docimo SG, Surer I et al (2001) A multi-institutional analysis of laparoscopic orchidopexy. BJU Int 87:484–489

Caldamone AA, Amaral JF (1994) Laparoscopic stage two Fowler–Stephens orchidopexy. J Urol 152:1253–1256

Chang B, Palmer LS, Franco I (2001) Laparoscopic orchidopexy: a review of a large clinical series. BJU Int 87: 490–493

Cisek LJ, Peters CA, Atala A et al (1998) Current findings in diagnostic laparoscopic evaluation of the non-palpable testis. J Urol 160:1145–1149 (discussion 1150)

Cortesi N, Ferrari P, Zambarda E et al (1976) Diagnosis of bilateral abdominal cryptorchidism by laparoscopy. Endoscopy 8:33–34

Docimo SG (1995) The results of surgical therapy for cryptorchidism: a literature review and analysis. J Urol 154:1148–1152

Elder JS (2004) Management of the abdominal undescended testicle. Presented at the American Association of Genito-urinary Surgeons. Amelia Island FL, April 2004

Esposito C, Lima M, Mattioli G et al (2003) Complications of pediatric urological laparoscopy: mistakes and risks. J Urol 169:1490–1492 (discussion 1492)

Fowler R, Stephens FD (1959) The role of testicular vascular anatomy in the salvage of high undescended testes. Aust N Z J Surg 29:92–106

Giuliani L, Carmignani G, Belgrano E et al (1984) Testis autotransplantation. Prog Reprod Biol Med 10:153–158

Huff DS, Hadziselimovic F, Duckett JW et al (1987) Germ cell counts in semithin sections of biopsies of 115 unilaterally cryptorchid testes. The experience from the Children's Hospital of Philadelphia. Eur J Pediatr 146(Suppl 2):S25–S27

Jordan GH, Winslow BH (1994) Laparoscopic single stage and staged orchiopexy. J Urol 152:1249–1252

Levitt SB, Kogan SJ, Engel RM et al (1978) The impalpable testis: a rational approach to management. J Urol 120:515–520

Lindgren BW, Franco I, Blick S et al (1999) Laparoscopic Fowler–Stephens orchiopexy for the high abdominal testis. J Urol 162:990–993 (discussion 994)

Oh J, Landman J, Evers A, Yan Y, Kibel AS (2002) Management of the postpuberal patient with cryptorchidism: an updated analysis. J Urol 167:1329–1333

Metwalli AR, Cheng EY (2002) Inguinal hernia after laparoscopic orchiopexy. J Urol 168:2163

Silber SJ, Kelly J (1976) Successful autotransplantation of an intra-abdominal testis to the scrotum by microvascular technique. J Urol 115:452–454

Wacksman J, Billmire DA, Lewis AG et al (1996) Laparoscopically assisted testicular autotransplantation for management of the intraabdominal undescended testis. J Urol 156:772–774

# Imaging the Undescended Testis

Eriz Özden, Ahmet T. Turgut, and Vikram S. Dogra

## Contents

E. Özden (✉)
Department of Urology,
Ankara University School of Medicine,
06100 Ankara, Turkey
e-mail: erizozden@yahoo.com

A. T. Turgut
Department of Radiology,
Ankara Training and Research Hospital,
06590 Ankara, Turkey

V. S. Dogra
Department of Imaging Sciences,
University of Rochester School of Medicine,
601 Elmwood Ave, Box 648,
Rochester, NY 14642, USA

**Abstract**

Undescended testis, i.e., cryptorchidism, implies failure of testicular descent into the scrotum with concomitant abnormality in testicular development. It represents an important clinical entity because of its close association with infertility and testicular malignancy. Abnormalities in anatomical and hormonal factors involved in embryogenesis and testicular descent may all have a role in the etiology of cryptorchidism, though the exact mechanism is not fully understood. The diagnosis of the entity depends mainly on laparoscopy and the role of imaging is controversial, though diagnostic imaging has been considered to be helpful particularly for the evaluation of patients with a nonpalpable undescended testis. US is the most common diagnostic imaging study employed in the evaluation of cryptorchidism. The technique is accepted as the first step after clinical evaluation, whereas MRI has been proposed as the modality of choice preoperatively when US findings are negative.

## 1 Incidence and Background

Undescended testis (UDT), i.e., cryptorchidism, implies failure of testicular descent into the scrotum with concomitant abnormality in testicular development. It is considered as an important clinical entity because of its close association with infertility and testicular malignancy. UDT is the most common abnormality in male infants with reported incidences of 2–8% for full term and 20–33% for preterm neonates (Burgu et al. 2010; Christensen and Dogra 2007;

M. Bertolotto and C. Trombetta (eds.), *Scrotal Pathology*, Medical Radiology. Diagnostic Imaging,
DOI: 10.1007/174_2011_195, © Springer-Verlag Berlin Heidelberg 2012

Virtanen et al. 2007). The higher frequency noted in preterm infants is attributed to the occurrence of birth before completion of the inguinoscrotal migration of the testes. Notably, the entity is usually unilateral and has a prediliction for the right side, with 70 and 30% of the cases being right- and left-sided, respectively (Burgu et al. 2010). Infrequently, both testes may be affected by the abnormality.

UDT can be divided into two major groups as palpable and nonpalpable testes (NPT), with the former group comprising undescended and ectopic testes. Furthermore, retractile testes can be included to palpable testes category (Burgu et al. 2010). On the other hand, about 20% of all UDT is nonpalpable, which includes intra-abdominally or inguinally located testes and absent testes (Christensen and Dogra 2007). It is suggested that 40–80% of NPT has an intra-abdominal or inguinal location, whereas the rest is believed to be atrophic or absent. However, the literature data regarding the frequencies of the aforementioned locations for NPT is variable. Importantly, the primary goal of imaging here is to find the location of the NPT. Although the exact mechanism resulting in cryptorchidism is not fully understood, abnormalities both in anatomical and hormonal factors involved in embryogenesis and testicular descent may all have a role in the etiology. For better understanding the mechanisms involved in the etiopathogenesis of cryptorchidism, the multistaged process of testicular migration to the scrotum including transabdominal and inguinoscrotal phases should be overviewed.

## 2 Phases of Testicular Descent

### 2.1 Transabdominal Descent Phase

The gonadal development starts during the 5–7th weeks after fertilization. The differentiated testis remains near the lower pole of the kidneys until 10–15th weeks of gestation. In the transabdominal phase the abdominal cavity enlarges, where the ascent of testes is prevented by regression of the cranial suspensory ligament and enlargement of the gubernaculum, with the testes remaining anchored to the inguinal area (Christensen and Dogra 2007; Virtanen et al. 2007). The gubernaculum, the key structure for testicular descent in humans, is the caudal ligament of the testis which is also

described as caudal genital ligament (Burgu et al. 2010; Hutson et al. 1997). It is believed to facilitate testicular descent by preventing cranial migration during abdominal phase. It is also suggested that the proximal gubernacular cord shortens during testicular descent, which may be an important part of the mechanism of positioning of the testis over the inguinal ring (Heyns and Hutson 1995). Additionally, the regression of the cranial suspensory ligament, which is an embryologic structure holding the urogenital tract near the developing diaphragm and fixating the testis to the kidney, plays a role in gonadal descent (Christensen and Dogra 2007; Hutson et al. 1997). The transabdominal phase of testicular descent lasts until about 15th week of gestational age (Hutson and Hasthorpe 2005a).

Although transabdominal descent is mainly regulated by gubernacular enlargement and regression of the cranial suspensory ligament, some endocrine factors such as mullerian inhibiting substance (MIS) (antimullerian hormone) and insulin-like hormone (INSL3) are also believed to be involved in the process.

### 2.2 Inguinoscrotal Descent Phase

After the transabdominal phase the testes remains stationary near the inguinal ring until the 7th month, when they begin to descend through the inguinal canal (Christensen and Dogra 2007). The inguinoscrotal migration which starts approximately at 28th week is completed at 36–40th weeks of gestation (Christensen and Dogra 2007; Virtanen et al. 2007). Notably rising abdominal pressure, processus vaginalis, androgen control and, especially significant movement of the gubernaculum are required for inguinoscrotal phase (Christensen and Dogra 2007; Hutson et al. 1997). The intrabdominal pressure rise has a direct impact on testis and particularly on formation of processus vaginalis, which serves as an intraperitoneal path for the descending testis (Hutson et al. 1995). It is noteworthy that the development of proccessus vaginalis and the inguinal canal is accepted to be a seperate phase of testicular descent by some authors (Burgu et al. 2010). The gubernaculum which reaches its maximum diameter during the 7th month of gestation induces the widening of the inguinal canal and the testis which is attached caudally to the gubernaculum, bulges beyond the external inguinal ring and descends further down to the scrotum through processus vaginalis (Heyns 1987; Hutson and Hasthorpe 2005; Moore and Persaud 1993; Virtanen et al. 2007). After the descent, the gubernaculum involutes and leaves a fibrous remnant known as the scrotal ligament. Finally, the processus vaginalis closes at 37–40th weeks of gestation (Christensen and Dogra 2007; Moore and Persaud 1993).

It has been reported that androgen production has a significant impact on the inguinoscrotal phase (Ritzen et al. 2007). Accordingly, it has been suggested that androgens may control the migration and growth of the gubernaculum via the sensory branch of genito-femoral nerve innervating the gubernaculum and its neurotransmitter calcitonin gene-related peptide (Hutson and Hasthorpe 2005a, b). In this regard, the migration of the gubernaculum beyond the inguinal region is believed to be absent in gonadotrophin–deficient animals and in animals who have complete androgen resistance (Kaplan et al. 1986).

## 3 Etiology

Cryptorchidism is simply the result of any abnormality affecting the aforementioned phases of testicular descent. Owing to the fact that the transabdominal phase is rarely affected, intrabdominal testes comprises only 5–10% of UDT (Hutson et al. 1997). On the contrary, the inguinoscrotal phase is affected more frequently and UDT is commonly located near the neck of the scrotum or outside the external ring in most cases (Hutson et al. 1997). From etiological point of view, four different type of abnormalities are suggested to be associated with cryptorchidism, namely hormonal abnormalities (androgen deficiency), mechanical abnormalities (inguinal canal obstruction associated with Prune belly syndrome or posterior urethral valve, abdominal wall defects resulting in lower abdominal pressure, processus vaginalis defects), neurological anomalies (genitofemoral nerve dysplasia), and acquired anomalies (retractile-ascending testis) (Christensen and Dogra 2007). Despite being multifactorial, the most common cause of UDT is thought to be a defect in prenatal androgen secretion (Hutson et al. 1997). Accordingly, abnormal action of hypothalamic- pituitary axis, abnormal testicular differentiation, deficient androgen production or action, and deficient

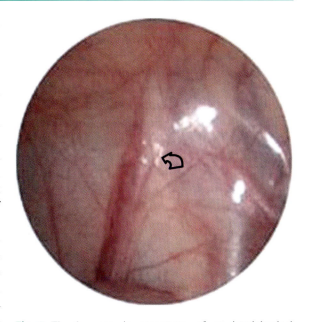

**Fig. 1** The laparoscopic appearance of an intrabdominal vanishing testes. It is very likely that the testes have developed and secreted hormones that caused ipsilateral regression of Müllerian structures and vanished due to a vascular problem. *Curved arrow* shows blind ending testicular vessels. Note that no scrotal nubbin can be palpated (*Courtesy* of Tarkan Soygür, MD, Ankara, Turkey)

action of INSL3 are among the endocrine disorders associated with UDT (Virtanen et al. 2007).

Failure in germ cell migration and induction may cause early developmental arrest resulting in the absence of the testis while late failure due to various factors like ischemia secondary to in utero torsion may lead to atrophy or absence of the testis (Christensen and Dogra 2007). The entity of absent testis may be categorized as vanishing testis and testicular agenesis. The detection of testicular vessels and a vas deferens in spite of the absence of the testis itself on surgical exploration reveals a vanishing testis (Fig. 1) (Burgu et al. 2010). The abnormality is believed to be the result of in utero infarction of a normal testis secondary to gonadal vessel torsion (Burgu et al. 2010). Testicular agenesis, on the other hand, results from failure of the testicular blood supply or from abnormal gonadal ridge differentiation (Burgu et al. 2010). Another abnormality, testicular dysgenesis syndrome, may be caused by chromosomal or endocrine factors at the time of sex determination (Christensen and Dogra 2007). Furthermore, several genetic disorders may cause maldescent of the testis. UDT is also common in some inherited syndromes and some specific urological disorders such as Prune belly syndrome and posterior urethral valves and patients with neural tube defects have also a high frequency of UDT (Hutson et al. 1997). In case of bilateral NPT, anorchidism and ambigious genitalia should be considered in the differential diagnosis and, an urgent and thorough evaluation must be performed to rule out life threatining congenital adrenal hyperplasia (Burgu et al. 2010).

## 4 The Retractile and Ascending Testis

As 3.8% of all boys demonstrate uni- or bilateral UDT at birth and most of them descend into the scrotum during the first 3 months, the final diagnosis should not be established before 6 months of age (Ritzen 2008). In this regard, the definition "ascending testis" refers to the testis which is normally located in the scrotum in infancy and located too high in later periods of childhood (Fenton et al. 1990). The term "retractile testis", on the other hand, implies a suprascrotal testis which can be manipulated into the scrotum, whereas those lacking this feature are called as "ascending testis" or "acquired cryptorchidism" (Christensen and Dogra 2007). Notably, a retractile testis is typically normal in size, whereas a true UDT may be smaller than a normal testis (Burgu et al. 2010). On the other hand, the laparoscopic finding of a testis moving in and out of the internal inguinal ring during laparoscopy is called "peeping" testis (Fig. 2).

The suggested etiology for acquired UDT is a short spermatic cord or strong cremasteric reflex. The latter term refers to cremasteric muscle contraction, and the stimulation of this reflex in low temperatures results in retraction of the testis from the scrotum to the inguinal region (Christensen and Dogra 2007; Hutson et al. 1997). This reflex, which is mediated by the cutaneous temperature receptors of the genitofemoral nerve, is usually weak at birth and becomes prominent between 3 and 10 years of age, followed by a period of gradual weakening (Hutson et al. 1997). It is proposed that the strength of the reflex is inversely proportional to androgen levels and becomes stronger than normal in androgen deficiency (Christensen and Dogra 2007; Hutson et al. 1997). Naturally, this results in a higher testicular position as the child grows. According to another theoretical mechanism for testicular ascent proposed by Agarwal et al. (2006), the spermatic cord

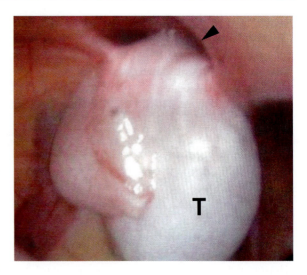

**Fig. 2** The laparoscopic appearance of a peeping testis. The testis (*T*) can be palpated when it is in the inguinal canal but becomes nonpalpable when peeps back to the abdominal cavity. *Arrowhead*, internal ring of the inguinal canal (*Courtesy* of Tarkan Soygür, MD, Ankara, Turkey)

may have a limited growth potential or a fibrous persistence, and the testis may move out of the scrotum as the spermatic cord of the ascending testis fails to keep up with the somatic growth.

In general, the management of retractile testes involves a clinical follow-up because the risk of ascent in a retractile testis may be as high as 32–50% (Agarwal et al. 2006; La Scala and Ein 2004). For the ascended testes that cannot be manipulated into the scrotum, orchiopexy has been accepted as the treatment of choice.

## 5 Risks and Clinical Significance of UDT

Infertility secondary to impairment of spermatogenesis and higher incidence of testicular cancer are considered as the major risks in UDT. Normally, the testis is located in the scrotum with an enviroment having a temperature lower than the normal body temperature (33°C, 91°F). It is believed that secondary degeneration of the UDT is related to higher temperature levels which decrease production of androgens and/or MIS and causes defective or delayed germ cell maturation, reduced number of germ and leydig cells and testicular atrophy in turn (Christensen and Dogra 2007). Due to a failure in the

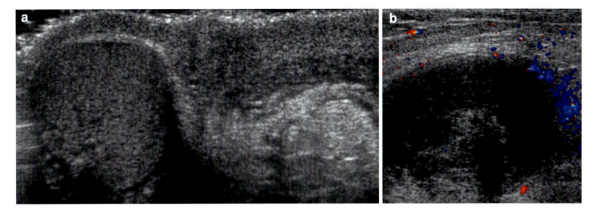

**Fig. 3** Torsion of a cryptorchid testis. **a** Gray-scale ultrasound scan demonstrating an undescended testis within the inguinal canal with the spermatic cord of a normal left testis. **b** Color Doppler ultrasound of the cryptorchid testis demonstrating absent intratesticular flow consistent with torsion. Adapted with permission from Christensen and Dogra (2007)

first step in postnatal spermatogenic developement, spermatogonia is deficient in infants with UDT (Huff et al. 1991, 1993). The decrease in germ cell number begins approximately at 4 months and becomes prominent after 6 months of age (Huff et al. 1991; Virtanen et al. 2007). After 2 years of life, the spermatogonia is found normal only in 10% of cryptorchid testes (Cortes 1998; Cortes et al. 2006). Inevitably, these findings neccessitate early surgical correction for UDT before 1 year of age.

Compared to the risk in the healthy population, a 4–7 fold increase has been noted for the risk of testicular malignancy in UDT, which is considered to be secondary to germ cell degeneration and dysplasia (Hutson et al. 1997; Whitaker 1988). Unfortunately, these degenerated germ cells are believed to be premalignant. Notably, the risk of malignancy is higher for intrabdominally located testes compared to those located in the inguinal canal. Interestingly, an increased incidence of malignancy has also been reported in the contralateral descended testis (Pincowzki et al. 1991). A single postpubertal biopsy of each testis at 18–20 years of age has been recommended for the identification of possible carcinoma in situ and malignant changes (Christensen and Dogra 2007; Giwercmann et al. 1989). Among the testicular tumors, seminoma is the most common malignancy seen in cryptorchid testes, whereas nonseminomatous tumors predominate following orchiopexy (Giwercmann et al. 1989). The patient age at the time of operation has a significant impact on malignancy risk. In a cohort study, it has been found that the risk of testicular cancer among men who were 13 years or older at the time they were operated was approximately twice that among men who underwent orchiopexy before the age of 13 (Pettersson et al. 2007). The authors also reported that the standardized incidence ratio for testicular cancer was 2.02 and 6.24 for those within the ranges of 0–6 and 16–19 years of age, respectively, during orchiopexy (Pettersson et al. 2007).

Testicular torsion which is believed to be caused by poor fixation or a persistent suspensory structure contiguos with the gubernaculum that fixates the epididymis to the testis, and inguinal hernia associated with a patent proccessus vaginalis are other entities believed to have higher incidences in patients with UDT (Fig. 3) (Christensen and Dogra 2007; Dogra et al. 2006; Lam et al. 2001). Owing to the fact that a tumoral mass and gonadal distortion may predispose to gonadal rotation resulting in vascular compromise, the likelihood of torsion is aggravated by the increased incidence of testicular malignancy in cryptorchid patients (Christensen and Dogra 2007; Dogra et al. 2006). Notably, surgical treatment of the cryptorchid testis by orchiopexy and inguinal hernia repair are performed in tandem, since they are almost always present concurrently (Christensen and Dogra 2007).

## 6 Treatment

Apart from observation, which may be the choice of management for patients younger than 1 year of age, the two major definitive treatment approaches for

UDT in older patients are surgery and hormonal treatment as spontaneous descent thereafter is uncommon and the risk of progressive gonadal dysgenesis increases (Christensen and Dogra 2007). The aim of surgery, which is the primary choice of treatment for most patients, is to locate and replace the testis into the scrotum and maintain the normal testicular function. Among the surgical options to locate a NPT are laparoscopy, open abdominal exploration, inguinal exploration, and retroperitoneal exploration (Desireddi et al. 2008; Elder 2002). It has been predicted that accuracy of locating a testis by laparoscopy, which is becoming the standard approach for the management of NPT, is approximately 97% in case the testis is present (Fig. 4) (Gatti and Ostlie 2007). Nevertheless, some surgeons still prefer initial scrotal exploration rather than initial laparoscopy to establish the diagnosis and facilitate the management of unilateral NPT (Snodgrass et al. 2007). The laparoscopic findings can provide guidance to other surgical approaches such as groin exploration, orchiectomy, orchiopexy, and laparoscopic mobilization (Gatti and Ostlie 2007). The most commonly preferred surgical approach for UDT is orchiopexy which can be performed either typically under laparoscopical guidance or with open exploration. Technically, orchiopexy involves mobilization of the UDT with its spermatic cord and vascular pedicle and delivering the testis into a pouch created within the scrotum (Christensen and Dogra 2007). In general, success rate of orchiopexy for inguinal testes has been reported to be greater than 95% in most series, while the relevant rate has been noted to be greater than 85–90% for abdominal testes (Taran and Elder 2006). On the other hand, orchiectomy may be performed when a nubbin, which can be defined as a vanished testis or a testicular remnant possibly following intrauterine torsion, is identified (Snodgrass et al. 2007). The timing of surgery is crucial for preventing degeneration and preserving testicular function. In this regard, early intervention before 1 year of age is recommended, though the surgery should not be performed within the first 6 months because of the high rate of spontanous descent during the first month (Ritzen 2008).

Medical treatment, which is based on the hormonal dependence of testicular descent phases, targets the hypothalamic-pituitary–gonadal axis and consists of exogenous administration of human choriogonadotropin (HCG) or gonadotropin-releasing hormone (GnRH)

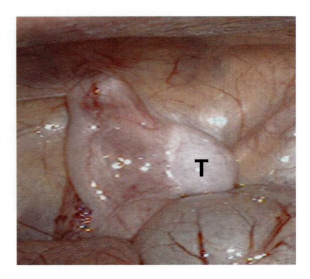

**Fig. 4** The laparoscopic appearance of an undescended intrabdominal testis (*T*), which is always nonpalpable (*Courtesy of* Tarkan Soygür, MD, Ankara, Turkey)

(Christensen and Dogra 2007). The hormonal therapy is most effective in infants with unilateral undescended testis within the inguinal canal, with a reported testicular descent success rate of roughly 65% (Giannopoulos et al. 2001). However, the overall efficacy of hormonal treatment alone for cryptorchidism is poor, with reported rates less than 20% and up to 25% of the testes have been reported to reascend to a suprascrotal position after hormonal treatment (Ong et al. 2005; Ritzen et al. 2007).

## 7 Radiological Evaluation

Imaging is useful both for localizing a NPT or visualizing the possible degenerative-malignant changes in a palpable UDT. A NPT which may be situated in the scrotum may be too small to palpate. Alternatively, it may be localized anywhere along the normal pathway of testicular descent, namely intrabdominal region, internal inguinal ring, inguinal canal, or external inguinal ring (Fig. 5). Although various locations have been reported for intrabdominal testes, the majority is located within a distance less than 2 cm from the internal inguinal ring (Burgu et al. 2010). A testis located in the inguinal canal can migrate to abdominal position intermittantly (peeping testis) or may be lacking (Nijs et al. 2007). Rarely, the

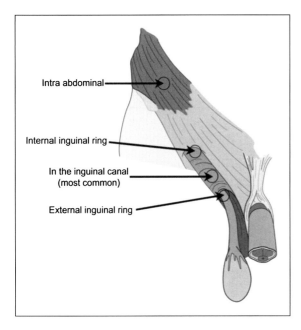

Fig. 5 *Line drawing* demonstrating common locations of cryptorchid testis. Adapted with permission from Christensen amd Dogra (2007)

testis may also have an ectopic location, and hence, be located at the perineum, femoral canal, superficial inguinal pouch, or contralateral hemiscrotum (Dogra et al. 2003). Among these, superficial inguinal pouch which is defined as a subcutaneous pocket in front of and lateral to the external ring, has been noted as the most common ectopic location (Dogra et al. 2003).

Apparently, an ideal imaging study should document the presence or absence of a testis and its location, and hence guide laparoscopy or inguinal or abdominal surgical approach. However, the role of imaging has become almost controversial because of the recent reports suggesting that the sensitivity of radiological tools for imaging a NPT is insufficient. Recently, imaging has been noted not to alter the decision for performing the surgery itself or for the choice regarding the surgical approach. In this regard, diagnostic imaging seems useless in cases of NPT. Hence, it has been recommended by some authors that laparoscopy or inguinal exploration should be performed regardless of the presence of the testis in the imaging studies, as the latter evaluation by imaging has a high false negative rate and the overall accuracy for localizing a NPT by magnetic resonance imaging (MRI) or ultrasonography (US) is less than 85% (Gatti and Ostlie 2007; Kanemoto et al. 1986;

O'Hali et al. 1997). The same authors also suggest that surgical exploration is necessary when the testis is not identified by imaging, and they propose exploration also for the situations where the testis is identified as exploration is also required for orchiopexy. In this regard, diagnostic imaging has recently been considered an unnecessary step as laparoscopic orchiopexy is becoming the standard operation. On the other hand, some surgeons still prefer knowing the exact location of the testis before laparoscopy, which can be possible by imaging studies. Furthermore, imaging may still be beneficial for preoperative planning in some cases. Not surprisingly, physical examination for an UDT has been noted to be difficult in overweight boys (Hutson et al. 1995). MRI, on the other hand, has been proposed for the same purpose as laparoscopy may be more difficult to perform and has a higher complication rate in obese children (De Filippo et al. 2000). Imaging may also be useful for the follow-up of cryptorchid boys who are not suitable for surgery because of comorbid conditions (Burgu et al. 2010). Notably, US has been found helpful in the newborn with genital ambiguity in which uterus, enlarged adrenals, and inguinal testes should be identified (Elder 2002).

## 7.1 US

Thanks to its well-known advantages such as wide availability, lack of ionizing radiation, and relatively shorter duration of the study, US has been accepted as an ideal imaging modality for children with UDT. It is the most common diagnostic imaging study employed in the evaluation of cryptorchidism. Routinely, the inguinal canal and lower abdomen must be scanned by US to visualize a NPT. On conventional gray scale US, an UDT is seen as a hypoechoic round or oval structure between 7 and 15 mm in maximum diameter (Fig. 6) (Cain et al. 1996; Christensen and Dogra 2007). For an exact diagnosis, the mediastinum testis, which is an invagination of the tunica albuginea posteriorly, must be identified as a linear hyperechogenicity within the testicular parenchyma (Fig. 7). Despite having a high accuracy for the detection of cryptorchid testes lying below the internal inguinal ring, US has an unacceptably low success for locating nonpalpable abdominal testes (Nijs et al. 2007; Wolverson et al. 1983). In a recent study, almost all

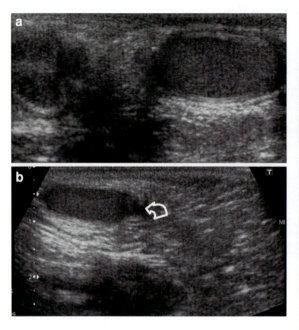

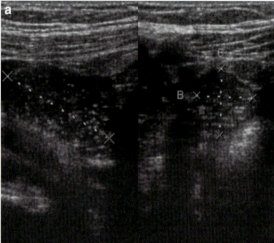

**Fig. 6** Five year-old male with cryptorchid left testis. **a** Transverse gray-scale ultrasound of the scrotum shows that the left testis is in its normal position in the left hemiscrotum, whereas the right scrotal sac is empty. **b** Longitudinal gray scale US of the right inguinal canal reveals an undescended testis which is elongated, relatively smaller in size, and having normal echogenecity (*curved arrow*)

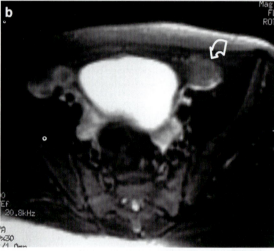

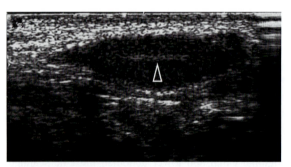

**Fig. 7** Longitudinal gray-scale ultrasound shows the mediastinum testis in the cryptorchid left testis as a linear hyperechogenicity (*arrowhead*) within the testicular parenchyma

**Fig. 8** 13 year-old male with, cryptorchid left testis. **a** Longitudinal (*left*) and transverse (*right*) ultrasound pelvic scans showing undescended left testis with multiple, tiny nonshadowing echogenecities randomly scattered throughout the testicular parenchyma implying microlithiasis **b** T2 W transverse pelvic MR image of the same patient demonstrating a well-defined, nodular soft tissue with left paravesical location consistent with intraabdominally located left undescended testis (*curved arrow*) (*Courtesy* of Suat Fitöz, MD, Ankara, Turkey)

viable inguinal testes were reported to be correctly located by US, whereas only half of the abdominal testes could be detected successfully by the technique (Nijs et al. 2007). In the same study, only 68% of the NPT were successfully localized by US (Nijs et al. 2007). In another study, the authors reported a sensitivity rate of 76%, a false negativity rate of 24%, and an accuracy rate of 84% for the diagnosis of NPT by US (Kanemoto et al. 1986).

US can also reveal testicular microlithiasis which may be an additional predisposing condition for testicular germ cell tumor in patients with UDT necessitating tighter surveillance of these patients (Fig. 8). However, controversy still exists regarding the cost-effectiveness of sonographic follow-up of these patients, though the incidence of testicular microlithiasis in UDT is comparable with the incidence in asymptomatic patients. Not surprisingly, it is very uncommon to visualize by US an intrabdominally located and atrophic testis. Difficulty in differentiating a UDT from a lymph node or the bulbous terminal part of the gubernaculum and inability to distinguish an atrophic testis from an agenetic one are the main limitations of US in the evaluation of UDT (Rosenfield et al. 1989). Finally, US has been recommended by some authors as the first step after clinical evaluation and MRI has been proposed as the modality of choice preoperatively when US is negative (Kanemoto et al. 1986).

## 7.2 CT

CT is mainly used for imaging the nonpalpable testis (Fig. 9). The sensitivity of CT for identifying testes in the inguinal canal is similar to US, whereas it is significantly higher for the detection abdominal testes with reported rates within the range of 94–100% (Lee and Glazer 1982; Wolverson et al. 1983). The typical finding for a NPT is a mass located in the inguinal canal or between the internal inguinal ring and lower pole of the pelvis with uniform enhancement after intravenous contrast administration (Christensen and Dogra 2007). The mediastinum testis cannot be depicted with CT, whereas the spermatic cord leading to testis can be traced (Rosenfield et al. 1989). The low body fat percent in infants may decrease the utility of CT as it technically depends on the presence of fat for imaging (Desireddi et al. 2008). Owing to the fact that CT lacks the sensitivity and specificity required for accurate diagnosis of testicular agenesis, nonvisualization of the testis does not preclude the need for surgery, as is the case for US (Christensen and Dogra 2007). Finally, inherent disadvantages of CT like radiation exposure and the requirement for iodinated intravascular contrast material limit the utility of the technique for the management of UDT.

## 7.3 MRI

Despite having the advantages of not involving ionizing radiation and higher soft tissue contrast compared to US and CT, the use of MRI for the evaluation of NPT has been limited by various drawbacks such as necessitating patient sedation in the pediatric age group and relatively higher cost. Moreover, bowel

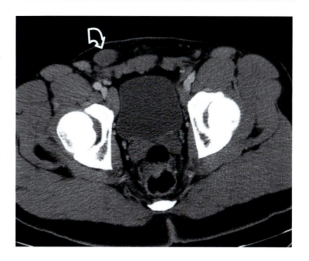

**Fig. 9** CT scan of pelvis shows a right-sided undescended testis (*curved arrow*)

movements obscuring the intrabdominally located testis which might hamper the differentiation of testis from nodal tissue might pose as a technical limitation (Desireddi et al. 2008). The proposed protocol for localizing a NPT involves evaluation from the level of the kidneys to the pelvic outlet using T1 W, T2 W, and gadolinium enhanced T1 W sequences in both axial and coronal planes (Christensen and Dogra 2007). On T1 W images the testis will be visualized as a hypointense ovoid mass while on T2 W and postcontrast images it will appear hyperintense (Fig. 10) (Christensen and Dogra 2007). Nevertheless, an atrophic testis may appear hypointense on T2 images (Rosenfield et al. 1989). The visualization of mediastinum testis, which has been reported as the only absolute finding that identifies a structure as an undescended testis is helpful for confirming the diagnosis, though it may not be seen always (Kier et al. 1988). Additionally, features of malign degeneration can also be detected by MRI. Based on a sensitivity of 79% and a specificity of 100%, MRI has been noted to be a reliable method for for the localization of nonpalpable undescended testes (Sarihan et al. 1998).

More recently, the sensitivity, specificity, and accuracy of the technique for the relevant evaluation were reported to be 86, 79, and 85%, respectively (Kanemoto et al. 1986). In the latter report, all false positive cases were noted to have been confused with the surrounding lymph node tissue, which was reported as a disadvantage for MRI. In another report

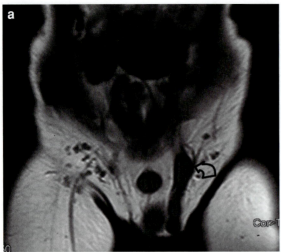

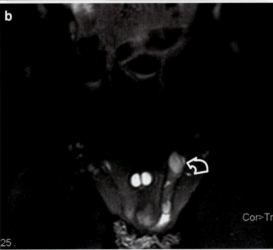

**Fig. 10** Left canalicular testis in 16 year-old boy (**a**, **b**) T1 W and T2 W coronal abdominal MR images showing unde-scended testis at the left side of the groin with respective hypointense and hyperintense appearences (*curved arrows* in **a** and **b**)

by Rosenfield et al. (1989), distal bulbous segment of the gubernaculum was reported to be of similar signal intensity with the normal testis on T1 W images and hypointense compared to normal testis on T2 W images, which could not be distinguished reliably from an atrophic ectopic testis. In the same study, it was also noted that the spermatic cord leading to the testis and distal bulbous part of gubernaculum have identical properties on MR imaging.

In another study by Lam et al. (2001) evaluating the adjunctive value of gadolinium-infusion magnetic resonance venography (MRV) to locate the impalpable testis, the technique was reported to be superior to

MRI in the detection of atrophic testes. Technically, MRV enables the determination of the testicular location by the detection of bright linear enhanced pampiniform venous plexus (Lam et al. 2001). In this regard, gadolinium enhanced MRV has been proposed as the only means for differentiating testicular agenesis from ectopia (Lam et al. 2001).

Recently, the application of magnetic resonance arteriography (MRA) and MRV after gadolinium administration has been noted by Desireddi et al. (2008) to be capable of identifying not only the spermatic vessels and pampiniform plexus during the delayed venous phase but also the testicular tissue itself. In the same report, the accuracy of MRI and MRA/MRV for identifying a viable testis was only 74 and 67%, respectively (Desireddi et al. 2008). Accordingly, the authors concluded that preoperative MRI or MRA/MRV should not be recommended for identification of NPT (Desireddi et al. 2008). However, MRA/MRV can be helpful for the diagnosis of a testicular nubbin by enabling the visualization of the spermatic cord vessels ending blindly, that is without visualization of the testicular parenchyma or ending in a nubbin of tissue (Desireddi et al. 2008). In another report, Eggener et al. (2005) noted that nubbin surgery can be avoided by means of MRA/MRV thanks to the high accuracy of MRA/MRV in identifying testicular nubbin and low risk of malignancy in the nubbin tissue. On the contrary, in the aforementioned report by Desireddi et al. (2008), it was noted that MRA/MRV could identify only three of nine nubbins, whereas the other six cases were incorrectly reported as viable testes. In this regard, the authors concluded that MRI can serve as a screening tool for NPT and aid in surgical planning but cannot exclude a testis if imaging is negative (Desireddi et al. 2008). On the other hand, Lam et al. (2001) proposed that, if the testis could not be found on MRI, the cause can be a vanishing testis or an unidentified intrabdominal testis, and the surgeon must proceed to laparoscopy as leaving an intrabdominal testis with significantly higher risk of malignant degeneration is unacceptable.

## 8    Conclusion

Cryptorchidism is an important clinical entity which is strongly associated with infertility and testicular malignancy. The diagnosis depends mainly on laparoscopy where the role of imaging is controversial. In general, US is accepted to be the initial study of choice for a palpable undescended testis, whereas CT and/or MRI may be required for localizing a nonpalpable one, particularly in cases where the US findings are negative. Nevertheless, applying directly diagnostic laparoscopy without performing imaging studies may be the method of choice in some centers.

**Acknowledgements** We would like to acknowledge our sincere thanks to Tarkan Soygür, MD for his providing Figs. 1, 2, and 4 and Suat Fitöz, MD for his providing Fig. 8.

# References

Agarwal PK, Diaz M, Elder JS (2006) Retractile testis is it really a normal variant? J Urol 175:1496–1499

Burgu B, Baker LA, Docimo SG (2010) Cryptorchidism. In: Gearhart JP, Rink RC, Mouriquand PDE (eds) Pediatric Urology, second edn. Elsevier, Philadelphia

Cain MP, Gara B, Gibbons MD (1996) Scrotal-inguinal ultrasonography: a technique for identifying the nonpalpable inguinal testis without laparoscopy. J Urol 156:791–794

Christensen JD, Dogra VS (2007) The undescended testis. Semin Ultrasound CT MRI 28:307–316

Cortes D (1998) Cryptorchidism-aspects of pathogenesis, histology and treatment. Scand J Urol Nephrol Suppl 196: 1–54

Cortes D, Thorup J, Petersen BL (2006) Testicular histology in cryptorchid boys- aspects of fertility. J Pediatr Surg Special 1:34–37

De Filippo RE, Barthold JS, Gonzales R (2000) The application of magnetic resonance imaging for the preoperative localization of nonpalpable testis in obese children: an alternative to laparoscopy. J Urol 164:154–155

Desireddi NV, Liu DB, Maizels M et al (2008) Magnetic resonance arteriography/venography is not accurate to structure management of the inpalpable testis. J Urol 180:1805–1809

Dogra VS, Gottlieb H, Oka M et al (2003) Sonography of the scrotum. Radiology 227:18–36

Dogra VS, Bhatt S, Rubens DJ (2006) Sonographic evaluation of testicular torsion. Ultrasound Clin 1:55–66

Eggener SE, Lotan Y, Cheng EY (2005) Magnetic resonance angiography for the nonpalpable testis: a cost and cancer risk analysis. J Urol 173:1745–1750

Elder JS (2002) Ultrasonography is unnecessary in evaluating boys with a nonpalpable testis. Pediatrics 110:748–751

Fenton EJM, Woodward AA, Hudson IL et al (1990) The ascending testis. Pediatr Surg Int 4:6–9

Gatti JM, Ostlie DJ (2007) The use of laparoscopy in the management of nonpalpable undescended testes. Curr Opin Pediatr 19:349–353

Giannopoulos MF, Vlachakis IG, Charissis GC (2001) 13 years' experience with the combined hormonal therapy of cryptorchidism. Horm Res 55:33–37

Giwercmann A, Brunn E, Frimodt-Moller C et al (1989) Prevalance of carcinoma in situ and other histopathological abnormalities in testes of men with a history of cryptorchidism. J Urol 142:998–1001

Heyns CF (1987) The gubernaculum during testicular descent in the human fetus. J Anat 153:93–112

Heyns CF, Hutson JM (1995) Historical review of theories in testicular descent. J Urol 153:754–767

Huff DS, Hadziselimovic F, Synder HM III et al (1991) Early postnatal testicular development in cryptorchidism. J Urol 146:624–626

Huff DS, Hadziselimovic F, Synder HM III et al (1993) Histologic maldevelopment of unilaterally cyrptorchid testes and their descended partners. Eur J Pediatr 152(suppl 2):10–14

Hutson JM, Hasthorpe S (2005a) Abnormalities of testicular descent. Cell Tissue Res 322:155–158

Hutson JM, Hasthorpe S (2005b) Testicular descent and cryptorchidism: the state of art in 2004. J Pediatr Surg 40:297–302

Hutson JM, Terada M, Zhou B et al (1995) Normal testicular descent and aetiology of cryptorchidism. Adv Anat Embryol Cell Biol 132:1–56

Hutson JM, Hasthorpe S, Heyns CF (1997) Anatomical and functional aspects of testicular descent and cryptorchidism. Endocr Rev 18:259–280

Kanemoto K, Hayashi Y, Kojıma Y et al (1986) Accuracy of ultrasonography and magnetic resonance imaging in the diagnosis of non-palpable testis. Int J Urol 12:668–672

Kaplan LM, Kolye MA, Kaplan GW et al (1986) Association between abdominal wall defects and cryptorchidism. J Urol 136:645–657

Kier R, McCarthy S, Rosenfield AT et al (1988) Nonpalpable testes in young boys:evaluation with MR imaging. Radiology 169:429–433

La Scala GC, Ein SH (2004) Retractile testes: an outcome analysis on 150 patients. J Pediatr Surg 39:1014–1017

Lam WWM, Tam PK, Ai VH et al (2001) Using gadolinium-infusion MR venography to show the impalpable testis in pediatric patients. Am J Roentgenol 176:1221–1226

Lee JK, Glazer HS (1982) Computed tomography in the localization of the nonpalpable testis. Urol Clin North Am 9:397–404

Moore KL, Persaud TVN (1993) The developing human: clinically oriented embryology. Saunders, Philadelphia

Nijs SMP, Eijbouts SW, Madern GC et al (2007) Nonpalpable testis: is there a relationship between ultrasonographic and operative findings? Pediatr Radiol 37:374–379

O'Hali W, Anderson P, Giacomantonio M (1997) Management of impalpable testes; indications for abdominal exploration. J Pediatr Surg 32:918–920

Ong C, Hasthorpe S, Hutson JM (2005) Germ cell development in the descended and cryptorchid testis and the effects of hormonal manipulation. Pediatr Surg Int 21:240–254

Pettersson A, Richiardi L, Nordenskjold A et al (2007) Age at surgery for undescended testis and risk of testicular cancer. N Engl J Med 356:1835–1841

Pincowzki D, McLaughlin JK, Lackgren G et al (1991) Occurence of testicular cancer in patients operated on for cryptorchidism and inguinal hernia. J Urol 146:1291–1294

Ritzen EM (2008) Undescended testis: a consensus on management. Eur J Endocrinol 159:87–90

Ritzen EM, Bergh A, Bjerknes R et al (2007) Nordic consensus on treatment of undescended testes. Acta Paediatr 96:638–643

Rosenfield AT, Blair DN, McCarthy S et al (1989) The pars infravaginalis gubernaculi: importance in the identification of the undescended testis. Am J Roentgenol 153:775–778

Sarihan H, Sari A, Abes M et al (1998) Nonpalpable undescending testis: value of magnetic resonance imaging. Minerva Urol Nefrol 50:233–236

Snodgrass WT, Yucel S, Ziada A (2007) Scrotal exploration for unilateral nonpalpable testis. J Urol 178:1718–1721

Taran I, Elder JS (2006) Results of orchiopexy for the undescended testis. World J Urol 24:231–239

Virtanen HE, Cortes D, De Meyts ER et al (2007) Development and descent of the testis in relation to cryptorchidism. Acta Paediatr 96:622–627

Whitaker RH (1988) 9 Neoplasia in crytorchid men. Semin Urol 6:107–109

Wolverson MK, Houttin E, Heiberg E et al (1983) Comparision of computed tomography with high resolution real-time ultrasound in the localization of the impalpable undescended testis. Radiology 146:133–136

# Incidental Scrotal Findings at Imaging-1: Calcifications

Michele Bertolotto, Marco M. Cavallaro, Ferruccio Degrassi, Micheline Djouguela Fute, and Pietro Pavlica

## Contents

### Abstract

Scrotal calcifications are commonly encountered in the clinical practice at ultrasound, and they may be occasionally identified also at CT and Rx ray examination performed for other purposes. Intra- or extra-testicular calcifications have different clinical relevance. Intratesticular calcifications are usually benign, but may also be found in tumors, or follow trauma, infarction, and inflammation. Testicular microlithiasis is increasingly encountered in otherwise healthy men. Currently, there is no evidence that it is either a premalignant condition or a causative agent for neoplasia, but a clear association exists between this condition, other testicular calcifications, and an increased risk of testicular malignancy. Extra-testicular calcifications are more frequent than intratesticular calcifications and are almost always benign. They include scrotal pearls, calcifications of the epididymis and appendages, and those involving the tunicae and the scrotal wall.

M. Bertolotto (✉) · M. M. Cavallaro · F. Degrassi ·
M. D. Fute
Department of Radiology, University of Trieste,
Ospedale di Cattinara, Strada di Fiume 447,
34124 Trieste, Italy
e-mail: bertolot@units.it

P. Pavlica
Servizio di Diagnostica per Immagini,
Villalba Hospital, Via di Roncrio 25,
40136 Bologna, Italy

## 1 Introduction

Scrotal calcifications are commonly encountered in the clinical practice (Dogra et al. 2003; Oyen 2002). They are usually incidental findings at ultrasound but, occasionally, they may be identified also with other imaging modalities. Differentiation between intratesticular and extratesticular calcifications is important, and can be obtained at ultrasound in virtually all cases.

M. Bertolotto and C. Trombetta (eds.), *Scrotal Pathology*, Medical Radiology. Diagnostic Imaging,
DOI: 10.1007/174_2011_196, © Springer-Verlag Berlin Heidelberg 2012

## 2    Testicular Calcifications

Calcified foci within the testis are readily identified at ultrasound against the normal homogeneous echotexture. Most of them are benign, either isolated, or in the context of testicular microlithiasis, but there is an established association between presence of testicular calcifications and increased risk of malignancy. Moreover, testicular calcifications may be encountered within benign or malignant testicular masses.

### 2.1    Testicular Microlithiasis

This condition is usually discovered incidentally during ultrasound investigation of the testis. Microlithiasis is not detected with MR imaging, but this technique may be helpful if there is concern for a coexisting mass. Incidental identification at CT is rare, also using MDCT equipment.

Histologically microliths consist of a central calcified core surrounded by concentric laminations of cellular debris, glycoprotein, and collagen. The etiology is unknown. It is thought that calcification in the seminiferous tubules results from the formation of microliths in degenerating cells and failure of the Sertoli cells to phagocyte the debris (van Casteren et al. 2009). Testicular microlithiasis is generally bilateral. Diffuse symmetrical distribution is the characteristic pattern, but the number and distribution of calcified foci may vary, and unilateral, or circumscribed cases can be encountered.

#### 2.1.1    Prevalence of Testicular Microlithiasis
Prevalence of testicular microlithiasis varies over a wide range. This may be explained by differences in the ethnic group, selection of patients, use of a wide variety of ultrasound transducers, and different classification of testicular microlithiasis itself (van Casteren et al. 2009). In particular, with the advancement of ultrasound equipment an increasing number of microliths is identified in the testis, and therefore the incidence of microlithiasis appears now higher than in the past.

Among different races, testicular microlithiasis has been reported as most prevalent in Afro-American (14.1%), followed by Hispanic (8.5%), Taiwanese (7.6%), Asian (5.6%), and Caucasian men (4.2%)

(Costabile 2007; Chen et al. 2010). Generally speaking, in healthy men the prevalence varies between 1.5 and 5.6% (van Casteren et al. 2009). Prevalence increases markedly in infertile patients (0.8–20.0%) and in those with cryptorchidism, Down syndrome (Vachon et al. 2006), varicocele, male pseudohermaphroditism, pulmonary alveolar microlithiasis, and Klinefelter syndrome (van Casteren et al. 2009; Cast et al. 2000). Testicular microlithiasis was reported also in otherwise healthy siblings, suggesting a common risk factor, and in siblings with fragile X and pseudoxanthoma elasticum.

#### 2.1.2    Clinical Significance of Testicular Microlithiasis
Despite a variety of studies on large number of patients, the clinical significance of testicular microlithiasis remains unclear. Early studies considered it a premalignant condition. Current epidemiological investigations show no evidence that testicular microlithiasis is either a premalignant condition or a causative agent in testicular neoplasia. Goede et al. (2009), for instance, reported a 2.4% prevalence of classic testicular microlithiasis in a series of asymptomatic boys, compared to the much lower incidence of testicular cancer. Serter et al. (2008) determined similar findings in adult asymptomatic men. Several studies showed that testicular cancer would not develop in the majority of men (more than 90%) with testicular microlithiasis. There is, however, an increasing body of literature associating testicular microlithiasis with testicular germ cell tumor. In particular, increasing evidence exists of an association between testicular microlithasis and carcinoma in situ (CIS), a precursor of overt malignancy (van Casteren et al. 2009).

A lot of confusion arises from analysis of the different studies regarding this argument which, as underlined before, are different regarding the characteristics of patients, study methodology, results, and conclusions. As a consequence, there is also a debate regarding the follow-up strategy, either clinical follow-up, annual or biannual sonographic surveillance along with periodic self-examination for the early tumor detection, or tissue biopsy.

A recent systematic review and meta-analysis of the body of publications on testicular microlithiasis in adults integrates the existing data and provides a more objective estimate of the tumor risk. Conclusions were that while testicular microlithiasis is relatively common in asymptomatic men, in otherwise healthy, asymptomatic individuals the absolute risk of concurrent or interval testicular germ cell tumor or CIS is very low (Tan et al. 2010). Based on these data, the authors conclude that further surveillance or close follow-up is unwarranted in asymptomatic men with incidentally discovered microlithiasis since the vast majority of them do not have and will not develop testicular cancer. In the presence of risk factors testicular microlithiasis is associated with germ cell tumor and CIS. Since cure rates for patients developing testicular germ cell tumor are very high, however, the survival benefits resulting from early, preclinical detection and treatment of them is uncertain, and probably the complications and morbidity associated with chosing an aggressive approach toward biopsy and radiotheraphy, if CIS is identified, is not justified (Tan et al. 2010). Practice patterns in some European countries favor biopsy (van Casteren et al. 2009; Derogee et al. 2001), whereas urologists in the United States generally avoid biopsies in the absence of a testicular mass. According to Dogra et al., in our clinical practice we perform an annual or biannual follow-up of patients with testicular microlithiasis (Dogra et al. 2003), depending on the presence or not of associated risk factors. While the cost of this approach is not considered acceptable in other countries (Costabile 2007; Dagash and Mackinnon 2007; Lam et al. 2007; DeCastro et al. 2008), it is probably the best suited strategy in our clinical environment.

### 2.1.3 Ultrasound Appearance of Testicular Microlithiasis

Ultrasound appearance of testicular microlithiasis is characteristic. Multiple tiny, highly reflective foci are identified within the testis, too small to produce acoustic shadowing (Bushby et al. 2002). Absence of acoustic shadowing could also be attributable to the multilayered envelope of the microliths (Dogra et al. 2003).

The number of microliths required to define testicular microlithiasis is debated. Some authors considered testicular microlithiasis as presence of any quantity of microliths within the testis (van Casteren et al. 2009), and most of them (Fig. 1) classify patients presenting with less than five foci per ultrasound view as having limited testicular microlithiasis,

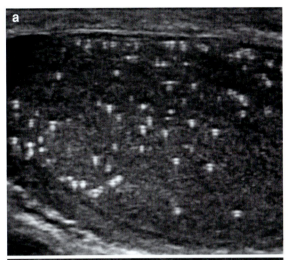

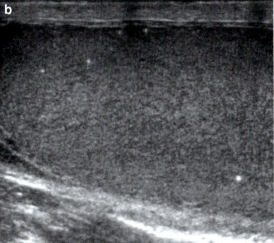

**Fig. 1** Testicular microlithiasis. **a** Longitudinal ultrasound image of the testis shows classic testicular microlithiasis. More than five microliths (*echogenic dots*) are scattered diffusely though the testis. **b** Longitudinal ultrasound image of the testis of a different patient shows limited testicular microlithiasis. Five microliths are visible in the ultrasound view

while patients having more than five foci as classic testicular microlithiasis (Middleton et al. 2002). Moreover, different degrees can be considered for classic testicular microlithiasis, depending on the number of microliths (Bennett et al. 2001).

Albeit generally accepted and widely used in the clinical practice distinction between limited and classic testicular microlithiasis is arbitrary, and, according to Middleton et al. (2002) there is no evidence of different risk of malignancy associated to them. Similarly, according to Sanli et al. (2008), the risk of malignancy does not change grading the

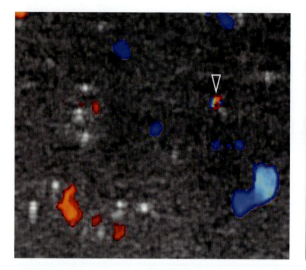

**Fig. 2** Twinkling artifact in a patient with classic microlithiasis. Color Doppler ultrasound image shows multiple microliths scattered in the parenchyma. One of them (*arrowhead*) displays the twinkling artifact, which presents as a mosaic of colors behind the microlith

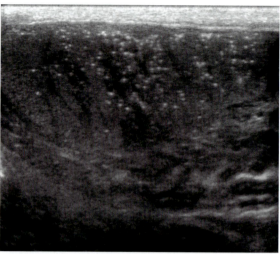

**Fig. 4** Classic testicular microlithiasis in hypothrophic testis. Longitudinal ultrasound image shows a hypothrophic testis with striated appearance and multiple microliths

microliths may display twinkling artifact (Fig. 2), but this finding is not common (Serter et al. 2008; O'Flynn and Sidhu 2009).

Besides identification of microliths, in patients with testicular microlithiasis, ultrasound has the role to seek for associated testicular masses (Fig. 3), or alterations of the parenchyma which may constitute risk factors for developing a germ cell tumor, such as abnormal echopattern, and hypotrophy (Fig. 4). A recent review, in particular, demonstrated that an irregular echopattern of the testis is suspicious for CIS (Lenz and Giwercman 2008).

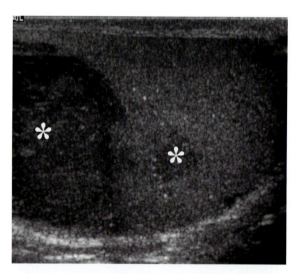

**Fig. 3** Testicular tumor with associated classic microlithiasis. Longitudinal ultrasound image shows two hypoechoic masses (*) pathologically proved to be seminomas. Multiple microliths are scattered throughout the testicular parenchyma. The contralateral testis showed classic testicular microlithiasis as well (*not shown*)

patients with classic testicular microlithiasis according to the number of microliths.

Color Doppler interrogation has a limited role in investigating patients with testicular microlithiasis. Pulsed Doppler interrogation does not show testicular vascular changes (Serter et al. 2008). Occasionally,

## 2.2 Other Testicular Calcifications

A recent study retrospectively investigated the prevalence of the different types of scrotal calcification in symptomatic patients complaining of testicular pain, lump in testis, sub-fertility, undescended testis, or suspected infection or torsion (Miller et al. 2007). In these patients, a significant association was found not only between the presence of testicular microlithiasis and tumor, but also between other types of testicular calcifications and tumor. The authors concluded that long-term follow-up deserves consideration also of patients with intratesticular calcification different from microlithiasis. Other factors, however, should be considered to stratify the risk of

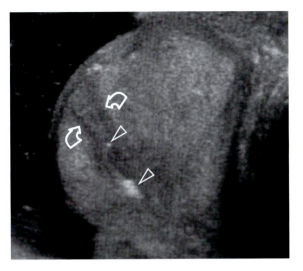

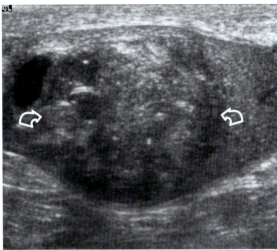

**Fig. 5** Chronic segmental testicular infarction in a patient with history of acute scrotal pain 6 years before. Grey-scale ultrasound shows a wedge-shaped hypoechoic area within the testis (*curved arrows*) containing calcification (*arrowheads*)

**Fig. 6** Calcification within a testicular mass. Longitudinal ultrasound image shows a testicular mass (*curved arrows*) containing microliths and coarse calcifications. A mature teratoma was proved pathologically

malignancy. In particular, calcifications should be evaluated by taking into account any accompanying scrotal sonographic or clinical finding, history of scrotal trauma, infection (Krone and Carroll 1985), and sports activities such as biking and horse riding. In fact, a high prevalence of testicular calcifications was found in equestrian (Turgut et al. 2005; Turksoy et al. 2006) and mountain bikers (Frauscher et al. 2001; Mitterberger et al. 2008), as a result of chronic microtraumas. It is conceivable that these patients would not have an increased risk for malignancy. Solitary punctate intratesticular calcific foci representing vascular calcifications are likely to not have pathological significance.

Chronic segmental testicular infarction often presents as a wedge-shaped hypoecoic peripheral area with punctuate or coarse calcifications representing areas of necrosis (Fig. 5). Differential diagnosis from a hypovascular tumor may be difficult. Patient history and comparison with previous investigations, whenever available, add important information which often lead toward differential diagnosis.

Many testicular tumors may contain calcification, especially mixed germ cell tumors, teratomas, and teratocarcinoma (Fig. 6). Large cell calcifying Sertoli cell tumors often present with coarse calcifications, or as an extensively calcified mass (Shin and Outwater 2007).

Dystrophic calcified nodule of the testicle is a rare lesion of unknown origin reported in a limited number of case reports (Goel et al. 2007). It presents at ultrasound and CT as a discrete calcified lesion. Malignancy, whether active or "burned out," can be excluded histologically by presence of a calcified lesion with no evidence of intratubular germ cell neoplasia and peripheral fibrous capsule. No alteration of the surrounding parenchyma is present.

Granulomatous disease and other benign testicular lesions, such as spermatic granuloma, can also present with a hypoechoic testicular mass containing areas of calcification (Bushby et al. 2002; Martin and Tubiana 1988). These lesions are difficult to differentiate from other calcific testicular masses.

## 2.3 Solid Masses with Associated Calcifications

As already discussed previously in this chapter, the most important role of imaging when testicular calcifications are identified is ruling out a testicular mass.

## 2.4 Cystic Masses with Associated Calcifications

Minimally complicated testicular cysts may present with wall calcifications and epidermoid cysts (Fig. 7) may present as a well demarcated hypoechoic mass

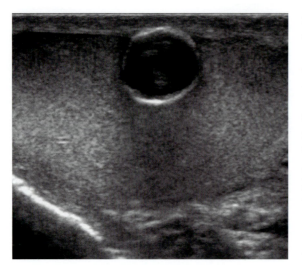

**Fig. 7** Testicular epidermoid cyst with calcified wall. Longitudinal ultrasound image shows a well demarcated hypoechoic testicular mass with echogenic central core and markedly echogenic wall (By courtesy of L.E. Derchi, Genova, Italy)

with a rim of calcification (Manning and Woodward 2010). Presence of intralesional calcified foci have been described in two surgically proved cases of epidermoid cyst in which the lesion presented as a calcified mass at ultrasound (Taghizadeh and Howlett 2000; Meiches and Nurenberg 1991). MR imaging may help differentiate these lesions from tumors because enhancement is lacking after gadolinium administration (Kim et al. 2007).

## 2.5    Isolated Macrocalcifications

Several case reports show that in patients presenting with retroperitoneal nodal metastases from germ cell tumor isolated calcific testicular foci, or clusters of small calcifications, may contain histological evidence of a regressed testicular neoplasm (Oyen 2002; Bushby et al. 2002; Comiter et al. 1996; Tasu et al. 2003). Although it is possible that regressed, "burned out" germ cell tumor might present in a similar way also in patients without secondary nodes, the vast majority of isolated coarse calcifications within the testis are encountered incidentally at ultrasound in otherwise healthy men, and are benign sequelae of trauma or infection. Differential diagnosis is possible histologically (Azzopardi et al. 1961), while no specific imaging criteria exist. History of trauma,

infection, or ischemia may help diagnosis of benign calcification.

## 3    Extra-Testicular Calcification

Calcifications within the extratesticular space are more frequent than intratesticular calcification and usually represents benign disease. They may involve all anatomical structures in the scrotum, or present as loose calcific bodies between the sheets of the tunica vaginalis.

### 3.1    Scrotal Calculi

Scrotal calculi, also known as scrotoliths or scrotal pearls, are solitary or multiple calcifications within the layers of the tunica vaginalis, usually associated with hydrocele (Namjoshi 1997; Artas and Orhan 2007). Histologically they are fibrinoid deposits around a central nidus of hydroxyapatite. Their origin is unclear. It was originally thought that scrotal pearls resulted from detachment of calcified twisted appendages (Linkowski et al. 1985), but this is unlikely because multiple scrotal calculi are identified in approximately 50% of patients and most of them do not have history of acute scrotal pain (Artas and Orhan 2007). Most authors currently think that scrotal calculi likely result from hematomas, inflammation, and repeated microtrauma. High prevalence in mountain bikers (Frauscher et al. 2001) and equestrians (Turgut et al. 2005) without previous history of acute scrotal pain supports this hypothesis.

At ultrasound scrotal pearls present typically as free-floating echogenic foci between the layers of the tunica vaginalis (Fig. 8). They are round or oval, with or without acoustic shadowing. A variable amount of fluid is usually associated. Movement of the pearls depend on their size and quantity of scrotal fluid. The larger the calculus, the less it moves (Artas and Orhan 2007).

### 3.2    Epididymal and Appendigeal Calcification

Calcifications in the epididymis are common finding (Fig. 9). They usually result from chronic epididymitis,

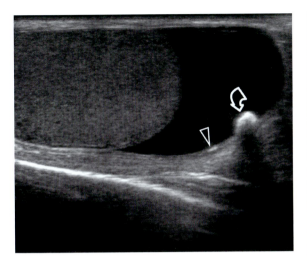

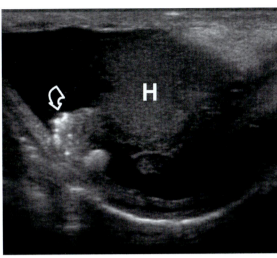

**Fig. 8** Scrotal pearl. Longitudinal ultrasound image shows hydrocele, and an echogenic calculus (*curved arrow*) with acoustic shadowing within the layers of the tunica vaginalis. A thin calcification of the outer layer of the tunica vaginalis (*arrowhead*) is also visible

**Fig. 10** Appendigeal calcification. Appendix epididymis (*curved arrow*) containing coarse and thin calcified foci (*H* = head of the epididymis)

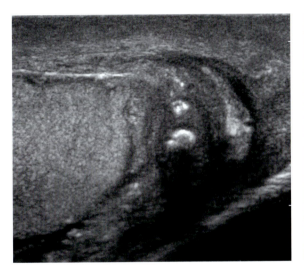

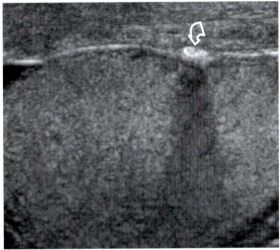

**Fig. 9** Epididymal calcification in a patient with history of epididymitis. Longitudinal ultrasound images showing enlarged epididymal tail containing coarse and thin calcifications

**Fig. 11** Tunical calcification. Localized calcification on the surface of the tunica albuginea (*arrowhead*)

but presence or history of tuberculosis and other granulomatous disease should be investigated (Bushby et al. 2002; Chung et al. 1997; de Cassio Saito et al. 2004). Epididymal calcifications may also be found in sperm granulomas, or may be posttraumatic.

Calcified appendix epididymis and appendix testis may be recognized at ultrasound by their characteristic position and shape (Fig. 10). They may follow atrophy or twisting (Sellars and Sidhu 2003), or may

result from inflammatory changes (Bushby et al. 2002).

## 3.3 Tunical Calcifications

Coarse calcifications of the tunica albuginea may follow scrotal trauma with missed albugineal rupture. Localized calcific foci secondary to minor traumas or

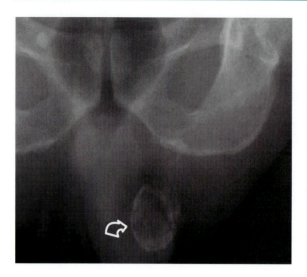

**Fig. 12** Plain X-ray showing extensive calcification of the tunica albuginea (*curved arrow*). [reprinted with permission from Elzevier et al. (2006)]

inflammation are occasionally encountered on the surface of the tunica albuginea (Fig. 11) and of the tunica vaginalis (De Luis Pastor et al. 2007). Extensive tunical calcification is very rare, and has been only reported in a limited numer of cases.

Extensive calcification of the tunica albuginea (Fig. 12) have been identified incidentally on plain radiography of the hip, and confirmed at ultrasound, in an elderly man with no history of orchitis, torsion, or trauma (Elzevier et al. 2006).

Extensive calcification of the inner surface of the tunica vaginalis may be encountered in patients with diffuse fibrous pseudotumor of the scrotum (Garriga et al. 2009). Calcification may also be secondary to chronic irritation in patients with long-standing hydroceles, especially from tuberculous infection. Intratesticular coarse calcifications may be associated (Fig. 13). A calcified hydrocele sac can be seen on plain radiography of the pelvis, and on CT. Ultrasound shows linear plaques with acoustic shadowing.

A recent case reported on a patient that developed eggshell calcification in both the tunica albuginea and the tunica vaginalis, associated to testicular ischemia, in a patient with prior severe epididymo-orchitis. At ultrasound, a double-layer echogenic line encircling the atrophic testis was found (Conkbayir et al. 2009).

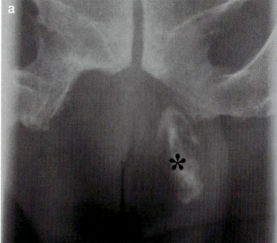

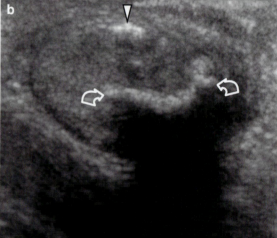

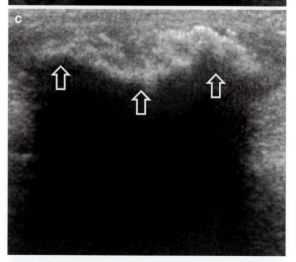

**Fig. 13** Patient with previous history of hydrocele and tuberculous epididymo-orchitis. (**a**) Plain X-ray showing tunical and testicular calcification (*). (**b, c**) Ultrasound confirms presence of coarse calcifications within the parenchyma (*curved arrows*), the tunica albuginea (*arrowhead*) and the tunica vaginalis (*arrows*)

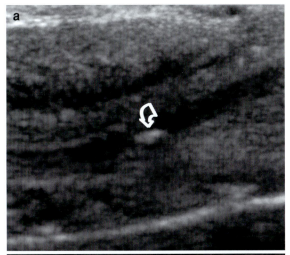

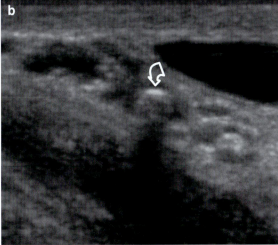

**Fig. 14** Phleboliths. Patients with varicocele (**a**) and hemangioma of the scrotal wall (**b**) showing intravenous echogenic foci consistent with calcifications (*curved arrows*)

## 3.4 Calcifications of the Scrotal Wall

Scrotal calcification may occur in infants secondary to meconium peritonitis, with leakage of meconium through the processus vaginalis during the fetal life.

Scrotal calcinosis is a rare benign condition characterized by multiple, firm, painless nodules of the scrotal wall in the absence of any systemic metabolic disorder. Histological examination reveals calcified epidermal inclusion cysts, some of which with partial or complete disintegration of their epithelial walls, associated with inflammatory infiltrate (Dubey et al. 2010; Shah and Shet 2007). Although this disorder may be encountered at any age, presentation is

prevalent between 20 and 40 years. Patients are usually asymptomatic, but may complain of itching, or discharge of white chalky material.

## 3.5 Phleboliths

Phleboliths are identified at CT as calcific foci, and at ultrasound as echogenic foci, usually with distal acoustic shadowing, within venous channels (Rastogi 2008). They are often encountered in genital hemangiomas (Fig. 14), which are benign malformations of enlarged dysplastic vascular channels with abnormal growth of endothelial cells. Rarely they may be encountered also in varicoceles.

## References

Artas H, Orhan I (2007) Scrotal calculi. J Ultrasound Med 26:1775–1779

Azzopardi JG, Mostofi FK, Theiss EA (1961) Lesions of testes observed in certain patients with widespread choriocarcinoma and related tumors. The significance and genesis of hematoxylin-staining bodies in the human testis. Am J Pathol 38:207–225

Bennett HF, Middleton WD, Bullock AD et al (2001) Testicular microlithiasis: US follow-up. Radiology 218:359–363

Bushby LH, Miller FN, Rosairo S et al (2002) Scrotal calcification: ultrasound appearances, distribution and aetiology. Br J Radiol 75:283–288

Cast JE, Nelson WM, Early AS et al (2000) Testicular microlithiasis: prevalence and tumor risk in a population referred for scrotal sonography. AJR Am J Roentgenol 175:1703–1706

Chen JL, Chou YH, Tiu CM et al (2010) Testicular microlithiasis: analysis of prevalence and associated testicular cancer in Taiwanese men. J Clin Ultrasound 38:309–313

Chung JJ, Kim MJ, Lee T et al (1997) Sonographic findings in tuberculous epididymitis and epididymo-orchitis. J Clin Ultrasound 25:390–394

Comiter CV, Renshaw AA, Benson CB et al (1996) Burned-out primary testicular cancer: sonographic and pathological characteristics. J Urol 156:85–88

Conkbayir I, Yanik B, Keyik B et al (2009) Eggshell calcification of the testis: ultrasonographic findings. J Ultrasound Med 28:1581–1583

Costabile RA (2007) How worrisome is testicular microlithiasis? Curr Opin Urol 17:419–423

Dagash H, Mackinnon EA (2007) Testicular microlithiasis: what does it mean clinically? BJU Int 99:157–160

de Cassio Saito O, de Barros N, Chammas MC et al (2004) Ultrasound of tropical and infectious diseases that affect the scrotum. Ultrasound Q 20:12–18

De Luis Pastor E, Villanueva Marcos A, Zudaire Diaz-Tejeiro B et al (2007) Scrotal ultrasound: pearls, patterns and pitfalls. Actas Urol Esp 31:895–910

DeCastro BJ, Peterson AC, Costabile RA (2008) A 5-year followup study of asymptomatic men with testicular microlithiasis. J Urol 179:1420–1423 discussion 1423

Derogee M, Bevers RF, Prins HJ et al (2001) Testicular microlithiasis, a premalignant condition: prevalence, histopathologic findings, and relation to testicular tumor. Urology 57:1133–1137

Dogra VS, Gottlieb RH, Oka M et al (2003) Sonography of the scrotum. Radiology 227:18–36

Dubey S, Sharma R, Maheshwari V (2010) Scrotal calcinosis: idiopathic or dystrophic? Dermatol Online J 16:5

Elzevier HW, Bevers RF, Wasser MN et al (2006) Testis calcification of the tunica albuginea. Eur Radiol 16:240–241

Frauscher F, Klauser A, Stenzl A et al (2001) US findings in the scrotum of extreme mountain bikers. Radiology 219:427–431

Garriga V, Serrano A, Marin A et al (2009) US of the tunica vaginalis testis: anatomic relationships and pathologic conditions. Radiographics 29:2017–2032

Goede J, Hack WW, van der Voort-Doedens LM et al (2009) Prevalence of testicular microlithiasis in asymptomatic males 0 to 19 years old. J Urol 182:1516–1520

Goel RK, Norman RW, Gupta R (2007) Dystrophic calcified nodule of the testicle: a case report. Can Urol Assoc J 1:402–403

Kim W, Rosen MA, Langer JE et al (2007) US MR imaging correlation in pathologic conditions of the scrotum. Radiographics 27:1239–1253

Krone KD, Carroll BA (1985) Scrotal ultrasound. Radiol Clin North Am 23:121–139

Lam DL, Gerscovich EO, Kuo MC et al (2007) Testicular microlithiasis: our experience of 10 years. J Ultrasound Med 26:867–873

Lenz S, Giwercman A (2008) Carcinoma-in situ of the testis—is ultrasound of the testes useful as a screening method? J Med Ultrasound 16:256–267

Linkowski GD, Avellone A, Gooding GA (1985) Scrotal calculi: sonographic detection. Radiology 156:484

Manning MA, Woodward PJ (2010) Testicular epidermoid cysts: sonographic features with clinicopathologic correlation. J Ultrasound Med 29:831–837

Martin B, Tubiana JM (1988) Significance of scrotal calcifications detected by sonography. J Clin Ultrasound 16:545–552

Meiches MD, Nurenberg P (1991) Sonographic appearance of a calcified simple epidermoid cyst of the testis. J Clin Ultrasound 19:498–500

Middleton WD, Teefey SA, Santillan CS (2002) Testicular microlithiasis: prospective analysis of prevalence and associated tumor. Radiology 224:425–428

Miller FN, Rosairo S, Clarke JL et al (2007) Testicular calcification and microlithiasis: association with primary intra-testicular malignancy in 3, 477 patients. Eur Radiol 17:363–369

Mitterberger M, Pinggera GM, Neuwirt H et al (2008) Do mountain bikers have a higher risk of scrotal disorders than on-road cyclists? Clin J Sport Med 18:49–54

Namjoshi SP (1997) Calculi in hydroceles: sonographic diagnosis and significance. J Clin Ultrasound 25:437–441

O'Flynn EA, Sidhu PS (2009) The sonographic twinkling artifact in testicular calcification. J Ultrasound Med 28:515–517

Oyen RH (2002) Scrotal ultrasound. Eur Radiol 12:19–34

Rastogi R (2008) Diffuse cavernous hemangioma of the penis, scrotum, perineum, and rectum–a rare tumor. Saudi J Kidney Dis Transpl 19:614–618

Sanli O, Kadioglu A, Atar M et al (2008) Grading of classical testicular microlithiasis has no effect on the prevalence of associated testicular tumors. Urol Int 80:310–316

Sellars ME, Sidhu PS (2003) Ultrasound appearances of the testicular appendages: pictorial review. Eur Radiol 13:127–135

Serter S, Orguc S, Gumus B et al (2008) Doppler sonographic findings in testicular microlithiasis. Int Braz J Urol 34:477–482 discussion 482–474

Shah V, Shet T (2007) Scrotal calcinosis results from calcification of cysts derived from hair follicles: a series of 20 cases evaluating the spectrum of changes resulting in scrotal calcinosis. Am J Dermatopathol 29:172–175

Shin SL, Outwater EK (2007) Benign large cell calcifying Sertoli cell tumor of the testis in a prepubescent patient. AJR Am J Roentgenol 189:W65–W66

Taghizadeh AK, Howlett DC (2000) Calcified epidermoid cyst in the testis: an unusual finding on ultrasound. Eur J Ultrasound 11:199–200

Tan IB, Ang KK, Ching BC et al (2010) Testicular microlithiasis predicts concurrent testicular germ cell tumors and intratubular germ cell neoplasia of unclassified type in adults: a meta-analysis and systematic review. Cancer 116(19):4520–4532

Tasu JP, Faye N, Eschwege P et al (2003) Imaging of burned-out testis tumor: five new cases and review of the literature. J Ultrasound Med 22:515–521

Turgut AT, Kosar U, Kosar P et al (2005) Scrotal sonographic findings in equestrians. J Ultrasound Med 24:911–917 quiz 919

Turksoy O, Ozcan N, Tokgoz H (2006) Extratesticular scrotal calcifications: their relationship with sports. J Ultrasound Med 25:141–142

Vachon L, Fareau GE, Wilson MG et al (2006) Testicular microlithiasis in patients with Down syndrome. J Pediatr 149:233–236

van Casteren NJ, Looijenga LH, Dohle GR (2009) Testicular microlithiasis and carcinoma in situ overview and proposed clinical guideline. Int J Androl 32:279–287

# Incidental Scrotal Findings at Imaging-2: Miscellaneous Benign Conditions

Ahmet T. Turgut and Vikram S. Dogra

## Contents

A. T. Turgut (✉)
Department of Radiology
Ankara Training and Research Hospital,
06590 Ankara, Turkey
e-mail: ahmettuncayturgut@yahoo.com

V. S. Dogra
Department of Imaging Sciences,
University of Rochester School of Medicine,
601 Elmwood Ave, Box 648, Rochester,
NY 14642, USA

## Abstract

High-frequency ultrasound is the imaging modality of choice for the evaluation of scrotal disorders. Infrequently, scrotal ultrasound may demonstrate a non-palpable lesion which may be detected incidentally during the examinations performed for indications such as scrotal pain, infertility, and trauma. Although most intratesticular masses are malignant, benign lesions can also occur within the testes. In the appropriate clinical setting, familiarity with the imaging features of various benign scrotal disorders may allow a prompt and accurate diagnosis thus helping to salvage the testis.

## 1   Introduction

The widespread use of ultrasonography (US) for the diagnostic evaluation of patients presenting with scrotal trauma, orchialgia, and infertility has allowed more frequent detection of incidental testicular and paratesticular lesions. Besides, current advances in US technology enable the detection of lesions as small as 1 mm and magnetic resonance imaging (MRI) has improved the diagnostic yield in equivocal cases. Apart from the relatively common disorders, various infrequently encountered entities should be considered for the differential diagnosis of scrotal lesions. Here, we review the diagnostic features of some less common benign scrotal lesions.

M. Bertolotto and C. Trombetta (eds.), *Scrotal Pathology,* Medical Radiology. Diagnostic Imaging,
DOI: 10.1007/174_2011_197, © Springer-Verlag Berlin Heidelberg 2012

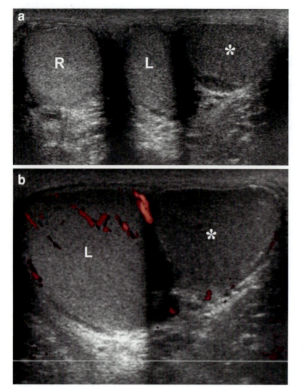

**Fig. 1** Polyorchidism. An extra testis is seen in the left hemiscrotum, which is located adjacent to the left testis (**a**), The supernumerary testis (*asteriks*) is found to have mild hypoechogenicity on gray-scale ultrasound with decreased vascularity on color flow Doppler (**b**). *R* right testis, *L* left testis (Courtesy of Mustafa Secil, MD, Izmir, Turkey)

## 2 Polyorchidism

Polyorchidism, which is a very rare developmental anomaly of the genitourinary system is defined as the presence of more than two testes within the scrotum (Öner et al. 2005). The anomaly results in supernumerary testes with a few more than 100 cases reported in the literature (Savas et al. 2010). The patients may present with a painless palpable scrotal mass on their initial evaluation, though the majority of reported cases were incidentally detected. Although triorchidism is the most common type of polyorchidism, polyorchidism involving more than three testes has been rarely reported in the literature (Amodio et al. 2004). Notably, the extra testis is predominantly on the left side (Savas et al. 2010). In about half of the cases, the anomaly is detected between 15 and 25 years of age. Embryologically, the testes develop

from a mesodermal band called the urogenital ridge, whereas the epididymis and vas deferens develop from mesonephric ducts. A developmental accident affecting any step in the union and division of the urogenital ridge and mesonephric ducts can result in a supernumerary testis (Hwang et al. 2005). In about 75% of the cases, the supernumerary testes are intrascrotal, whereas the remaining may be either inguinal or retroperitoneal (Savas et al. 2010). Importantly, the supernumerary testes are associated with an increased risk for torsion and malignancy.

On US, supernumerary testis usually appears as a homogeneous, well-defined mass which is similar in echogenicity to normal testis, although this appearance can be variable (Carkaci et al. 2010). Likewise, color Doppler US usually reveals a normal testicular flow pattern, though decreased vascularity can also be seen (Fig. 1). MRI is helpful for making a definitive diagnosis, particularly in cases with equivocal US findings. Laparoscopy, on the other hand may enable the identification of polyorchia, especially in cases with an intra-abdominally located proximal testis (Savas et al. 2010).

## 3 Tubular Ectasia of the Rete Testis

Tubular ectasia of the rete testis, also known as cystic transformation of rete testis is a benign condition resulting from partial or complete obliteration of the efferent ducts resulting in ectasia of the rete testis. This is usually associated with epididymal obstruction secondary to prior inflammation or trauma (Akin et al. 2004). Ischemia is also believed to have a role in the etiology (Nistal et al. 1996). Tubular ectasia occurs usually in men older than 50 years and is frequently bilateral and asymmetric. The entity is characterized by numerous, small spherical, or tubular anechoic structures in the region of the mediastinum testis (Fig. 2). This appearance can also extend beyond the testis in patients who have had a vasectomy (Dogra et al. 2003).

US demonstrates bilateral, multiple cystic, fluidfilled tubular structures in or adjacent to the mediastinum testis, which is very specific for its diagnosis. Color Doppler US reveals the absence of flow in these small tubular cystic structures within the rete testis, which are without calcifications or solid components. This appearance does not change much over time.

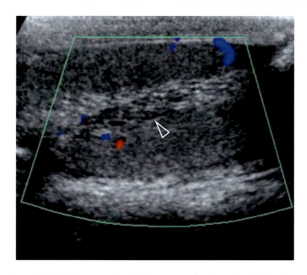

**Fig. 2** Tubular ectasia of the rete testis. Longitudinal color Doppler ultrasound image showing multiple channels with no evidence of color flow in the region of mediastinum testis consistent with mild cystic transformation of the rete testis (tubular ectasia) (*arrowhead*)

On MRI, the appearance of non-enhancing serpiginous tubular structures of low T1- and high T2-weighted signal intensity in the vicinity of the rete testis implies tubular ectasia of the rete testis (Coakley et al. 1998). The entity is commonly associated with the presence of epididymal cysts or spermatoceles, which is helpful for distinguishing it from malignant cystic testicular tumors (Bree and Hoang 1996). Cystic malignant tumors, being most commonly the teratomas, are characterized by the presence of frequently unilateral, multiple cystic areas, often surrounded by a soft tissue rind, and not limited to mediastinum (Bhatt et al. 2010). Additionally, serum tumor markers may be helpful for further confirmation. The differential diagnosis includes epididymal cystadenoma, adenocarcinoma of the rete testis, non-Hodgkin's lymphoma, and dilatation of the seminiferous tubules secondary to testicular tumor (Coakley et al. 1998). Obviously, the differentiation of this benign entity from malignant cystic tumors of the testis is crucial as this may help avoid unnecessary orchidectomy.

# 4 Testicular Fibrosis

The fibrosis of the testis manifesting as seminiferous tubule sclerosis and interstitial fibrosis may occur secondary to aging, trauma, orchitis, cryptorchidism,

inflammation, or incomplete testicular torsion. Besides, the entity may also be caused by radiation therapy (Aguado et al. 2005) and post-biopsy changes (Yagan 2000). Interestingly, inguinal hernia repair has been noted to cause testicular ischemia and fibrosis in turn. Morphologically, the fibrosis of the testis is associated with a small or normal sized testis.

On US, a striated pattern of the testicle characterized by multiple hypoechoic bands radiating from the mediastinum testis, testicular enlargement, diffuse heterogeneity of the testicular parenchyma, focal hypoechoic masses, or unilateral or bilateral focal hyperechoic masses can be detected (Fig. 3) (Yagan 2000; Kim 2002; Cohn et al. 1996; Harris et al. 2000; Einstein et al. 1992). Owing to the significant overlap in the sonographic appearance of benign fibrotic lesions and testicular malignancies, care should be taken to make an accurate diagnosis. In this regard, failure to palpate a mass in the presence of a sonographically heterogeneous or focal hypoechoic lesion and negative tumor markers should lead the clinician to consider an open biopsy with frozen section analysis rather than proceeding directly to orchiectomy (Einstein et al. 1992). On the other hand, homogeneously hyperechoic masses can be considered benign and do not require surgery (Einstein et al. 1992).

# 5 Fibrous Pseudotumor of the Testis

A fibrous pseudotumor, which is the second most common mass in the testicular adnexa after adenomatoid tumors, is a painless tumor that clinically mimics testicular and paratesticular neoplasms. Almost three-fourths of these pseudotumors arise from the tunica vaginalis, whereas the remainder affects the testis, epididymis, spermatic cord, or tunica albuginea (Rubenstein et al. 2004; Akbar et al. 2003). The etiology for the entity is not known exactly. A reactive nature is suggested in some cases by a history of trauma, surgery, infection, or inflammatory hydrocele, though this history is absent in many cases (Rubenstein et al. 2004). Fibrous pseudotumor of the testis is considered as a benign fibroinflammatory reaction resulting in the formation of one or more nodules, diffuse thickening, or a plaque-like process of the testicular capsule rather than a neoplasm (Woodward et al. 2003). The peak incidence is in the

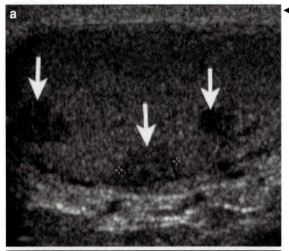

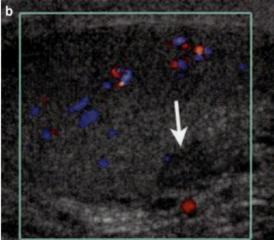

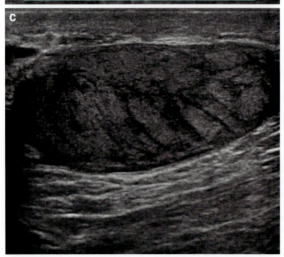

**Fig. 3** Testicular fibrosis. A 63-year-old male with previous history of left orchiectomy for a seminoma and history of radiation therapy. Gray-scale (**a**), color flow Doppler (**b**) ultrasound show normal-sized testis with multiple avascular hypoechoic masses (*arrows*), which were found to be stable on follow-up ultrasound. Gray-scale sonogram of the testis in a 85-year-old male (**c**) depicting age related testicular fibrosis resulting in a striated pattern. [**a** and **b**, Reprinted from Bhatt et al. (2010) with permission]

third decade of life, though these lesions occur within a wide age range. Although the patients are usually asymptomatic, they may present with a painless scrotal lump of widely varying sizes or unilateral scrotal swelling.

On US, the appearance of fibrous pseudotumors is widely variable and depends upon the fibrous and cellular tissue present. Fibrous pseudotumors can appear as a well-defined hyperechoic or hypoechoic mass on US without another specific appearance (Fig. 4) (al-Otaibi et al. 1997; Germaine and Simerman 2007). In this regard, single or multiple nodules ranging from 0.5 to 8 cm may occasionally detach from the tunical surface and give rise to floaters or scrotal pearls in the tunical space (Rubenstein et al. 2004). Less commonly, US may reveal plaques or slight focal thickening in the tunica albuginea without abnormalities in the testicle (Rubenstein et al. 2004). MRI, on the other hand, reveals low signal intensity on T1- and T2-weighted MRI images (Coakley et al. 1998). Because of the fibrous pseudotumor's sonographic similarity to malignant neoplasms, the diagnosis of these patients may be challenging necessitating surgery through an inguinal incision (Rubenstein et al. 2004).

## 6 Testicular Hamartomas in Cowden's Disease

Cowden's disease, also known as multiple hamartoma syndrome is a rare disease marked by increased cellular proliferation of ectodermal, mesodermal, and endodermal tissues (Lloyd and Dennis 1963; Weary et al. 1972). The associated hamartomas, which may be benign or malignant may arise from any of the germ cell layers and can occur anywhere in the body.

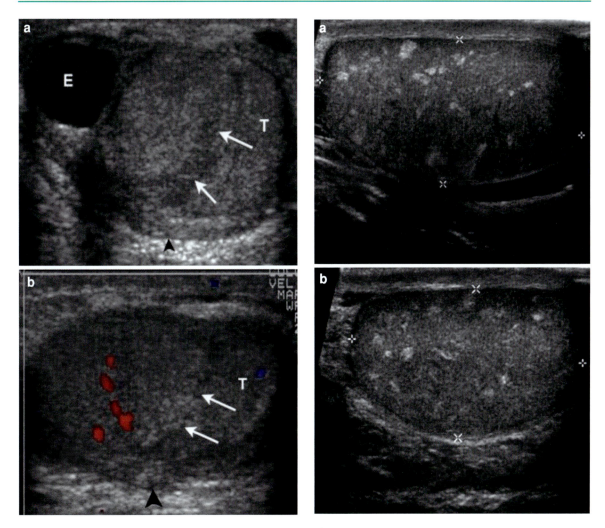

**Fig. 4** Fibrous pseudotumor of the testis (surgically confirmed). A 59-year-old male with a palpable left testicular mass. Transverse gray scale (**a**), and longitudinal color flow Doppler ultrasound image (**b**) of the left testis and epididymis showing variable echotexture with areas of hypoechogenicity within the testicular parenchyma (*arrows*). The testis is surrounded by a rind of soft tissue (*arrowhead*) in the expected location of the tunica albuginea. *T* testis; *E* epididymal cyst. Small areas of parenchymal scarring with a markedly thickened capsule composed of dense collagenous fibrous tissue was detected by histopathological analysis. Notably, scarring and atrophy of the testicular parenchyma adjacent to the thickest portion of the capsule was noticed. [Reprinted from Bhatt et al. (2010) with permission]

Multiple testicular lesions have been reported to be a very frequent occurrence in Cowden's disease, which represent histopathologically lipomatosis of the testis

**Fig. 5** Testicular hamartomas in Cowden disease. A 38-year-old male presenting with mucocutaneous lesions and mild testicular pain. Longitudinal gray-scale images of the *left* (**a**) and *right* (**b**) testis demonstrate multiple hyperechoic lesions without acoustic shadowing in the testicular parenchyma bilaterally. [Reprinted from Bhatt et al. (2010) with permission]

(Woodhouse and Ferguson 2006; Lindsay et al. 2003). In a recent series by Woodhose and Ferguson, these lesions were all noted to be impalpable incidentalomas found while investigating subfertility (Woodhouse and Ferguson 2006). They have no impact on fertility or testicular biochemical function (Woodhouse et al. 2005). Rarely, testicular lipomas are reported as singular lesions (Harper et al. 2002;

Honore 1979). Testicular lipomatosis, on the other hand, is not described outside the context of Cowden's disease and apparently considered as pathognomonic for the disease (Woodhouse and Ferguson 2006).

The sonographic and MRI features of testicular hamartomas in Cowden disease were first described by Lindsay et al. (2003). On US, the presence of multiple, discrete, non-shadowing hyperechoic foci in both testes, varying in size from 1 to 6 mm implies Cowden's disease (Fig. 5) (Bhatt et al. 2010). On color Doppler US, these lesions do not demonstrate any vascularity (Woodhouse and Ferguson 2006). On MRI, they demonstrate a high signal on a T1-weighted sequence, supporting a fatty component to the lesions (Lindsay et al. 2003). Testicular microlithiasis, presenting as multiple, bilateral, non-shadowing hyperechoic lesions, is the main differential consideration during the US evaluation of these patients (Dogra et al. 2003). Nevertheless, the lesions associated with testicular microlithiasis are often punctate and varies from 1 to 3 mm in size, which may be helpful for a proper distinction between two entities (Woodhouse and Ferguson 2006). Furthermore, the aforementioned lesions associated with microlithiasis may not be visible on MRI (Heinemann et al. 2003).

# 7    Congenital Testicular Adrenal Rests

Testicular adrenal rest tissue involves aberrant adrenocortical cells in the testis, which responds to high levels of circulating adrenocortical hormone (ACTH) and produces a benign, hypoechoic mass or masses in the testis (Dogra et al. 2003; Avila et al. 1996; Seidenwurm et al. 1985). They are seen in 8–29% of patients with congenital adrenal hyperplasia, which is an autosomal recessive disorder due to the absence of adrenocortical enzymes, particularly 21-hydroxylase an enzyme of the adrenal cortex (Akin et al. 2004; Dogra et al. 2003; Dogra et al. 2004a; Proto et al. 2001). In these patients, an increase in adrenocorticotropic hormone (ACTH) levels causes hyperplasia of adrenal remnants in the testes (Willi et al. 1991) resulting in the development of intratesticular masses. Besides, these lesions can be found in patients with Addison's disease, Cushing's syndrome, and Adrenogenital syndrome

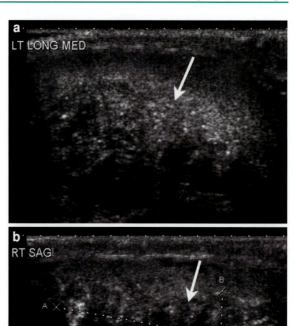

**Fig. 6** Congenital testicular adrenal rests. A 39-year-old male presenting with infertility. Gray-scale ultrasound images of the *left* (**a**) and *right* (**b**) testes demonstrate bilateral hypoechoic masses (*arrows*) with some posterior acoustic shadowing. These lesions were found to be stable in both size and appearance by follow-up ultrasound examinations at one and six month. [Reprinted from Dogra et al. (2004a) with permission]

(Akin et al. 2004). On US, these masses appear as bilateral, multiple, hypoechoic intratesticular masses, with or without posterior acoustic shadowing, depending on the degree of fibrosis (Dogra et al. 2004a; Hamm 1997). They are mostly typically located in the region of the mediastinum testis (Proto et al. 2001). Although these lesions require no further work-up, they should be differentiated from Leydig cell tumors as 10% of these are malignant (Akin et al. 2004). Notably, adrenal rests secrete cortisol and regress with the administration of prednisone.

Ultrasound is the modality of choice for the diagnosis of this entity. On US, these masses appear as bilateral, multiple, hypoechoic intratesticular masses, with or without posterior acoustic shadowing, depending on the degree of fibrosis (Fig. 6)

(Dogra et al. 2004a; Hamm 1997). They are typically located in the region of the mediastinum testis (Proto et al. 2001). Besides, focal areas of hyperechogenicity associated with fibrosis can be detected in the lesions (Seidenwurm et al. 1985; Vanzulli et al. 1992). MRI, as a problem-solving modality, can aid in the diagnosis in some cases. In this regard, testicular adrenal rests appear isointense on T1- and hypointense on T2-weighted images with a diffuse enhancement pattern after gadolinium administration (Dogra et al. 2004b; Avila et al. 1999; Stikkelbroeck et al. 2003). Testicular adrenal rest tissue may be mistaken for malignancy and results in unnecessary orchiectomy as bilateral, synchronous testicular tumors are the main differential consideration in bilateral testicular masses. However, it should be kept in mind that bilateral, synchronous testicular tumors are extremely rare (about 1%) (Dieckmann et al. 1986). Finally, congenital adrenal rests must be considered in patients with congenital adrenal hyperplasia and US follow-up is required to demonstrate stability of these lesions over time, keeping in mind that these masses typically regress with treatment (Bhatt et al. 2010).

## 8 Sarcoidosis

Sarcoidosis is a multisystemic chronic inflammatory disease presenting with pulmonary manifestations in the majority of the cases, though it may have variable systemic presentations (Hurd and Olsen 2000; Opal et al. 1979). The pathological hallmark of the entity is the formation of non-caseating granulomas (Lee et al. 2008). Sarcoidosis can involve any organ system, and the urologic manifestations are seen in only 5% of autopsy specimens (Woodward et al. 2003). Scrotal involvement by the entity, which may be unilateral or bilateral, is rare and may be seen without coexisting pulmonary involvement; when it occurs the epididymis is more likely to be involved than the testis. Clinically, these patients are usually asymptomatic or present with symptoms of epididymitis or with a painless mass. It may also present as epididymoorchitis (Dogra et al. 2003). Testicular involvement by sarcoidosis is particularly common in the African–American population (Woodward et al. 2003).

On US, sarcoid granulomas appear as single or multiple hypoechoic nodules within the testes and epididymis, and may calcify (Fig. 7) (Lee et al. 2008;

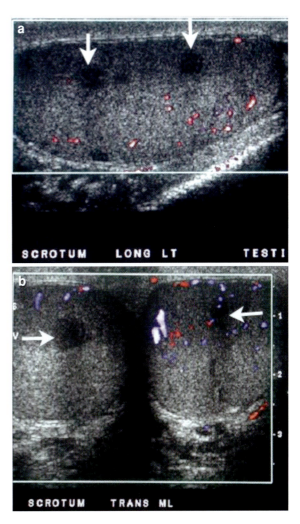

**Fig. 7** Sarcoidosis of testes. A 66-year-old white male having a past history of pulmonary sarcoidosis presented with right scrotal numbness and pain. Longitudinal (**a**), and transverse (**b**) color flow Doppler ultrasound images of the testes demonstrate multiple, avascular, hypoechoic nodules (*arrows*) in the testes and epididymides bilaterally (*not shown*). The lesions were found to be stable at follow-up ultrasound examination at one year. [Reprinted from Bhatt et al. (2010) with permission]

Bhatt et al. 2006). The epididymis may be enlarged and heterogeneous (Woodward et al. 2002; Warshauer and Lee 2004). Interestingly, testicular sarcoidosis appearing as testicular appendices has also been described (Obinata et al. 2007). Although the aforementioned nodular involvement of testes and epididymis may mimic tumors, the presence of multiple bilateral lesions with the simultaneous involvement of the epididymis and testes, in conjunction with other systemic presentations such as pulmonary or abdominal involvement should raise the suspicion of sarcoidosis and may enable a proper differentiation of the two entities. Nevertheless, surgical exploration may be required in equivocal cases.

## 9    Epidermoid Cyst

Epidermoid cysts, also known as keratocysts, are uncommon benign tumors of germ cell origin ranging in size from 1 to 3 cm. Histopathologically, they are composed of an outer layer of fibrous tissue with an inner lining of squamous epithelium with the cystic center containing flakes of keratin (Akin et al. 2004; Dogra et al. 2003). Epidermoid cysts of the testis are relatively uncommon and account for less than 1% of all testicular neoplasms. The patients most commonly present with painless testicular mass, at routine physical examination or with pain as the chief complaint (Shah et al. 1981). On physical examination a discrete mass or nodule is the cardinal finding, though enlargement of the whole testis can be detected as well (Rubenstein et al. 2004). Epidermoid cysts usually present between 20 and 40 years of age (Woodward et al. 2002). Bilateral epidermoid cysts are rare (Sanderson et al. 1995). Epidermoid cysts are usually spherical and deeply embedded within the testicular parenchyma, though they may occasionally protrude through the tunica albuginea (Rubenstein et al. 2004).

These solid intratesticular lesions always require further evaluation and US is a necessary part of the patient management. The US appearance of epidermoid cyst varies with the maturation, compactness, and quantity of keratin within the cyst (Dogra et al. 2003). In general, a well circumscribed, ovoid lesion with variable echogenicity can be detected on US (Cohen et al. 1984; Maxwell and Mamtora 1990). However, the appearance of an "onion-ring" pattern with alternating concentric hyperechoic and hypoechoic layers is considered characteristic of an epidermoid cyst and corresponds to its natural evolution (Fig. 8) (Langer et al. 1999; Dogra et al. 2001a). Nevertheless, this appearance has also been reported to be seen in teratomas (Maizlin et al. 2005). A target appearance involving a halo with a central area of increased echogenicity, a sharply defined

mass with a rim of calcification and a solid mass with an echogenic rim are other appearances described for epidermoid cysts (Langer et al. 1999; Dogra et al. 2001a). On color or pulsed Doppler US, there is no blood flow within the lesion. Testicular epidermoid cyst can often be differentiated from other germ cell tumors by the combination of an onion-ring configuration, negative tumor-marker status, and avascularity in the lesion (Dogra et al. 2001a). MRI may aid in the relevant differentiation by characterizing the fatty component of an epidermoid cyst. The management of these patients relies on excisional biopsy findings that provide the final diagnosis and suggest the treatment. A conservative approach involving enucleation can be followed for an epidermoid cyst of less than 3 cm in size with negative tumor markers provided that frozen sections confirm the diagnosis and that two biopsies of the surrounding parenchyma show no testicular involvement (Loya et al. 2004).

## 10    Intratesticular Varicocele

Contrary to extratesticular varicocele being present in 15–20% of men, intratesticular varicocele is a rare and relatively new entity, reported in fewer than 2% of symptomatic men undergoing scrotal US (Das et al. 1999; Mehta and Dogra 1998). An intratesticular varicocele can occur in association with an extratesticular varicocele, though intratesticular varicoceles are more commonly found alone (Das et al. 1999). Their location may be subcapsular (under the tunica albuginea) or adjacent to mediastinum testis (Kessler et al. 2005). Clinically, patients with an intratesticular varicocele may have pain related to passive congestion of the testis, eventually stretching the tunica albuginea (Rubenstein et al. 2004).

Sonographically, the appearance of an intratesticular varicocele is similar to that of an extratesticular varicocele (Rubenstein et al. 2004). On gray-scale US, multiple, tubular, or serpentine structures more than 2 mm in diameter with a positive Valsalva maneuver can be seen, confirming the venous origin (Mehta and Dogra 1998; Weiss et al. 1992). Color flow and duplex Doppler US facilitates the visualization of

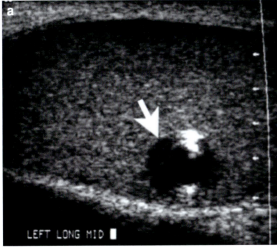

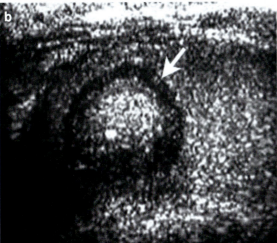

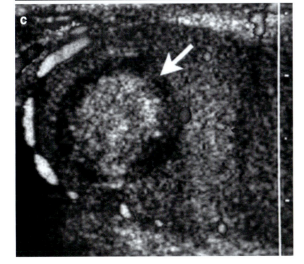

◀**Fig. 8** Epidermoid cysts. A 25-year-old male presenting with palpable mass in the left testis (**a**). Longitudinal gray-scale ultrasound of the testis showing the characteristic appearance of the epidermoid cyst (*arrow*), which is seen as an onion ring configuration due to alternating layers of hypo- and hyperechogenicity. Atypical ultrasound appearance of epidermoid cyst in a 16-year-old male presenting with a hard tender nodule in right testis. [Reprinted from Dogra et al. (2001b) with permission]. Gray-scale ultrasound image demonstrating target appearance involving a smooth (**b**), spherical, well-circumscribed nodule with a hypoechoic rim (*arrow*) and a hyperechoic center. Corresponding color Doppler ultrasound image revealing only peripheral vascularity associated with the lesion (**c**). [Reprinted from Bhatt et al. (2010) with permission]

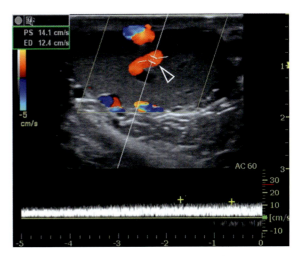

**Fig. 9** Intratesticular varicocele. A young male patient presenting with scrotal pain. Longitudinal color Doppler ultrasound image of the left testis during valsalva maneuver demonstrating presence of prominent color flow within the dilated intratesticular cystic-tubular structures with spectral venous flow pattern (*arrowhead*)

intratesticular varicoceles by demonstrating the venous flow pattern with a characteristic venous spectral waveform that increases during a Valsalva maneuver (Fig. 9) (Mehta and Dogra 1998). Notably, intratesticular varicoceles adjacent to the mediastinum testis may mimic tubular ectasia and color flow Doppler is also helpful for the differentiation between the two entities (Dogra and Bhatt 2004).

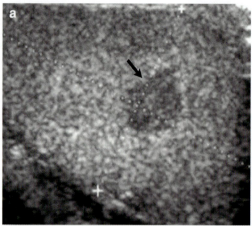

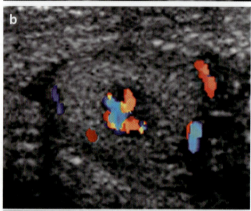

◀**Fig. 10** Intratesticular arterio-venous malformation (AVM). A 32 year-old male presenting with left scrotal pain. Gray-scale image (**a**) of the testis demonstrates a hypoechoic lesion (*arrow*), which fills with a mixture of colors and shows an arterialized–venous waveform pattern on the corresponding color flow (**b**), and spectral (**c**) Doppler images; the findings were consistent with an AVM. [Reprinted from Dogra et al. (2004a) with permission]

## 11  Intratesticular Arteriovenous Malformation

Intratesticular arteriovenous malformation (AVM) is an extremely rare vascular malformation with a benign course (Dogra and Bhatt 2004). It may be congenital or post-traumatic (Dogra et al. 2004a). On gray-scale US, it may appear hypoechoic with a characteristic arterialized venous spectral waveform (Fig. 10) (Kutlu et al. 2003). The main differential diagnosis of an AVM is arteriovenous type of an intratesticular hemangioma (Ricci et al. 2000), though testicular tumor, intratesticular varicocele, and tubular ectasia of rete testis should also be considered (Skiadas et al. 2006).

## 12  Conclusion

Although differential diagnosis of scrotal disorders solely based on US criteria may be challenging, several imaging features may favor the diagnosis of various benign entities and may enable a more proper management of the patients by precluding the need for an immediate surgery. In this regard, the radiologist's familiarity with the imaging features of the aforementioned entities is very important for early diagnosis and more appropriate management.

**Acknowledgments** We would like to acknowledge our sincere thanks to Mustafa Secil, MD for his providing Fig. 1.

## References

Aguado A, Grant TH, Miller FH et al (2005) Radiation-induced fibrosis of the spermatic cord: sonographic and MRI findings. AJR Am J Roentgenol 184:S102–S103

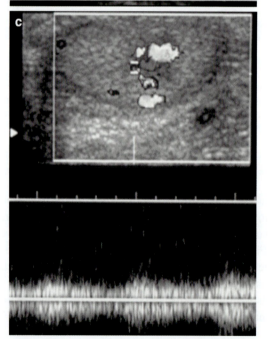

Akbar SA, Sayyed TA, Jafri SZ et al (2003) Multimodality imaging of paratesticular neoplasms and their rare mimics. Radiographics 23:1461–1476

Akin EA, Khati NJ, Hill MC (2004) Ultrasound of the scrotum. Ultrasound Q 20:181–200

al-Otaibi L, Whitman GJ, Chew FS (1997) Fibrous pseudotumor of the epididymis. AJR Am J Roentgenol 168:1586

Amodio JB, Maybody M, Slowotsky C et al (2004) Polyorchidism: report of 3 cases and review of the literature. J Ultrasound Med 23:951–957

Avila NA, Premkumar A, Shawker TH et al (1996) Testicular adrenal rest tissue in congenital adrenal hyperplasia: findings at gray scale and color Doppler US. Radiology 198:99–104

Avila NA, Premkumar A, Merke DP (1999) Testicular adrenal rest tissue in congenital adrenal hyperplasia: comparison of MR imaging and sonographic findings. AJR Am J Roentgenol 172:1003–1006

Bhatt S, Rubens DJ, Dogra VS (2006) Sonography of benign intrascrotal lesions. Ultrasound Q 22:121–136

Bhatt S, Jafri SZ, Wasserman N, et al. (2010) Imaging of non-neoplastic intratesticular masses. Diagn Interv Radiol. doi: 10.4261/1305-3825

Bree RL, Hoang DT (1996) Scrotal ultrasound. Radiol Clin North Am 34:1183–1205

Carkaci S, Ozkan E, Lane D et al (2010) Scrotal sonography revisited. J Clin Ultrasound 38:21–37

Coakley FV, Hricak H, Presti JC Jr (1998) Imaging and management of atypical testicular masses. Urol Clin North Am 25:375–388

Cohen EL, Mandel E, Goodman JD et al (1984) Epidermoid cyst of testicle. Ultrasonographic characteristics. Urology 24:79–81

Cohn EL, Watson L, Older R et al (1996) Striated pattern of the testicle on ultrasound: an appearance of testicular fibrosis. J Urol 156:180–181

Das KM, Prasad K, Szmigielski W, Noorani N (1999) Intratesticular varicocele. evaluationusing conventional and Doppler sonography. AJR Am J Roentgenol 173:1079–1083

Dieckmann KP, Boeckmann W, Brosig W et al (1986) Bilateral testicular germ cell tumors. Report of nine cases and review of the literature. Cancer 57:1254–1258

Dogra V, Bhatt S (2004) Acute painful scrotum. Radiol Clin North Am 42:349–363

Dogra VS, Gottlieb RH, Rubens DJ et al (2001a) Testicular epidermoid cysts: sonographic features with histopathologic correlation. J Clin Ultrasound 29:192–196

Dogra VS, Gottlieb RH, Rubens DJ, Liao L (2001b) Benign intratesticular cystic lesions: US features. Radiographics 21(Spec No):S273–S281

Dogra VS, Gottlieb RH, Oka M et al (2003) Sonography of the scrotum. Radiology 227:18–36

Dogra V, Nathan J, Bhatt S (2004a) Sonographic appearance of testicular adrenal rest tissue in congenital adrenal hyperplasia. J Ultrasound Med 23:979–981

Dogra VS, Rubens DJ, Gottlieb RH et al (2004b) Torsion and beyond: new twists in spectral Doppler evaluation of the scrotum. J Ultrasound Med 23:1077–1085

Einstein DM, Paushter DM, Singer AA et al (1992) Fibrotic lesions of the testicle: sonographic patterns mimicking malignancy. Urol Radiol 14:205–210

Germaine P, Simerman LP (2007) Fibrous pseudotumor of the scrotum. J Ultrasound Med 26:133–138

Hamm B (1997) Differential diagnosis of scrotal masses by ultrasound. Eur Radiol 7:668–679

Harper M, Arya M, Peters JL et al (2002) Intratesticular lipoma. Scand J Urol Nephrol 36:223–224

Harris RD, Chouteau C, Partrick M et al (2000) Prevalence and significance of heterogeneous testes revealed on sonography: exvivo sonographic-pathologic correlation. AJR Am J Roentgenol 175:347–352

Heinemann V, Frey U, Linke J et al (2003) Testicular microlithiasis—one case and four points to note. Scand J Urol Nephrol 37:515–518

Honore LH (1979) Fatty metaplasia in a postpubertal undescended testis: a case report. J Urol 122:841–842

Hurd DS, Olsen T (2000) Cutaneous sarcoidosis presenting as a testicular mass. Cutis 66:435–438

Hwang S, Aronoff DR, Leonidas JC (2005) Case 82: polyorchidism with torsion. Radiology 235:433–435

Kessler A, Meirsdorf S, Graif M et al (2005) Intratesticular varicocele: gray scale and color Doppler sonographic appearance. J Ultrasound Med 24:1711–1716

Kim R (2002) Clinical importance of a unilateral striated pattern seen on sonography of the testicle. AJR Am J Roentgenol 178:927–930

Kutlu R, Alkan A, Soylu A et al (2003) Intratesticular arteriovenous malformation: color Doppler sonographic findings. J Ultrasound Med 22:295–298

Langer JE, Ramchandani P, Siegelman ES et al (1999) Epidermoid cysts of the testicle: sonographic and MR imaging features. AJR Am J Roentgenol 173:1295–1299

Lee JC, Bhat S, Dogra VS (2008) Imaging of the epididymis. Ultrasound Q 24:3–16

Lindsay C, Boardman L, Farrell M (2003) Testicular hamartomas in Cowden disease. J Clin Ultrasound 31:481–483

Lloyd KM, Dennis M (1963) Cowden's disease. A possible new symptom complex with multiple system involvement. Ann Intern Med 58:136–142

Loya AG, Said JW, Grant EG (2004) Epidermoid cyst of the testis: radiologic-pathologic correlation. Radiographics 24(Suppl 1):S243–S246

Maizlin ZV, Belenky A, Baniel J et al (2005) Epidermoid cyst and teratoma of the testis: sonographic and histologic similarities. J Ultrasound Med 24:1403–1409

Maxwell AJ, Mamtora H (1990) Sonographic appearance of epidermoid cyst of the testis. J Clin Ultrasound 18:188–190

Mehta AL, Dogra VS (1998) Intratesticular varicocele. J Clin Ultrasound 26:49–51

Nistal M, Mate A, Paniagua R (1996) Cystic transformation of the rete testis. Am J Surg Pathol 20:1231–1239

Obinata D, Yamaguchi K, Hirano D et al (2007) Intrascrotal involvement of sarcoidosis presenting like testicular appendices. Int J Urol 14:87–88

Öner AY, Sahin C, Pocan S et al (2005) Polyorchidism: sonographic and magnetic resonance image findings. Acta Radiol 46:769–771

Opal SM, Pittman DL, Hofeldt FE (1979) Testicular sarcoidosis. Am J Med 67:147–150

Proto G, Di Donna A, Grimaldi F et al (2001) Bilateral testicular adrenal rest tissue in congenital adrenal hyperplasia: US and MR features. J Endocrinol Invest 24:529–531

Ricci Z, Koenigsberg M, Whitney K (2000) Sonography of an arteriovenous-type hemangioma of the testis. AJR Am J Roentgenol 174:1581–1582

Rubenstein RA, Dogra VS, Seftel AD et al (2004) Benign intrascrotal lesions. J Urol 171:1765–1772

Sanderson AJ, Birch BR, Dewbury KC (1995) Case report: multiple epidermoid cysts of the testes-the ultrasound appearances. Clin Radiol 50:414–415

Savas M, Yeni E, Ciftci H et al (2010) Polyorchidism: a three-case report and review of the literature. Andrologia 42:57–61

Seidenwurm D, Smathers RL, Kan P et al (1985) Ultrasound diagnosis of testicular masses secondary to hyperplastic adrenal rests diagnosed by ultrasound. Radiology 155:479–481

Shah KH, Maxted WC, Chun B (1981) Epidermoid cysts of the testis: a report of three cases and an analysis of 141 cases from the world literature. Cancer 47:577–582

Skiadas V, Antoniou A, Primetis H et al (2006) Intratesticular arteriovenous malformation. Clinical course, ultrasound and MRI findings of an extremely rare lesion on a 7 year follow-up basis. Int Urol Nephrol 38:119–122

Stikkelbroeck NM, Suliman HM, Otten BJ et al (2003) Testicular adrenal rest tumours in postpubertal males with congenital adrenal hyperplasia: sonographic and MR features. Eur Radiol 13:1597–1603

Vanzulli A, DelMaschio A, Paesano P et al (1992) Testicular masses in association with adrenogenital syndrome: US findings. Radiology 183:425–429

Warshauer DM, Lee JK (2004) Imaging manifestations of abdominal sarcoidosis. AJR Am J Roentgenol 182: 15–28

Weary PE, Gorlin RJ, Gentry WC Jr et al (1972) Multiple hamartoma syndrome (Cowden's disease). Arch Dermatol 106:682–690

Weiss AJ, Kellman GM, Middleton WD et al (1992) Intratesticular varicocele: sonographic findings in two patients. AJR Am J Roentgenol 158:1061–1063

Willi U, Atares M, Prader A et al (1991) Testicular adrenal-like tissue (TALT) in congenital adrenal hyperplasia: detection by ultrasonography. Pediatr Radiol 21:284–287

Woodhouse J, Ferguson MM (2006) Multiple hyperechoic testicular lesions are a common finding on ultrasound in Cowden disease and represent lipomatosis of the testis. Br J Radiol 79:801–803

Woodhouse JB, Delahunt B, English SF et al (2005) Testicular lipomatosis in Cowden's syndrome. Mod Pathol 18:1151–1156

Woodward PJ, Sohaey R, O'Donoghue MJ et al (2002) From the archives of the AFIP: tumors and tumorlike lesions of the testis: radiologic-pathologic correlation. Radiographics 22:189–216

Woodward PJ, Schwab CM, Sesterhenn IA (2003) From the archives of the AFIP: extratesticular scrotal masses: radiologic-pathologic correlation. Radiographics 23:215–240

Yagan N (2000) Testicular US findings after biopsy. Radiology 215:768–773

# Nuclear Medicine Methods in Scrotal Imaging

Giuseppe Caruso, Giuseppe Salvaggio, Artor Niccoli Asabella,
Santo Carluccio, and Giuseppe Rubini

## Contents

### Abstract

In patients with acute scrotal pain scrotal scintigraphy can be used to exclude torsion of the testicle, which presents with unilateral decrease in activity on the affected side. The role of nuclear medicine methods, however, faded in the last years after the introduction of high performance color Doppler ultrasound equipment. Lymphoscintigraphy can be used in patients with testicular cancer to demonstrate the lymphatic drainage pathway of the neoplasm. Several studies suggest that 18FDG-PET/CT might have a role in the staging germ cell tumors, in identification of recurrent/residual disease, to monitor the treatment response and during the follow-up. Other investigations, however, did not confirm these results.

## 1 Introduction

The field of nuclear medicine is a broad one, with an extensive array of studies spanning virtually all aspects of medicine. Although some studies are routine, others are performed only rarely, in large hospitals with various clinical units and emergency care.

Studies may be performed infrequently for a variety of reasons. For example, the condition they assess may be rare, imaging evaluation may not be routinely required for the given condition, and there may be alternative imaging modalities (MacDonald and Burrell 2009). Testicular scintigraphy is one of these infrequent studies, since gray-scale ultrasonography in combination with color or power Doppler imaging is a well-accepted technique for assessing

G. Caruso (✉) · G. Salvaggio
Department of Radiology, University of Palermo,
Via del Vespro 129, 90127 Palermo, Italy
e-mail: carusogi@unipa.it

A. N. Asabella · G. Rubini
Department of Nuclear Medicine, University of Bari,
Piazza Giulio Cesare 11, 70124 Bari, Italy

S. Carluccio,
Department of Nuclear Medicine, Villa Sofia Hospital,
Viale Strasburgo 233, 90146 Palermo, Italy

M. Bertolotto and C. Trombetta (eds.), *Scrotal Pathology,* Medical Radiology. Diagnostic Imaging,
DOI: 10.1007/174_2011_198, © Springer-Verlag Berlin Heidelberg 2012

scrotal lesions and testicular perfusion (Aso et al. 2005).

The majority of men who present with acute scrotal pain and/or swelling have nonsurgical conditions, most often epididymitis or torsion of the appendix testis (MacDonald and Burrell 2009; Aso et al. 2005; Paltiel et al. 1998). Because the clinical appearances of these conditions are frequently indistinguishable from that of testicular torsion, imaging is often done to assist with diagnosis and avoid unnecessary surgery (Paltiel et al. 1998). Ultrasounds, and in particular the color Doppler ultrasonography, allow differentiation between lesions that require urgent surgery (testicular torsion, malignant tumors, and traumatic rupture) and those that can be managed conservatively (e.g. epididymo-orchitis, and torsion of the testicular appendages) (Aso et al. 2005). Moreover, despite the ability to distinguish scrotal inflammation from testicular ischemia with scintigraphy, the use of nuclear medicine is limited by its relatively poor spatial resolution, and use of ionizing radiation. Nevertheless, testicular scintigraphy is a very important diagnostic tool in Nuclear Medicine Departments with 24 h diagnostic service or ready on call service organized to manage emergency situations (Paltiel et al. 1998).

## 2    Scrotal Scintigraphy

The role of scrotal scintigraphy in patients with painful scrotum is predicated on assessing the blood flow to the scrotum and contents. The aim of these procedures is to exclude torsion of the testicle, a condition requiring emergency surgery to untwist the testicle and prevent necrosis. Scrotal scintigraphy no longer has a role in the diagnosis of testicular tumors. In fact, ultrasound is the best technique in defining the presence and nature of these conditions. Moreover, scintigraphic appearance of tumors is only occasionally encountered because these conditions rarely cause a painful scrotum.

Scrotal scintigraphy was introduced by Nadel et al. (1973) in order to differentiate the non-perfused testicle of acute torsion from the hyperaemic tissues seen in epididymo-orchitis. While simply in principle, effective use of scrotal scintigraphy is dependent on a number of factors, including an adequate history and physical examination, accurate positioning and

marking of the patient, and reliable acquisition of data and proper interpretation.

### 2.1    Positioning

No specific patient preparation is required for this study. After a clear and detailed interview is conducted and an explanation of the scan is given, the patient is asked to lie supine on the imaging table, with his legs abducted and feet together in a frog-leg position to decrease background activity from the thighs. The penis should be taped over the pubis to avoid overlap with the scrotum. A towel may be draped under the scrotum and over the thighs, acting as a sling to raise the scrotum. Proper positioning is vital for a proper diagnosis, and with detailed instruction the patient is usually more than willing to assist (MacDonald and Burrell 2009).

### 2.2    Radiotracer and Protocol

The radiopharmaceuticals, usually $^{99m}$Tc-pertecnetate, are injected intravenously in small volume bolus [555 MBq (15 mCi), with a minimum of 185 MBq (5 mCi) for the pediatric population] with the acquisition started immediately to ensure the flow portion of the study is not missed, although this phase of the examination often does not add significant information to the static studies. The study includes dynamic imaging at 2–5 s/frame for 1–2 min of the anterior pelvis, with further static imaging after the flow portion for at least 500,000 counts (500 K) per static image.

### 2.3    Imaging

In the normal testicular scan, blood flow is demonstrated in the iliac and femoral arteries, in the penis, and symmetrically and faintly in the scrotum and testicles.

Static images should clearly display a unilateral decrease in activity on the affected side (Fig. 1). In the early phase of torsion, inflammation in the surrounding scrotum is insignificant and no hyperemic rim is visible. If the testicle spontaneously untwists before imaging, there may actually be increased flow to the testicle due to hyperemia.

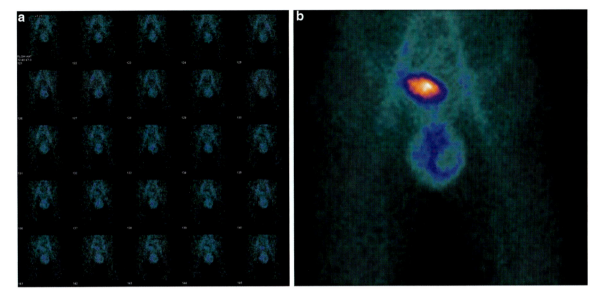

**Fig. 1** $^{99m}$TcO$_4$-testicular scintigraphy in a patient with complete testicular torsion. Dynamic (**a**) and static (**b**) acquisition showing asymmetric radiopharmaceutical distribution in scrotum with reduced flow and perfusion in left scrotum, associated with a photopenic area at the left testicle surrounded by hyperemic edge

In epididymo-orchitis the onset of symptoms is usually more gradual than in testicular torsion, developing over 1–2 days. Scintigraphic findings are opposite of those seen in testicular torsion. However, physicians must be aware of the clinical presentation, including which side is painful, because asymmetry may be due to abnormally increased uptake on one side, in case of epididymo-orchitis, or abnormally decreased uptake on the other side, in case of testicular torsion.

## 3 Lymphatic Mapping and Sentinel Node Biopsy

The concept of sentinel lymph node relates to the existence and subsequent identification of specific lymph node centers that predict the nodal status of patients with a malignancy. Sentinel lymph node biopsy could help physicians provide the best staging and better define prognosis. It also permits to minimize the surgical approach for the loco regional lymph node excision. The purpose of lymphoscintigraphy for lymphatic mapping is to demonstrate the lymphatic drainage pathway of neoplasm. Lymphatic mapping enables accurate staging because the pathologist receives the lymph node at greater risk of harboring metastatic disease.

Linking the transit of radiolabeled microparticles from a primary neoplastic site to a sentinel lymph node ideally is based on the visualization of lymphatic channels that lead to a sentinel node. Retention of radiolabeled particles within sentinel lymph nodes is required for the identification of these nodes at subsequent surgical exploration (usually 1–3 h after imaging was completed) aided by the handheld gamma probe.

At least three aspects may be of importance in this respect: particle size, number of particles, and dosage of the radiopharmaceutical. Particle size is a major factor that affects the entrance of particles into the lymphatic system, their rate of transit, and their degree of retention by lymph nodes; therefore, optimization of imaging and identification of sentinel nodes intraoperatively is dependent on choice of suitable particle size of the radiocolloidal agent (Goldfarb et al. 1998).

Numerous radiopharmaceuticals have been used for sentinel node lymphoscintigraphy. For testicular cancer, before the sentinel node era, lymphoscintigraphy using intratesticular injection of colloidal gold ($^{198}$Au) was described in the literature (Tanis et al. 2002). Actually, $^{99m}$Tc-nanocolloid is used with a dose ranging between 50 and 135 MBq. A single dose of small volume of radiopharmaceutical (0.2 ml) is injected directly in the testicular parenchyma using a fine needle; this procedure can be performed with or without local anesthesia with a funicular block using lidocaine 2%. The intratesticular injection leads to the visualization of the lymph nodes of the para-aortic region.

## 4    Gallium Scintigraphy

The degree of [67]Gallium ([67]Ga) uptake in metastatic testicular carcinomas has been reported to vary according to cell type. [67]Ga scan sensitivity results ranged from 93% for seminomas (Paterson et al. 1976) to 74% for metastatic embryonal cell carcinomas and only 25% for teratomas (Sauerbrunn et al. 1978). Although shown to concentrate in embryonal cell carcinoma and seminoma, currently [67]Ga is infrequently used as a staging tool in testicular carcinoma. Prior surgery may reduce specificity due to [67]Ga uptake at surgical site (Jackson et al. 1976), while initiation of treatment prior to scanning may reduce sensitivity (Symmonds and Tauxe 1972).

[67]Ga scintigraphy has an important role in the evaluation of residual masses after radiation therapy or chemotherapy: the presence of a residual mass after treatment on CT examination may not always indicate residual disease. In the study of Uchiyama et al. (1994) the postsystemic therapy CT examination showed residual masses in 3/3 extragonadal seminoma sites, and in 5/8 gonadal seminoma sites. However, [67]Ga imaging returned to normal immediately in 10/11 indicating an absence of active tumor, an observation supported by clinical follow-up ranging from 6 to 72 months. One patient who maintained a positive [67]Ga scan after chemotherapy received adjuvant radiation therapy and subsequently remained disease free. Authors concluded that [67]Ga imaging may be useful in confirming the absence of active tumor in patients with residual radiologic masses after treatment. However, other studies reported that while a positive gallium scan remains highly suggestive of recurrence, a negative scan does not seem to conclusively rule it out (Bekerman et al. 1984; Warren and Einhorn 1995). The failure of [67]Ga uptake to predict which posttherapy patients will recur severely limits utility of this potential application.

Moreover, it should be remembered that many other conditions such as infection and inflammatory processes may result in gallium uptake, so, the interpretation of scrotal [67]Ga uptake should be considered in the clinical context. Further improvement of nuclear medicine consisted of the introduction of [68]Ga as a positron emission radiopharmaceutical associated with PET/CT technique in the detection of testicular tumor.

## 5    2-18Fluoro-2-Deoxy-D-Glucose (18FDG) PET

Clinical staging of low-stage testicular germ cell tumors is inaccurate, especially in patients with clinical stage I nonseminoma in which even CT misses about 30% of low-volume metastases. To improve the imaging modality in clinical staging, 18FDG-PET/CT has been extensively used in the staging of testicular cancer (Figs. 2 and 3).

In the study of Albers et al. (1999) 18FDG-PET/ CT staging was equivalent to CT staging in patients with nonseminomatous clinical stage I germ cell tumors. Conversely, in patients with nonseminomatous clinical stage II germ cell tumors CT showed four false-positive results as shown by surgical staging, whereas 18FDG-PET/CT was able to correctly classify all of them. Authors's conclusions were that 18FDG-PET/CT is able to identify viable cancer in clinical stage II lesions with the exception of teratoma. In fact, mature lesion, such as teratoma, was not 18FDG-PET/CT avid, consistent with their low metabolic rate.

Results of preliminary experiences demonstrated 18FDG-PET/CT to be a potentially useful diagnostic tool for initial staging in patients with stage I–II germ cell tumors, even if 18FDG-PET/CT was not able to identify mature teratoma (Albers et al. 1999; Spermon et al. 2002; Tsatalpas et al. 2002; Hain et al. 2000). In particular, 18FDG-PET/CT might be helpful to identify stage IIA in clinical stage I non-seminomatous germ cell tumors. These preliminary results were considered sufficient to suggest that a large prospective study was mandatory. A Medical Research Council trial has recently started to evaluate the role of 18FDG-PET/CT in stage I non-seminomatous germ cell tumors.

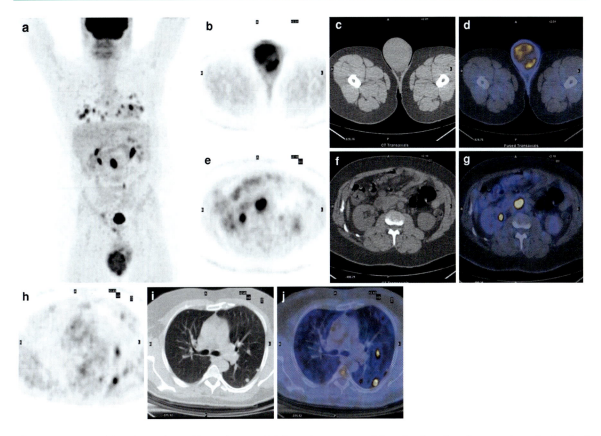

**Fig. 2** 18FDG-PET/CT of a patient with seminoma of right testicle. **a** Whole-body PET image. **b–d** Transaxial PET (**b**), CT (**c**) and fusion (**d**) images of the right testicular tumor. **e–g** Transaxial PET (**e**), CT (**f**) and fusion (**g**) images of interaortocaval lymphnodes, site of metastasis at the level of L2–L3. **h–j** Transaxial PET (**h**), CT (**i**) and fusion (**j**) images at the pulmonary's bases in which are evident metastases

18FDG-PET/CT has been evaluated in patients with residual masses after chemotherapy in seminomatous and non-seminomatous germ cell cancer with promising, but heterogeneous, results (Stephens et al. 1996; Nuutinen et al. 1997; Cremerius et al. 1998, 1999; Sugawara et al. 1999).

The accurate prediction of residual masses after chemotherapy is still a major diagnostic challenge in patients with germ cell tumors. Conventional diagnostic procedures such as CT or MR imaging are not able to predict the viability of residual masses with clinically acceptable accuracy (Toner et al. 1990; Stomper et al. 1991). 18FDG-PET imaging seems to be a promising method to predict the viability of residual masses on the basis of its ability to visualize and quantify glucose metabolism in tumor tissue (Strauss and Conti 1991).

In the study of Hain et al. (2000) a 18FDG-PET/CT was performed in patients following chemotherapy with elevated serum tumor markers. They found a positive predictive value of 18FDG-PET/CT equivalent to that of markers (96 vs. 94%), while the negative predictive value was higher than that of markers (90%). 18FDG-PET/CT, moreover, had the advantage of identifying the site of residual/recurrent testicular carcinoma.

However, different results were found in seminomatous and non-seminomatous germ cell tumors: In an analysis by De Santis et al. (2001), 2004) in patients with pure seminoma, a sensitivity of 100% and a specificity of 80% in patients with residual masses larger than 3 cm were reported. In the seminoma patients of the German multicenter PET trial, this high sensitivity was confirmed, although the specificity and the positive predictive value were considerably lower

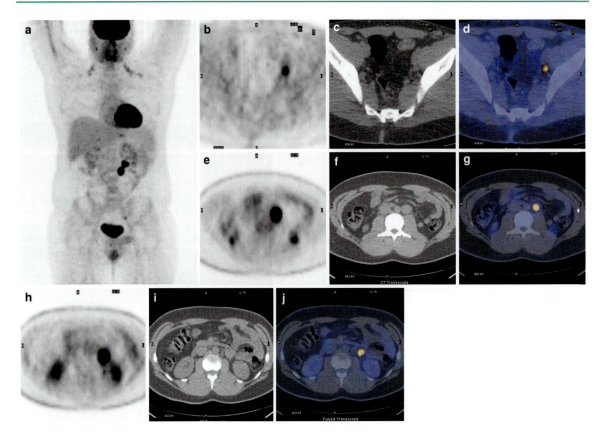

**Fig. 3** 18FDG-PET/CT of a patient who underwent right orchiectomy. **a** Whole-body PET image. **b–d** Transaxial PET (**b**), CT (**c**) and fusion *(**d**) images to the pelvis with left iliac lymph node metastases. **e–j** Transaxial PET (**e, h**), CT **f, i** and fusion (**g, j**) images with two metastases in left para-aortic lymphnodes near the kidney

with 47 and 25%, respectively (Hinz et al. 2008). In case of non-seminomatous germ cell tumors, a multicenter study (Oechsle et al. 2008) demonstrated that 18FDG-PET/CT is not able to give additional clinically relevant information and clinical benefit to standard diagnostic procedures (CT and serum tumor markers), for the common presence (55%) of vital carcinoma and mature teratoma in residual masses.

**Acknowledgment** The authors thank Vincenzo Allegri, Valentina Ambrosini and Stefano Fanti of the Department of Nuclear Medicine, S. Orsola Malpighi Hospital, Bologna, for their contribution.

# References

Albers P, Bender H, Yilmaz H et al (1999) Positron emission tomography in the clinical staging of patients with Stage I and II testicular germ cell tumors. Urology 53:808–811

Aso C, Enriquez G, Fite M et al (2005) Gray-scale and color Doppler sonography of scrotal disorders in children: an update. Radiographics 25:1197–1214

Bekerman C, Hoffer PB, Bitran JD (1984) The role of gallium-67 in the clinical evaluation of cancer. Semin Nucl Med 14:296–323

Cremerius U, Effert PJ, Adam G et al (1998) FDG PET for detection and therapy control of metastatic germ cell tumor. J Nucl Med 39:815–822

Cremerius U, Wildberger JE, Borchers H et al (1999) Does positron emission tomography using 18-fluoro-2-deoxyglucose improve clinical staging of testicular cancer? Results of a study in 50 patients. Urology 54:900–904

De Santis M, Bokemeyer C, Becherer A et al (2001) Predictive impact of 2–18fluoro-2-deoxy-D-glucose positron emission tomography for residual postchemotherapy masses in patients with bulky seminoma. J Clin Oncol 19: 3740–3744

De Santis M, Becherer A, Bokemeyer C et al (2004) 2–18fluoro-deoxy-D-glucose positron emission tomography is a reliable predictor for viable tumor in postchemotherapy seminoma: an update of the prospective multicentric SEMPET trial. J Clin Oncol 22:1034–1039

Goldfarb LR, Alazraki NP, Eshima D, et al (1998) Lymphoscintigraphic identification of sentinel lymph nodes: clinical evaluation of 0.22-micron filtration of Tc-99 m sulfur colloid. Radiology, 208:505–509

Hain SF, O'Doherty MJ, Timothy AR et al (2000a) Fluorodeoxyglucose PET in the initial staging of germ cell tumours. Eur J Nucl Med 27:590–594

Hain SF, O'Doherty MJ, Timothy AR et al (2000b) Fluorodeoxyglucose positron emission tomography in the evaluation of germ cell tumours at relapse. Br J Cancer 83:863–869

Hinz S, Schrader M, Kempkensteffen C et al (2008) The role of positron emission tomography in the evaluation of residual masses after chemotherapy for advanced stage seminoma. J Urol 179:936–940 discussion 940

Jackson FI, Dierich HC, Lentle BC (1976) Gallium-67 citrate scintiscanning in testicular neoplasia. J Can Assoc Radiol 27:84–88

MacDonald A, Burrell S (2009) Infrequently performed studies in nuclear medicine: part 2. J Nucl Med Technol 37:1–13

Nadel NS, Gitter MH, Hahn LC et al (1973) Preoperative diagnosis of testicular torsion. Urology 1:478–479

Nuutinen JM, Leskinen S, Elomaa I et al (1997) Detection of residual tumours in postchemotherapy testicular cancer by FDG-PET. Eur J Cancer 33:1234–1241

Oechsle K, Hartmann M, Brenner W et al (2008) [18F]Fluorodeoxyglucose positron emission tomography in nonseminomatous germ cell tumors after chemotherapy: the German multicenter positron emission tomography study group. J Clin Oncol 26:5930–5935

Paltiel HJ, Connolly LP, Atala A et al (1998) Acute scrotal symptoms in boys with an indeterminate clinical presentation: comparison of color Doppler sonography and scintigraphy. Radiology 207:223–231

Paterson AH, Peckham MJ, McCready VR (1976) Value of gallium scanning in seminoma of the testis. Br Med J 1:1118–1121

Sauerbrunn BJ, Andrews GA, Hubner KF (1978) Ga-67 citrate imaging in tumors of the genito-urinary tract: report of cooperative study. J Nucl Med 19:470–475

Spermon JR, De Geus-Oei LF, Kiemeney LA et al (2002) The role of (18)fluoro-2-deoxyglucose positron emission tomography in initial staging and re-staging after chemotherapy for testicular germ cell tumours. BJU Int 89:549–556

Stephens AW, Gonin R, Hutchins GD et al (1996) Positron emission tomography evaluation of residual radiographic abnormalities in postchemotherapy germ cell tumor patients. J Clin Oncol 14:1637–1641

Stomper PC, Kalish LA, Garnick MB et al (1991) CT and pathologic predictive features of residual mass histologic findings after chemotherapy for nonseminomatous germ cell tumors: can residual malignancy or teratoma be excluded? Radiology 180:711–714

Strauss LG, Conti PS (1991) The applications of PET in clinical oncology. J Nucl Med 32:623–648 discussion 649-650

Sugawara Y, Zasadny KR, Grossman HB et al (1999) Germ cell tumor: differentiation of viable tumor, mature teratoma, and necrotic tissue with FDG PET and kinetic modeling. Radiology 211:249–256

Symmonds RE, Tauxe WN (1972) Gallium-67 scintigraphy of gynecologic tumors. Am J Obstet Gynecol 114:356–369

Tanis PJ, Horenblas S, Valdes Olmos RA et al (2002) Feasibility of sentinel node lymphoscintigraphy in stage I testicular cancer. Eur J Nucl Med Mol Imaging 29:670–673

Toner GC, Panicek DM, Heelan RT et al (1990) Adjunctive surgery after chemotherapy for nonseminomatous germ cell tumors: recommendations for patient selection. J Clin Oncol 8:1683–1694

Tsatalpas P, Beuthien-Baumann B, Kropp J et al (2002) Diagnostic value of 18F-FDG positron emission tomography for detection and treatment control of malignant germ cell tumors. Urol Int 68:157–163

Uchiyama M, Kantoff PW, Kaplan WD (1994) Gallium-67-citrate imaging in extragonadal and gonadal seminomas: relationship to radiologic findings. J Nucl Med 35:1624–1630

Warren GP, Einhorn LH (1995) Gallium scans in the evaluation of residual masses after chemotherapy for seminoma. J Clin Oncol 13:2784–2788

# Contrast Enhanced US of the Scrotum

Michele Bertolotto, Massimo Valentino, and Paul S. Sidhu

## Contents

M. Bertolotto (✉)
Department of Radiology, University of Trieste,
Ospedale di Cattinara, Strada di Fiume 447,
34124 Trieste, Italy
e-mail: bertolot@units.it

M. Valentino
S.S.D. Radiologia d'Urgenza, Dipartimento di Radiologia e
Diagnostica per Immagini Azienda Ospedaliera,
Universitaria di Parma Ospedale Maggiore,
Via Gramsci 14, 43100 Parma, Italy

P. S. Sidhu
Department of Radiology, King's College London,
King's College Hospital, Denmark Hill,
London, SE5 9RS, UK

**Abstract**

High performance contrast specific modes are currently implemented for superficial probes, and an increasing interest is now rising for use of contrast enhanced ultrasound (CEUS) in evaluation of scrotal pathologies. Microbubble contrast agents are highly sensitive in assessing presence or absence of vascular flow. While use in evaluation of patients with high degree torsion has limited clinical application, at least in adults, since this pathological condition can be effectively evaluated with conventional color Doppler ultrasound alone, diagnosis of segmental testicular infarction is improved. Virtually all scrotal tumors are vascularized at CEUS. This technique does not allow differentiation among different histotypes, but provides a useful instrument for the differential diagnosis between tumors with cystic components and complex benign cysts. In inflammation, abscesses are clearly defined, and in trauma patients viability of the testicular parenchyma is assessed. Preliminary investigation suggests use of microbubble contrast agents to evaluate infertile patients with varicocele, and for therapeutic applications.

## 1 Introduction

Contrast enhanced ultrasonography (CEUS) of superficial organs has long been considered unlikely because the main resonance frequency of microbubbles commonly used in the clinical practice is in the range of abdominal ultrasound applications. Ultrasound contrast agents, however, contain microbubbles

M. Bertolotto and C. Trombetta (eds.), *Scrotal Pathology*, Medical Radiology. Diagnostic Imaging,
DOI: 10.1007/174_2011_199, © Springer-Verlag Berlin Heidelberg 2012

of different sizes whose resonance frequency range covers the whole range of frequencies used for ultrasound imaging (Greis 2004). In particular, in microbubble distribution there is a substantial tail of small bubbles which resonate at high frequencies.

High performance contrast specific modes are currently implemented in many ultrasound equipment for imaging superficial structures. While relatively low frequencies of approximately 4–5 MHz have been initially used to collect signal from a larger percent of resonating bubbles, small-part transducers operating at frequencies of 7 MHz or higher are now used, with a substantial improvement of spatial resolution. Preliminary investigations on superficial structures show that CEUS may provide clinically useful information in small bowel, carotid artery, superficial nodes, joints, and other areas (Bertolotto and Catalano 2009).

Ultrasonography is the imaging modality of choice for examination of the scrotum, and other imaging modalities are rarely necessary.

Occasionally, however, ultrasound findings are equivocal. Differential diagnosis between hypovascular and avascular lesions, for instance, may be difficult at color Doppler interrogation, and a detailed evaluation of vessel morphology may be desired. CEUS is a practical problem-solving technique in these cases because it is inexpensive, easy to use, and can be performed immediately after the conventional Doppler study. An increasing interest is, therefore, rising for use of microbubble contrast agents in evaluation of scrotal pathologies as well (Shah et al. 2010).

## 2 Microbubble Contrast Agents

Ultrasound contrast agents consist of microbubbles of gas stabilized by a protein, lipid, or polymer shell which are small and stable enough to traverse the pulmonary circulation following peripheral venous injection. Their typical half-life in blood is of few minutes. Microbubbles are blood pool agents, and cannot move through the vascular endothelium into the interstitium. They respond to the ultrasound beam by changing their size, rapidly contracting and expanding in response to the pressure changes of the sound wave. Like all oscillating systems, microbubbles of ultrasound contrast agents have a natural or resonant frequency, at which their response is greatly enhanced.

When properly insonated with an ultrasound beam of appropriate power and frequency microbubble oscillation becomes nonlinear. Increased diameter in the rarefaction phase of the acoustic cycle exceeds its compression in the pressure phase, a consequence of the bubble's increased stiffness as the gas within it is compressed. These asymmetric oscillations result in nonlinear echoes containing overtones, or harmonics, of the driving frequency. It is this phenomenon that makes "non-destructive" contrast-specific imaging in real time possible. At a higher power of the ultrasound beam microbubble oscillation becomes so pronounced that the bubbles are disrupted and emit a strong, highly nonlinear, transient echo.

A variety of contrast specific ultrasound modes have been developed by the different manufacturers, optimized to detect nonlinear signal arising either from microbubble disruption (destructive modes) or from microbubble harmonic oscillation (non-destructive modes). Contrast specific non-destructive modes, in particular, represent the state-of-the-art in ultrasound imaging with microbubbles and in the clinical practice replaced nearly completely destructive techniques. The major advantage of non-destructive imaging is the possibility to image vascularity of organs and lesions in real time.

Microbubble contrast agents are not nephrotoxic and can be used safely in patients with impaired renal function.

## 3 Examination Technique

In our clinical practice we use SonoVue (BR1, Bracco, Milan, Italy), a sulfur hexafluoride-filled microbubble contrast agent licensed for imaging of abdominal organs in most European countries. Other latest generation microbubbles, however, such as Definity (Bristol-Myers Squibb Medical Imaging, N. Billerica, Massachusetts, USA), or Sonazoid (Daiichi-Sankyo, Tokyo, Japan) have similar use.

After a preliminary grey-scale and color Doppler evaluation, the equipment is set for contrast examination. The power of the US beam is set to obtain minimum microbubble destruction with the available equipment. Typically, non-destructive contrast-specific imaging is obtained by setting the mechanical index

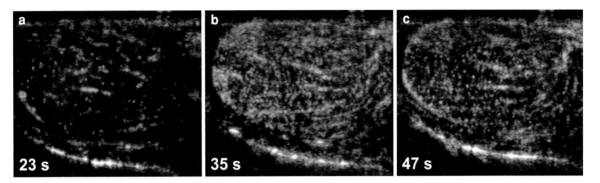

**Fig. 1** Normal testicular anatomy at CEUS. Testicular arteries enhance first (**a**) followed within few seconds by complete fill-in of the parenchyma (**b**). A progressive washout is then appreciable (**c**). Enhancement typically fades within about 3 min

between 0.2 and 0.06, depending on the equipment used. A SonoVue bolus of 2.4–4.8 mL is injected using a 20-gauge cannula, followed by a 10 mL normal saline flush. Digital cine-clips should be registered during all contrast-enhanced examination to allow accurate retrospective evaluation.

## 4 Normal Scrotal Anatomy

After microbubble administration testis and epididymis enhance quickly and intensively. The arteries enhance first, followed within few seconds by complete fill-in of the parenchyma (Fig. 1). Scrotal wall enhancement is less pronounced. Signal from microbubbles is independent from the angle of insonation. Adequate evaluation of organ perfusion is obtained with a spatial resolution approaching that of conventional grey-scale ultrasound imaging. There is no significant accumulation of microbubbles in the parenchyma of scrotal structures, and enhancement typically fades within about 3 min.

## 5 High Degree Testicular Torsion

Microbubble contrast agents are extremely effective in assessing presence or lack of organ perfusion. In principle, this technique is able to detect and display echoes from individual bubbles (Wilson and Burns 2010), and therefore, it is able to assess whether an organ is completely avascular or not.

The potential use of CEUS in the diagnosis of testicular ischemia has been investigated with experimental studies in rabbit since 1996 (Coley et al. 1996;

O'Hara et al. 1996). Coley et al. (1996) showed that in adult rabbits with unilateral low-degree torsion (360°) contrast-enhanced power Doppler imaging provides higher flow grades than unenhanced investigation. Microbubble administration might, therefore, increase the difference between torsed and normal testes, but might also mask subtle perfusion differences in case of low degree torsion (Coley et al. 1996). O'Hara et al. examined 17 prepuberal rabbits with unilateral spermatic cord ligation. After microbubble injection the false positive test results for ischemia decreased from 53 to 6%.

On these experimental basis, CEUS can be considered as a possible problem-solving technique especially in children with small testes in whom conventional Doppler imaging methods provide a suboptimal assessment of flow (Paltiel et al. 2006). CEUS might also decrease operator-dependent variability in the assessment of testicular ischemia. Using current ultrasound equipment, however, the sensitivity of conventional Doppler techniques in the diagnosis of high degree testicular torsion in children is high and microbubble contrast agents are not currently licensed for pediatric clinical use.

Despite promising experimental results, only few studies report cases of testicular torsion in men investigated with CEUS, and there is no evidence that microbubble injection might add significantly to color Doppler ultrasound. Cosgrove et al. (2000) present a case of testicular torsion investigated with contrast-enhanced power Doppler imaging. Microbubble injection increased the operator's confidence in diagnosis. Catalano et al. (2004) evaluated six patients with high degree and one patient with low degree testicular torsion. CEUS confirmed absence of

**Fig. 2** High-degree testicular torsion. **a** Color Doppler ultrasound shows avascular testis and slightly increased peritesticular flows. **b** CEUS confirms complete testicular ischemia and better demonstrates peritesticular hyperemia. Compared to conventional color Doppler ultrasound, however, no additional clinically relevant new information is obtained

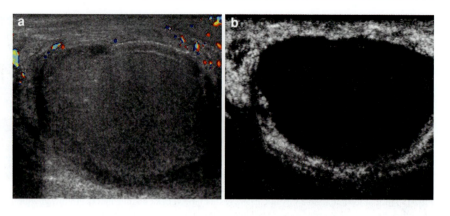

vascularization in the ischemic testes, but failed to add any relevant adjunctive information to unenhanced color Doppler ultrasound. Cochlin presented two cases of spermatic cord torsion concluding that CEUS is extremely effective in assessing lack of testicular perfusion. The diagnostic benefit over conventional Doppler modes, however, has not been discussed (Cochlin 2005). Moschouris et al. (2009) found that both the conventional power Doppler investigation and CEUS equally diagnosed testicular ischemia in four cases of testicular torsion, one of which of low degree.

As results from the current evidence, which, however, is largely anecdotal, based on a very limited number of case reports, CEUS failed to add any relevant information in complete testicular torsion of adult (Fig. 2). Studies on children are lacking, the patient group which most likely develop spermatic torsion and benefit from the use of microbubble ultrasound contrast agents (Cochlin 2005).

## 6    Low Degree Testicular Torsion

The ability of color Doppler ultrasound to show incomplete or partial torsion remains problematic. Arterial testicular flows can be present, principally near the hilum but occasionally also in a more peripheral distribution, with variable waveform characteristics depending on the severity and duration of torsion.

The potential use of CEUS in the diagnosis of low degree testicular torsion has been investigated in rabbits by Paltiel et al. (2006). Noninvasive quantification of testicular blood flow with CEUS correlated with radiolabeled microsphere-based perfusion measurements, and different levels of testicular perfusion

are qualitatively distinguished better with CEUS compared to conventional Doppler techniques.

Since low-degree torsion is uncommon in the clinical practice, its appearance at CEUS is reported only anecdotally in men. Moschouris et al. (2009) reported on a case in which CEUS showed a clear difference in the degree of enhancement between the normal and the affected side.

## 7    Segmental Testicular Infarction

The appearance of acute segmental testicular infarction at grey-scale and color Doppler ultrasound may be variable, but often allows one to establish the benign nature of the lesion and to guide diagnosis. According to Bilagi et al. (2007), a typical segmental testicular infarction presents as a solitary solid wedge shaped or round area in the testis, hypoechoic or with mixed echogenicity, with markedly diminished or absent vascularity. Differential diagnosis from a tumor less vascularized than the surrounding testicular parenchyma may be problematic in rounded lesions and when vascularity is not completely absent at color Doppler interrogation. CEUS improves characterization of segmental infarction (Fig. 3) showing one or more ischemic parenchymal lobules separated by normal testicular vessels (Bertolotto et al. 2011). Subacute segmental infarction characteristically shows a perilesional rim of enhancement (Fig. 4), while appearance of chronic infarction is not characteristic as the lesion presents as an hypovascular nodule. Changes in lesion shape, vascular features, and size reduction compared with the previous examinations are necessary to reach the diagnosis (Fig. 5).

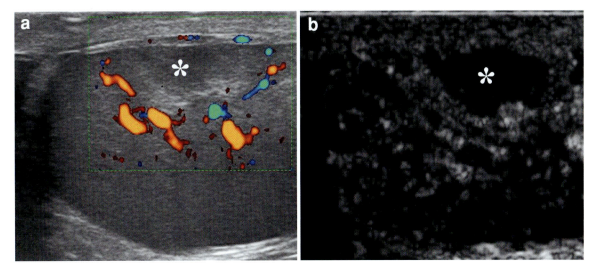

**Fig. 3** Acute segmental testicular infarction. Conventional color Doppler (**a**) and CEUS (**b**) images obtained within 24 h after the onset of acute scrotal pain. An inhomogeneously isoechoic area (*asterisks*) lacking vascularity at color Doppler interrogation is identified surrounded by a perilesional hyperemia. CEUS confirms that the lesion is completely avascular, allowing differential diagnosis with a hypovascular testicular tumor. There is no perilesional rim of enhancement

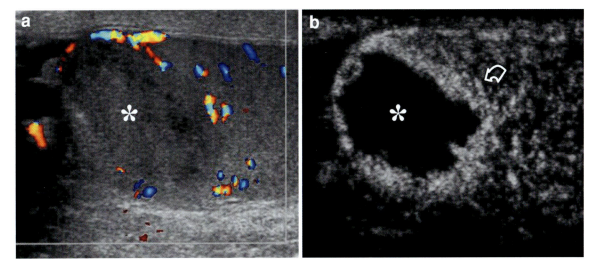

**Fig. 4** Subacute segmental testicular infarction. Conventional color Doppler (**a**) and CEUS (**b**) images obtained within 7 days after the onset of acute scrotal pain show an inhomogeneously hypoechoic area (*asterisks*) lacking vascularity at color Doppler interrogation surrounded by a perilesional hyperemia. CEUS confirms that the lesion is completely avascular, and identifies a perilesional rim of enhancement (*curved arrow*)

## 8    Tumors

Although the sensitivity of newest equipment allows identification of vascular signals in an increasing number of small testicular masses, several lesions less than 1.5 cm may still appear avascular at color Doppler interrogation and cannot be distinguished effectively from non-neoplastic lesions. In our experience virtually all testicular and extratesticular tumors display vascularization at CEUS. Cystic components in mixed tumors, and areas of necrosis or hemorrhage present as areas lacking contrast enhancement.

In patients with scrotal tumors CEUS does not allow a reliable differentiation among different histotypes (Fig. 6). This limitation, however, is not

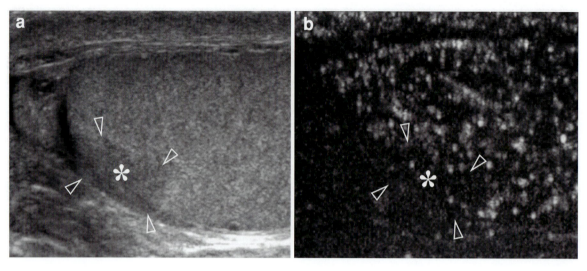

**Fig. 5** Chronic segmental testicular infarction. Grey-scale (**a**) and CEUS (**b**) images obtained 1 year after the episode of acute scrotal pain. Same patient of Fig. 4. Grey scale ultrasound shows a slightly hypoechoic, wedge-shaped area, changed in shape and markedly reduced in size compared to lesion appearance during the subacute phase. A few microbubble signals are identified within the lesion at CEUS

**Fig. 6** Testicular tumors. Surgically proved seminoma (**a**) and pure choriocarcinoma (**b**) presenting with similar appearance at CEUS

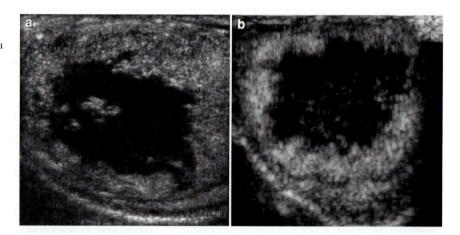

clinically relevant because all lesions require surgical removal.

CEUS may also ease identification of small testicular tumors barely visible at grey-scale ultrasound in patients with no testicular masses on conventional ultrasound and metastases containing germinal cells (Fig. 7).

## 9 Complex Cystic Lesions

Simple testicular cysts can be categorized as benign, but presence of any complexity should raise the possibility of a cystic testicular tumor (Bhatt et al. 2006; Winter 2009). In most of cases, however, echogenic content within the cysts does not represent vegetations, but amorphous material such as mucoid or keratinous fluid (Woodward et al. 2002). Content mobilization allows diagnosis of debris, and presence of color signal is diagnostic for vegetation. Intracystic amorphous content, however, is often not mobile, and absence of flows at color Doppler interrogation is not sensitive enough to rule-out vegetations.

Some urologists claim that all testicular lesions that do not meet at ultrasound the criteria for simple cysts must be removed surgically. In our experience tumors, enclosed mature teratomas, are vascularized after microbubble injection (Fig. 8), while complicated not neoplastic cysts do not (Fig. 9).

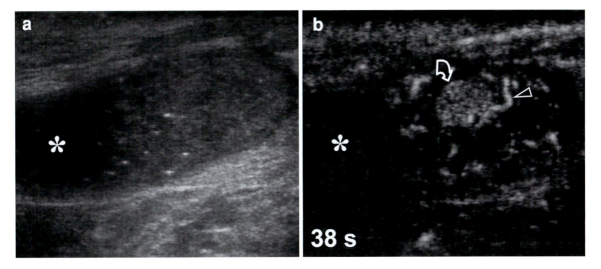

**Fig. 7** Patient with biopsy-proved retroperitoneal nodal metastases from seminoma. **a** Grey-scale ultrasound shows hypothrophic testis with microliths and hypoechoic upper pole (*asterisks*), consistent with ischemia. No distinct masses are identified. **b** CEUS. Images obtained 38 s after microbubble injection show the tumor (*curved arrow*) and its feeding vessel (*arrowhead*). Ischemia of the upper pole of the testis is confirmed (*asterisks*)

**Fig. 8** Hypovascular testicular tumor. **a** Color-Doppler ultrasound shows a testicular nodule (*curved arrows*) with cystic areas and calcifications. The lesion is avascular at color Doppler interrogation. **b** CEUS shows intralesional vascularization, leading to the diagnosis of hypovascular tumor. A mature teratoma was found at surgery

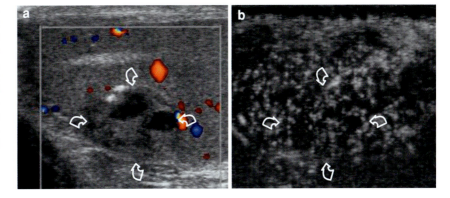

Besides simple and complicated cysts other testicular non-neoplastic conditions that should be differentiated from hypovascular tumors are epidermoid cyst and spontaneous intratesticular hemorrhage.

Epidermoid cyst can be treated performing a testis sparing enucleation rather than orchiectomy. Conservative treatment is particularly important in patients with bilateral presentation. The classic ultrasound appearance of epidermoid cyst is the "onion ring" pattern, consisting in alternating rings of low and high echogenicity, which represent layers of keratinized squamous epithelium. Unfortunately epidermoid cysts may present with atypical appearance as well. No matter the imaging features, epidermoid cysts do not demonstrate internal flow at Doppler interrogation nor enhancement after microbubble administration (Fig. 10) (Shah et al. 2010).

Spontaneous intratesticular hemorrhage is an extremely rare entity with few described reports in the literature (Sinclair et al. 2003; Chong and Flynn 1998; Gaur et al. 2011). Sonographically the lesion presents as an heterogeneous mass with cystic areas lacking vascularization at color Doppler interrogation. On serial examination, the mass will tend to show changes in echo texture as clot resolution occurs. As for post-traumatic intratesticular hematoma, spontaneous

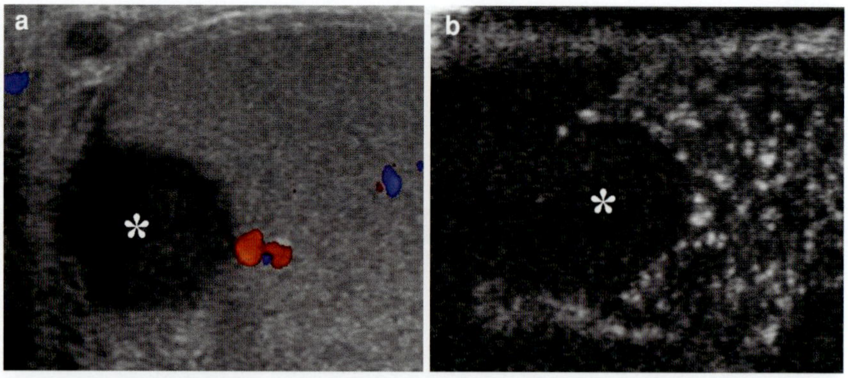

**Fig. 9** Complex testicular cyst. **a** Color-Doppler ultrasound shows a testicular cystic lesion with echogenic content (*asterisks*) **b** CEUS confirms absence of enhancing mural nodules, and of enhancing intralesional areas, leading to a confident diagnosis of benign intratesticular spermatocele

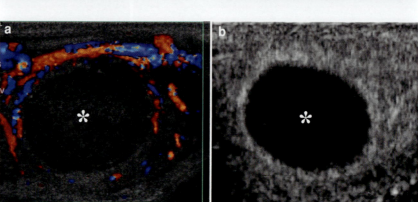

**Fig. 10** Surgically proved epidermoid cyst. **a** Color-Doppler ultrasound shows hypoechoic testicular lesion lacking vascularization at color Doppler interrogation (*asterisks*) **b** CEUS confirms complete absence of enhancement, leading to a confident diagnosis of benign lesion, which was enucleated. An epidermoid cyst was found at surgery

testicular hemorrhage can be managed conservatively (Gaur et al. 2011; Purushothaman et al. 2007). Lacking history of trauma, however, a confident differential diagnosis from a hypovascular tumor is difficult with conventional grey-scale and Doppler techniques, and orchiectomy is usually performed. Lack of microbubble enhancement differentiates spontaneous testicular hemorrhage from hypovascular tumors (Gaur et al. 2011).

## 10    Inflammation

Diagnosis of epididymo-orchitis is usually straightforward based on clinical features and presentation at color Doppler ultrasound. CEUS, however, offers an higher definition in the visualization of testicular and epididymal abscesses (Fig. 11) and can provide additional clinically useful information in patients with severe inflammation (Moschouris et al. 2009). Besides identification of small abscesses that may be overlooked at grey-scale ultrasound, also in large abscesses CEUS may have a role to better assess the

extension of the disease and the relationships with adjacent structures.

## 11    Traumas

In patients with scrotal trauma color Doppler ultrasound is the imaging modality of choice to assess the extent of injury and the viability of testicular parenchyma. However, the extent of hematomas and hemorrhagic areas within the testis is often underestimated at grey-scale ultrasound because their echogenicity can be similar to the normal testis and testicular vascularity can be globally reduced in trauma patients due to edema. Fracture lines often cannot be seen directly.

As reported by Moschouris et al. (2009) CEUS has an exceptional capability in demonstrating parenchymal vascularization and its changes in the injured testis. This method clearly depicts fracture lines and intratesticular hematomas. It can assess exactly the amount of viable testis, allowing the urologist to decide on rescue or removal of it (Fig. 12).

**Fig. 11** Scrotal inflammation. Testicular (**a**) and epididymal (**b**) abscesses presenting as parenchymal areas lacking enhancement (*asterisks*) surrounded by hyperemic viable parenchyma

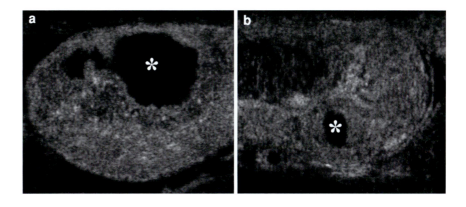

**Fig. 12** Testicular rupture in a monorchid patient. **a** Color Doppler ultrasound shows contour irregularity of the testis and nearly complete absence of flow in the injured parenchyma, suggesting ischemia. **b** CEUS shows that the lower pole of the testis (*asterisks*) is still viable. The testis was rescued at surgery

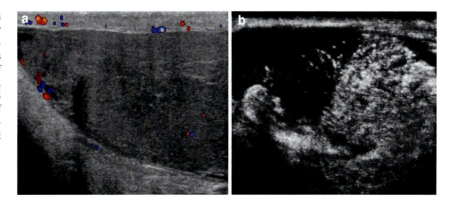

## 12 Varicocele

The exact mechanism by which varicocele affects fertility only in some men is unknown. It has been suggested that hydrostatic pressure may exceed pressure in the intratesticular arterial microcirculation resulting in relative hypoxia of the testicular tissues and ischemic damage (Gat et al. 2003). A recent study on 90 patients with left varicocele, 50 with oligospermia, and 40 with normozoospermia confirms this mechanism (Caretta et al. 2010). Testicular microcirculation has been evaluated noninvasively with CEUS after bolus injection of 2.5 mL Sonovue, and time intensity curves processed automatically using a dedicated software designed for ultrasound signal quantification (Fig. 13). A negative linear correlation was found between total sperm count and left mean transit time. In particular, a mean transit time greater than 36 s was an independent predicting parameter for oligospermia with 78% sensitivity and 58% specificity. If these data will be confirmed in larger studies, CEUS could provide a more appropriate indication for surgical or interventional treatment, compared to those that are currently available.

## 13 Therapeutic Applications

Multiple diagnostic and therapeutic clinical applications are being investigated for use of targeted microbubbles carrying bioactive materials such as drugs or genes to specific sites. When microbubbles reach the target site, for compounds of small molecular size intracellular delivery can occur with the contribution of endocytosis, while sonoporation (i.e., ultrasound-induced formation of pores in cell membranes) is the predominant mechanism for larger molecules and plasmids (Bertolotto and Catalano 2009).

A great challenge in sonoporation is to open the blood barriers in a reversible way. An experimental study investigated rats receiving luciferase without microbubbles and rats receiving intravenous injection of luciferase-loaded microbubbles while ultrasound was applied to the right testis (Bekeredjian et al. 2007). The testes that received ultrasound and

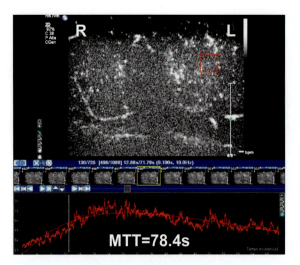

**Fig. 13** Time-intensity curve analysis of testicular perfusion in a patient with varicocele. Transversal scan. Both right (*R*) and left (*L*) testis are displayed. Signal intensity changes over time were calculated on a region of interest (*red square*) within the left testis using a commercially available dedicated software (QLAB, Philips, NH). A mean transit time (MTT) of 78.4 s was calculated automatically, consistent with oligospermia, which was confirmed at sperm analysis. The parameters of the time-intensity curve were similar in the contralateral testis (*not shown*)

luciferase-loaded microbubbles showed about twofold greater luciferase activity compared with testes without ultrasound or without microbubbles. The authors' conclusion was that CEUS is a safe and feasible technique to augment delivery of bioactive substances to the testis as well.

## References

Bekeredjian R, Kuecherer HF, Kroll RD et al (2007) Ultrasound-targeted microbubble destruction augments protein delivery into testes. Urology 69:386–389

Bertolotto M, Catalano O (2009) Contrast-enhanced ultrasound: past, present and future. 4:339–367

Bertolotto M, Derchi LE, Sidhu PS et al (2011) Acute segmental testicular infarction at contrast-enhanced ultrasound: early features and changes during the follow-up. Am J Roentgenol 196:834–841

Bhatt S, Rubens DJ, Dogra VS (2006) Sonography of benign intrascrotal lesions. Ultrasound Q 22:121–136

Bilagi P, Sriprasad S, Clarke JL et al (2007) Clinical and ultrasound features of segmental testicular infarction:

six-year experience from a single centre. Eur Radiol 17:2810–2818

Caretta N, Palego P, Schipilliti M et al (2010) Testicular contrast harmonic imaging to evaluate intratesticular perfusion alterations in patients with varicocele. J Urol 183:263–269

Catalano O, Lobianco R, Sandomenico F et al (2004) Real-time, contrast-enhanced sonographic imaging in emergency radiology. Radiol Med 108:454–469

Chong J, Flynn JT (1998) Spontaneous anticoagulant-induced testicular haemorrhage mimicking a testicular tumour. Br J Urol 81:777

Cochlin D (2005) Acute testicular pain. Imaging 17:91–100

Coley BD, Frush DP, Babcock DS et al (1996) Acute testicular torsion: comparison of unenhanced and contrast-enhanced power Doppler US, color Doppler US, and radionuclide imaging. Radiology 199:441–446

Cosgrove DO, Kiely P, Williamson R et al (2000) Ultrasonographic contrast media in the urinary tract. BJU Int 86(Suppl 1):11–17

Gat Y, Zukerman ZV, Bachar GN et al (2003) Adolescent varicocele: is it a unilateral disease? Urology 62:742–746 discussion 746–747

Gaur S, Bhatt S, Derchi L et al (2011) Spontaneous intratesticular hemorrhage: two case descriptions and brief review of the literature. J Ultrasound Med 30:101–104

Greis C (2004) Technology overview: SonoVue (Bracco, Milan). Eur Radiol 14(Suppl 8):P11–P15

Moschouris H, Stamatiou K, Lampropoulou E et al (2009) Imaging of the acute scrotum: is there a place for contrast-enhanced ultrasonography? Int Braz J Urol 35:692–702 discussion 702–695

O'Hara SM, Frush DP, Babcock DS et al (1996) Doppler contrast sonography for detecting reduced perfusion in experimental ischemia of prepubertal rabbit testes. Acad Radiol 3:319–324

Paltiel HJ, Kalish LA, Susaeta RA et al (2006) Pulse-inversion US imaging of testicular ischemia: quantitative and qualitative analyses in a rabbit model. Radiology 239:718–729

Purushothaman H, Sellars ME, Clarke JL et al (2007) Intratesticular haematoma: differentiation from tumour on clinical history and ultrasound appearances in two cases. Br J Radiol 80:e184–e187

Shah A, Lung PF, Clarke JL et al (2010) Re: New ultrasound techniques for imaging of the indeterminate testicular lesion may avoid surgery completely. Clin Radiol 65:496–497

Sinclair J, Ferucci P, Lovell MA et al (2003) Spontaneous testicular hemorrhage in an adolescent. J Urol 169:303–304

Wilson SR, Burns PN (2010) Microbubble-enhanced US in body imaging: what role? Radiology 257:24–39

Winter TC (2009) There is a mass in the scrotum-what does it mean? Evaluation of the scrotal mass. Ultrasound Q 25:195–205

Woodward PJ, Sohaey R, O'Donoghue MJ et al (2002) From the archives of the AFIP: tumors and tumorlike lesions of the testis: radiologic-pathologic correlation. Radiographics 22:189–216

# Index

M. Bertolotto and C. Trombetta (eds.), *Scrotal Pathology*, Medical Radiology. Diagnostic Imaging,
DOI: 10.1007/978-3-642-12456-3, © Springer-Verlag Berlin Heidelberg 2012

Printing and Binding: Stürtz GmbH, Würzburg